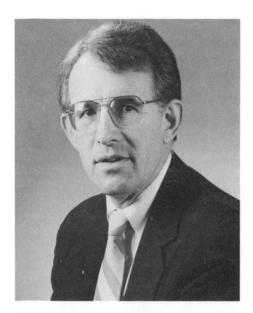

M. Winston Egan

M. Winston Egan is currently Director of Graduate Professional Degree Programs in the Department of Special Education at the University of Utah. His professional interests include teacher education, behavior disorders in children and youth, parent training, and distance education via telecommunications technologies. He also serves as the executive secretary for Educational Tele-Communications (ETC), an organization that specializes in providing training for television instruction, developing instructional materials and programs for low efficiency learners, conducting research, and delivering quality educational programs to rural/remote communities. Educational Tele-Communications was honored in 1989 by the American Council on Rural Special Education with the Research and Technology Award for its utilization of telecommunications technologies in reaching and teaching prospective rural educators.

Dr. Egan and his wife, Linda, are the parents of Daniel, Amy Dott, Mary Ann, and Marcia. The Egan family operates The Dotted Line in Salt Lake, a retail store that specializes in unique wooden products for children and other decorative accessories for the home.

Win Egan's hobbies include youth development, event planning, and sports of all kinds. His favorite pastimes include playing tennis and basketball, canoeing the Snake River in Wyoming, rafting on the Colorado River, exploring Indian dwellings in the Four Corners Area, mountain biking, and engaging in water activities of all kinds.

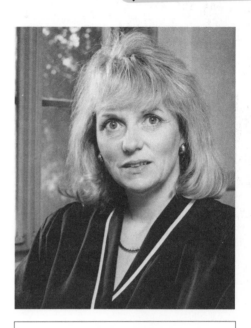

Barbara Wolf

Barbara Wolf is Associate Dean of the Faculties at Indiana University in Bloomington. She is appointed to the Honors Faculty and teaches jointly in the Department of Special Education. For more than a decade, she has taught the introductory course in special populations. Dr. Wolf has been the recipient of numerous teaching awards. In 1984, she received the highest recognition for Distinguished Teaching at Indiana, and recently she was honored on a national level by the American Association for Higher Education.

Dr. Wolf has published numerous articles on policy and practice in special education teacher preparation programs. Correspondingly, she chaired the National Task Force on Quality Professional Preparation for Undergraduate Special Education. Her other research projects and publications focus on programmatic accessibility for the disabled as she works with professionals in museums, zoos, parks, and gardens to plan program options that integrate disabled and nondisabled visitors.

In the community, Barbara Wolf works on the homeless project and volunteers as a fundraiser for the Leukemia Society. She finds enjoyment in quiet times shared with family and friends, getting about in her eighteen-year-old car, listening to all types of music (from rock to opera), and continuing to teach her sheepdog and springer spaniel how to hop.

Human
Exceptionality

Human Exceptionality

Society, School, and Family

THIRD EDITION

MICHAEL L. HARDMAN *University of Utah*

CLIFFORD J. DREW *University of Utah*

M. WINSTON EGAN *University of Utah*

BARBARA WOLF *Indiana University*

ALLYN AND BACON
Boston   London   Sydney   Toronto

Managing Editor: Mylan Jaixen
Series Editor: Ray Short
Developmental Editor: Elizabeth Brooks
Production Administrator: Rowena Dores
Editorial Assistant: Carol Craig
Cover Administrator: Linda Dickinson
Composition Buyer: Linda Cox
Manufacturing Buyer: Tamara Johnson
Text Designer: Margaret Ong Tsao

Copyright © 1990, 1987, 1984 by Allyn and Bacon
A Division of Simon & Schuster, Inc.
160 Gould Street, Needham Heights, Massachusetts 02194

Library of Congress Cataloging-in-Publication Data

Human exceptionality: society, school, and family / Michael L.
    Hardman . . . [et al.].—3rd ed.
        p.   cm.
    Includes bibliographical references.
    ISBN 0-205-12372-4
    1. Handicapped.   2. Exceptional children.   3. Handicapped—
Services for.   4. Learning disabilities.   I. Hardman, Michael L.
HV 1568.H37   1990
362—dc20
                                                89-29101
                                                CIP

Photo Credits
Pages xxviii and 270, Bob Daemmrich/Stock Boston; Page 18, © by Blair Seitz/FPG; Pages 54
and 212, Michal Heron/Woodfin Camp & Associates, Inc.; Page 86, © Richard Hutchings/
Photo Researchers, Inc.; Pages 88, 128, 174, 214, 238, 310, 344, 380, and 422, John Telford;
Page 126, Suzanne Szasz/Photo Researchers, Inc.; Page 172, © by Ulrike Welsch/Photo Re-
searchers, Inc.; Pages 236 and 488, © Will & Deni McIntyre/Photo Researchers, Inc.; Page 272,
© Thomas Craig/The Picture Cube; Page 308, © Mikki Ansin/The Picture Cube; Page 342,
© Glyn Cloyd/Taurus Photos; Page 378, © Alan Carey/Photo Researchers, Inc.; Page 420,
© J. Myers/FPG International; Page 456, © Peter Menzel/Stock Boston; Page 458, © David
Schaefer/The Picture Cube; Page 490, William Lupardo

Printed in the United States of America

10 9 8 7 6 5 4 3 2 1   95 94 93 92 91 90

Brief Contents

Contents

3

4

5

6

7

12

13

CHILDREN AND YOUTH WHO ARE GIFTED, CREATIVE, AND TALENTED   421

14

FAMILY IMPACT   457

15

Features

Foreword

There is probably no joy in life that compares to the happiness that comes with the anticipation and entry of a newborn into the family constellation. Parents, relatives, and friends all have preconceived notions of what life will be like with the new child around. Great plans and hopes for the child's future often dominate the parents' thinking. But can you imagine what happens to the family when the "bundle of anticipation" is born with unique problems?

A little over nineteen years ago, I well remember the physician coming out of the delivery room to announce to this excited new father that "It is a girl and [all in the same sentence] we have a problem." Even though I had been a professional special educator for several years, having a child with unique problems was something that happened to other families, not to mine.

During the next several days there were numerous unbelievable emotional and psychological adjustments that had to be made, while simultaneously trying to respond to the medical professionals, as well as additional extraordinary requirements that came so unexpectedly to a set of new parents. The changes in our lives that began early on that Tuesday morning in January would be long lasting. New adjustments were required on a regular basis, and they soon became almost automatic. The desire for more information in order to understand the health condition was a driving force. At the same time, there emerged within our family a keen appreciation and value for life that we had never before known.

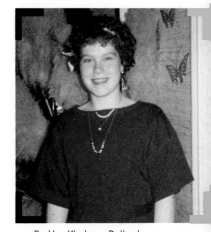

Brekke Khyleen Bullock

The years passed very quickly, and almost every one of them can be remembered with some unusual special joys as well as some very challenging events. We have recently completed a full life cycle with our daughter, Brekke Khyleen. It has been only a few years since this very bright and special young lady left us for her eternal future. Her optimism, cheerful attitude, and personal determination were her most obvious characteristics. Although she presented the medical profession and her parents with unusual challenges, she maintained that her physical limitation was only a nuisance with which she had to contend. She made it quite clear that the limitation was in no way to interfere with her productivity and zest for life. As a result of the personal characteristics she possessed, medical assistance, and parental understanding and caring, Brekke became a highly independent young lady, who in a few short years contributed significantly to the lives of others.

For our family, one of the critical elements in helping our daughter was the continuous search for knowledge that would heighten our understanding of the situation and that would guide us in ensuring her independence and personal growth. The book that you are beginning to read and study is a valuable source of information that will enhance your knowledge and understanding of exceptional individuals and the families in which they live. Within each chapter you will find vignettes about special individuals, which will enable you to relate your learning to actual cases.

You will find the book to be written in a scholarly, yet practical, manner. The book represents current research on the major exceptionalities and examines critical issues that impact upon providing appropriate interventions for exceptional persons. You will want to keep this book in your library as a future reference.

As a person involved in the helping profession, you will have numerous opportunities to work with individuals who present unusual challenges. However, you will want to remember that special individuals are first of all "individuals" and second, "individuals with special and unique characteristics." The knowledge and understanding that you develop about these persons will enable you to interact positively with them and to facilitate opportunities that will enable them to become contributing members of society. It has been my experience that special individuals bring many personal returns, "blessings," to those who interact with them. They give to us much more than they require of us.

Careful attention to the contents of this book will significantly affect your future as you have the opportunity to become acquainted with exceptional persons and their families. Knowledge facilitates our understanding and our ability to care.

Lyndal M. Bullock
Professor, Special Education, North Texas State University, Denton, Texas, and a Past President of the International Council for Exceptional Children

Preface

There is hope, I believe, in seeing the human adventure as a whole and in the shared trust that knowledge about mankind sought in reverence for life, can bring life.
MARGARET MEAD

As you begin your study of the third edition of *Human Exceptionality: Society, School, and Family,* we would like to provide some perspective on those features that continue from our second edition as well as on what is new and different. It is important to remember that this text is about people. It is about people with diverse needs, characteristics, and lifestyles. It is about people who for one reason or another are called exceptional. What does the word *exceptional* mean to you? For that matter what do the words, *disordered, deviant,* or *handicapped* mean to you? Who or what influenced your knowledge and attitudes about these terms and the people behind them? It is likely that you were influenced most by life experiences and not by formal training. You may have a family member, friend, or casual acquaintance who is exceptional in some way. It may be that you are a person with exceptional characteristics. Then again, you may be approaching a study of human exceptionality with little or no background on the topic. You will find that the study of human exceptionality is the study of being human. Perhaps you will come to understand yourself better in the process.

ORGANIZATIONAL FEATURES

In addition to providing you with current and informative content, we are committed to making your first experience with the area of exceptionality interesting, enjoyable, and productive. To accomplish this, we have incorporated some features within the third edition of the text that should greatly enhance your desire to learn more and become acquainted with exceptional people.

To Begin With . . .

"To Begin With . . ." boxes, found at the beginning of each chapter, are designed to introduce and stimulate interest on topics. They offer a variety of fascinating and current quotes, facts, and figures related to each subject area.

Chapter Vignettes

Beginning with Chapter 3, we present at least one vignette, or short case study, of an exceptional individual in every chapter. The purpose of these vignettes is to provide you with some insight into the needs, characteristics, and lifestyles of exceptional people. These vignettes are, however, in no way representative of the range of characteristics associated with a given area of exceptionality. At best, they simply provide you with a frame of reference for your reading. They let you know we are talking about real people who deal with life in many of the same ways.

Windows

"Windows" is a series of personal statements found throughout the text that focus on critical issues affecting the lives of exceptional people. The purpose of windows is to share with you some personal insights into the lives of these people. These insights may come from teachers, family members, friends, peers, and professionals, as well as from the exceptional individual. We believe you will find windows to be one of the most enriching aspects of your introduction to exceptionality.

In the News

Scattered throughout the book are "In the News" boxes that highlight current events relating to various exceptionalities. For example, Chapter 9 features an article on the Gallaudet University student protest. These boxes are designed to keep you up-to-date on issues and people who are making news.

Reflect on This

Every chapter includes at least one section entitled "Reflect on This." Each reflect highlights a piece of interesting and relevant information that will add to your learning and enjoyment of the chapter content. These reflect sections give you a temporary diversion from the chapter narrative, while providing you with some engaging facts about a variety of subjects. These may include misconceptions regarding people with Down syndrome; information on the development of artificial arms, ears, and eyes; or a letter to the mother of a child who stutters.

Debate Forum

Every chapter in this third edition concludes with a debate forum. The purpose of these forums is to broaden your view of the issues concerning exceptional people. The debate forums in each chapter focus on issues about which there is some philosophical difference of opinion, such as labeling, federal involvement in education, the role of a professional working with an exceptional individual, and the appropriateness of an intervention strategy. For each issue discussed, there is a position taken (*point*) and an alternative to that position (*counterpoint*). Remember, the purpose of the debate forum is not to establish right or wrong answers, but to help you better understand the diversity of issues concerning the exceptional individual.

IMPROVING YOUR STUDY SKILLS

Each chapter in this text is organized in a systematic fashion. Here are some brief suggestions that will increase your learning effectiveness.

Survey the Chapter.   In the margins of each chapter you will find a series of focus questions that should guide your reading. Survey the focus questions before reading the chapter. Each question highlights important information to be learned. After surveying the focus questions, examine key chapter headings to further familiarize yourself with chapter organization.

Ask Questions.   Using the focus questions as a guide, ask yourself what it is you want to learn from the chapter material. After reviewing chapter headings and the focus section, write down any additional questions you may have and use them as a supplement to guide your reading. Now organize your thoughts and schedule time to actively read the chapter.

Read.   Again using the focus questions as your guide, actively read the chapter.

Recite.   After you have completed your reading of the chapter, turn back to the focus questions and respond orally and in writing to each question. Develop a written outline of the key points to remember.

Review.   Each chapter in this text concludes with a section entitled review. Each focus question for the chapter is repeated in this section along with key points to remember from the material presented. Compare your memory of the material and your written outline to the key points addressed in the review section. If you forgot or misunderstood any of the important points, return to the focus question in the chapter and reread the material. Follow this process for each chapter in the book. In addition, you may consider developing your own short-answer essay tests to further enhance your understanding of the material in each chapter.

A Study Guide is available to help you master the information included in *Human Exceptionality*. Each chapter of the Study Guide includes an overview of the important points, learning objectives, exercises for mastering key terms, multiple choice practice tests, fill-in-the-blank study sections, and activities that encourage further exploration into various topics of interest.

The study of human exceptionality is relatively young and unexplored. For those of you who may be seeking careers in fields concerned with exceptional people, we believe this book will serve you well as a guidepost for future exploration. If after reading this book you are excited and encouraged to study further in this area, then we have met our primary goal. We would be unrealistic and unfair if we said this book will provide you with everything you ever wanted to know about people who are exceptional. What it does provide, however, is an overview on the lives of exceptional people within their own communities, at school, and as family members.

ACKNOWLEDGMENTS

We wish to genuinely thank our colleagues from around the country who provided in-depth and constructive feedback on various chapters within this new third edition. We extend our gratitude to the following national reviewers: William E. Davis, University of Maine; Thomas P. DiPaola, Providence College; Deborah Gartland, Towson State University; Ramon Rocha, SUNY-Geneseo; Stuart E. Schwartz, University of Florida; and Kathlene S. Shank, Eastern Illinois University. We would also like to thank Lani Florian of The University of Maryland for her invaluable assistance in obtaining the most current demographic information available on Public Law 94–142.

Our special thank you to the faculty and students at the University of Utah and Indiana University who taught us a great deal about writing textbooks. Many of the changes incorporated into this third edition are a direct result of critiques from students in our introductory classes.

We are indebted to Editor Ray Short and his Editorial Assistant Carol Craig at Allyn and Bacon for the many hours they spent helping us to shape the manuscript for this third edition. Ray's knowledge of the needs and interests of professors and students in the field of education and psychology helped us to cast this edition into a comprehensive text for the 1990s. We cannot express enough appreciation to Elizabeth Brooks, our Developmental Editor, who consistently kept our focus on quality issues and extended our creative thinking on a daily basis. A significant amount of credit for the final manuscript of this text belongs to Beth Brooks. Her thoughtful and in-depth reviews of each chapter provided us with the most constructive criticisms we have ever received as authors. We would also like to thank Rowena Dores, our Production Administrator. Her painstaking editorial work on the final manuscript assured the publication of a quality textbook.

To Jayne Leigh and Carolyn Osterman, we express our appreciation for the painstaking keyboarding, copying, and mailing of the manuscript. Thank you for caring so much about the calibre of the finished product. To John

Telford, who brings life to our words through his photographs, we thank you once again for going the extra mile.

To those professors who have chosen this book for adoption, and to those students who will be using this book as their first information source on human exceptionality, we hope this volume meets your expectations.

Michael L. Hardman

Clifford J. Drew

M. Winston Egan

Barbara Wolf

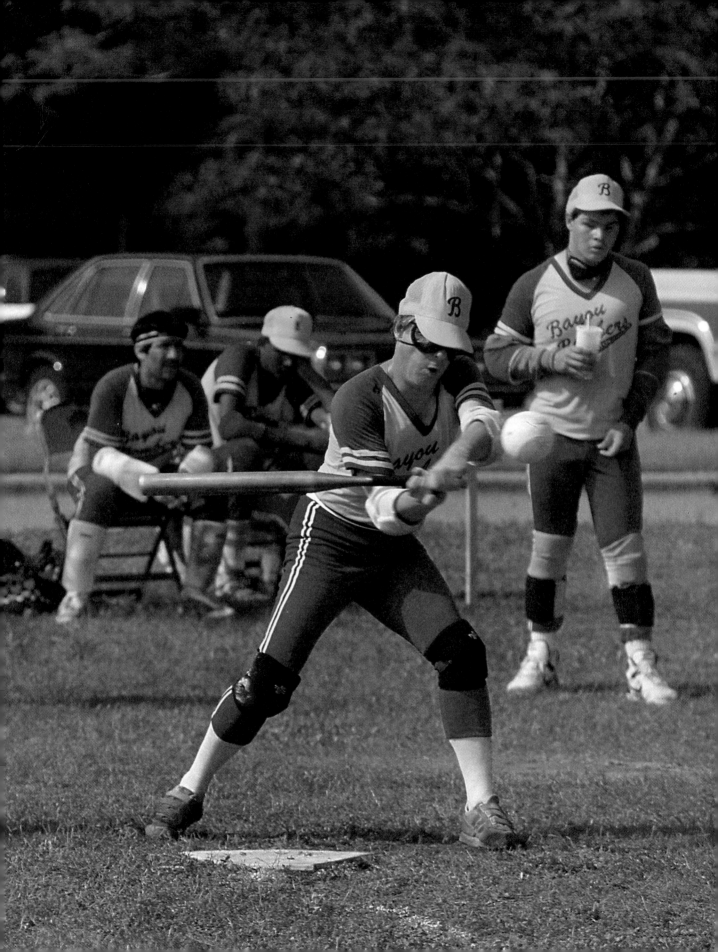

1 Understanding Human Differences

To Begin With...

- "Where nature has created great and fundamental differences in abilities . . . these must not be allowed to determine the individual's chances in life but rather, society should intervene to restore the balance" (Myrdol, 1971, p. 17).

- Current Census figures total 37,034,000 people in the United States with physical disabilities, making this the largest American minority. Comparatively, the census count was 29,000,000 Blacks and 17,000,000 Hispanics (U.S. Bureau of the Census, 1984–85, p. 144).

- We now have a generation of young people who, because of their public school experience with disabled classmates, are more comfortable with the handicapped. Most older Americans simply have not had this kind of exposure (Teltsch, 1989, pp. 1, 9).

INTRODUCTION

Whether your career goals lie in the field of education, the behavioral and social sciences, medicine, or law, it is important that you view the exceptional individual from a broader perspective than that projected by a single profession. Exceptional people live and function in many contexts, not just the school. Their differences affect them as they try to adjust to their environments, but the differences also have a significant impact on their families and society at large.

Although exceptionality is sometimes described as a human problem, we prefer to characterize it as just being human. Exceptionality may present certain obstacles for the individual, but it should not be viewed as always being difficult to deal with or to understand.

> Peter is twelve years old and in the seventh grade at McAllister School. In the basic subjects of reading, writing, and arithmetic, Peter's performance is as expected for a boy of his age. Achievement tests indicate that Peter is at approximately the seventh grade level in all his subject areas. Recently, Peter took a test that indicated he has an intelligence quotient of 106. Peter has 20/20 vision and no measurable hearing loss. He is physically active and healthy, with no serious medical problems. Emotionally, he has developed appropriate family and peer relationships.

Is Peter normal? We can say that Peter meets the basic medical, educational, and social criteria of normalcy. But what is normal, and how do we determine who is and who is not "normal"?

Normal is a relative term that is defined within the context of any given culture. Every society develops procedures to define what is normal. In every culture, the vast majority of individuals fall within the range of accepted physical and behavioral criteria. There are, however, individuals who exhibit differences that do not meet the cultural expectations of normalcy. These differences may be physical, such as **blindness** or an inability to walk. They can also be overt behaviors, as in the child who has a discipline problem, or the child who does not learn the same way or at the same rate as his or her siblings or friends.

How does society deal with these human differences? Everyone is in some way different from everyone else. Therefore, it is not a matter of merely being different; it is a matter of the type and extent of the difference. Every society creates descriptors to identify people who differ significantly from the accepted norm. This process is called **labeling.**

PEOPLE WITH DIFFERENCES

FOCUS 1
What are two functions of a label?

Labels are an attempt to describe, identify, and distinguish one person from another. A sociologist labels to describe people who are socially deviant; educators and psychologists label to identify students with learning, physical, and behavioral differences who need specialized instructional service; and physicians label to distinguish the sick from the healthy. Labels are only rough approximations and consequently their effects differ from person to person. Some labels are permanent, others are temporary. Some are positive, others are negative.

Labels communicate whether or not a person meets the expectations of the culture. A society establishes criteria that are easily exceeded by some but cannot be met by others. For example, a society may value creativity, innovation, and imagination. Someone with these attributes is then valued and rewarded with positive labels, such as bright, intelligent, or **gifted.** However, anyone whose ideas drastically exceed the limits of conformity may be branded with negative labels, such as radical, extremist, or rebel. There is a fine line between the application of a positive or a negative label. For example, a high school student may be labeled a conformist. From the school administration's point of view this is a positive characteristic, but by the student's peer group it may have strong negative connotations. What are the effects of using labels to describe people? Reynolds, Wang, and Walberg (1987) contend that the use of categorical labels, such as **learning disabled** and **emotionally disturbed,** has been mixed at best. On the one hand, these labels have been the basis for access to educational services, but they have also been unreliable. "The boundaries of the categories have shifted so markedly in response to legal, economic, and political forces as to make diagnosis largely meaningless" (Reynolds et al., p. 396). Roos (1982) indicates that the label **mentally retarded** has been a mixed blessing. This label has been the basis for developing and providing services to people, but it has also promoted stereotyping, discrimination, and exclusion. This view is shared by Leitch and Sodhi (1986), who indicate that the practice of labeling children for services has perpetuated and reinforced both the label and the behaviors implied by the label.

Labeling People with Differences

If labels can have negative consequences, why are they used so extensively? One reason we label people is that the current funding of many social services and educational programs for exceptional individuals is based on the use of a label to distinguish who is eligible for a service and who is not. To illustrate, Rick is a child with a hearing problem. By federal and state law, Rick must be assessed and defined as a **hearing impaired** child before specialized educational or social services can be made available to him as a **handicapped** child. A second reason for the use of labels is that they assist professionals in communicating effectively with one another and provide a common ground for evaluating research findings. A third reason is that labeling helps us to identify the specific needs of a group of people. We are thus able to more clearly differentiate between the needs of various categories of individuals, such as blind people versus those with **cerebral palsy.**

FOCUS 2
What are three reasons we label people?

Who Uses Labels?

Labels may be applied by both "official" and "unofficial" labelers (Feldman, 1978). Official labelers are sanctioned by society. The criminal justice system, including the arresting officer, jury, and court judge, labels the person who

FOCUS 3
Distinguish between official and unofficial labels.

commits a crime as a criminal. A criminal may be incarcerated in a penal institution and is consequently labeled a convict. Besides the term *criminal,* other official labels might include gifted and talented, mentally ill, mentally retarded, blind, and so forth. An official label changes our perception of the individual and in turn may change the individual's self-concept. Additional examples of official labelers include doctors, educators, and behavioral and social scientists. Official labelers have the sanction of their society, as when a court judge pronounces sentence upon a convicted felon on behalf of all who live in the community.

An unofficial labeler is usually some significant other, such as a family member, friend, teacher, or peer, and the applied label is meaningful only to this person or a restricted group. Unofficial labels may be expressed in a number of ways. They can be derogatory slang terms, such as *stupid, cripple, fat,* or *crazy.* Some unofficial labels reflect more favorably on the individual than do others. These may include such terms as *witty, smart,* or *cool.* Other labels, such as *ambitious* or *conformist,* are open to individual interpretation.

Approaches to Labeling

FOCUS 4
What are three approaches that can be used to describe the nature and extent of human differences?

Significant physical and behavioral differences are found infrequently in every society. The vast majority of people in any given culture conform to the established standards of that culture. Conformity—people doing what they are supposed to do—is practiced by most people most of the time (Baron & Byrne, 1987). For the most part, people look the way they are expected to look, behave the way they are expected to behave, and learn the way they are expected to learn. However, when someone deviates substantially from the expectations, a number of approaches can be used to describe the nature and extent of the differences.

The Developmental Approach.   This approach to labeling is based on deviations in the course of development from what is considered normal physical, social, or intellectual growth. Human differences are the result of an interaction of biological and environmental factors. To understand these differences, we must first establish what is normal development. According to the developmental view, normal development can be described statistically. We observe large numbers of individuals and look for those characteristics that occur most frequently at a specific age. For example, the average three-month-old infant should be able to follow a moving object visually. *Average* is a statistical term based on observations of the behavior of three-month-old infants. An individual child's growth pattern is then compared to the group average. Differences in development (either advanced or delayed) are labeled accordingly.

The Cultural Approach.   This approach defines what is normal according to the standards established by a given culture. Whereas a developmental approach measures only the frequency of behaviors to define differences, cultural definitions suggest that differences can also be explained by examining the values inherent within a culture. What constitutes a significant difference changes over time, from culture to culture, and among the various social classes within a culture. Edgerton (1976) states that people everywhere follow cultural rules, even though the rules are often arbitrary and vary dramatically from one society to the next. For example, in the United States intelligence is often described in terms of how

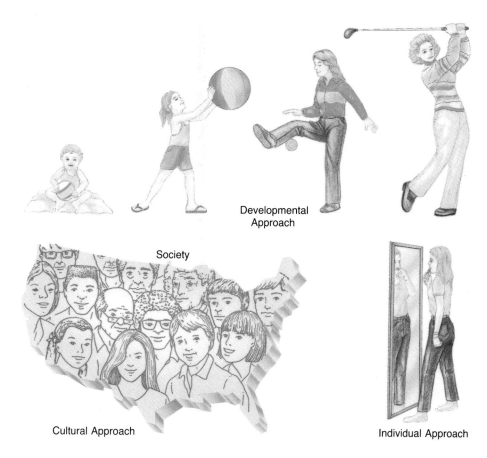

Developmental
Approach

Society

Cultural Approach

Individual Approach

Figure 1–1
Approaches to Labeling:
What Is "Normal"?

well one scores on a test measuring a broad range of abilities, while in Africa it may relate much more to how skillful one is at hunting.

The idea that human beings are the product of their culture has received its greatest thrust from anthropology. This field has emphasized "the diverse and arbitrary nature of man's rules about dress, food, sex, religion, etiquette, marriage, politics" (Edgerton, 1976, p. 8). The human infant is so flexible that it is possible for the child to adjust to nearly any environment.

The Individual Approach.   All people engage in a self-labeling process that is not recognized by others. Self-imposed labels are a reflection of how we perceive ourselves, although those perceptions may not be consistent with how others see us. The opposite may also occur: The culture uses a label to identify a person, but the cultural label is never accepted by that person. Such was the case with Thomas Edison. While the schools labeled Edison as an intellectually incapable child, he eventually recognized that he was an individualist whose strength was in marching to a different drummer.

The Effects of Labeling

Several studies have indicated that reactions to a label differ greatly from one person to another (Aloia & MacMillan, 1983; Bak, Cooper, & Siperstein, 1987;

FOCUS 5
What is a self-fulfilling prophecy?

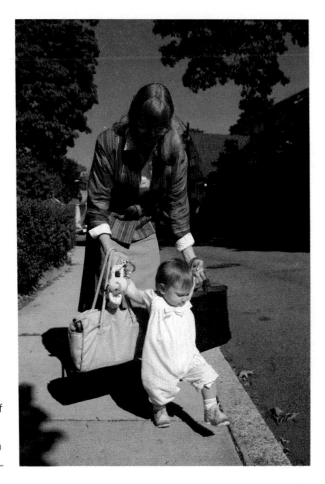

According to the developmental approach to labeling, this child would not be considered normal if her motor abilities were far behind that of her peers.
(John Coletti/The Picture Cube)

Fiedler & Simpson, 1987; Freeman & Algozzine, 1980; Graham & Dwyer, 1987; Van Bourgondien, 1987). However, researchers have been unable to draw consistent conclusions about how labeling a person influences our view of that person. Rosenthal and Jacobsen (1968) examined this issue in a well-known study involving intelligence. A group intelligence test was administered to elementary-age school children. Teachers were informed that this test was an effective method for determining intellectual potential. The teachers were then provided with a list of about 20 percent of the children who had taken the test. They were told that these children had the greatest potential for intellectual growth. The list was in fact composed of children who had been randomly selected from the entire elementary school population. The test was administered again later in the school year, and the children who had been identified to the teachers as having the greatest potential scored significantly higher than the rest of the children in the school. The researchers concluded that teacher expectations contributed to the differences in scores. This effect is known as the **self-fulfilling prophecy,** or "you become what you are labeled" (Merton, 1948).

Unfortunately, the research of Rosenthal and Jacobsen contains many methodological flaws and has not been consistently replicated. In recent years, the

Reflect on This 1–1

So Who's Right?

To see how cultures can truly differ, look at some interesting facts from a study done by noted anthropologist Ruth Benedict. She compared the very different values of two Native American cultures in the areas of fasting, torture, dancing, initiative, death, war, and suicide. Are any of the beliefs of the two cultures consistent with what you value? So who's right?

	Plains Indians	Pueblo Indians
Fasting	Fasting is a way to induce visions.	Fasting is a means of preparing for ritual activity.
Torture	Self-torture is used for visions and protection.	Self-torture is absent.
Dancing	Dancing is employed to induce ecstatic states and is often wild.	Dancing is monotonous and is intended to promote crop growth.
Initiative	Value is placed on the self-reliant person of initiative, who wins honor and prestige.	The ideal person is mild mannered and tries not to stand out from the crowd.
Death	Death promotes uninhibited grief, and mourning is prolonged and involves self-torture.	Death promotes sorrow, but little is made of the event.
War	The war hero is honored and envied.	The war hero must be purified of the impurities brought about by killing.
Suicide	Men often vow suicide if they have been failures or shamed.	Tales about suicide cannot be taken seriously.

Source: Adapted from John J. Collins, *Anthropology: Culture, Society, and Evolution*, p. 214. Copyright © 1975 Prentice-Hall, Inc., Englewood Cliffs, N.J. Reprinted by permission.

investigation has stimulated considerable controversy (Rosenthal, 1987; Wineburg, 1987). Several authors (Becker, 1974; Keogh & Levitt, 1976; MacMillan & Becker, 1977; Palmer, 1980) suggest that the theory is without foundation when viewed in relation to everyday experience. "It would seem foolish to propose that stick-up men stick up people simply because someone has labeled them stick-up men, or that everything a homosexual does results from someone having called him homosexual" (Becker, p. 24).

Teacher bias as a function of *negative* labels has also been a focus of investigation (Aloia & MacMillan, 1983; Foster, Ysseldyke, & Reese, 1975; Neubauer, 1986; Ysseldyke & Foster, 1978). Foster et al. studied the expectations of special education teacher trainees relative to children labeled **emotionally disturbed.** They found that the trainees held preconceived negative stereotyped expectations concerning these children. Ysseldyke and Foster, in a study of elementary schoolteachers, reported that negative labels (e.g., emotionally disturbed

Reflect on This 1–2

I Am Not Mentally Retarded

Thomas Alva Edison was labeled intellectually slow during his childhood, but never accepted the label. On the contrary, Tom Edison sought throughout his life to prove otherwise. The following excerpts from Edison biographies provide us with some real insight into Thomas Edison as a young boy.

Alva appears to have been a perplexing problem for which Sam was unable to find a solution. The boy's active, inquisitive mind led him into places and predicaments a less vigorous mentality would not have considered. His great curiosity, his continuous flow of questions, caused many people, including his father, to think the boy was of low mentality. It appears that in those days a boy who asked countless questions was considered stupid.

Apparently his father—a frequent target of the constant flow of puzzling questions—maintained a similar opinion of him. Perhaps this opinion was confirmed when, following his father's frequent "I don't know," the boy began countering with "Why don't you know?"*

Tom Edison caught scarlet fever and it was not until 1855, at the age of eight and a half, that he began attending the white school house. Here he showed what has almost become a sign of genius: after only three months he returned home in tears, reporting that the teacher had described him as "addled." This was in fact no cause for alarm. Leonardo da Vinci, Hans Anderson and Niels Bohr were all singled out

in their youth as cases of retarded development; Newton was considered a dunce; the teacher of Sir Humphry Davy commented, "While he was with me I could not discern the faculties by which he was so much distinguished"; and Einstein's headmaster was to warn that the boy "would never make a success of anything." As youths, all had one characteristic in common: each was an individualist, saw no need to explain himself and was thus listed among the odd men out.†

---

* *Source:* Reprinted, by permission of the publisher, from L. A. Frost, *The Thomas A. Edison Album* (Seattle: Superior Publishing Co., 1969), p. 23.
† *Source:* Reprinted by permission from R. S. Clark, *Edison: The Man Who Made the Future* (New York: G. P. Putnam's Sons, 1977), p. 9.

---

and **learning disabled**) "generated initial negative stereotypes, which were retained in the observance of behaviors inconsistent with the labels" (p. 615). Aloia and MacMillan (1983), in a study of regular-classroom teachers, found similar results with mentally retarded children, who were being educated in a regular class program. Neubauer studied kindergarten teachers in Australia and found their behavior was negatively influenced toward children labeled as aggressive. (It is important to note here that although we have focused on teachers in our discussion of self-fulfilling prophecy, the phenomenon can happen with anyone.)

Two other effects of labeling need to be addressed at this point: (1) The person and the label may become one and the same, and (2) the environment may influence our perceptions of the individual.

Separating the Person and the Label. Once a label is affixed, the person and the label may become inseparable. For example, instead of saying that Ruth

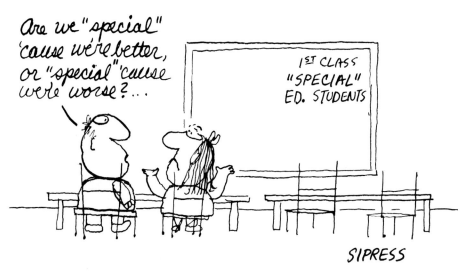

1ST CLASS "SPECIAL" ED. STUDENTS

Are we "special" 'cause we're better, or "special" 'cause we're worse?...

SIPRESS

Source: From *Is It Really Only Monday?* by David Sipress. Copyright © 1981 by Fearon Teacher Aids, Simon & Schuster Supplementary Education Group.

does not possess age-appropriate intellectual or socialization abilities, Ruth may be referred to as a retardate. We lose sight of the fact that Ruth is a human being with exceptional characteristics. If we treat Ruth as a label rather than a person with special needs we are doing an injustice not only to Ruth but to everyone else as well.

Environmental Bias.   The environment can clearly influence our perceptions of another person. For example, it can be said that if you are in a mental hospital, you must be insane. Rosenhan (1973) investigated this premise by having himself and seven other sane individuals admitted to a number of state mental hospitals across the country. Once the experimenters were in the mental hospitals, they behaved normally. The question was whether the staff would perceive them as healthy people instead of mentally ill patients. Rosenhan reported that the pseudopatients were never detected by the hospital staff, although several of the "real" patients recognized the experimenters as imposters. Throughout their hospital stays, these pseudopatients were incorrectly labeled and treated as schizophrenics. In fact, when a staff nurse observed one experimenter writing she noted, "Patient engages in writing behavior." Rosenhan's investigation shows that the perception of what is normal can be biased by the environment in which the observations are made.

THE STUDY OF HUMAN DIFFERENCES

In order to gain a broader understanding of the nature and extent of human differences, let us briefly examine several fields of study concerned with the exceptional individual. These fields include medicine, psychology, sociology, and education. Each of these fields is unique in its approach to exceptionality, which is reflected in the labels used to describe a person with exceptional characteristics. Figure 1–2 provides the common terminology associated with each field.

Medicine

FOCUS 6
What are the two dimensions of the *medical model?*

The medical model has two dimensions: normal and pathological. Normal is defined as the absence of a biological problem; **pathology,** as alterations in the organism caused by disease. The emphasis is on defining the nature of the disease and its pathological effects on the individual. Disease is a state of ill health that interferes with or destroys the integrity of the organism.

The medical model, often referred to as the disease model, focuses primarily on biological problems. The model is universal and does not have values that are culturally relative. It is based on the value that being healthy is better than being sick, regardless of the culture in which one lives.

When diagnosing a problem, a physician carefully follows a definite pattern of procedures that includes questioning the patient and obtaining a history, a physical examination, laboratory studies, and in some cases surgical exploration.

Figure 1–2
Common Terminology of Fields of Study Concerned with Exceptional Individuals

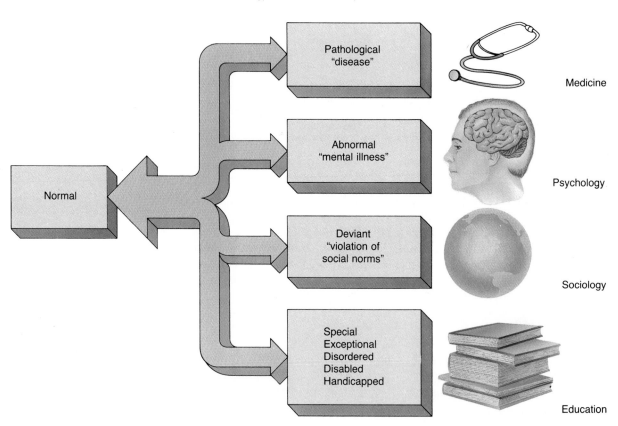

The person who has a biological problem is labeled the patient, and the deficits are then described as the patient's disease.

Psychology

Modern psychology is the science of human and animal behavior, the study of the overt acts and mental events of an organism that can be observed and evaluated. Broadly viewed, psychology is concerned with every detectable action of an individual. Behavior is the focus of psychology, and when the behavior of an individual does not meet the criteria of normal, it is labeled abnormal.

FOCUS 7
Distinguish between abnormal behavior as a physical illness and as a social problem.

One cannot live in society without encountering the dynamics of **abnormal behavior.** The media are replete with stories of murder, suicide, sexual aberrations, burglary, robbery, embezzlement, child abuse, and other incidents that display behavioral disorders. Each case represents a point on the continuum of personal maladjustment that exists in our society. This continuum ranges from behaviors that are slightly deviant or eccentric but still within the confines of normal human experience, to **neurotic disorders** (partial disorganization characterized by combinations of anxieties, compulsions, obsessions, and phobias), to **psychotic disorders** (serious disorders resulting in loss of contact with reality and characterized by delusions, hallucinations, or illusions).

or combinations thereof

The History of Study of Abnormal Behavior.   The study of abnormal behavior is historically based in philosophy and religion in Western culture. Until the

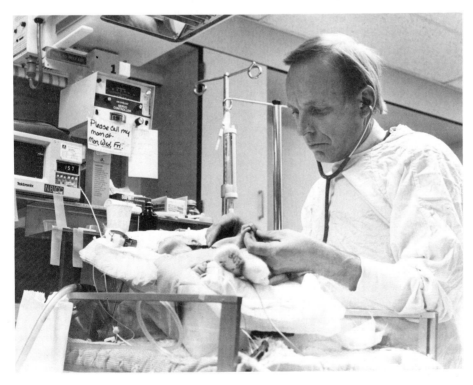

In the medical model of exceptionality, a physician is responsible for defining the nature of a disease and its effect on the individual. (John Telford)

Middle Ages, psychological disturbance was believed to be a result of divine intervention. The disturbed or mad person was thought to have made a pact with the devil, and the psychological affliction was a result of divine punishment. Psychological disturbances were a function of devils, witches, or demons residing within the person. The earliest known treatment for mental disorders, called trephining, involved drilling holes in a person's skull to permit evil spirits to leave (Carlson, 1987). During the sixteenth and seventeenth centuries, people who were disturbed continued to be viewed as mad persons, fools, and public threats who had to be removed from society.

Our knowledge of medicine expanded in the eighteenth century and abnormal behavior then became associated with physical disease. The disturbed individual was considered ill; thus the origin of the term **mental illness.** A person with mental illness became a patient, and in many cases was sent to a mental hospital to be cured.

Throughout the first half of the twentieth century, medicine was considered the most logical and most scientific approach to understanding abnormal behavior. Goldberg (1977) indicated that medicine "laid to rest all of the myths giving demonological explanations of disordered behavior" (p. 27). In addition, the public was more accepting of the view that psychologically disturbed people were sick and not fully responsible for their problems. As such they deserved the same kind of care as people who were physically ill.

In the latter part of the twentieth century, several professionals (for example, Cowen, 1973; Lain, 1967; Szasz, 1961) emerged with an alternative viewpoint on the nature of abnormal behavior. This perspective is sometimes referred to as the ecological approach. Professionals espousing the ecological approach view abnormal behavior more as a result of the interaction of an individual with the environment than as a disease within the individual. They theorize that social and environmental stress, in combination with the individual's inability to cope, lead to psychological disturbances. Bogdan (1986) indicated that there is "symbolic meaning" in what "society honors and what it degrades" (p. 351). In this context, abnormal behavior is a social problem and therefore should be examined within the context of both psychology and sociology.

Sociology

FOCUS 8
What are the four principles that guide us in determining who will be labeled socially deviant?

Psychology and sociology are similar in that both fields are concerned with the study of human behavior. Sociology is the science of social behavior, whereas psychology emphasizes the person as a separate being. Sociology is concerned primarily with modern cultures, group behavior, societal institutions, and intergroup relationships. It examines the individual in relation to the physical and social environment. When individuals meet the social norms of the group, they are considered normal. When individuals are unable to adapt to social roles or to establish appropriate interpersonal relationships, their behaviors are labeled **deviant.** Unlike medical pathology, social deviance cannot be defined in universal terms. Instead, it is defined within the context of the culture, in any way the culture chooses to define it. "Group norms can establish almost any form of behavior, from the most innocent to the most harmful, as deviant" (Dinitz, Dynes & Clarke, 1975, pp. 3–4).

There are four principles that serve as guides in determining who will be labeled socially deviant. First, normal behavior must meet societal, cultural, or group expectations. Deviance is defined as a violation of social norms. Second, social deviance is not necessarily an illness. Failure to conform to societal norms does not imply that the individual has pathological or biological deficits. Third, each culture determines the range of behaviors that are defined as normal or deviant. These norms are enforced by the culture. Those people with the greatest power within the culture can impose their criteria for normalcy on the less powerful. Fourth, social deviance may be caused by the interaction of several factors, including genetic makeup and individual experiences within the social environment. One social environment in which deviance becomes most visible is the school.

Education

As children progress through formal schooling, their parents, teachers, peers, and others expect they will learn and behave according to established patterns. Most children move through their educational programs in about the same way, requiring the same level of service, and within similar time-frames. Children and youths who do not meet educational expectations of normal growth and development are labeled according to the type and extent of their deviation. They are provided services and resources that are different from those required for the normal population. These differences in educational service patterns are reflected in the numerous terms used to describe these students: **special, disabled, disordered, handicapped,** and **exceptional.**

FOCUS 9
Distinguish between the educational labels of special, disordered, disabled, handicapped, and exceptional.

Educational Labels.   Historically, *special* is the most widely used educational descriptor for students with differences. It is also used extensively to describe the nature of the education services these students require. *Special* is defined as unusual, peculiar, unique, and distinctive. A special person has physical and behavioral characteristics that differentiate that person from the normal peer group and therefore establish the need for special education services. As an educational label, *special* has traditionally communicated a feeling of isolation or separatism. In fact, in the not-too-distant past, all special education programs were segregated from regular education services. Many students with significant differences were not merely separated from regular education; they were excluded from all public education programs. Even today, many teachers are still trained in separate programs of higher education and students are taught in separate classrooms in public schools; in some cases, in separate school buildings.

Other terms that describe physical and behavioral differences include *disorder, disability,* and *handicap.* These terms are not synonymous. A disorder is the broadest of the three terms and refers to a general malfunction of mental, physical, or psychological processes. It is defined as a disturbance in normal functioning. A disability is more specific than a disorder and results from a loss of physical functioning (such as the loss of sight, hearing, or mobility) or difficulties in learning and social adjustment that significantly interfere with normal growth and development. A handicap is a limitation imposed on the individual by environmental demands and is related to the individual's ability to adapt or adjust to those demands. For example, a person who is confined to a wheelchair has a physical disability, the inability to walk. The individual is dependent on the wheelchair for mobility. When the physical environment does not accommodate the wheelchair (e.g., in a building without ramps, accessible only by stairs), the person's disability becomes a handicap.

As an educational label, handicapped has a narrow focus and a negative connotation. The word *handicapped* literally means "cap in hand" and originates from a time when the disabled begged in the streets in order to survive (Avoiding Handicapist Stereotypes, 1977, p. 1). The term *handicapped* describes only those individuals who are deficient in or lack ability. The term *exceptional* is much more comprehensive and may describe any individual whose physical or behavioral performance deviates so substantially from the norm, either higher or lower, that additional educational and other services may be necessary to meet the individual's needs. An exceptional person is not necessarily a handicapped person.

Persons with exceptional characteristics are identified for additional educational, social, or medical services on the basis of physical and behavioral characteristics that deviate substantially from what is considered normal. These differences can be—

1. **learning and behavioral disorders,**
2. **speech and language disorders,**
3. **sensory disorders,**
4. physical and other health disorders, or
5. gifts or talents.

It is important to remember that an exceptional person is not necessarily a handicapped person. (© Michal Heron/Woodfin Camp & Associates)

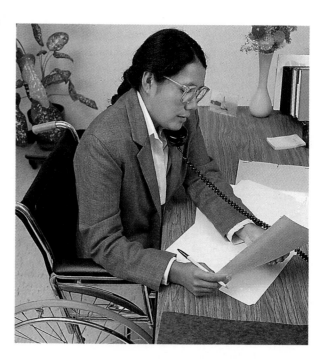

In subsequent chapters of this book we explore each of the above areas of exceptionality. We study how to describe exceptional people, their physical, social, and intellectual characteristics, and what services are needed to assist them in living a full life from the early childhood years through the transition to adult life. We examine the effects an exceptional person may have on his or her family, as well as the important area of multicultural education. In the next chapter we continue our study of human exceptionality with a history of human services.

REVIEW

FOCUS 1: What are two functions of a label?

☐ Labels describe, identify, and distinguish one person from another.

☐ Labels communicate whether or not a person meets the expectations of the culture.

FOCUS 2: What are three reasons we label people?

☐ Many social and educational services require that an individual be labeled in order to determine who is eligible to receive special services.

☐ Labels help professionals to communicate more effectively with each other and provide a common ground for evaluating research findings.

☐ Labels enable professionals to differentiate more clearly the needs of one group of people from another.

FOCUS 3: Distinguish between official and unofficial labels.

☐ Official labelers have the approval of society when applying a label to any individual.

☐ Official labels include such terms as *criminal, gifted, mentally ill, mentally retarded,* and *deaf.*

☐ An official label changes our perception of a person and in turn can change the labeled person's self-concept.

☐ Unofficial labels are usually applied by significant others in a person's life, such as family, friends, or peers.

☐ Unofficial labels can be expressed in several ways, including derogatory slang expressions.

☐ Unofficial labels can also reflect positively on the individual (e.g., bright, cool, witty).

FOCUS 4: What are three approaches that can be used to describe the nature and extent of human differences?

☐ The developmental approach is based on differences that occur in the course of human development from what is considered normal physical, social, and intellectual growth.

☐ In the developmental approach, human differences are the result of an interaction between biological and environmental factors.

☐ According to the developmental view, normal growth can be explained by observing large numbers of individuals and looking for characteristics that occur most frequently at any given age.

☐ The cultural approach to describing human differences defines normal according to established cultural standards.

☐ The cultural view suggests that human differences can be explained by examining the values of any given society.

☐ Using the cultural approach, what is considered different changes over time and from culture to culture.

☐ The individual approach to labeling suggests that labels can be self-imposed.

☐ Self-imposed labels are a reflection of how we perceive ourselves, although the perceptions may not be consistent with how others see us.

☐ It is also possible for a culture to label a person but the label is rejected by the individual.

FOCUS 5: What is a self-fulfilling prophecy?

☐ The self-fulfilling prophecy suggests that you will become what you are labeled.

☐ Teachers may contribute to a self-fulfilling prophecy by lowering their expectations for certain children, based upon preconceived negative stereotypes.

☐ It is possible for a person and a label to become inseparable (e.g., "Mary *is* mentally ill" as opposed to "Mary is a person *with* an illness").

☐ Environmental factors can influence our perceptions of another person.

FOCUS 6: What are the two dimensions of the medical model?

☐ One dimension of the medical model is normal, which is defined as the absence of biological problems.

☐ Pathology is the other dimension of the model and is defined as the alteration of an organism produced by disease.

FOCUS 7: Distinguish between abnormal behavior as a physical illness and as a social problem.

□ Abnormal behavior as a physical illness is linked to the belief that a disturbed individual is physically ill, thus the origin of the term *mental illness.*

□ As a social problem, abnormal behavior results from the interaction of the individual and the environment.

□ Abnormal behavior as a social problem results from environmental stress in combination with an individual's inability to cope.

FOCUS 8: What are the four principles that guide us in determining who will be labeled socially deviant?

□ Normal behavior must meet societal, cultural, or group expectations.

□ Social deviance is not necessarily a physical illness.

□ Each culture determines the range of behaviors that will be defined as normal or deviant.

□ Social deviance may be caused by the interaction of several factors, including genetic makeup and individual experiences within the environment.

FOCUS 9: Distinguish between the educational labels of special, disordered, disabled, handicapped, and exceptional.

□ People defined as special have unusual, peculiar, unique, and distinctive characteristics that differentiate them from the normal peer group.

□ The term *disordered* refers to an individual with a general malfunction of mental, physical, or psychological processes.

□ The term *disabled* is more specific and describes the individual who has a loss of physical functioning (sight, hearing, legs, arms) or difficulties in learning and social adjustment that significantly interfere with normal growth and development.

□ A handicap is a limitation imposed on the individual by environmental demands and is related to the individual's ability to adapt or adjust to those demands.

□ The term *handicapped* usually describes only those individuals who are deficient in or lack ability.

□ The term *exceptional* is comprehensive and describes any individual whose physical or behavioral performance deviates so substantially from the norm, either higher or lower, that additional educational and other services may be necessary to meet the individual's needs.

Debate Forum

Label Jars, Not People—or, A Rose by Any Other Name

We put labels on people for many reasons. However, there is evidence that labeling is detrimental to an individual's self-image. So why do we continue to use labels? Isn't there a better way?

No label, no money

Point You have to label people who are in need of special services or they will not get the help they need. Funding for social service and educational programs requires labels. People qualify for these services based on labels. It is important for an agency to clearly distinguish between mentally retarded and non–mentally retarded people. If one does not distinguish between groups, then people who do not deserve the service may get it. In other words, no label, no money. Besides, labels help the general public more clearly distinguish between various categories of handicapped individuals. Labels help us distinguish blind people from deaf people, retarded people from those who have normal intelligence, and so forth. Without labels, how would we know who is who?

Counterpoint You are saying the reason we label is because the present bureaucracy says this is the way we have always done it and so this is the way we will always do it. Your concern is not with the individual who is labeled, but with how we can make the system run efficiently. We put people in boxes because that is the most convenient way to make sure that the right people, those who truly need help, get the service. So your logic for continuing to label people is founded on tradition. It is also based on the premise that public attitudes are inalterable. For many years the general public has developed conditioned responses to various social labels. Consequently, people in general react more to stereotyped characteristics of a group (e.g., physically handicapped people) than to the individual needs of the human beings that make up that group. You can argue that grouping people on the basis of some set of generalized characteristics ensures that services will be made available to those within the group. However, you can never be sure that the service provided to the group really meets the needs of any single individual so labeled.

How are we going to talk to each other?

Point We need labels so that professionals can communicate effectively with one another. Labels assist professionals in talking to each other about which populations need specialized medical, social, or educational services. Labels are also necessary so that research findings can be shared across several fields of study (e.g., medicine, psychology, etc.) using common criteria based on a label.

Counterpoint Once again your rationale for using labels is based on groups of people and not on the individual who is labeled. Your assumption that professionals across several fields of study all use the same labels when talking about people with exceptional characteristics is not accurate. For example, a physician's perception of a handicapping condition reflects the terminology of his or her field, namely medicine. Using a medical criterion, a physician may describe an individual as severely handicapped. An educator assessing the same individual may say he or she has a mild problem. Besides, if you read this chapter you know that the labels used by any given professional mirror the terminology of their specific field of study. So each professional may use different labels to describe the same person. You say abnormal, I say deviant. You say pathological, I say disabled. You say disordered, I say handicapped.

A label by any other name is still a label.

Point The direction you seem to be taking in this discussion is that we should get rid of all the labels we use on people and stick to labeling peanut butter jars. However, dumping the labels we currently use simply results in new and different labels. A new label will always be there to replace the old one. A label of some kind is necessary to communicate the nature of human differences. Over the years we've seen how

labels have evolved, and the fact is every time we stop using one label a new one appears to take its place. Historically, we have used many different labels to describe mentally retarded individuals, including feebleminded, moron, idiot, and imbecile. These labels were modernized to educable and trainable mentally retarded, but even they have become dated. Which will it be? Minimal brain dysfunction or learning disabilities? Deaf and dumb or hearing impaired? Insane or behavior disordered? Cripple or physically handicapped?

Counterpoint Your point seems to be that we are simply dealing in word games. Perhaps; but the words used in the game may mean a great deal to the person who is on the receiving end of a label. It is true that getting rid of one label may simply result in a new one. But maybe the new label or word will be less derogatory than the last. Many professionals don't use the labels moron, idiot, or imbecile to describe mentally retarded people, because they are no longer a part of our everyday language. They are used derogatorily to make fun of someone: "You stupid moron." I've tried to make the point that labels promote stereotyping. The labeled individual is viewed as part of a group (e.g., the physically handicapped) and not as an individual with unique characteristics. Let me end our discussion with an example of how stereotyping works.

> Suppose that most of the persons around you believe that you have a violent temper and are both moody and emotional. Further, imagine that the basis for these beliefs is simple: you possess red hair. Will these views, which can be seen as part of a widely held stereotype about redheads, exert any impact upon your behavior? The chances are good they might. Because others perceive you as possessing certain traits, they may treat you in specific ways. For example, they may lean over backwards to avoid making you angry. And such treatment, in turn, may well shape your own behavior. After all, if others expect you to act like an emotional volcano, you may be strongly tempted to do so. That is, you may often "blow your stack" in response to mild provocations. To the extent you come to behave in this fashion, of course, you will confirm the view that redheads really are emotional and moody (Baron & Byrne, 1984, p. 174).

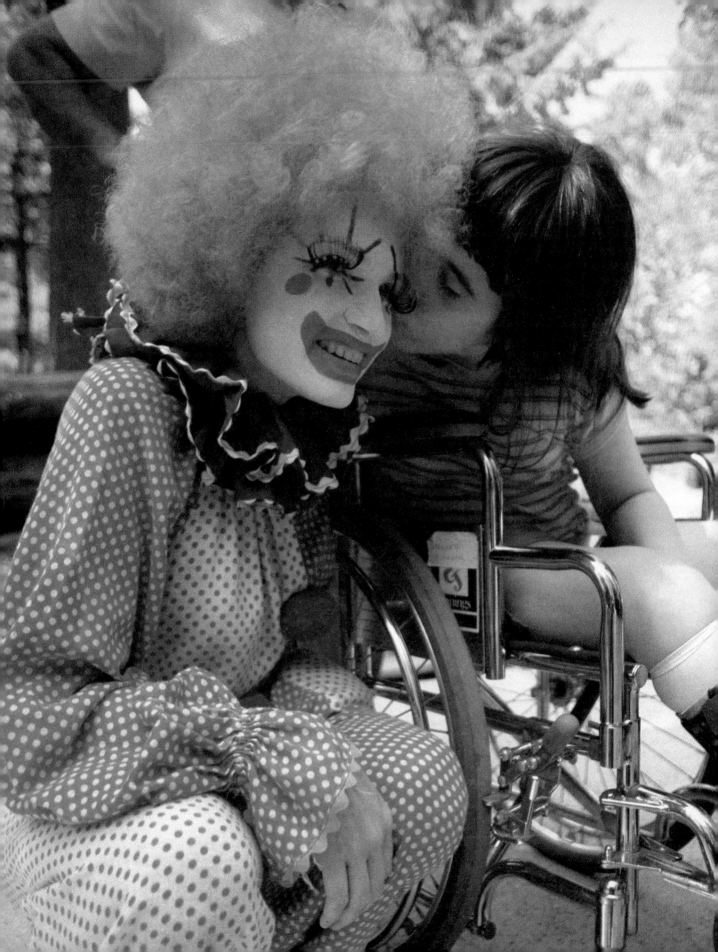

2 Human Services: Past and Present

To Begin With...

■ In a Senate debate on June 18, 1975, Senator Robert Stafford argued: "We can all agree that all handicapped children should be receiving an education. We can all agree that education should be equivalent, at least to the one those children who are not handicapped receive. The fact is, our agreeing on it does not make it the case. There are millions of children with handicapping conditions who are receiving no services at all" (Weiner & Hume, 1987).

■ To: The Access Committee
   Attention: Handicapped Romeo

   There is now a suitable ramp installed at my balcony.

                              Impatiently,
                              Miss Juliet
                              (Baird & Workman, 1986)

INTRODUCTION

The 1980s have been witness to some of the most significant legal, technological, and attitudinal changes in the treatment of exceptional individuals in the history of this country. Our reaffirmation of the rights of exceptional people is the result of a long evolutionary process. Today's services are actually the products of seeds planted centuries ago. Some of these seeds have yielded humane, healthy, and productive human service models. However, some models have not fully attended to the needs and rights of the exceptional individual.

History is a valuable resource that can help us determine which human service models are appropriate for the exceptional individual in today's society. We can learn from those who have preceded us.

THE HISTORY OF INDIVIDUALIZED TREATMENT AND EDUCATION

An Early Treatment Model: Itard and Victor

FOCUS 1
How did the work of Jean-Marc Itard contribute to our understanding of people with differences?

We must go back at least 200 years to find the first documented attempts to personalize a treatment program to the needs of exceptional individuals. During the seventeenth and eighteenth centuries, many professionals contributed to the understanding of human differences. Jean-Marc Itard (1775–1838) epitomizes the orientation of professionals during this period, and his work is reflected in our modern medical, psychological, social, and educational intervention models.

In 1799 Itard, a young physician and authority on diseases of the ear and the education of the deaf, was working for the National Institute of Deaf-Mutes in Paris. Itard believed that the environment in conjunction with physiological stimulation could contribute to the learning potential of any human being. Itard was influenced by the earlier work of Philippe Pinel and John Locke. Pinel advocated that people characterized as insane or idiots needed to be treated humanely. However, Pinel's teachings emphasized that such individuals were essentially incurable and that any treatment to remedy their disabilities would be fruitless. Locke's philosophy was contrary to that of Pinel. Locke described the mind as a blank slate that could be opened to all kinds of new stimuli. The positions of Pinel and Locke represent the classic "nature versus nurture" controversy: What are the roles of heredity and environment in determining a person's capabilities?

Itard tested the theories of Pinel and Locke in his work with Victor, the so-called wild boy of Aveyron. Victor was twelve years old when he was found in the woods by hunters. He had not developed any language, and his behavior was virtually uncontrollable, described as savage or animal-like. Ignoring Pinel's diagnosis that the child was an incurable **idiot,** Itard took responsibility for Victor and put him through a program of sensory stimulation that was intended to cure his condition. After five years Victor developed some verbal language and became more socialized as he grew accustomed to his new environment. Itard's work with Victor documented for the first time that learning is possible even for individuals described by most professionals as totally hopeless.

Reflect on This 2–1

Itard in the 1990s

Historians have recognized the contributions of Jean-Marc Itard as among the most visible landmarks in the development of education and treatment for handicapped people. Many of Itard's contributions are still evident today in our education programs.

1. *A developmental approach to instruction.* An intervention is based on the interaction of biological/genetic characteristics and the physical environment. In order to initiate treatment effectively, the professional must clearly identify where in the normal developmental sequence the individual is currently functioning.

2. *Individualized instruction.* An intervention is based on assessment of the needs, characteristics, and functioning level of the individual.

3. *Sensory stimulation.* An intervention is directed toward the remediation of deficits in the basic sensory systems: vision, hearing, touch, kinesthesis, smell, and taste.

4. *Systematic instruction.* An intervention begins with tasks the child is capable of performing and then gradually builds to more complex learning. The sequence builds from concrete or real objects to more abstract concepts or ideas.

5. *The functional-life curriculum.* An intervention is directed toward the development of independent living skills wihin the individual's immediate environment. All content areas (e.g., self-care, motor, language, and academic instruction) are intended to assist the handicapped individual to function independently.

Itard's work was instrumental in early nineteenth-century treatment programs. His ideas about appropriate treatment were continued and expanded on by many individuals. The contributions of notable physicians and educators of this period are highlighted in Table 2–1.

Psychology's Contribution to Understanding the Individual

During the nineteenth century European countries established special schools and segregated living facilities for people with handicaps (e.g., the **feebleminded, deaf, blind,** and **insane**). As explained by McCleary, Hardman, and Thomas (1989), expertise and knowledge about people with disabilities was extremely limited. Most programs during this period focused on care and management rather than treatment and education. Although many professionals had demonstrated that positive changes in the development of the individual were possible, they had not been able to "cure" such conditions as insanity or idiocy.

In the late nineteenth and early twentieth centuries, a new school of thought emerged: the science of the mind. Modern psychology, as we know it today, is about one hundred years old. In 1879, Wilhelm Wundt defined psychology as the science of conscious experience. The definition was based on the principle of **introspection**—looking into oneself to analyze experiences. William James expanded Wundt's conceptions of conscious experience, in his treatise *The Principles*

FOCUS 2
Identify two major contributions of modern psychology to our understanding of human differences.

TABLE 2–1 Contributions of Physicians and Educators Concerned with Treatment of Exceptional Individuals (Seventeenth Through Nineteenth Centuries)

	Profession	Major Contributions
John Locke (1632–1704)	English philosopher	Distinguished between idiocy (mental retardation) and insanity (mental illness) (1690). Advocated the idea that there is no basic human nature, that our minds at birth are a blank slate.
Philippe Pinel (1742–1826)	French physician	Classified mental illness as a disease. Advocated humane treatment for the mentally ill.
Jean-Marc Itard (1775–1838)	French physician/educator	Believed that idiocy could be treated through educational intervention (1799). Advocated individualized intervention, sensory stimulation, systematic instruction.
Thomas Hopkins Gallaudet (1787–1851)	American minister/educator	Established first American residential school for the deaf (1817).
Samuel Gridley Howe (1801–1876)	American physician/educator	Involved in education of the blind and the deaf. Founded the Perkins Institute for the Blind (1832). As a social reformer, advocated public financial support for education and treatment of exceptional populations.

of *Psychology* (1890), to include learning, motivation, and emotions. In 1913, John B. Watson shifted the content of psychology from conscious experience to observable behavior and mental events.

In 1920, Watson conducted an experiment with an eleven-month-old child named Albert. Albert showed no fear of a white rat when initially exposed to the animal. He saw the rat as a toy and played with it freely. Watson then introduced a loud, terrifying noise directly behind Albert each time the rat was presented. After a period of time the boy became frightened by the sight of any furry white object, even though the loud noise was not present. Albert had learned to fear rats through **conditioning.** Conditioning is the process in which new objects or situations elicit responses that were previously elicited by other stimuli. Watson thus demonstrated that abnormal behavior could be learned through the interaction of the individual with environmental stimuli. The contributions of other notable nineteenth- and twentieth-century psychologists are highlighted in Table 2–2.

The early twentieth century was marked by contrasts in the treatment of exceptional individuals. On the positive side, the **scientific method** was being applied to the measurement of intelligence, as with the Binet-Simon Intelligence Test, developed in 1905. Services that had been denied to exceptional individuals for centuries were becoming more accessible. Special classes in urban public schools were being developed for children with learning problems as well as those with visual and hearing impairments. As the twentieth century began,

	Profession	Major Contributions
Dorothea Dix (1802–1887)	American educator	As a social reformer, secured reforms in U.S. mental institutions, making them professionally administered hospitals for the "sick" rather than punishment-oriented facilities (prisons).
Louis Braille (1809–1852)	French educator	Developed a system of reading and writing for the blind (1834).
Eduoard Seguin (1812–1880)	French physician/educator	Developed physiological method of treatment: intervention through sensory motor development. Established first school for the intellectually retarded in Paris (1837). Helped establish first residential facility for the retarded in the U.S. (1854).
Maria Montessori (1870–1952)	Italian physician/educator	Involved in education of the mentally retarded. Developed theory and curricula for early-childhood education of normal and exceptional populations.

public sentiment was aroused and more federal, state, and local monies were being channeled into human services.

By contrast, many misconceptions during the early twentieth century resulted in fear of handicapped people and a movement to isolate them from society. Many people believed that the mentally and morally defective were defiling the human race: "We must come to recognize feeble-mindedness, idiocy, **imbecility,** and insanity as largely communicable conditions or diseases, just as the ordinary physician recognizes smallpox, diphtheria, etc., as communicable" (Sprattling, 1912; cited in Wolfensberger, 1975).

SOCIAL SEGREGATION

Henry Herbert Goddard, an American psychologist, believed that inferior intelligence was caused solely by hereditary factors. He attempted to convince the scientific and lay community that feeblemindedness was indeed transmitted from generation to generation (Goddard, 1912). He later hypothesized that there is an irrefutable link between intelligence and social deviance: The less intelligence people have, the less responsible they are for their actions. Therefore, less intelligent people are more likely to exhibit socially deviant or unacceptable behavior (Goddard, 1914). Goddard's definition of social deviates included criminals,

FOCUS 3
In the early part of the twentieth century, what role were hereditary factors thought to play in regard to intelligence and social deviance?

TABLE 2–2   Contributions of Professionals Concerned with Human Behavior (Late Nineteenth Through Early Twentieth Century)

	Profession	Major Contributions
Wilhelm Wundt (1832–1920)	German psychologist trained in physics, physiology, and philosophy	Defined psychology as the science of conscious experience. Developed system of psychology known as structuralism: discovering the structure or anatomy of conscious experience (what and how something happens). Established first laboratory for the scientific study of psychology (1879).
William James (1842–1910)	American psychologist	Extended study of psychology beyond conscious experience to a functional and applied psychology (functionalism: why something happens). Published *Principles of Psychology* in the U.S. (1890).
Sigmund Freud (1856–1939)	Viennese physician	Concerned with motivation and dynamics of personality. Saw mental life as more than consciousness, that there is an underlying force labeled the *unconscious*. As the father of psychoanalysis, developed a theory of personality, a philosophical view of human nature, and a method of treating disturbed individuals. Constructed a vocabulary of the mind (i.e., the id, ego, and superego). Published basic ideas on psychoanalysis in *Die Traumdeutung*.
Ivan Pavlov (1849–1936)	Russian physiologist	Discovered a technique called *classical conditioning*, the principle that a neutral stimulus paired with a stimulus that already evokes a response will eventually evoke a response by itself. In Russian, published results of his studies on classical conditioning.
The Gestaltists (1912) Wolfgang Köhler Kurt Koffka Max Wertheimer	German psychologists	Responsible for what is known as Gestalt psychology: Behavior cannot be divided into discrete elements. Components must be brought together and examined as a pattern or whole; the whole is greater than the sum of its parts.
John B. Watson (1878–1958)	American psychologist	Shifted study of psychology away from conscious-experience orientation of structuralists and fundamentalists to the study of observable behavior. Advocated that psychology be studied in a rigorous, objective, and experimental manner. Advocated that virtually all human behavior is learned. Changed the course of American psychology with paper on behaviorism (1913).
B. F. Skinner (1904–)	American psychologist	Described the basic principles of operant behavior and their influence on people. Advocated an interpretation of behavioral principles that led to a treatment approach commonly referred to as *behavior modification*.

alcoholics, the sexually immoral, **mongoloids, epileptics,** the mentally ill, and the feebleminded. Goddard's thesis was widely accepted by American and European psychologists in the 1920s and 1930s, although it is no longer accepted by contemporary professionals in psychology or sociology (Drew, Logan, & Hardman, 1988).

Many professionals (e.g., Barr, 1915; Fernald, 1915; Johnson, 1908) supported Goddard's theory that mental and moral deviance were hereditary and that intellectual deficiencies were primarily fixed and incurable. The outcome of this theory was a widespread movement toward selective breeding and the overall prevention of deviance. This brought about an extended period of alarm and fear of, as well as an indictment against, many handicapped people. In the latter half of this century we have come to recognize that hereditary factors play a less significant role in the causes of mental and social deviance than was once thought, especially when compared to maternal health and sociocultural factors (Westling, 1986).

The focus of early twentieth-century preventive measures was the passage of state legislation that prohibited "mental and social deviates" from marrying. Eventually such legislation was expanded to include sterilization of such individuals. Compulsory surgical **sterilization** became widespread, and laws were passed throughout the Nation in an effort to reduce the number of deviates. Karier (1973) estimates that over 8500 persons were sterilized in twenty-one states between 1907 and 1928. Sterilization laws in some states contained provisions for sterilizing mentally retarded people, individuals with epilepsy, the sexually promiscuous, and criminals. In addition to marriage and sterilization laws, large numbers of individuals were moved from their communities into isolated, special-care facilities whose sole purpose was care and maintenance. These facilities became widely known as **institutions.**

The Meaning of An Institution

An institution is defined as an establishment or facility governed by a collection of fundamental rules. The five principal types of institutions may be described as follows:

FOCUS 4
What are the five principal types of institutions?

1. Institutions for persons who are both "incapable" and "harmless"; for example, schools for people who are blind, nursing homes, and orphanages

2. Institutions for persons who are "incapable" and who unintentionally pose a threat to the community, such as mental hospitals, leper colonies, and TB sanitariums

3. Institutions for persons who intentionally endanger the community: prisons and jails

4. Institutions established for some instrumental task: army barracks, boarding schools, and work campuses

5. Institutions that are retreats from the secular world: abbeys, monasteries, convents, and cloisters (Goffman, 1975).

Institutions for deviant populations have had many different labels: school, hospital, colony, prison, and asylum. The term *institution* did not originate with the facilities of early twentieth-century America. Asylums, prominent in many parts of Europe in the seventeenth century, were used to segregate, dehumanize, and punish moral defectives. Through the work of Pinel, in France, and Benjamin Rush, the father of American psychiatry, an era of humanitarian reform began in the last half of the eighteenth century.

The early nineteenth century brought a period of optimism concerning the treatment and eventual cure of people described as deviant. However, hope eventually eroded into despair and fear of these people, because social and mental deviance was not being cured. Because deviance continued to be a major social problem, many professionals were convinced that it was necessary to segregate large numbers of both mental and social deviates. By 1868, over 4000 people resided in fifteen institutions throughout the United States (McCarver & Cavalier, 1983).

Institutions became more and more concerned with social control as they grew in size and financial resources became scarce. These facilities had to establish rigid rules and regulations in order to manage large numbers of individuals with a limited financial base. In many cases, these rules stripped away the individuals' identity and forced them into group regimentation. For example, individuals could have no personal possessions. They were forced to wear institutional clothing and were given an identification tag and number.

FOCUS 5
What are the seven characteristics of institutions?

Characteristics of Institutions.   Institutions, whether they are called mental hospitals, asylums, state prisons, or colonies for mentally retarded people, share a number of characteristics:

1. All aspects of life are conducted in the same place and under the same single authority.
2. Each phase of the member's daily activity is carried on in the immediate company of a large batch of others, all of whom are treated alike and required to do the same thing together.
3. All phases of the day's activities are tightly scheduled, the whole sequence of activities being imposed from above by a system of explicit formal rulings and a body of officials.
4. Social mobility between the two strata is grossly restricted; social distance is typically great and often formally prescribed.
5. There exists a work ideology which the institution may define as treatment, **rehabilitation,** punishment, or the like.
6. There exists a system of rewards and punishments which takes in the total life situation of the "inmate."
7. There exists a "mortification" or "stripping" process, where "desocialization" or "disculturation" takes place and "resocialization" begins (Goffman, 1975, p. 410).

By the early 1920s, all states had hospitals for mentally ill people, and the number of large, isolated residential facilities for mentally retarded people was growing rapidly (Fernald, 1984). For the most part, these facilities remained

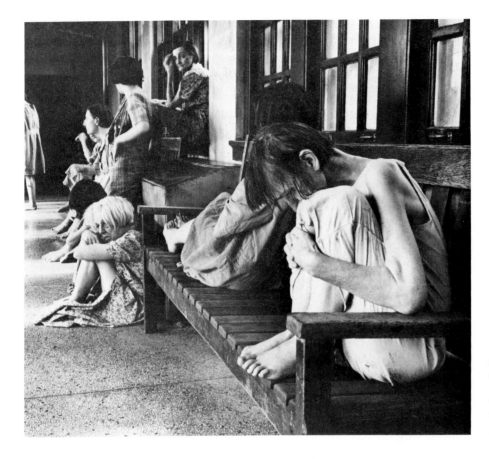

Segregation and dehumanization characterize many institutions of the twentieth century. (© J. Cooke/Photo Researchers)

largely custodial and were characterized by locked living units, barred windows, and high walls surrounding the facility. Organized treatment programs declined, and "terminal," uncured patients accumulated. This forced even more expansion and the erection of new buildings. In addition, public and professional pessimism concerning the value of treatment programs meant diminishing funds for mental health care.

This alarming situation remained unchanged for nearly five decades and declined even further during the depression years of the 1930s. By the early 1950s there were more than 500,000 persons committed to mental hospitals throughout the Nation.

Reform of Institutions. In the early 1950s, the first attempts to reform mental hospitals were initiated by the American Psychiatric Association, which led efforts to inspect and rate the nation's 300 mental hospitals and called attention to the lack of therapeutic intervention and deplorable living conditions. In 1950, parents of mentally retarded children organized, and the National Association for Retarded Children (now known as the Association for Retarded Citizens—USA) was founded. The purpose of this association is "to promote the general welfare of the mentally retarded of all ages everywhere: at home, in the communities, in institutions, and in public, private, and religious schools" (Residential services, Position statements of the ARC, 1976, p. 3). This parent movement in the United States was paralleled by many others in countries around the world, as families organized to lobby policymakers for more appropriate services (McCleary et al., 1989).

Over the next two decades (1950–1970), the philosophy regarding segregation underwent some important changes. Institutional practices were severely criticized by many professionals (such as Blatt & Kaplan, 1966), and the general public became more aware that many institutions did not have any provision for treatment and **habilitation.** Legal action was taken, and several law-suits were brought against states for operating inadequate facilities. We explore some of the more important court cases in detail in the next section.

The Right to Treatment in an Institution

FOCUS 6
Identify four primary issues in the right-to-treatment cases that have come before the courts in the latter half of the twentieth century.

Several court cases of the past three decades have been significant in reforming state institutions for mentally retarded and mentally ill people. In 1966, the ruling in *Rouse* v. *Camerson* established that institutions must provide treatment. Although the treatment need not be curative, the court ruled that a legitimate attempt must be made to improve the individual's condition. In that same year, *Lake* v. *Camerson* ruled that in addition to institutions there must be options (e.g., community mental health centers) for all individuals labeled as mentally ill. A U.S. district court ruled, in the case of *Wyatt* v. *Stickney* (1972), that the mentally retarded patients at an institution in Alabama were being deprived of the right to individual treatment that would give them a realistic opportunity for habilitation. This case was the first major court action on behalf of mentally retarded people residing in public institutions (Cavalier & McCarver, 1981). The court described the institutional facilities as human warehouses steeped in an atmosphere of psychological and physical deprivation. It further specified that the state must make changes to ensure a therapeutic environment. The court stipulated that patients have a right to (1) privacy and dignity; (2) manage their own affairs (including marriage, divorce, and voting privileges); (3) have visitors, make phone calls, and receive confidential mail; (4) be free from physical restraint and isolation; (5) wear their own clothes and keep personal possessions; (6) an adequate medical program; and (7) be free from experimental research without informed consent.

The case of *Halderman* v. *Pennhurst* (1977) began as a suit on behalf of the residents of a Pennsylvania state institution alleging inhumane and dangerous conditions, unnecessary physical restraints, and lack of habilitative programs in the **least restrictive environment.** However, in a 1981 review of the case, the U.S. Supreme Court found that current law does not create substantive rights to treatment in the least restrictive environment. Current law does no more than establish a national policy to improve treatment of mentally retarded people and to provide financial incentives to induce states to do so. It does not require states to expend their financial resources to provide specific kinds of treatment.

Reflect on This 2–2

Did You Know That . . . ?

The late president John F. Kennedy played a significant role in the expansion of services to people with disabilities, particularly those with mental retardation. As both family member and statesman John Kennedy was a powerful impetus toward social reform.

■ He (and the entire Kennedy family) openly acknowledged that his sister Rosemary was mentally retarded, thus focusing public attention on the needs of disabled people.

■ He focused the Nation's attention on family and community living for all people with disabilities.

■ He established the President's Committee on Mental Retardation in 1961, to examine critical social and educational issues affecting people with mental retardation.

■ He strongly supported the Community Mental Health Center Construction Act of 1963, which was intended to reduce the size of the country's institutions and to promote prevention of both mental illness and mental retardation.

In 1982, the case of *Youngberg* v. *Romeo* dealt with the question of whether physical restraint or lack of safe conditions in a state institution was a violation of **due process.** Nicholas Romeo suffered either self- or externally inflicted injuries on at least seventy different occasions while a resident at the Pennhurst State School and Hospital. The court held that appropriate training for the mentally retarded person is necessary to ensure safety and freedom from restraint. This decision is significant because it is the first time the Supreme Court has found that retarded people in institutions have a limited right to treatment. However, the larger issue of a general constitutional right to treatment has yet to be considered by the Supreme Court.

In the case of *Homeward Bound* v. *The Hissom Memorial Center* (1988), a U.S. district court ruled that because they were institutionalized, persons with mental retardation residing at Hissom State School and Hospital had been denied opportunities for a quality life. The court directed the State of Oklahoma to close the school within a four-year period, and to create community alternatives for people with mental retardation using the following guiding principles:

1. All persons are capable of growth and development.
2. All persons deserve to be treated with dignity.
3. All persons have value.
4. All persons must be involved in and carry the primary responsibility for the decisions that affect their lives.
5. All persons should live and work in the most natural settings.
6. All children should live with their families.
7. All persons should live in and be a part of the community.

The Effects of Institutionalization

FOCUS 7
Identify two possible effects
of institutionalization on an
individual.

A number of investigations (e.g., Balla, 1976; Blatt, Ozolins & McNally, 1979; Butterfield, 1976; Lakin, Bruininks & Sigford, 1981; Rotegard, Hill, & Bruininks, 1983; Rothman & Rothman, 1984; Staff Report, 1985; and Zigler, 1973) have shown that present-day institutions continue to range from dehumanizing warehouses that have a deleterious effect on the cognitive and physiological development of their residents, to facilities that, through systematic treatment and a noninstitutional atmosphere, attempt to bring about some positive behavioral changes.

Some institutions have attempted to normalize the environment of the residents by providing homelike living arrangements. Such efforts may include private or semiprivate bedrooms, family dining facilities, homelike furnishings, a choice of clothing and hairstyles, encouraging individual possessions, access to everyday household risks such as hot water and electrical appliances, and individualized educational or therapeutic programs. The most harmful aspect of institutionalization is related to a restrictive regimen with little regard for individual needs or desires.

What constitutes a good institution continues to be a matter of legal and moral debate. Objective criteria have not been agreed on by parents or professionals. We do know that the original rationale for the social-segregation model in the early twentieth century is not valid. Institutional accomplishments of the past eighty years can be summed up in a few rather negative statements. In this century institutions became isolate asylums concerned more with social management and regimentation than with education or treatment. The large institution in many cases became a place where residents were subject to physical abuse and emotional neglect (Blatt & Kaplan, 1967; Blatt, Ozolins & McNally, 1979; *Homeward Bound* v. *Hissom*, 1988; *Wyatt* v. *Stickney*, 1972; *Youngberg* v. *Romeo*, 1982). The civil rights of individuals were often ignored. Lakin and Bruininks (1985) summarized the research on large public and private institutions: These facilities, "once virtually the only model of extrafamilial care of handicapped persons, are both aberrant social settings and have debilitating effects that increase the probability of segregated living" (p. 12).

Large institutions, originally intended to stop the spread of deviance, did not prevent mental or social problems, as some early twentieth century professionals predicted. Menolascino, McGee, and Casey (1982) discussed the need for alternatives beyond the institutional model:

> There is abundant information and research data available to support the contention that: (1) prolonged institutionalization has destructive developmental consequences . . . , (2) appropriate community-based residential settings are generally more beneficial than institutional placements . . . , and (3) mentally retarded individuals with a wide spectrum of disabilities—including the severely and profoundly retarded—can be successfully served in community-based settings. (p. 65)

As evidence that this country is moving away from institutionalization, note that the number of people residing in these facilities has declined dramatically since the late 1960s. Braddock, Hemp, and Howes (1984) report that less than 100,000 people resided in institutions in the early 1980s, a 50-percent decline in less than two decades. We are moving away from the era of social segregation

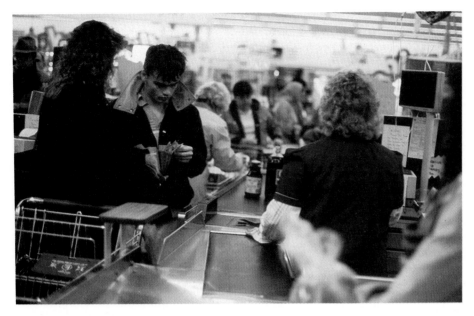

The United States is moving away from a policy of social segregation to one of social integration. Today, people with disabilities are living and working in their own communities more than ever before. (The Institute for the Study of Developmental Disabilities at Indiana University)

to one of social integration. People with handicaps are living and working in their own communities more than they have for many years.

SOCIAL INTEGRATION

Defining the Least Restrictive Environment

The concept of the least restrictive environment, or LRE, is central to the expansion of social integration for people with handicaps. Bachrach (1985) suggests that LRE deals with a question that is basic to the care of all handicapped people: How are we going to ensure that the services provided in community settings are humane, relevant, and responsive to the needs of the individual?

The LRE doctrine states that persons with exceptional characteristics should receive services in an environment that is consistent with individual needs. Court cases have progressively clarified the basis for the application of the LRE doctrine to social, medical, and educational services. The following are three of the doctrine's major components:

1. *There must be available a range of services capable of meeting an individual's developmental needs. The more restricted the range, the greater the probability that gaps will exist, thus forcing individuals into inappropriate environments.* This position is contrary to the segregation model, where institutionalization was routine for many individuals. In many cases the maintenance of segregated services resulted in a failure to develop community-based alternatives.

FOCUS 8
Identify three major components of the concept of least restrictive environment.

2. *The least restrictive environment is defined by individual need and not by the range of services available.* Thus every effort should be made to expand environmental alternatives to meet individual needs. If the needs of a person do not match the services available, then the services must be altered in order to accommodate the individual. This position also emphasizes that a setting defined as "restrictive," such as a state hospital or institution, should be employed only if individual need warrants such a placement.

3. *The LRE concept establishes that all environmental alternatives are fluid. Placement in any social or educational service pattern is not terminal or irreversible but must be continuously reassessed.* This position reaffirms that individuals are not to be placed and then forgotten. In order to meet the intent of LRE, there must be an ongoing evaluation of individual growth. This process can be accomplished only through the interaction of the individual, his or her parents, and professionals. This approach provides for a comprehensive evaluation, including medical, social, and educational factors.

Developing Community Resources

FOCUS 9
What are the three types of services that must be available to ensure that an individual is living in the least restrictive environment?

The intent of the LRE concept is to have comprehensive services (such as educational programs, public transportation, restaurant access, or religious activities) available to an individual within or as close as possible to family and community life. An individual should also be able to purchase additional services: dental examinations, medical treatment, life insurance, and so forth. The purpose of such services is to allow the person an opportunity to achieve community integration. In order to accomplish integration, several factors should be taken into account, including the developmental level of the individual; the individual's ability, with appropriate training, to adapt to societal expectations; and the willingness of society to adapt to and accommodate the individual with differences.

Medical Services.   Appropriate medical care is essential for people with exceptional characteristics. In many cases, the physician is the first professional with whom parents have contact concerning their child's disability. This is particularly true when the child's problem is identifiable immediately after birth or during early childhood. The physician is the family advisor and communicates with parents regarding the medical prognosis and recommendations for treatment. However, too often, physicians assume that they are the family's only counseling resource (Drew, Logan, & Hardman, 1988; Hardman & Drew, 1980). They should be aware of additional resources within the community, including other parents, social workers, mental health professionals, and educators.

Medical services are often taken for granted simply because they are readily available for most people. This is not true for many exceptional people. It is not uncommon for a pediatrician to suggest that parents seek treatment elsewhere for their exceptional child even when the problem is a common illness such as a cold or a sore throat (Levine, 1982).

It would be unfair to stereotype medical professionals as unresponsive to the needs of exceptional people. On the contrary, medical technology has prevented many disabilities and enhanced the quality of life for handicapped people. However,

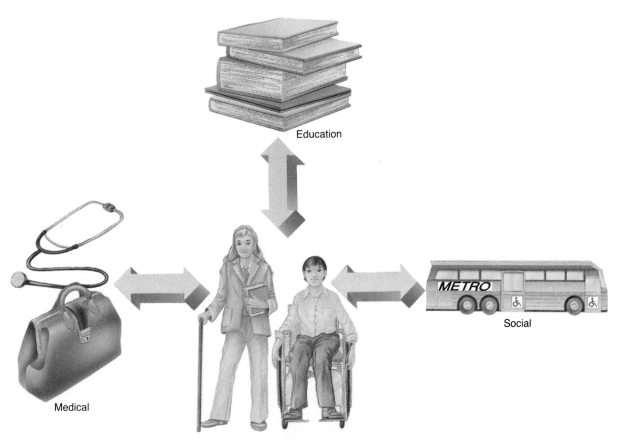

Figure 2–1
Community Services

in order for handicapped people to receive comprehensive medical services in a community setting, several factors must be considered. The physician in community practice (general practitioners, pediatricians, etc.) must receive more medical training in the medical, psychological, and educational aspects of handicapping conditions. This training could include: (1) knowledge regarding developmental milestones, (2) attitudes regarding handicapped children, (3) knowledge of handicapping conditions, (4) prevention, (5) screening, diagnosis, and assessment, (6) interdisciplinary collaboration, (7) working effectively with parents, (8) long-term medical and social treatment programs, and (9) community resources. Physicians must be more willing to treat handicapped patients for common illnesses when the treatment is irrelevant to the patient's disability. Physicians need not become disability specialists, but they must have enough knowledge to refer the patient to an appropriate specialist when necessary. Finally, they must be aware of and willing to refer the patient to other community resources such as social workers, educators, or psychologists.

The medical profession must continue to support physician specialists and other allied health personnel who are well equipped to work with disabled

In the News 2–1

They'll Astonish You!

. . . in the years since losing one of my legs to cancer [at the age of thirteen], I have gained something worth far more than a leg—a firsthand understanding of the torment, condescension and discrimination that millions of disabled men, women and children endure each day, not because of their disability but because of society's denial of reasonable opportunities for them to reach their potential and lead satisfying lives.

Now, of course, I realize those feelings—of pity and drastically reduced expectations—are the very attitudes that people who are mentally and physically challenged are fighting to change. I have come to know, firsthand, that the most severe limitation people with a disability often face is lack of opportunity—lack of opportunity to participate fully in society, to be regarded by others as an equal and have access to things we all take for granted, like getting a job or living independently in the community.

People with disabilities deserve opportunities to participate in all that life has to offer, including the arts. Unfortunately, our society does not place as high a priority on the arts as many other countries do. Often, when there are budget cuts, the arts are among the first to go. Arts programs for people with disabilities are in even greater jeopardy of being eliminated. I am not an artist myself, but I have seen the new worlds that can be opened up when a disabled child first learns to paint a picture, sing a song, recite a poem, or perform a dance.

A few weeks ago, I was reminded again of the influence the arts can have on the life of a person with a disability. Though I have been deeply involved with the organization called Very Special Arts for several years, I am always moved, as if for the first time, when one individual achieves a goal that seems to embody our essential purpose. Willie Britt's story is one of those.

Willie Britt's now-famous "Sandals" poster hangs over my desk at home. It depicts row after row of brightly colored but otherwise identical sandals, with one askew. I think it conveys a powerful message about individuality. So, I thought I knew the Willie Britt story. Last month, however, I learned that William Britt—who had spent his first 34 years in the Willowbrook State School, an institution for the mentally re-

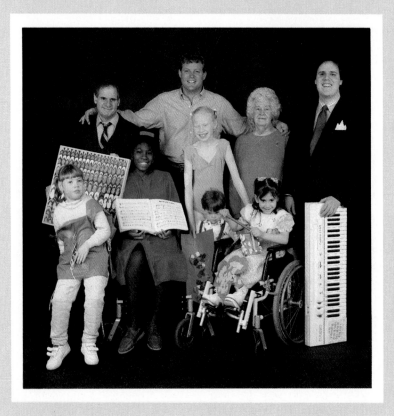

(Barbra Walz)

tarded—had just graduated from Westchester Community College in New York at the age of 53. I was overwhelmed. I knew that when he had first left Willowbrook in 1974 for the Margaret Chapman School in Hawthorne, N.Y., the prospects for meaningful rehabilitation seemed poor. His counselors reported that he was angry, withdrawn and given to long periods of solitude. Fortunately, shortly after entering the Chapman School, Willie discovered his love for painting. That love soon became consuming, and Willie found his "canvases" everywhere—on the backs of discarded cardboard boxes and on crumpled pieces of construction paper. His talent blossomed.

It didn't take long for the school's director, Eileen Bisordi, to enroll Willie in the state's Very Special Arts program, enabling him to receive formal instruction in art. The talent which had gone unrecognized all his life now found its full expression. Soon his paintings, often of New York landmarks like the State Capitol and the Statue of Liberty, painted from postcards or photographs, were exhibited at the state's Very Special Arts festivals. Then, as part of a community outreach program initiated by the organization, Mrs. Bisordi enrolled Willie in Westchester Commuity College's fine arts program. For several years, Willie took art courses leading to the diploma he received last month. I am sure that few graduates anywhere this year were more deserving, tenacious or courageous than William Britt in achieving their goal.

... Willie's story is remarkable but not unusual. In this country, there are millions of children and adults with disabilities for whom the arts have special meaning. They may not have such exceptional talents, but they benefit from participation in the arts, which can foster independence and self-esteem. This is so important for those who must rely on others to do everyday things people take for granted. The creative process itself plays a role, since it involves making choices and taking control of a situation, a process which generalizes to other aspects of life.

... Michael Naranjo, for example, is a sculptor of extraordinary ability and accomplishment. When a grenade exploded near Michael in Vietnam in 1968, it ended his eyesight but not his vision. He returned home to the Santa Clara Pueblo in New Mexico, determined to make sculpting his life's work. At first, he got little encouragement, and his rehabilitation counselors urged him to pursue a vocation where he could more easily earn a living. At the time, employment statistics for disabled veterans were grim. However, Michael persevered, and today his sculptures sell internationally for up to $30,000. ...

Of course, not all of the artists ... have attained the recognition that Michael has. Many are young adults with a great deal of talent and a promising future, like Denise Shipler of Burt, Iowa, a gifted 19-year-old singer. Denise was born with phocomelia, which means that several of her limbs were only partially formed. Like other young people with a disability, she often experienced the cruelty of other children who ridiculed and shunned her.

Denise feels that it was music which saved her from despair during those difficult times and gave her a new basis for relating to her classmates. She has won ovations for her performances at the Iowa State Fair, and when she sings at our international festival, people from all around the world will join in celebrating her accomplishments.

Often, one of the most important factors in a person's adjustment to a disability, especially if it comes later in life, is the love and encouragement received from family and friends. I've spoken with several people who became paralyzed as adults from spinal-cord injuries, and all reported experiencing a very dark period of despair when the only thing that kept them going was the support and encouragement of others. Once this period was over, passion for their work—especially where it involved the creative process in some way—was the most important link to participating fully in life again.

I know this was true for Corrie van Hugten, who lost the use of her legs 12 years ago because of a debilitating illness. Previously, Corrie had been a ballet dancer. Even when she learned that she'd never walk again, she was determined to continue dancing. She felt that rhythm is the essential element of dance and that people confined to chairs may have lost the use of their legs but not their sense of rhythm. With her partner, Ondine, she has introduced ballroom dancing, wheelchair style, throughout the Netherlands. There are now 75 official wheelchair dancing groups and 300 qualified instructors in the Netherlands, thanks to Corrie's efforts. Last year, Very Special Arts brought Corrie to the Cotting School in Lexington, Mass.—a school for kids with physical and learning disabilities—to give wheelchair dancing lessons. Since they were having their senior prom the next week, it was an incredible experience and a great success.

. . . I think it goes to show you how important and universal this movement is. On the walls of the Kennedy Center, where the festival will be held, there is a quote of President Kennedy's that I am always reminded of in my work with Very Special Arts. It reads: "I am certain that after the dust of centuries has passed over our cities, we, too, will be remembered not for victories or defeats in battle or in politics, but for our contribution to the human spirit."

Source: From "They'll Astonish You!" by Ted Kennedy, Jr., *Parade*, June 11, 1989, pp. 4–6. Excerpts reprinted with permission from Parade, copyright © 1989.

people. These specialized health professionals include **geneticists** and **genetic counselors,** physical and **occupational therapists,** public health nurses, and nutritional and dietary personnel.

Social Services. The integration of exceptional people into a community setting depends on the accessibility of appropriate social services. These services include community mental health centers, access to public buildings and transportation, community living alternatives, recreation and leisure-time activities, and employment opportunities.

Community mental health centers provide psychological services and early-intervention programs in a local setting. Such centers have provisions for both in-patient and out-patient care. Services provided by the centers include psychological evaluation, intensive treatment programs, and referrals to other agencies when appropriate. There are also provisions for crisis intervention on a twenty-four-hour-a-day basis, and rehabilitation services to help people restore physical, social, or vocational functioning.

Access to adequate housing and **barrier-free facilities** is essential for people with physical disabilities. A barrier-free environment may mean renovating some facilities and incorporating barrier-free designs in new buildings and public transportation. Those in wheelchairs or on crutches need entrance ramps to and within public buildings; accessibility to public telephones, vending machines, and restrooms; and lifts for public transportation vehicles. Available community living environments could include specialized boarding homes, supervised apartments, group homes, and foster home placement.

Recreation and leisure-time opportunities within the community vary substantially according to age and the severity of the individual's disability. Thus the availability of these services must also vary from community to community. Many families may not have access to such services as dance and music lessons, tumbling, swimming, or scouting; yet all these services are generally available for other children within the community. Similar problems exist for adolescents and adults with exceptional characteristics: Many have not been able to adapt to the community because they cannot use their leisure time constructively. Adults may do little with their leisure time beyond watching television. Recreational programs must be developed to assist individuals in developing worthwhile leisure-time activities and a more satisfying lifestyle. Therapeutic recreation is a profession concerned specifically with this goal: using recreation to help people adapt their physical, emotional, or social characteristics to take advantage of leisure-time activities more independently in a community setting.

Employment opportunities are essential to a successful lifestyle for adults, including those with disabilities. Yet many individuals with disabilities are unable to gain employment during the adult years. A recent Harris Poll (International Center for the Disabled, 1986) found that two-thirds of disabled people between the ages of sixteen and sixty-four were not working; and that 66 percent of those not working, and of working age, indicated they would like a job. A comparison of working and nonworking disabled individuals revealed that working individuals were more satisfied with life, had more money, and were less likely to blame their disability for preventing them from reaching their potential.

A report by the Organization for Economic Cooperation and Development (OECD, 1986) suggested that the common denominator around the world is "the lack of flexibility of systems which on occasion discourage the search for employment. A further feature of many [countries] is that benefits cease when employment is found, but are not easily obtained again if the individual is unemployed" (p. 18). For the individual with a disability, the messages are indeed mixed. One government entity urges that people with disabilities should strive to be contributing members of society, while another supports their dependence. OECD concluded that the proper role of governments may be to stimulate opportunities for people with disabilities in both the private and public sectors. This role would include legislation and policy development, a mandated process for interagency coordination, strategies to change public attitudes, and the dissemination of information regarding effective model programs that enhance community living and participation.

Educational Services. The right of handicapped students to a **free and appropriate public education** has been mandated by state and national legislation. Because much of this legislation has excluded gifted and talented students, the more narrowly defined term *handicapped* is used. However, a movement toward appropriate education for *all* exceptional students is gaining momentum.

Schools are faced with the challenge of educating a diverse population of students. This means greater emphasis on precise and individualized instruction, effective use of professionals in several disciplines (e.g., psychologists, social workers, and medical personnel), and a more clearly defined role for the educator. In order to understand why education has an expanded role in the 1990s, we must first review the history of special education services in this country.

EDUCATING EXCEPTIONAL STUDENTS

A Beginning: 1900–1920

The education of exceptional children in the United States began in the early 1900s with the efforts of many dedicated professionals. These efforts consisted of programs that were usually separate from the public schools. Many instructional programs took place in special schools and were concerned with educating children who were visually disordered, hearing disordered, mentally retarded, or emotionally disturbed.

FOCUS 10
What educational services were available for handicapped children at the beginning of the twentieth century?

Initially, the objective of these programs was to return the individual to a more normal environment, including public schools. Unfortunately, this objective was seldom realized. Although there were some special classrooms established for mentally retarded children as early as 1896 (Hoffman, 1972), the public schools of the early 1900s were not prepared for the nontraditional learner. Most children who could not keep up with peers academically or were discipline problems either dropped out of school by choice or were excluded. The major emphasis for most students was on learning the basics and then leaving school.

By 1910 several urban areas across the Nation had made some provisions for mentally retarded children in the schools, though local school officials could choose who would and would not be served. The majority of these early special education services were for slow-learning children and were primarily in segregated classrooms. Special education meant segregated education. In addition, the child's deviation from nonhandicapped peers could not be too substantial or the student would be excluded from public education entirely.

Because the schools needed to have some way of determining who would or would not receive a public education, an assessment device was developed to determine who was intellectually capable of attending school. The result was an individual test of intelligence developed by Alfred Binet and Theodore Simon (1905). This test was first used in France to predict how well a student would function in school. In 1908 it was translated into English. The **Binet-Simon Scales,** revised and standardized by Lewis Terman at Stanford University, were published in 1916 as the **Stanford-Binet Intelligence Scale.** This test provided a means of identifying children who deviated significantly from the average in intellectual capability, at least in terms of what the test actually measured.

Maintaining the Status Quo: 1920–1960

FOCUS 11
Why is the period from 1920 to 1960 described as maintaining the status quo?

From 1920 to 1960 the availability of public school programs for exceptional children continued to be sporadic and selective. Some states, such as New York, New Jersey, and Massachusetts, enacted mandatory education for mildly (educable) retarded children. However, most states only *allowed* for special education; they did not *require* that the services be made available. Services to children with mild emotional disorders (discipline problems) were initiated in the early 1930s, but mental hospitals continued to be the only alternative for most individuals with more severe emotional problems.

Special classes for children with physical disabilities were also started in the 1930s. These programs were for children with crippling conditions, heart defects, and other health-related problems that interfered with the ability to participate in regular education programs. Separate schools became very popular for these children during the late 1950s. These schools were specially equipped to accommodate the needs of the physically disabled, including elevators and ramps, and modified doors, toilets, and desks.

During the 1940s special-school versus regular-school placement for handicapped students emerged as an important policy issue. Polloway (1984) asserts that during this period educators were determined to find the most effective placement for handicapped students as well as to ensure that handicapped people had the opportunity for normal social interactions.

By the 1950s many countries began to expand educational opportunities for students with handicaps in special schools and classes funded through public education. McCleary, Hardman, and Thomas (1989) believe that two separate events had a significant impact on the evolution of education for students with handicaps:

> First, in many countries parents of handicapped children organized as a constituent group to lobby policymakers for more appropriate social and educational services for their children. Second, professionals from both behavioral and medical science became more interested in services for individuals with handicaps, thus enriching knowledge through research into effective practice. This provided the setting for the current period in which significant departures from past practice have been initiated.

An Era of Self-Examination: 1960–1970

During the late 1950s there was an increase in the number of public school classes for mildly retarded and emotionally disturbed children. For the most part, these children continued to be educated in an environment that isolated them from nonhandicapped peers. The validity of these segregated special classes continued to be an important issue in the field of education. Several studies (e.g., Ainsworth, 1959; Baldwin, 1958; Cassidy & Stanton, 1959; Johnson, 1961; Jordan, 1959; Thurstone, 1959) examined the efficacy of special classes for mildly retarded children. Johnson (1962), summarizing this research, suggested that there were no differences in academic achievement between retarded learners in special or regular education classes, although the retarded child's social adjustment was not harmed by the special class program. Dunn (1968) again cited the efficacy research and declared that most special classes for the mildly retarded could not be justified and should be abolished:

> In my view, much of our past and present practices are morally and educationally wrong. We have been living at the mercy of general educators who have referred their problem children to us. And we have been generally ill prepared and ineffective in educating these children. Let us stop being pressured into continuing and expanding a special education program that we know now to be undesirable for many of the children we are dedicated to serve (p. 5).

Although several authors (e.g., MacMillan & Becker, 1977; Robinson & Robinson, 1976) have suggested that many of the efficacy studies were poorly designed, they had already resulted in a movement toward an expansion of services beyond the special class in the public schools. One outcome was the development of a model where a child could remain in the regular class program for the majority, if not all, of the school day, receiving special education when and where it was needed. This concept became widely known as **mainstreaming**.

The 1960s were a period for other major changes in the field of special education as well. The federal government took on an expanded role in the education of exceptional children. University teacher-preparation programs received federal financial support and initiated programs to train special education teachers throughout the United States. The Bureau of Education for the Handicapped (BEH) in the U.S. Office of Education was created as a clearinghouse for information

FOCUS 12
Why was the effectiveness of special classes for mildly handicapped children questioned during the late 1950s and early 1960s?

at the federal level. Demonstration projects were funded nationwide to establish a research base for the education of handicapped students in the public schools.

The 1960s also saw the advent of a new special education category: specific **learning disabilities.** This category of exceptionality emerged in response to a need to identify children who require special education services but are not mentally retarded or emotionally handicapped. Their achievement in some subject areas, particularly reading and mathematics, is so far below their age-group that some type of additional service is required beyond the regular education program.

Reaffirming the Right to Education: 1970–1990

FOCUS 13
What were the principal issues in each of the right-to-education cases that led to eventual passage of the Education for All Handicapped Children Act (Public Law 94–142)?

The 1970s are often described as a decade of revolution in the field of special education. Many of the landmark cases in the right to education for handicapped students were brought before the courts during this period. In addition, major pieces of state and federal legislation were enacted to reaffirm the handicapped individual's right to a free public education. What is often overlooked is that the rights of handicapped individuals came to the public forum as a part of a larger social issue—the civil rights of all minority populations in the United States. The Civil Rights Movement of the 1950s and 1960s awakened the public to the issues of discrimination in employment, housing, access to public facilities (such as restaurants and transportation), and public education.

Education was reaffirmed as a right and not a privilege by the U.S. Supreme Court in the landmark case of *Brown* v. *Topeka, Kansas, Board of Education* in 1954. In its decision the Court ruled that education must be made available to everyone on an equal basis. A unanimous Supreme Court stated, "In these days, it is doubtful that any child may reasonably be expected to succeed in life

The rights of children with handicaps to an appropriate education have been reaffirmed by state and federal legislation. (The Institute for the Study of Developmental Disabilities at Indiana University)

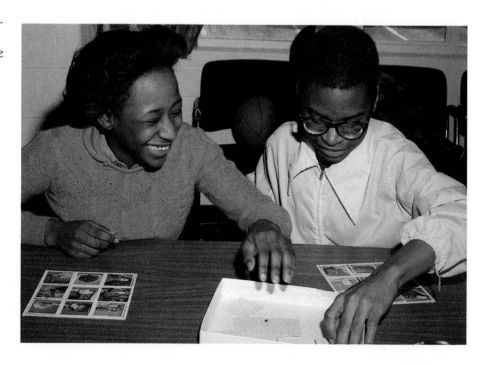

if he is denied the opportunity of an education. Such an opportunity, where the state has undertaken to provide it, is a right which must be made available to all on equal terms" (*Brown* v. *Topeka Board*, 1954).

This decision set a major precedent for the education of handicapped children in the United States. Unfortunately, it was nearly twenty years before federal courts were confronted with the issue of a free and appropriate education for handicapped children.

In 1971, the Pennsylvania Association for Retarded Citizens filed a class-action suit on behalf of resident retarded children who were excluded from public education on the basis of intellectual deficiency (*Pennsylvania Association for Retarded Citizens* v. *Commonwealth of Pennsylvania*, 1971). This suit charged that more than 50,000 retarded children in the state were being denied their right to a free public education. The plaintiffs claimed that retarded children can learn, if the educational program is adjusted to meet their individual needs. The central issue was whether public school programs should be required to accommodate the intellectually different child. The court ordered Pennsylvania schools to provide a free public education to all retarded children, ages six to twenty-one commensurate with their individual learning needs. In addition, pre-school education was to be provided for retarded children if the local school district was providing it for other children.

Later that same year, the case of *Mills* v. *District of Columbia* (1972) expanded the Pennsylvania decision to include all handicapped children. District of Columbia schools were ordered to provide a free and appropriate education to every school-age handicapped child. The court further ordered that when regular public school assignment was not appropriate, alternative educational services must be made available.

Thus, the right of handicapped children to an education was reaffirmed. The *Pennsylvania* and *Mills* cases served as catalysts for several court cases and pieces of legislation in the years that followed. Table 2–3 summarizes precedents that were established in the court cases and legislation from 1954 to 1986.

A National Mandate to Educate Handicapped Children.   In 1975 the U.S. Congress saw the need to bring together the various pieces of state and federal legislation into one comprehensive national public law. **The Education of All Handicapped Children Act, Public Law 94–142,** was passed by an overwhelming majority of both the House and the Senate.

Public Law (P.L.) 94–142 makes available a free and appropriate public education for all handicapped children in the United States. This law provides for:

FOCUS 14
Identify the four major components of Public Law 94–142.

1. **Nondiscriminatory and multidisciplinary assessment** of educational needs
2. Parental involvement in developing each child's educational program
3. Education in an environment suited to individual needs
4. An **individualized education program (IEP)**

Nondiscriminatory and Multidisciplinary Assessment.   Several provisions related to the use of nondiscriminatory testing procedures in labeling and placement

TABLE 2–3 Major Court Cases and Federal Legislation Focusing on the Right to Education for Handicapped Individuals (1954–1986)

Court Cases and Federal Legislation	Precedents Established
Brown v. Topeka, Kansas, Board of Education (1954)	Segregation of students by race held unconstitutional. Education is a right that must be available to all on equal terms.
Hobsen v. Hansen (1969)	The doctrine of equal educational opportunity is a part of the law of due process, and denying an equal educational opportunity is a violation of the Constitution. Placement of children in educational tracks based on performance on standardized tests is unconstitutional and discriminates against poor and minority children.
Diana v. California State Board of Education (1970)	Children tested for potential placement in a special education program must be assessed in their native or primary language. Children cannot be placed in special classes on the basis of culturally biased tests.
Pennsylvania Association for Retarded Citizens v. Commonwealth of Pennsylvania (1971)	Pennsylvania schools must provide a free public education to all school-age retarded children.
Mills v. Board of Education of the District of Columbia (1972)	Declared exclusion of handicapped individuals from free, appropriate public education is a violation of the due process and equal protection clauses of the Fourteenth Amendment to the Constitution. Public schools in the District of Columbia must provide a free education to all handicapped children regardless of their functional level or ability to adapt to the present educational system.

of children for special education services were incorporated into P.L. 94–142. These safeguards include:

1. The testing of children in their native or primary language whenever possible
2. The use of evaluation procedures selected and administered to prevent cultural or racial discrimination
3. The use of assessment tools validated for the purpose for which they are being used
4. Assessment by a **multidisciplinary team** utilizing several pieces of information to formulate a placement decision.

Handicapped students have too often been placed in special education programs on the basis of inadequate or invalid assessment information. One result of these procedures has been a disproportionate number of ethnic minority children and children from lower socioeconomic backgrounds being placed in special education programs.

Parent Involvement in the Educational Process. P.L. 94–142 describes the role of parents in the education of their children. Parents have the right to:

1. Consent in writing before the child is initially evaluated

Court Cases and Federal Legislation	Precedents Established
Public Law 93–112, Vocational Rehabilitation Act of 1973, Section 504 (1973)	Handicapped individuals cannot be excluded from participation in, denied benefits of, or subjected to discrimination under any program or activity receiving federal financial assistance.
Public Law 93–380, Educational Amendments Act (1974)	Authorized financial aid to the states for the implementation of programs for exceptional children, including the gifted and talented. Established due process requirements (procedural safeguards) to protect rights of handicapped children and their families in special-education placement decisions.
Public Law 94–142, Education for All Handicapped Children Act (1975)	A free and appropriate public education must be provided for all handicapped children in the U.S. (Birth to five year olds may be excluded in some states.)
Public Law 99–457, Education of the Handicapped Act Amendments (1986)	A new authority extending free and appropriate public education for all handicapped children ages three to five, and a new early intervention program for infants and toddlers.
Public Law 99–372, The Handicapped Children's Protection Act (1986)	Authorizes reimbursement of attorneys' fees and expenses to parents who prevail in administrative proceedings or court actions.

2. Consent in writing before the child is initially placed in a special education program

3. Request an independent education evaluation if they feel the school's evaluation is inappropriate

4. Request an evaluation at public expense if a due-process hearing decision is that the public agency's evaluation was inappropriate

5. Participate on the committee that considers the evaluation, placement, and programming of the child

6. Inspect and review educational records and challenge information believed to be inaccurate, misleading, or in violation of the privacy or other rights of the child

7. Request a copy of information from their child's educational record

8. Request a hearing concerning the school's proposal or refusal to initiate or change the identification, evaluation, or placement of the child, or the provision of a free appropriate public education (Federal Register, August, 1977).

These safeguards protect the child and family from decisions that could adversely affect their lives. In addition, families can be more secure in the knowledge that every reasonable attempt is being made to educate their child appropriately.

WINDOW 2–1

I Enjoy Working with Parents

As a special education teacher for the past five years, I have to say one of the most satisfying aspects of my career has been working with some of the parents of the handicapped children in my class. As a parent of a normal seven-year-old, I have to admit that it seems to me that, for the most part, the schools have done little to encourage parent involvement in education. The only time I hear from my child's teacher outside of the two ten-minute parent conferences held each year is when there is a problem. I guess you could say that from where I sit "no news is good news" from the school. For the handicapped children in my class, this is simply not true. The parents of students in my class are involved at every phase of their child's program. They work on the development of goals for their child and participate in activities at home that encourage learning. Sure, it's true that at first I resented being told where parents had to be involved and why. The law seemed to be telling me how I should run my classroom. Now, I not only work with my parents because the law says that is what I am supposed to do, I value having parents involved. It is very true that not all of my parents choose to be actively involved. However, for those who do, it has made a big difference in the development of appropriate educational experiences for their handicapped child. It has also taught me a lot about how important parent participation is to a good educational program for all children.

Roxanne, *special education teacher in an elementary school*

Education in the Least Restrictive Environment.   All children have the right to learn in an environment consistent with their academic, social, and physical needs. P.L. 94–142 mandated that handicapped children receive their education with nonhandicapped peers to the maximum extent possible. In order to meet this mandate, schools have developed services ranging from placement in regular classrooms with support services, to homebound and hospital programs. An educational services model is presented in Figure 2–2.

At Level I in the continuum, a student remains in the regular classroom, with no additional support services. Adaptations necessary for a given student should be handled by the classroom teacher. Consequently, a student's success depends on a teacher who has skills in developing and adapting programs to meet individual needs. A student placed at Level II also remains in the regular classroom, but **consultive services** are available to both the teacher and student. These services may be provided by a variety of professionals, including special educators, speech and language specialists, behavior specialists, physical education specialists, occupational therapists, physical therapists, school psychologists, and social workers. Services may range from assisting a teacher in the use of tests or modification of curriculum, to direct instruction with students in the classroom setting.

The student placed at Level III continues in the regular classroom for a majority of the school day but also attends a **resource room** for specialized instruction. A resource-room program is under the direction of a qualified special educator, and the amount of time a student spends there varies according to student need. The range of time is from as few as thirty minutes to as many as

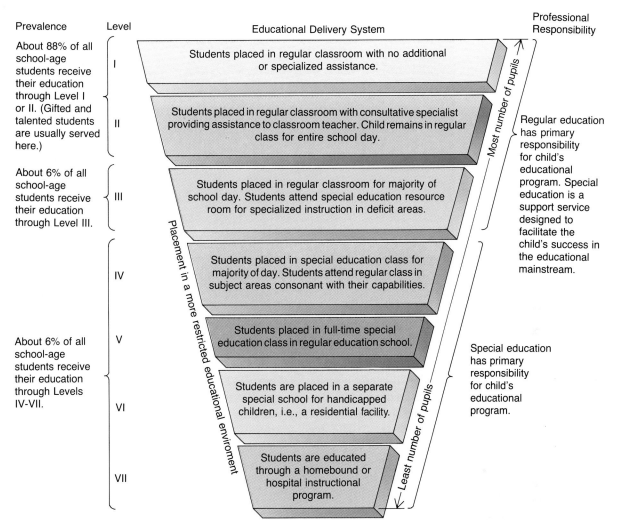

Figure 2–2
Educational Service Options for Exceptional Students

three hours a day. Instruction in a resource room is intended to reinforce or supplement the student's work in the regular classroom. The student receives necessary assistance to ensure his or her placement with regular education peers. About 6 percent of all school-age children are served in a resource-room setting. It is the most widely used public school setting for handicapped students. At Levels I, II, and III, the primary responsibility for the students' education lies with the regular class teacher. Consultive services, including special education, are intended to support the student's regular class placement.

Students placed at Level IV are in a **special education classroom** for the majority of the school day. At this level, there are provisions for a student to

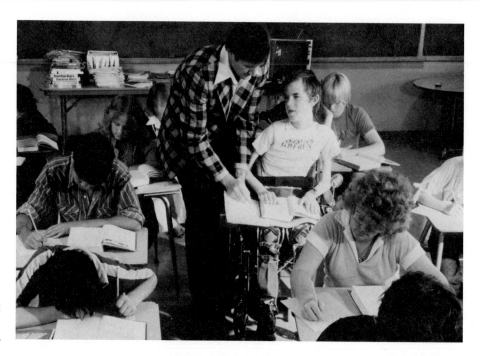

What are the advantages of interaction between children with disabilities and their peers who are not disabled? (John Telford)

be integrated with regular education peers, whenever possible and consistent with the student's learning capabilities. For more moderately to severely handicapped students, integration is usually for nonacademic subject areas. Level V placement involves full-time participation in a special education class. The student is not integrated with regular education students for formalized instructional activities. However, some level of social integration may take place at recess periods, lunch assemblies, field trips, or during tutoring. Placement at Level VI involves removing a student from the regular education facility to a classroom in a separate facility specifically for handicapped students. These facilities include **special day schools** where the educational program is one aspect of a comprehensive treatment program. Some students, because of the severity of their handicaps, are unable to attend any school program and must receive services through a homebound or hospital program (Level VII). Placement at Level VII generally indicates a need for an **itinerant teacher** who visits an incapacitated student on a regular basis to provide tutorial assistance. Some students with chronic conditions, such as certain types of cancer, may be placed at this level indefinitely, whereas others are served while recuperating from a short-term illness.

The issue of placement in the least restrictive environment continues to be a matter of public and private debate. Public Law 94–142 creates a clear presumption in favor of educating students in regular education settings. The law mandates that students with handicaps are to be educated with their nonhandicapped peers to the maximum extent possible. A recent examination of the placement of children with handicaps in segregated environments (Danielsen & Bellamy, 1989) suggests that about 6 percent of all handicapped students receive their education in a segregated school. Approximately 24 percent of all handicapped students are educated in separate special education classes. These authors also

Reflect on This 2–3

Meeting Children's Needs: An Analysis of the Success of P.L. 94–142

The Robert Wood Johnson Foundation completed a five-year collaborative study of children with special needs in an attempt to document whether the procedural guarantees of P.L. 94–142 are securely in place. The study was conducted in five large metropolitan school districts located throughout the Nation. Some of the findings are as follows:

The Positive Side

- Parents are generally satisfied with the services their disabled children receive. In fact, the researchers believe that parents of special education students are more satisfied with the public schools than are parents of school children in general.
- Schools are committed to the principle of serving disabled children in the least restrictive environment. The vast majority of special education students are in the mainstream, attend-

ing regular schools and spending at least part of the day with regular classes.

- Schools remain the major site of identification for most children with special needs. Physicians do, however, identify between 15 and 25 percent of children with learning disabilities, speech impairments, emotional disorders, and hyperactivity.
- Many therapeutic services are now provided in schools. Nearly half of all children in special education receive speech or hearing therapy.
- Most handicapped children have a regular source of health care, although they may not see the same physician at every medical visit.

The Negative Side

- Although parents are generally favorable regarding special edu-

cation services for their child, less than half actually attend their child's IEP meeting.

- On average, special education costs nearly twice as much as regular education. The concern is whether special programs for handicapped children can be maintained against the onslaught of cost-containment pressures facing school districts.
- Serious gaps still exist in services. Some children find themselves in a kind of "gray area" with respect to defining their problems and meeting their needs. Specifically, handicapped students who remain in school until they reach age twenty-one rarely have access to services that help them make the transition to adult life.

Source: Serving Handicapped Children: A Special Report, 1988, Princeton, N.J.: The Robert Wood Johnson Foundation.

reported that in spite of the law's strong preference for integrated placements, the use of "separate educational environments has been relatively stable over the 10 years in which the Department of Education has collected national data" (p. 452).

An Individualized Education Program.   P.L. 94–142 provides a vehicle for the development of an education program based on multidisciplinary assessment and designed to meet the individual needs of the exceptional student. This vehicle is an Individualized Education Program, or IEP. The IEP provides an opportunity for parents and professionals to join together in providing an appropriate educational experience for the handicapped child. The result should be more continuity in the delivery of educational services for exceptional children on a daily as well as an annual basis. The IEP process also promotes more effective communication between school personnel and the home.

An example of an IEP form is shown in Figure 2–3. All IEP forms contain some common elements: (1) the child's present level of performance, (2) a statement of annual goals, (3) short-term instructional objectives, (4) **related services,** (5) percent of time in regular education, (6) beginning and ending dates for special education services, and (7) an annual evaluation.

FOCUS 15
Identify the major components of Public Law 99–457, The Education of the Handicapped Act Amendments of 1986.

The 1986 Amendments to the Education of the Handicapped Act (Public Law 99–457). This important legislation, signed into law on October 8, 1986, extended the authority of Public Law 94–142 by (1) establishing a new mandate

Figure 2–3
Individualized Education Program

PRIMARY CLASSIFICATION Behavior Disorder
SECONDARY CLASSIFICATION ____________

STUDENT NAME Diane
DATE OF BIRTH 5-3-79 CA 11
SCHOOL Hamilton Elementary School GRADE 5
PRIMARY LANG: HOME English STUDENT English
DATE OF IEP MEETING April 27, 1989
ENTRY DATE TO PROGRAM April 27, 1989
PROJECTED TERMINATION DATE April 27, 1990

SERVICES REQUIRED: Specify amount of time in educational and/or related services per day or week

RESOURCE ____________
RES. SELF CONT. ____________
SELF CONTAINED 6 Hours daily
REG. CLASS ____________
RELATED SERV. group 45 min. 2x weekly
P.E. PROG. 45 min. daily
OTHER Individual Counseling 1 hour 1x weekly

TEAM SIGNATURES	IEP DATE	REVIEW DATE
LEA REP.		
PARENT		
SP. ED. TCHR.		
GUID. SPEC.		
COUNSELOR		
SP-LANG PATH.		
STUDENT		
OTHER		

JUSTIFICATION FOR PLACEMENT: Student needs indicated specialized placement and curriculum to deal with behavioral problems

TESTS UTILIZED
INTELLECTUAL WISC-R
EDUCATIONAL Key Math Woodcock Reading
BEHAVIORAL/ADAPTIVE Burks
SPEECH/LANGUAGE ____________
OTHER ____________
VISION Within Normal limits HEARING Within Normal limits
CLASSROOM OBSERVATION DONE ________ (Date) ________ (By Whom)

STRENGTHS: (INDICATE PRESENT LEVEL OF FUNCTIONING)
1. Polite to teachers and peers
2. Helpful and cooperative in the classroom
3. Good grooming skills
4. Good in sports activities

LIMITATIONS: (INDICATE PRESENT LEVEL OF FUNCTIONING)
1. Limited interaction skills with peers and adults 90%
2. Excessive tics and grimaces 70%
3. Difficulty with on task behaviors 60%
4. Difficulty expressing feelings
5. Below grade level in Math 3.9
6. Below grade level in Reading 4.3

ANNUAL REVIEW: DATE: ____________
COMMENTS/RECOMMENDATIONS ____________

IEP – ANNUAL GOALS AND SHORT TERM OBJECTIVES	PERSONS RESPONSIBLE	OBJECTIVE CRITERIA AND EVALUATION PROCEDURES
#1 ANNUAL GOAL: Diane will improve her interaction skills with peers and adults.	Classroom teachers guidance	classroom data target behavior
S.T. OBJ. Diane will initiate conversation with peers during an unstructured setting 2x daily.		
S.T. OBJ. When in need of assistance, Diane will raise her hand and verbalize her needs to teachers or peers		
S.T. OBJ. without prompting 80%.		
#2 ANNUAL GOAL: Diane will increase her ability to control hand and facial movements.	Teachers guidance	Data: classroom observation
S.T. OBJ. During academic work, Diane will keep her hands in an appropriate place and use writing		
S.T. OBJ. materials correctly 80%.		
S.T. OBJ. Diane will maintain a relaxed facial expression with teacher prompt 80%.		
#3 ANNUAL GOAL: Diane will improve on task behaviors.	Teachers guidance	Classroom observation and data
S.T. OBJ. Diane will work independently on an assigned		
S.T. OBJ. task with teacher prompt 80% of time.		
S.T. OBJ. Diane will complete academic work on time 90% as specified by teacher.		
#4 ANNUAL GOAL: Diane will improve her ability to express her feelings	Teachers guidance	Data observation
S.T. OBJ. When asked how she feels, Diane will give an		
S.T. OBJ. adequate verbal description of her feelings or moods with teacher prompting 80%		
S.T. OBJ. Given a conflict or problem situation, Diane will state her feelings to teachers and peers 80%.		
#5 ANNUAL GOAL: Diane will improve math skills from a 3.9 grade level.	Teachers	Precision teaching Addison Wesley Math Program
S.T. OBJ. Diane will improve rate and accuracy in oral		
S.T. OBJ. 1 digit division facts to 80 ppm without errors		
S.T. OBJ. Diane will improve her ability to solve word problems involving + - x ÷ 8/10.		
#6 ANNUAL GOAL: Improve reading skills from a 4.3 grade level	Teachers	Precision teaching Barnell + Loft materials
S.T. OBJ. Diane will answer progressively more difficult		
S.T. OBJ. comprehension questions in level D+E specific skills series with 80% accuracy.		
S.T. OBJ. Diane will increase her rate and accuracy of vocabulary words to 80 wpm without errors.		

Figure 2–3
(continued)

to provide a free and appropriate education for all handicapped children ages three through five; and (2) establishing a new early intervention program for infants and toddlers ages birth through two.

Under Public Law 99–457, all the rights and protection extended to school-age children (ages 5 through 21) are extended to preschoolers. This law requires that all states receiving funds under P.L. 94–142 must assure that three- to five-year-old children are receiving a free appropriate public education by the 1990–1991 school year. One significant difference, however, between the requirements of P.L. 94–142 and this new law is that states are not required to report preschool children by handicapping category (e.g., learning disabilities, mental retardation, deafness, etc.). Public Law 99–457 is administered directly through the state and local education agencies. To support states in meeting the requirements of this law, several new initiatives were enacted, including the establishment of demonstration and outreach programs for preschool-age handicapped children, the authorization of early childhood institutes to generate and disseminate research findings on early childhood education, and projects to demonstrate cost effective methods of delivering educational services.

Another provision of P.L. 99–457 is establishment of a state grant program for handicapped infants and toddlers ages birth through two years. Infants and toddlers who are developmentally delayed, as defined by each state, are eligible for services that include a multidisciplinary assessment and an **individualized family service plan,** or IFSP. This plan is to be cooperatively developed by a multidisciplinary team that includes parents. Although this provision does not mandate that states must provide services to all infants and toddlers who are developmentally delayed, it does establish strong financial incentives for state participation.

REVIEW

FOCUS 1: How did the work of Jean-Marc Itard contribute to our understanding of people with differences?

☐ Influenced by the work of Pinel, Itard emphasized that people with disabilities should be treated humanely.

☐ Itard also demonstrated that an individual with a severe disability could learn new skills through physiological stimulation.

FOCUS 2: Identify two major contributions of modern psychology to our understanding of human differences.

☐ Abnormal behavior can be learned through the interaction of the individual and the environment.

☐ Intelligence can be measured by applying the principles of the scientific method.

FOCUS 3: In the early part of the twentieth century, what role were hereditary factors thought to play in regard to intelligence and social deviance?

☐ One theory linked inferior intelligence solely to hereditary factors.

☐ Less intelligent people were also thought more likely to exhibit socially deviant and unacceptable behavior.

☐ The theory of social deviance led to widespread fear of handicapped people and a movement toward selective breeding, social isolation, and prevention.

FOCUS 4: What are the five principal types of institutions?

☐ Institutions may be established for those who are both incapable and harmless; those who unintentionally pose a threat to society; those who intentionally endanger the community; those who are to perform a specific task (e.g., military personnel); and those who seek to retreat from the secular world.

FOCUS 5: What are the seven characteristics of institutions?

☐ Institutions are characterized by all aspects of life being conducted in the same place and under a single authority; daily activities that are carried on in the immediate company of many others who are treated in similar ways; tightly scheduled activities; restricted social mobility; a work ideology defined by the institution as treatment; a system of rewards and punishments; and a stripping process that desocializes the individual from the outside community.

FOCUS 6: Identify four primary issues in the right-to-treatment cases that have come before the courts in the latter half of the twentieth century.

☐ Individuals residing in institutions were being deprived of the right to individual treatment that would give them a realistic opportunity for habilitation.

☐ People cannot be held against their will and without treatment if they pose no threat to society.

☐ Current law establishes a national policy to improve treatment and provides financial incentives to induce states to do so.

☐ Appropriate training is necessary to ensure safety and freedom from restraint for the handicapped individual.

FOCUS 7: Identify two possible effects of institutionalization on an individual.

☐ The most harmful aspect of institutionalization is a restrictive regimen with little regard for individual needs or desires.

☐ Institutions may become places where residents are subjected to physical abuse and emotional neglect.

FOCUS 8: Identify three major components of the concept of least restrictive environment.

□ The LRE concept indicates that an individual should receive services in an environment that is consistent with individual needs.

□ There must be a range of available services capable of meeting the needs of the individual.

□ The services for any individual can never be terminal or irreversible.

FOCUS 9: What are the three types of services that must be available to ensure that an individual is living in the least restrictive environment?

□ Appropriate medical services include screening, diagnosis, and assessment of the handicapped child; working effectively with parents; long-term medical and social treatment programs; and knowledge of community resources beyond medical ones.

□ Appropriate social services include community mental health centers, access to buildings and transportation, community living alternatives, recreation and leisure-time activities, and employment.

□ Every handicapped child, regardless of the severity or type of condition, must have access to an appropriate educational program.

FOCUS 10: What educational services were available for handicapped children at the beginning of the twentieth century?

□ Educational programs at the beginning of the twentieth century were primarily taught in separate special schools, and focused on the education of children with visual disorders, hearing disorders, mental retardation, and emotional disturbance.

□ The purpose of these educational programs was to return the child to a more normal environment, including the public schools.

FOCUS 11: Why is the period from 1920 to 1960 described as maintaining the status quo?

□ The availability of educational programs for handicapped students continued to be sporadic and selective.

□ Special education was allowed in many states but required in only a few.

FOCUS 12: Why was the effectiveness of special classes for mildly handicapped children questioned during the late 1950s and early 1960s?

□ Research on the efficacy of special classes for mildly handicapped children suggested that there was little or no benefit in removing the child from the regular education classroom.

FOCUS 13: What were the principal issues in each of the right-to-education cases that led to eventual passage of the Education for All Handicapped Children Act (Public Law 94–142)?

□ Education was reaffirmed as a right and not a privilege by the Supreme Court in the case of *Brown* v. *Topeka, Kansas, Board of Education.*

□ In a Pennsylvania case, the court ordered the schools to provide a free public education to all retarded children ages six to twenty-one.

□ The *Mills* case extended the right of a free public education to all school-age handicapped children.

FOCUS 14: Identify the four major components of Public Law 94–142.

□ The labeling and placement of a handicapped student in an educational program requires the use of non-discriminatory and multidisciplinary assessment.

□ Parent involvement in the educational process includes consent for testing and placement, and participation as a team member in the development of an IEP. Procedural safeguards (e.g., due process) are included in the law to protect the child and family from decisions that could adversely affect their lives.

□ All children have the right to learn in an environment that is consistent with their academic, social, and physical needs. The law mandates that handicapped children receive their education with nonhandicapped peers to the maximum extent possible.

□ Each child must have an individualized education program.

FOCUS 15: Identify the major components of Public Law 99–457, The Education of the Handicapped Act Amendments of 1986.

□ This law establishes a federal mandate to provide a free and appropriate public education to preschool-age children from three to five years of age.

□ States do not have to report eligible preschool-age children by disability category.

□ New initiatives are established to support implementation of the law, including demonstration programs, early childhood institutes, and projects on cost-effective methods of service delivery.

□ A state grant program for infants and toddlers is also established under P.L. 99–457.

Debate Forum

Federal Involvement in the Education of Handicapped Children

For many years the debate has raged over the federal role in the education of this Nation's children. With the passage of Public Law 94–142, the issue has been extended to the education of handicapped children and youth. The following are two differing points of view on the role of the federal government in the education of handicapped children.

Eileen Gardner, *Policy Analyst*
The Heritage Foundation

Point Vital debate is now taking place over the proper role of the federal government in education. The best documented and most compelling arguments show that increased federal involvement has all but destroyed quality in education. . . . During the past two decades, control of education has been centralized in Washington, D.C., where unelected and unaccountable special interest groups have skillfully maneuvered Congress into creating for them federal programs from which stunningly successful lobby efforts have been launched.

. . . Public Law 94–142 requires that states and local districts afford every handicapped child within its jurisdiction a "free and appropriate public education" in the least restrictive environment. In one of the sharpest intrusions of the federal government into the details of the teaching practice, every teacher of a handicapped child is required to write an Individualized Education Program for that child.

. . . The most costly requirements of P.L. 94–142 require that school districts provide services necessary to make learning possible. This includes everything from providing transportation, to eliminating architectural barriers, to hiring specially trained personnel, to paying private school tuition for those children who cannot be in public school, to whatever else the courts decide the school district is responsible for.

. . . Laws for the education of the handicapped . . . have drained resources from the normal school population, probably weakened the quality of teaching, and falsely labeled normal children. In a misguided effort to help a few, the many have been injured. Yet, the handicapped constituency displays a strange lack of concern for the effect of their regulations upon the welfare of the general population—the very population upon whom the well-being of these children ultimately depends.*

Madeleine Will, *Former Assistant Secretary*
Office of Special Education and Rehabilitative Services
U.S. Department of Education

Counterpoint When the National Commission on Excellence in Education published its report ("A Nation at Risk"), the nation was riveted. . . . The commission report stated that the federal government had primary responsibility for identifying the national interest in education. It stated further that the federal government must provide national leadership to ensure the nation's public and private resources are marshaled to address the issues discussed in the report. However, its underlying and most basic premise . . . is that the concept of excellence in education applies to all students, and excellence means striving to reach one's utmost potential.

. . . The past decade has produced results for students with disabilities that were considered unobtainable and unthinkable only a few years earlier. Little more than a decade ago, many children were left completely out of the nation's school systems. When Congress passed legislation creating an entitlement to education, severely and multiply handicapped children entered the schools across the nation. . . . The passage of this legislation ushered in the most creative period in the history of special education.†

Sources:
* E. Gardner, Fall, 1983, "The Federal Role in Education," *Backgrounder*, Washington, D.C.: The Heritage Foundation.
† From "Let Us Pause and Reflect—But Not Too Long," by M. Will, *Exceptional Children, 51*(1984), 11–16. Copyright 1984 by The Council for Exceptional Children. Reprinted with permission.

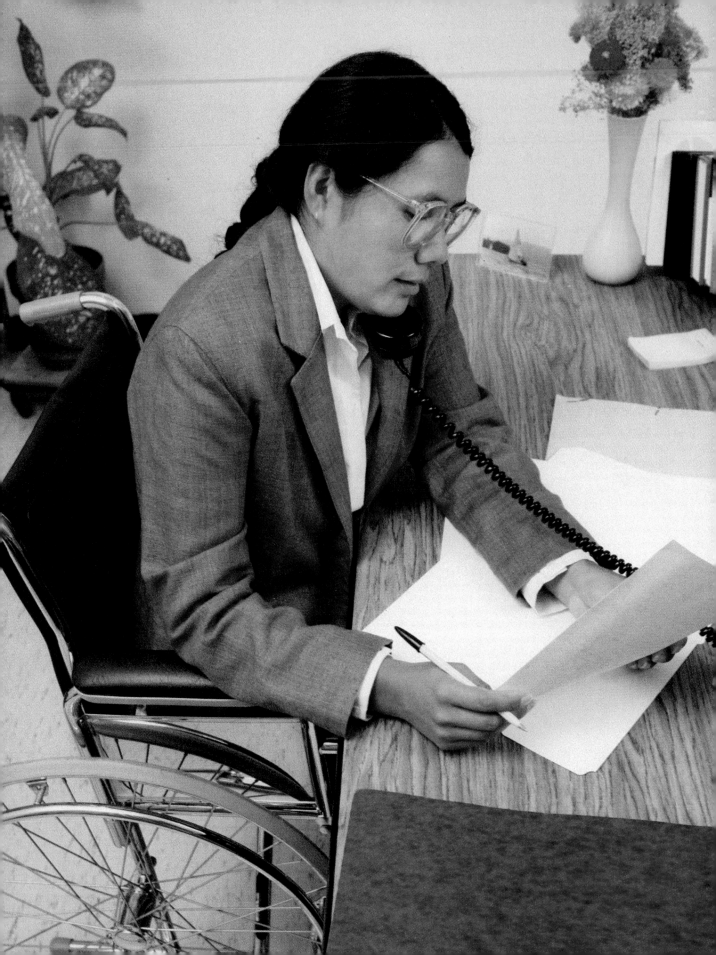

3 Education through the Lifespan

To Begin With...

- People with developmental disabilities are now living longer, well into their seventies and eighties and some into their nineties. This means that practitioners must understand and be able to serve the needs of elderly disabled persons and the changes in life-style that age brings. Those over age 60 constitute approximately 10 percent of the mentally retarded developmentally disabled population (Janrchi & Wishiewski, 1985).

- Approximately two million children in the United States under six years of age are considered to be "at risk" and are likely to experience problems in their physical, intellectual or emotional development (Peterson, 1987).

- In 1987, an estimated 300,000 special education students who exited the public schools had little to no prospects for employment or community participation (U.S. Department of Education, 1986).

INTRODUCTION

In this chapter, we continue our overview of education services with a presentation of issues that focus on exceptional children from birth through high school. Our discussion of educational services in the last chapter highlighted the major components of Public Law 94–142 (the Education for All Handicapped Children Act) and Public Law 99–457 (the 1986 Amendments to the Education of the Handicapped Act). This chapter, while still attending to many of the basic constructs of these laws, addresses intervention strategies as the individual moves from the early-childhood years into school, and eventually into adult life.

Schooling is successful for children and adolescents with exceptionalities, as it is for everyone, when it provides the skills and experiences necessary to participate in a heterogeneous world. Such participation may be evaluated using four standards: personal autonomy, social integration, lifestyle choice, and economic self-sufficiency. Each of these standards relates to different outcomes, depending on the age of the individual. For the young child (prior to age five), the world is defined primarily through family and a small, same-age peer group. As the child progresses chronologically, the world expands to the neighborhood, the school, and eventually to a larger heterogeneous group we call the *community*. For the field of education, the question is: How can we structure an exceptional student's educational program to effectively foster full participation in society? From this starting point, we then move into subsequent chapters in this book that address not only the educational interventions, but medical and social services as well, for each area of exceptionality.

THE EARLY-INTERVENTION YEARS

Anita was elated. She had just discovered that she was going to have twins. Based on the preliminary scans, they appeared to be girls. As the delivery date neared, she thought about the fun that would be hers in dressing them and taking them on walks in the double stroller that she would certainly purchase. The delivery date arrived and passed with no action. Nevertheless, in less than a week from her due date, she found herself in the hospital bearing down to greet the first of her two twins. The first little girl arrived without a hitch. The second little girl arrived, but there was something different about her; it was immediately discernable. She didn't have the same body tone as her sister. Within a couple days, the second twin was diagnosed as having cerebral palsy, with the prognosis that she would have significant learning problems. Her head and the left side of her body seemed to be affected most seriously. The attending physicians immediately referred the parents to Disabled Children's Services, a division of the state health department. Further testing was done, and Yvonne was placed in an early-intervention program for infants with developmental problems. At the age of three, Yvonne's parents enrolled her in a preschool program where she would have the opportunity to interact with both nondisabled and disabled children of her own age. As neither of the parents had any previous direct experience with a child with a disability, they were uncertain of how to help Yvonne. Would this program really help her that much, or should they only be working with her at home? It was hard for them to begin this little girl's schooling so very early.

Definitions and Concepts

Early-childhood special education is an integral component of any service-delivery system for children with a disability. The early experiences of at-risk infants and children provide the basis for subsequent learning, growth, and development (Bricker & Iacino, 1977; Palmer & Siegel, 1977; Ramey & Baker-Ward, 1982; Ramsey & MacPhee, 1985). The first years of life are critical to the overall

FOCUS 1
Why is it so important to provide early-intervention services to students at risk as early in the child's life as possible?

Figure 3–1
Education through the Lifespan

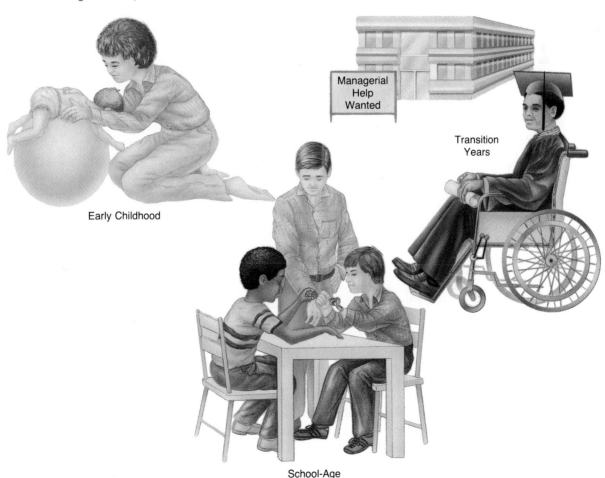

Early Childhood

Managerial Help Wanted

Transition Years

School-Age

development of all children, including those defined as being at risk (Akers, 1972; Bloom, 1964; Fowler, 1975; Hunt, 1961; White, 1975). Moreover, classic studies in the behavioral sciences from the 1960s and '70s indicate that early stimulation is critical to the later development of language, intelligence, personality, and a sense of self-worth (Bloom, 1964; Hunt, 1961; Piaget, 1970; White, 1975). Advocates of early-childhood special education believe that intervention should begin as early as possible in an environment that is free of the more traditional categorical labels (such as *mental retardation* and *behavior disorders*), particularly if there is any uncertainty about the permanency of the present assessment of the child's condition. Carefully selected interventions have the potential to lessen the long-term impact of the disability, as well as to counteract the negative effects of waiting to intervene. The postponement of services may, in fact, undermine a child's overall development, as well as the acquisition of specific skills (Peterson, 1987).

FOCUS 2
Define early-childhood special education.

Definitions. Early-childhood special education is concerned with infants and children with all types and degrees of at-risk conditions. Many of these children have multiple problems (such as motor, language, or hearing) across a variety of domains. Some may be severely delayed in their development, not because of inherent physical or mental problems, but because their home or community environments place them at risk. Diversity is the word to describe children who need early-intervention services.

Legislation. Of the federal legislation in the area of early intervention that has been enacted over the past two decades, three laws stand out as having a significant impact on the development of services to young children and infants at risk. In 1968, Congress passed the Children's Early Assistance Act to provide funding for demonstration programs, replication of validated practice, state implementation grants, and technical assistance for planning and program development. The Education of the Handicapped Act Amendments of 1983 (Public Law 98–199) focuses on developing statewide plans and programs to meet the needs of disabled children, birth through age three. Public Law 99–457, the most significant piece of legislation to date regarding early-childhood services for disabled infants and preschool-age children, assists states in providing funding for family training, counseling, home visits, specialized services and instruction, speech therapy, **occupational therapy, physical therapy,** psychological and diagnostic medical services, and **case management** services. An integral part of this law is the development of an **Individualized Family Service Plan (IFSP).** This plan is very similar to the content of the IEP (Individual Education Plan) that is an essential part of Public Law 94–142 (discussed in Chapter 2). The plan includes statements about the young child's present levels of development (physical, cognitive, language, psychosocial, etc.); a statement of the family's strengths and needs; statements regarding the major outcomes of the plan; a delineation of the specific interventions and delivery systems for accomplishing the outcomes; the projected dates for the initiation and duration of the services; the name of the case manager, and a transition plan for the infant or young child. Because of Public Law 99–457, infants and preschool-age children with disabling conditions have the same access to educational services as school-age children who are disabled.

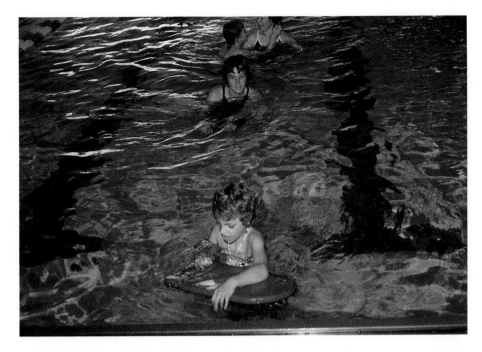

Public Law 99–457, passed in 1986, provides funds for a wide range of early-intervention services, including family training, counseling, and physical therapy. (The Institute for the Study of Developmental Disabilities at Indiana University)

Early-Intervention Services

Increasingly, technology is contributing to the number of at-risk infants who survive birth. Infant intensive-care specialists working with sophisticated medical technologies are preserving the lives of infants who years ago would have died in the first days or weeks of life. This technology is a major reason for the increased demand for trained early-childhood special education personnel.

Early prevention or intervention pays substantial dividends to affected infants and preschool-age children, as well as to their families and society at large. In all likelihood, many infants who have grown up to be disabled could clearly have developed normally if appropriate preventative steps had been taken early in their lives (Peterson, 1987). Additionally, people with disabilities would be far less disabled if effective interventions were applied from birth.

The intent of intervention programs for at-risk infants and preschool-age children is multifaceted. Goals include diminishing the effects of the disabling condition on the child's growth and development and preventing as much as possible the aggravation or worsening of the at-risk condition. The timing is critical in the delivery of the interventions. The maxim "the earlier, the better" is very true. Moreover, early intervention may in the long run be less costly and more effective than providing services later in the individual's life (Antley & DuBose, 1981; Casto & Mastropieri, 1985; Casto & White, 1984; Reaves & Burns, 1982; White, Mastropieri, & Casto, 1984).

According to Peterson (1987), interventions for at-risk or disabled infants and young children must be "intensive, comprehensive, continuous, and focused upon the individual needs of each child" (p. 74). *Intensity* refers to the frequency and amount of time an infant or child is engaged in intervention activities. About

FOCUS 3
What are some of the outcomes associated with early prevention and intervention for children at risk?

FOCUS 4
What is the purpose of early-childhood special education services?

four to five times a week, the child should participate in intervention activities that involve two to three hours of contact each day if the intensity requirement is to be met.

Comprehensive intervention services are broad in scope. They address the needs of the whole child based on the Individualized Family Service Plan (IFSP). Targets of intervention may include nutritional support, varied kinds of medical treatment (such as medication, surgery, and physical therapy), speech and language therapy, parent and family training, and cognitive development. Given the breadth of these services, the intervention team must include professionals with many experiential backgrounds (such as speech and language, physical therapy, nursing, and education). The coordination of early-intervention services is critical if the goals of the program are to be realized.

The academic-year programming of approximately nine months that is common to many public school programs is not in the best interests of at-risk infants and preschool-age children. Continuity is essential. Services must be provided throughout the early years, without significant periods of interruption. The four-to five-day regimen, with small breaks for holidays, is central to bringing about long-term growth and preparing these children for movement into less restrictive environments (Peterson, 1987).

In summary, early-childhood special education is designed to:

1. Teach infants and very young children very specific skills, such as how to eat, how to walk, how to talk, and how to play successfully with other children

2. Lessen the impact of conditions that may worsen or become more severe without timely and adequate treatment

3. Provide specialized therapies for speech, language, and motor problems

4. Prevent children from developing other, secondary disabling conditions

5. Prepare children as early as possible for meaningful experiences with their same-age peers

6. Teach children who exhibit troublesome behaviors (**noncompliance**, aggressiveness, etc.) that interfere with schooling more adaptive behaviors

7. Provide children with the preacademic skills necessary for further learning.

These goals are not achieved without consistent family participation and professional collaboration. We discuss the importance of this collaboration in Chapter 14, Family Impact.

THE SCHOOL-AGE YEARS

FOCUS 5
What is meant by "adaptive fitting" for students with disabilities?

Yvonne left her preschool program at five to attend her neighborhood elementary school. From kindergarten through sixth grade, she divided her day between a regular education classroom with her nondisabled friends and a special education class. Her educational program during the elementary years focused on developing basic academic skills, learning to manage her own personal affairs, and socialization activities with her friends. Yvonne's rate of academic learning was significantly slower than other children her age, and she required extensive specialized instruction in reading and arithmetic. She also needed assistance in such areas as developing age-appropriate personal hygiene skills, managing her time, socially interacting with her peers, and participating in recreation and leisure activities.

As we move from the preschool period (prior to age five) into the elementary school years, the emphasis is on whether the child with a disability is able to adapt (academically, behaviorally, or physically) to the regular education environment. The degree to which the child is able to cope with the demands of the educational environment depends on the type and severity of the disability, as well as how effectively the school can accommodate the student's needs. A student with a mild disability may be viewed as a discipline problem, slow learner, or a poorly motivated child. The differences are more pronounced for students with moderate and severe problems, and require more extensive educational interventions. The performance deficits of these individuals are evident in several environmental settings, including the home, community, and school.

In the educational setting, the degree to which an individual is able to cope with the requirements of a school setting is described as **the adaptive fit.** Cassell (1976) describes adaptive fitting as a dynamic and continuous process of negotiation between an individual and the environment intended to secure mutual coexistence. The individual is expected to modify his or her behavior to meet the standards of the system. The system, when confronted with the unique attributes of the individual, is also expected to make the appropriate adjustments. Adaptive fitting describes the attempts of students who are exceptional to meet the expectations of various learning environments. These individuals may find that the requirements for success within public education are beyond their adaptive capabilities and that the system is not able to accommodate their academic, behavioral, physical, sensory, or communicative differences. The result is the development of negative attitudes toward the educational environment. Buchanan and Wolf (1981) explain:

> Imagine what it would be like to be in an environment which gives you nothing but negative feedback most of the time—a place you hate, activities which are difficult and at which you frequently fail, a setting in which the other people involved emphasize your negative qualities—your inability to do something or your lack of knowledge. How would you feel about entering that environment six hours a day, five days a week, approximately 180 days a year for many years to come? (p. 119)

Wang (1981) developed a program for students with learning and behavior disorders that is based on the concept of adaptive fitting. The purpose of the **Adaptive Learning Environments Program (ALEM)** is to implement a classroom structure that can adapt to individual differences while teaching students with learning and behavior problems to develop self-management skills. These management skills help them profit from their school experiences. The specific components of this adaptive-fitting program include:

1. A series of highly structured and hierarchically organized curricula for academic skills development

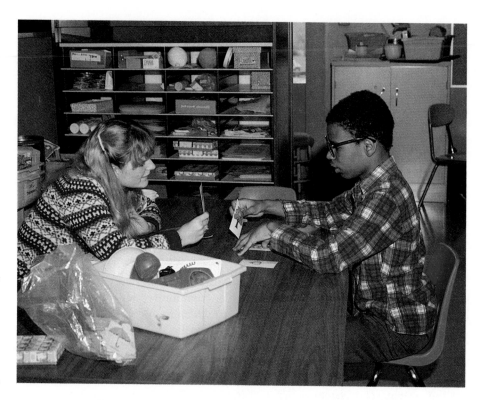

Adaptive fitting describes the attempts of students to meet the expectations of the educational system, and, conversely, the attempts of professionals working in the system to meet the needs of the individual. (The Institute for the Study of Developmental Disabilities at Indiana University)

2. An exploratory learning component that includes a variety of learning options

3. A classroom management system designed specifically to teach students self-management skills

4. A family-involvement program that attempts to reinforce the integration of school and home experiences

5. A multi-age and team-teaching organization that increases flexibility. (p. 205)

For years, the regular classroom teacher has had to assist students with disabilities, without any effective support systems. In many of today's schools, this is no longer the case. The emergence of collaborative efforts between the classroom teacher and the specialists available within the public schools represents a major breakthrough in the education of these individuals.

Coordinating Educational Services

FOCUS 6
Distinguish between the consulting teacher, the resource-room program, the self-contained special class, and the special school for students with disabilities.

There are several models of collaboration within the public schools to enhance the student's educational opportunities. We discuss four of these models: the **consulting teacher,** the **resource-room teacher,** the **self-contained special education classroom,** and the special school. Each of these models views the classroom teacher as being primarily responsible for the student's education. The services provided through each of the collaborative models is intended to support the regular education curriculum. We first discuss the consulting-teacher model.

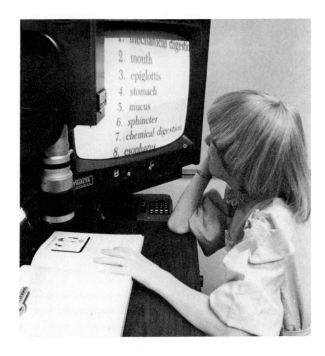

In the resource room, students receive specialized instruction to supplement their regular classroom education. (John Telford)

The Consulting Teacher.   The regular classroom teacher, particularly at the elementary level, is expected to teach nearly every school-related subject area. The elementary classroom teacher is responsible for teaching the basic subjects, including reading, writing, and arithmetic. In addition, the teacher is supposed to be developing within the student an appreciation for the arts, good citizenship, and maintenance of a sound physical body. The teacher is trained as a generalist, acquiring general knowledge of every subject area. When regular classroom teachers are confronted with instructional problems that are beyond their experience and previous training, however, the result is often frustration for the teacher and failure for the student. Given the present structure of public education (large class sizes), it is unrealistic and unnecessary for classroom teachers to become specialists in every school subject.

Many school districts offer support to classroom teachers through professionals who have extensive background in specific curriculum areas. These include specialists in reading, arithmetic, language, motor development, or the arts. These professionals are usually referred to as *consulting teachers*, although the terms **curriculum specialist, master teacher,** or **itinerant teacher** may also be used. These professionals are responsible for providing support to regular classroom teachers and their students. They may assist the teacher in further defining and refining the nature of a student's problem and may recommend appropriate assessment devices and intervention strategies. The effective consultant has several important characteristics, as indicated in Reflect on This 3–1. The consulting-teacher model includes the training and support of regular classroom teachers and an emphasis on modifying the regular education environment to accommodate exceptional students, rather than having these individuals removed to separate

Reflect on This 3-1

Characteristics of an Effective Consultant

1. Has state-of-the-art knowledge in the problem areas in which consultation is needed, has a reputation for the ability to diagnose and outline alternatives for treatment (instruction), and has built up experience and uses it well.

2. Makes sure all potential clients know in general how the process of consultation works. Offers services in a way that minimizes anxiety and does not stigmatize the recipient.

3. Is honest, spontaneous, courageous, and open to all facts, and makes no exclusions.

4. Is genuinely positive and authentic in expectations of constructive motives about people's competencies and is able to build mutually trusting relationships.

5. Is sensitive and responsive to others and has good knowledge of social dynamics.

6. Is interested in learning with others and communicating about processes of learning through consultation experiences.

7. Has a knack for being concrete and specific about approaches to problems, yet is also able to structure problems in broader, theoretical terms.

8. Lacks the need for "professional distance"; prefers co-equal relationships even though he or she is much more experienced than most others in the area of consultation. Finds rewards in successful performance by other persons, particularly by consultees or clients. Is noncompetitive and mature. Other people notice the maturity and feel comfortable with the consultant.

9. Has good research abilities and is able to access resources efficiently.

Source: M. C. Reynolds & J. W. Birch, 1988, *Adaptive Mainstreaming*, New York: Longman, Inc.

settings (Reynolds & Birch, 1982, 1988). In a class of twenty-five to thirty students, approximately one or two of these youngsters usually make it necessary for the classroom teacher to utilize the services of a consulting teacher.

The Resource Room. In the resource-room teacher model, the student receives specialized instruction in a classroom that is separate from the regular education setting, but still within the same school building. While still receiving the majority of instruction in their regular education classroom, students with learning and behavior difficulties come to the resource room for short periods during the day to supplement their school curricula. The resource room is not intended to be a study hall, where students come to do their homework or spend time catching up on other classwork. This room is under the direction of a qualified special education teacher, whose role is to provide individualized instruction in academic or behavioral areas that negatively affect the student's chances for success in the regular classroom. The resource-room teacher, in collaboration with an educational team that includes the student's regular classroom teacher, identifies high-risk skill areas. The team then develops and implements instruction intended to increase proficiency to a level where the student is competitive with classmates.

It can be anticipated that approximately one or two students in a classroom of twenty-five to thirty, or about 6 percent of the school-age population, need the additional instructional services offered by the resource-room program. In many states, because a student is receiving direct special education services, there is a requirement that the individual be labeled exceptional in order to fund the resource-room program through federal and state special education funds. Therefore, in order to adhere to the concept of the least restrictive environment, students receiving instruction through the resource-room program, by definition, have problems that require assistance beyond that offered by the consulting-teacher model. Although the problems are still of a mild nature, these students need instructional assistance in a more restricted setting than the regular classroom.

The resource-room model has some important features that differ from traditional special education role patterns. It allows students to remain with age-mates for the majority of the school day, while removing a great deal of the stigma associated with segregated special education classrooms. It also provides support to the regular classroom teacher, who despite realizing that these students have potential for success in the regular classroom, finds it extremely difficult to provide the appropriate individualized instruction to one or two students.

The resource-room program has been the predominant instructional approach for students with disabilities over the past decade. The approach used in the resource-room model is commonly referred to as **pull-out**—removing the student with a disability from the regular classroom to a separate class (usually a resource room) for at least part of the school day. There is a growing group of both regular and special educators that argue that although there have been some accomplishments in the pull-out programs, there have also been some negative effects or obstacles to the appropriate education of students with disabilities (Allington & McGill-Franzen, 1989; Gartner & Lipsky, 1987; 1989; Reynolds & Lakin, 1987; Will, 1986). The proponents of **shared responsibility** (sometimes referred to as the **regular education initiative**) between regular and special education argue that:

1. Pull-out programs result in a fragmented approach to the delivery of special education programs, with little cooperation between regular and special educators.

2. Students in pull-out programs are stigmatized when segregated from their nondisabled peers.

3. Placement decisions are often a battleground for parents and educators.

The proponents of shared responsibility also argue that placement in regular education classrooms with a partnership between regular and special educators results in an environment and curricula that are diverse and rich, rather than just a series of discrete programming slots and funding pots. A partnership between regular and special education personalizes each child's instructional program and brings the program to the child in the least restrictive environment, rather than bringing the child to a separate program. Additionally, special educators are more effective in a partnership because they can bring their knowledge and resources to assist regular educators in developing intervention strategies that are directly oriented to student need, in the natural setting of the regular education classroom.

Opponents of the shared-responsibility approach argue that:

1. Regular education has little expertise to assist students with learning problems and is already overburdened with large class sizes and inadequate support services.

2. Special educators have been specifically trained to develop instructional strategies and use teaching techniques (e.g., behavior management) that are not part of the training of regular education teachers.

3. More specialized academic and social instruction can be provided in a pull-out setting, and such settings can more effectively prepare the student to return to the regular education classroom.

4. Specialized pull-out settings allow for a centralization of both human and material resources.

The Self-Contained Special Education Classroom.   For some students with a disability, neither the consulting-teacher model nor the resource room may be appropriate. These students require more intensive and specialized educational services. The self-contained special education classroom employs the expertise of a qualified special education teacher to work with these students the majority of the school day, while still promoting integration with nondisabled peers wherever and whenever possible. These students can still be integrated in many ways, including some academic and nonacademically oriented classes, lunch, playground, school events, peer tutor programs, and so forth.

The Special School.   Students with a disability may also be placed in special schools. Proponents of this arrangement argue that special schools provide services for large numbers of disabled students and therefore provide greater homogeneity in the grouping and programming for children. They also support this type of arrangement because it allows teachers to specialize in their teaching areas. For example, one individual might decide to teach art, another physical education, and a third math. In smaller programs in which there are only one or two teachers, these individuals may be required to teach everything from art and home economics to academic subjects. Proponents also argue that special schools provide for the centralization of supplies, equipment, and special facilities.

Opponents argue that research studies on the efficacy of special schools do not support the above rationale. Several authors (Brinker, 1985; Stainback & Stainback, 1985; Wehman & Hill, 1982; Wilcox & Bellamy, 1982) contend that, regardless of the severity of their disabling condition, children benefit from placement in a regular education facility, where opportunities for integration with nondisabled peers are systematically planned and implemented.

Role of the Regular-Education Classroom Teacher.   Today's classroom teachers are confronted with the challenge of educating all students for the complex demands of our society. They are, at the same time, faced with an increased responsibility to meet the needs of certain students who require additional instructional support in order to succeed in school. The integration of exceptional students into a regular-education school and/or classroom may be met with frustration, anger, or refusal on the part of teachers. These reactions are symptomatic of the confusion surrounding the term **mainstreaming.** Mainstreaming, in many educational circles, has been synonymous with dumping; that is, returning the exceptional student to regular education without any support service to the classroom teacher and at the expense of other students in the class. Placing exceptional students in regular-education classrooms without needed support services is widely opposed by professionals and parents alike. Students with disabilities should be placed in regular classes only when the following conditions have been fulfilled:

1. The exceptional student has been appropriately assessed by a multidisciplinary team of professionals, and the regular classroom has been determined to be the least restrictive environment.

2. The classroom teacher has been adequately trained in how to meet the learning and behavioral needs of the exceptional student.

3. Appropriate support personnel and instructional materials are readily available to the teacher.

All these factors must be present if an exceptional student is to have a reasonable chance for success.

A multidisciplinary approach to assessment and educational planning is not only sound educational practice but also a legal mandate for disabled children receiving services under federal legislation (see Chapter 2). Swanson and Willis (1979) defined the team approach as an opportunity for various professionals to:

FOCUS 7
What is the role of the regular classroom teacher as a member of the multidisciplinary team?

> Evaluate, collaborate, and cooperate with each other in planning the provision of appropriate services for an exceptional child. The team may include any combination of the following—or other needed—professionals: educators (special, regular, administrative), medical personnel, psychologists and/or **psychometrists,** social workers, speech pathologists, physical therapists, **vocational rehabilitation specialists.** Parents are also very important and necessary contributors to the team (p. 13).

The student's educational program is developed using data accrued by this multidisciplinary team. The role(s) of each professional in relation to program planning, intervention, and evaluation of program effectiveness should be clearly described in the student's educational plan. Table 3–1 highlights possible roles for members of the multidisciplinary team.

In the case of students with mild disabilities, the regular classroom teacher has the primary responsibility for implementing an appropriate educational program, with consulting or resource-room teachers providing the necessary support.

In order to meet the needs of exceptional students and to function as an informed team member, regular teachers must receive expanded training at the preservice level. The National Advisory Council on Education Professions Development (1976) suggests that regular classroom teachers need to understand how a disorder affects a student's ability to acquire academic skills or cope socially in the educational environment. Teachers need to be able to recognize problems and to prescribe and implement individualized programs. They must

TABLE 3–1 Roles of Multidisciplinary Team Members

Team Member	Roles
Regular classroom teacher	Initially identifies students who may be in need of specialized services
	May initiate referral for testing and evaluation of students who may need specialized services
	Works with team members to develop and implement exceptional student's individualized educational program in the regular classroom
	Evaluates student progress in regular classroom in relationship to instructional goals
	Maintains on-going communication with parents
Special education teacher	Assesses educational needs of child
	Works with team to determine child's eligibility and placement into special education services
	Develops and implements exceptional student's individualized educational program
	Evaluates student progress in relationship to instructional goals
	Maintains on-going communication with parents
Parents	May initiate referral of their child
	Provide consent for evaluation and placement, if necessary, into special education services
	Provide information to team on child's needs and skills outside of school setting
	Work with team on development and implementation of child's individualized educational program
	Maintain on-going communication with team regarding child's performance in settings outside of school
Principal, school administrator	Coordinates team activities
	Calls team meetings
	Ensures appropriate information is available prior to decisions regarding child's educational program
	Works with team on development of child's individualized educational program
	Ensures that team decisions are implemented in an effective and timely fashion

Other team members may include school psychologists, physical education specialists, social workers, speech and language specialists, school counselors, school nurse, occupational therapists, physical therapists, vocational specialists, representatives from the courts, media specialists, and so on.

develop an understanding of mainstreaming and be aware of the kind of assistance support personnel can give.

There is also an important role for the regular classroom teacher with regard to students who have more moderate and severe disabilities. Although these students may not be mainstreamed into the regular education classroom, they are members of the school's student body. An important component of these students' success in the regular education facility is the cooperative relationship between regular-class and special-class teachers. Hamre-Nietupski (1980) found that this cooperative relationship is a critical factor in the successful integration of these students in regular school programs and activities. The role of the regular classroom teacher is to assist the special education teacher in creating *opportunities* for interaction between disabled and nondisabled students. Stainback and Stainback (1985) discuss the role of the regular classroom teacher in relationship to students with severe disabilities:

> Regular-class teachers can help facilitate integration by accepting students with severe handicaps into their classrooms during selected activities such as home-room, art, music, recess, holiday celebrations, birthday parties, show-and-tell times, and rest periods. . . . They can encourage their nonhandicapped students to visit the special education classroom(s) to work as tutors, or simply to spend a little time with a friend who experiences a severe handicap. In addition, regular class teachers can join with special class teachers in providing opportunities for interaction . . . in the school cafeteria, on the playground, at assembly programs, in the hallways, and at the bus loading and unloading zones (p. 13).

An Instructional Decision-Making Model

Learning is a continual process of adaptation for students with disabilities as they attempt to cope with the demands of school. These students learn to adapt to the limited time constraints placed on them by the educational system. They do not learn as quickly or as efficiently as their classmates and are constantly fighting a battle against failure. They must somehow learn to deal with a system that is often rigid and allows little room for learning or behavior differences. Students with mild disorders must also be able to adapt to a teaching process that may be oriented toward the majority of students within the regular classroom, not based on individualized assessment of needs or personalized instruction. In spite of major obstacles, however, these students can learn not only to survive in the education environment but also to develop personal/social and academic skills that can orient them toward striving for success rather than toward fighting failure. Success can be achieved only if the teacher remains flexible, adapting to meet the needs of these students.

An educational team plays an important role in creating the adaptive fit between the school environment and student needs. This team makes critical decisions concerning educational goals and objectives, the appropriate curricula, and the least restrictive environmental alternatives. The magnitude of these decisions is illustrated in Figure 3–2 (see page 72), a three-dimensional model for instructional decision making. The first dimension of this model is the curricular approaches that may be used in teaching students with disabilities. The second dimension focuses on the processes involved in teaching, including assessment,

FOCUS 8
Identify three curricular approaches that can be used in teaching students with learning and behavior disorders.

Reflect on This 3–2

Working as a Team Member—What's My Role?

A multidisciplinary team, as defined in the Education for All Handicapped Children Act (Public Law 94–142), is a group of professionals along with parents who join together to plan and implement an appropriate educational program for a handicapped child. *Multidisciplinary* suggests that team members may be trained in different areas of study, including education, health services, speech and language, school administration, and so on. The idea, however, is that these individual people sit down together and coordinate their efforts to help the student, regardless of where or how they were trained. In order for this effort to work, each team member must clearly understand his or her role and responsibilities as a member of the team. Let's visit with some multidisciplinary team members and have them share their perceived role in relationship to working with a handicapped child.

Special Education Teacher

It's my responsibility to coordinate the student's total program. I work with each member of the team to assist in selecting, administering, and interpreting appropriate assessment information. I maintain on-going communication with each team member to ensure that we are all working together to help the child. It's my job to compile, organize, and maintain good, accurate records on each student. I design the special education programming alternatives for the student and implement the recommended educational programs. To carry this out, I locate or develop the necessary curriculum materials to meet each student's specific needs. I work directly with the student's parents to ensure that they are familiar with what is being taught at school and can reinforce school learning experiences at home.

Parents

We are advocates for our child. We work with each team member to make sure that our child is involved in an appropriate educational program. We give information to the team about our child's life outside of school, and we suggest educational experiences that might be relevant to the home and the community. We sometimes

planning, implementation, and evaluation of a program. The third dimension is temporal: There is only so much instructional time available from the early-childhood through secondary years. Difficult decisions relating to what must be taught and when to teach it are critical in determining an appropriate educational experience for a child.

Three curricular approaches may be used in teaching students. The major approach may be termed *the learning of basic skills*, which stresses that the student must learn a specified set of skills that are sequenced, each a prerequisite to the next step. This process can be exemplified by briefly analyzing the foundation approach to teaching reading. Hansen and Eaton (1978) define the reading process as "a blend of many separate skills working in harmony. If one skill or cluster of skills is missing, the entire process breaks down and the child is unable to read or comprehend" (p. 41). The teaching of basic reading skills can be divided into three phases: (1) the development of readiness skills (such as left to right sequencing, visual and auditory discrimination skills, and memory skills), (2) word-recognition or decoding skills (breaking the code and correctly identifying the abstract symbols in sequence), and (3) reading comprehension (giving symbols meaning). The **basic-skills approach,** whether in reading or any other content also work with our child at home to reinforce what is learned in school. As members of the team, we give our written consent for any evaluations of our child and any changes in our child's educational placement. We also sign our child's individualized educational program.

School Psychologist

I select, administer, and interpret appropriate psychological, educational, and behavioral assessment instruments. I consult directly with the special education teacher, parents, and other team members regarding the student's overall educational development. It is also my responsibility to directly observe the student's performance in the classroom and assist in the design of appropriate behavioral management programs in the school and at home.

School Administrator

As the school district's representative, I work with the team to ensure that the resources of my district are used appropriately in providing services to the handicapped student. I am ultimately responsible for ensuring that the team's decisions are implemented properly.

Regular Classroom Teacher

I work with the team to develop and implement appropriate educational experiences for the handicapped student during the time that he or she spends in the regular classroom. I ensure that the student's special education experiences are consistent with the programming the student receives in my classroom. In carrying out my responsibilities, I keep an accurate and continuous record of the

student's progress. I am also responsible for referring any other students in my classroom who may need special education services to the school district for an evaluation of their needs.

The above individuals generally constitute the core members of the multidisciplinary team, but the team is not limited to these people. Depending on the needs of the student, many other professionals sometimes serve as members of the team, including speech and language specialists, social workers, the school counselor, the school nurse, occupational or physical therapists, the adaptive physical education teacher, vocational rehabilitation counselors, juvenile court authorities, physicians, and school media coordinators.

area, lays the groundwork for further development and higher levels of functioning. However, not all children learn basic skills within the time-frame dictated by the schools.

Educators have available to them several alternatives that assist students who do not learn in the traditional way or within the specified time-frame. One alternative is to remediate the gaps in the student's repertoire of skills. The **remediation approach** identifies the specific gaps by determining what skills the student does or does not have and then locating appropriate materials and instructional approaches to correct the problem. This approach focuses on "changing the learner in some way so that he or she may more effectively relate to the educational program as it is provided and administered for all students" (Marsh, Gearheart, & Gearheart, 1978, p. 85). Gaps in information may be the result of either poor teaching or lack of ability on the part of the student. Therefore, it is doubtful that the learner's behavior can be changed by simply repeating that which resulted in failure—asking the student to try harder in other words. Teaching must be more systematic and precise if deficits are to be remediated.

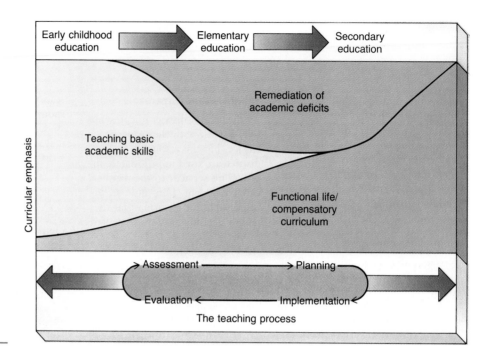

Figure 3-2
An Instructional Decision-Making Model

Another alternative for educators is to teach basic skills using a **functional life/compensatory curriculum.** This approach teaches only those skills that facilitate the student's accommodation to society. "The focus is on changing the learning environment or the academic requirements so that the student may learn in spite of a fundamental weakness or deficiency" (Marsh et al., 1978, p. 85). Content areas within a functional life/compensatory curriculum might include daily living skills (such as self-care, consumer financing, and community travel), person-social skills (including learning socially responsible behaviors), communication

WINDOW 3-1

What Will I Do with These Kids?

I remember the first year I taught third grade and someone mentioned to me that there would undoubtedly be at least one or two handicapped students in my class. I thought to myself, No kidding? I don't have the training, background, or experience to be dealing with handicapped students. What on earth will I do with these kids? It didn't take long for me to find out that these two students, labeled *learning disabled* and *behavior disordered,* could and should be in my classroom with their nonhandicapped peers. Oh, I've needed help, but through the assistance of our school's special education consultant these kids are progressing right along with the rest of my third graders. Marie, our special education consultant, has given me some terrific ideas about behavior management, adapting instructional programs, and dealing with my students' questions about children who don't learn in the same way they do. These handicapped students belong in my class, and they deserve the support that will help them stay there. I know that neither they nor I would have it any other way.

Tricia, *third-grade teacher*

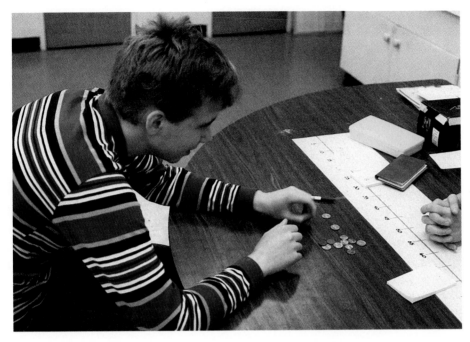

The functional life/compensatory curriculum focuses on skills that will facilitate a person's accommodation to society. In addition to handling money, what other consumer skills will this student need to be able to make purchases? (The Institute for the Study of Developmental Disabilities at Indiana University)

skills, and occupational/vocational skills. This approach is based on the premise that if these practical skills are not taught through formal instruction, they will not be learned. Most students do not need to be taught these functional skills because they have already learned them through everyday experience. However, the functional life/compensatory curriculum may need to be the primary emphasis for students who cannot learn through basic or remedial approaches to instruction. This does not mean that students being taught with a functional-life approach are not learning basic academic skills such as reading, arithmetic, and handwriting. These academic skills may be taught, but not in the same sequence as in the basic-skills approach. For example, a functional-life reading approach would initially teach words that are high-use words and necessary for survival within the environment (including *danger, exit,* and *restrooms*). These words are paired immediately with an environmental cue. It is possible to combine curricular approaches; they are not mutually exclusive. The basic-skills approach may be utilized in conjunction with a functional-life orientation in some skill areas.

The educational team is confronted with some difficult decisions about how to teach and what to teach. These decisions must take into account such factors as the student's age, previous learning history, and the available resources. In addition, decisions regarding a student's educational experience must encompass the constraints of time. Instructional time in the classroom is limited, and decisions have to be made concerning how to use the available time efficiently. Figure 3–2, the curricular decision-making model, illustrates that the time factor can be separated into three educational dimensions: the early-childhood, elementary years, and secondary years. The curricular emphasis is different for each dimension.

The elementary-school years are a time when the emphasis is on learning academic and socialization skills. For most children, these skills are learned quickly and eventually become tools that expand the child's knowledge in all

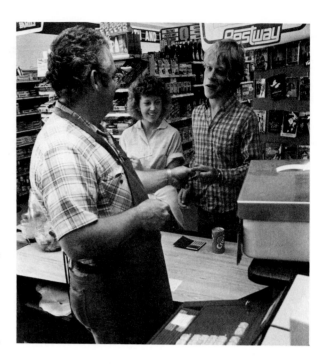

Once students in a functional life/compensatory curriculum have learned the basic skills in the classroom, they are given opportunities to practice them in the community. (John Telford)

content areas. However, the student with learning and behavior disorders will still be struggling with basic academics and appropriate social skills long after his or her peers have become proficient in these areas.

Secondary-school educators also have to determine appropriate curricular emphases for the student, based on the skill level he or she has attained during the elementary years. An adolescent may have acquired enough foundation skills to function successfully in some content areas, such as social studies, algebra, history, and chemistry; and the primary instructional emphasis may have to be on career education, vocational training, personal management, and use of recreation/leisure time. These areas of emphasis are not mutually exclusive; an intervention may be a combination of all of the above.

THE TRANSITION YEARS: FROM SCHOOL TO ADULT LIFE

FOCUS 9
Give four reasons why it is important to study the relationship between what is taught in school and the needs of an individual during the adult years.

For many years, the development and implementation of appropriate services for people with exceptionalities has focused primarily on school-age children and youth. As we begin the second decade of the national mandate to educate disabled children, one of the most critical issues parents and professionals face is, "What is the relationship between what is taught in school and the needs of the individual during the adult years?" There are some substantial reasons why this issue is receiving such attention. Follow-up studies of students with disabilities leaving the public schools indicate that they are not adequately prepared for employment, and that they generally do not have access to the necessary resources and services that would enhance their participation in the community.

The increasing emphasis on transition from school to adult life has altered many of our previously held perceptions about people who are exceptional,

Reflect on This 3–3

Objectives for a Functional Reading Program

Functional reading programs focus on using reading as a tool in the everyday environment. The following are some examples of objectives that could be included in a student's individualized reading program.

- The student will identify his or her name, address, and phone number when it is written.
- The student will carry out the directions written on grocery items, toys, games, or specific items that require assembly.

- The student will use a telephone directory to locate needed information on another person.
- The student will respond appropriately to written information found on employment forms, work time cards, check stubs, grocery store receipts, and so on.

- The student will locate needed information on restaurant menus and place an order with a waitress.
- The student will respond appropriately to directions written on simple notes.
- The student will respond appropriately to public restroom signs and safety signs.

particularly those we would define as handicapped or disabled. Without question, we have significantly underestimated the potential of adults with disabilities. Thorough study of disabled people as they move through adult life is one of the most important and challenging areas for professionals in the remaining years of this century.

Yvonne is now twenty-two and is leaving school for adult life. During most of her high school years, she was in special education classes, receiving extra assistance and tutoring in reading and math. During the last term of high school, she attended a class dealing with jobs, although the rest of her courses still focused on reading and math. The job class was required for graduation but it didn't make much sense to Yvonne, since she had never had anything like that before, and it didn't seem to be related to her other schoolwork.

Yvonne wants to get a job now that she is out of school but she hasn't had much success. She does not have a driver's license, and her parents don't have much time to take her around to apply for a job. The business people she has approached are close by her home and know her well. They say they are unable to give her a job even though several have signs in their windows saying "Help Wanted." Yvonne's parents are not very enthusiastic about her finding employment because they are afraid she might lose some of the benefits she is receiving from social services. Yvonne is able to go to movies but only with her parents. She is lonesome for her old friends from school.

This vignette should raise some questions for you. Why was Yvonne's vocational preparation limited to one term, while the rest of her schooling was

In the News 3–1

The Eden Express, a Restaurant with a Mission as Well as a Menu, Teaches the Disabled to Fend for Themselves

It is early morning, and the Eden Express seems much like any other unpretentious little eating house in the blue-collar town of Hayward, California. The 82-seat restaurant buzzes with the chatter of the breakfast crowd as the youthful, well-scrubbed staff moves about among the butcher-block tables. Two newcomers take a seat by the window, and Sean, a heavyset waiter in a striped apron, ambles over to hand them their menus. "Thank you," they say. "You're welcome," he replies, and he means it.

Returning to take the order, Sean pulls a notepad from his pocket, squints at the page and laboriously writes E-G-G-S. But the second customer wants something more complicated. "I'd like the eggs scrambled on the muffin," he says, "not poached, and I want them dry." A look of mild panic flashes in Sean's blue eyes. A subtle kick under the table, from his companion, prompts the diner to simplify his request. He asks for toast instead, and Sean breathes a little inward sigh of relief.

As the tabletop placards explain, the Eden Express is unlike any other restaurant in America.

Sean, 20, is learning-disabled, and his co-workers are afflicted with manic depression, deafness, schizophrenia and other disabilities. Founded in 1980, the restaurant is headquarters for a groundbreaking project in which students like Sean are trained to live in the mainstream and rescued from a life of hopelessness. "We give these kids a chance to start dreaming again, to start believing they have a chance to make it out there," says director Barbara Lawson. "The majority of them had given up on themselves."

Celebrating its eighth anniversary this week, the program has turned out more than 400 graduates, 90 percent of whom have moved on to paying jobs. But the Express's most significant achievement has more to do with pride than with paychecks. In afterwork seminars and counseling sessions, Sean and his classmates are learning the intricacies of proper social interaction, grooming, personal budgeting, math and reading—all of the skills they will need in the marketplace. Armed with new confidence, they will have a chance to shake the wrenching sense of failure that often plagues

the disabled. "My kids are really proud of me," reports Denise, a 33-year-old learning- and hearing-impaired graduate who passed through Eden's gate and now works as a baker's assistant at Safeway. A single mother of two, she had never held a regular job before she was hired by the supermarket chain in July. "When I got my first paycheck, I was real excited—I went and framed it," she says. "Now my dream is to move from where I'm living into a nicer neighborhood."

Not surprisingly, the program has the enthusiastic support of the mental health community. Wrote psychiatrist and author Dr. Maryellen Walsh in her 1985 book *Schizophrenia*: "To call Eden Express another rehab project is to call Paris another town, Picasso another artist, and Dietrich just another pretty face. . . ."

still focusing on reading and math, with graduation so near? Where were the vocational counseling and transition support during her last years of school?

The transition to adult life for people with disabilities presents some perplexing but interesting issues. The vignette above does not represent unusual circumstances. Fortunately, transition services and adult support systems for people with disabilities are undergoing considerable change.

For many years, professionals working with disabled people focused their efforts on young children. Concern with adolescents, the transition to adulthood, and older disabled individuals was nearly nonexistent. Interest in this area has emerged rather recently, partially prompted by an interest in aging in general. However, over the years, professionals have become more conscious that disabled individuals do not disappear after they leave the school system.

The increased attention to adult and elderly people also requires reflection on some fundamental questions if research and service are to progress effectively. For example, the notions of *transition, adult, aging,* and *old* need serious examination. Most of us have some idea about the meaning of these terms, but our concepts are often quite personal and very fluid. As children, we typically thought of our parents as being old even though they may have been in their mid-thirties or early forties, an age most adults do not view as old, and some think is rather young. Aging is a fluid concept. There is considerable variation in terms of what age represents adulthood or elderly status. Definitions of age have presented considerable difficulty for both researchers and service providers (Siegel, 1980).

In recent years, professionals and parents have begun to address some of the critical issues facing adolescents with disabilities as they prepare to leave school and face life as adults in their local communities. Currently, over a quarter of a million disabled youths are finishing school each year. Since the advent of Public Law 94–142, schools have made significant strides in preparing disabled youths for adult life, but much remains to be done. Many of the current graduates from special education programs, like Yvonne, are neither adequately prepared for employment nor able to access other critical services necessary for them to succeed in their local communities (Brodsky, 1983; Hasazi et al., 1985). Long waiting lists for vocational and housing services await many of these individuals (McDonnell, Wilcox, & Boles, 1985).

In this section, we discuss some of the issues surrounding the transition from school to the adult years. First, we define the components of a transition process. We then focus on the role of the schools and adult-service agencies in developing an appropriate transition system. Finally, we address what parents should expect as their son or daughter makes the transition to adult living.

Defining Transition

The **transition from school to adult life** is a complex process that may begin as the individual enters the high school years, or even before. The process involves a series of choices about what experiences disabled students should have in their remaining school years, to better prepare them for what lies ahead in the adult world. Will (1984) defines transition as a "bridge between the security and structure offered by the school and adult life" (pp. 6–7). This bridge requires a sound preparation program during high school, support for individuals as they finish school, and opportunities to access services when needed during the adult years. While there is some disagreement about the specific programs that are necessary to bridge the gap between school and adult life, there is a consensus about the principal components of a transition system. These components include:

FOCUS 10
Give three factors involved in the definition of *transition.*

1. Effective high school programs that reference instruction to community activities and demands

2. An array of adult services that can meet the unique vocational, residential, and leisure needs of disabled youth

3. A cooperative system of transition planning that ensures access to needed postschool services (McDonnell & Hardman, 1985).

Transition is obviously much more than the mere transfer of administrative responsibility for an individual from school to an adult service agency. It is a process that involves many agencies and the family in developing activities and services that are appropriate to the individual.

The Role of the School

FOCUS 11
What are five aspects of the school's role in preparing a student for life during the adult years?

Vincent is twenty-two years old and a student at Monument Valley High School. This is Vincent's final year in school. As a student in a program for adolescents with disabilities, he has been spending the past three years preparing for the transition to adulthood. His vocational training experiences have included working in three different jobs in his local community, with support from school staff and people from the State Vocational Rehabilitation Agency. During the past two years, much of Vincent's educational program has taken him out of the classroom and into the malls, grocery stores, parks, theaters, and restaurants in his neighborhood.

Transition begins with a solid foundation on which to build. The school is that foundation. High school programs must provide those activities that lead directly to outcomes facilitating success for the individual during the adult years. For Vincent, these activities included learning to shop in a neighborhood grocery store and training for a job in the community. What, then, are the expected outcomes for youths with disabilities as they enter adulthood? First, adults should be able to function as independently as possible in their daily lives—their reliance on others to meet their needs should be minimized. These individuals should also be involved in the economic life of the community. There should be opportunities for both paid and unpaid work. Working in the community is of value to the disabled individual both for the monetary benefits it offers and for the opportunities for social interaction, personal identity, and contribution to others. Finally, an adult should be able to participate in social and leisure activities that are an integral part of community life.

High schools are in the unique position of being able to coordinate activities during the school years that enhance student participation in the community and link students such as Vincent with needed services. The school has many roles in the transition process, including the assessment of individual needs, developing transition plans for each student, coordinating transition planning with adult service agencies, and participating with parents in the planning process.

Assessing Individual Needs. The needs of a disabled adult vary according to the functioning level of the individual in relationship to the requirements of the environment. People with more severe disabling conditions may require significant and long-term support from society in order to be involved in activities

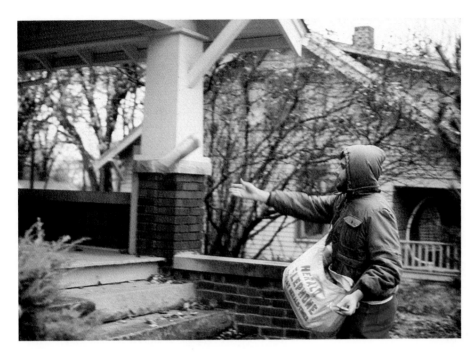

Working in the community offers monetary benefits as well as opportunities for social interaction, personal identity, and contribution to others. (The Institute for the Study of Developmental Disabilities at Indiana University)

within their communities. Adults with mild disabilities may need only short-term assistance or no support system whatsoever during their adult years. However, Brolin (1977; 1982) suggests that while in school even students with mild disabilities must receive more than vocational training experiences. Schools must broaden their focus on vocational preparation to include career education. Clark (1979) indicates that career education includes preparation for life skills and personal social skills, in addition to occupationally related instruction. Career education systematically coordinates all school, family, and community components. Thus, the disabled individual's potential for economic, social, and personal fulfillment is greatly enhanced. Given the range of disabled individuals who may need assistance during the adult years, a transition planning system must take into account the level of support necessary for successful participation in a given community. In order to identify the levels of support that an individual will require, parents and the schools must be able to assess the individual during the high school years across a variety of performance areas (including self-care, work, residential living, recreation, and leisure time). In the area of self-care, for example, assessments should be made for activities such as riding buses, using grocery stores, keeping a time schedule, crossing streets, and the like.

Developing Transition Plans. Once individual needs have been determined, schools should initiate a formal transition-planning process that allows the disabled youth, parents, and professionals to review options for services during the adult years. McDonnell and Hardman (1985) suggest that the purpose of the **transition plan** is to (1) identify the range of services needed by the individual to participate in the community, (2) identify activities that must occur during the high school

| Student: _____ Bob Robins _____ | | Meeting Date: _____ 10/15/89 _____ |
| | | Graduation Date: _ 6/7/91 _ |

Participants:

Parents(s) _____ Mrs. Robins _____
School _____ William B. _____
DSH Casemanager _____ Susan L. _____
DVR Casemanager _____ N/A _____

Planning Area: Vocational Services	*Responsible Person*	*Timelines*
Transition Goal		
Bob will initiate work training in Wasatch Work Crew Program	William B.	12/15/89
Support Activities		
1. Complete application process	Mrs. Robins Susan L.	11/1/89
2. Obtain UTA bus pass	Mrs. Robins	11/1/89
3. Teach bus route to Wasatch business office	William B.	11/14/89
4. Establish planning meeting with Wasatch WCP director	Susan L.	1/10/90

Figure 3–3

High School Transition Plan for a Severely Handicapped Student (*Source:* Adapted from J. McDonnell and M. L. Hardman, "Planning the Transition of Severely Handicapped Youth from School to Adult Services: A Framework for High School Programs," *Education and Training of the Mentally Retarded* [December 1985])

years to facilitate the individual's access to an adult-service program, and (3) establish timelines and responsibilities for completion of these activities.

Working with Adult-Service Agencies.   A critical component of the transition process is coordination between the schools and **adult-service agencies.** Adult-service agencies focus on providing the necessary services to assist individuals with disabilities to become more independent. These agencies may include vocational rehabilitation, social services, and mental health services. It is important for these agencies to become involved early in the student's high school program in order to begin targeting the services that will be needed once the student leaves school. This involvement includes direct participation in the development of the student's transition plan. Adult-service professionals should collaborate with the disabled student, parents, and school in establishing transition goals and identifying appropriate activities for the student during the remaining school years. Additionally, adult-service professionals must be involved in developing information systems that can effectively track students as they leave school programs and monitor the availability and appropriateness of services provided during the adult years (McDonnell & Hardman, 1985; Wehman, Kregel, & Barcus, 1985).

They really didn't prepare me for this. The job is incredible, it's satisfying—no, more than that—it's downright fun! But in a lot of ways the professors didn't prepare me for all that I have to do. When you think about it, though, there's really no way they could do any more than they did. All they could do was train me with the general skills of counseling, analysis of individual needs, program development, provide some examples and practical experience, and tell me to be creative in my approach to helping clients. They did a fantastic job of these things, and actually I had the very best preparation available. It's just that there is so much to do.

Let me back up a second. I have a job that is called "transition specialist" for the State Division of Health and Human Services. I work with young handicapped individuals who are in the process of leaving high school or have already graduated. I find employment and housing, arrange for transportation, and sometimes help with personal problems. So at one time or another during the week I'm working with prospective employers and lining up others, counseling and advising clients, meeting with politicians and community groups arguing for more services, and arranging for recreation events. I guess I'm a jack-of-all-trades, so to speak. Things are never boring, and each individual's case needs are different. It's really fun to see some of these people having successes that I guess were never thought of a few years ago. It's also wonderful to see some of the community people respond to what handicapped adults can accomplish in a work environment. More and more, they are calling me and wanting "my people" on the job. It isn't always like that, but when it is, there's nothing like it.

So what am I complaining about? Really nothing. I guess I wouldn't change much at all. It's exciting to be a part of these people's lives, and sometimes I wake up really early in the morning with a new idea for some aspect of the program. When I say they didn't prepare me for this, I'm really referring to the wide variety of things I do and the fact that I enjoy it so much that I don't think about much else. There isn't any way to prepare a person for all of that. Would I recommend to others that they go into the training program and this profession? Only if they want to get "hyped" by their job and do something that helps others at the same time!

Doreen, *transition specialist*

Involving Parents in the Transition Process. When a student with a disability leaves school and enters the adult world, many parents receive a considerable shock. First, there is the realization that the services their child was entitled to during the school years are no longer mandated by law. As such, there may be a significant loss of service from school to adult years. Second, many parents know very little, if anything at all, about adult-service systems. Consequently, during the student's high school years parents must be educated in critical components of adult-service systems. These components include the characteristics of adult-service agencies, criteria for evaluating adult-service programs, and potential as well as current service alternatives for their child. McDonnell and Hardman (1985) suggest two strategies for getting information to parents. First, school districts need to offer on-going in-service programs for parents, to acquaint them with the issues involved in the transition from school to adult life. Second, every school district should develop and use a transition-planning guide to help parents complete critical planning activities.

From early childhood to the high school transition years, the issues in delivering quality educational services to students with disabilities are varied and complex. With the information in this chapter as background, we now move into the chapters that focus on each of the areas of exceptionality: learning and behavior disorders, communication and sensory disorders, physical and health disorders, and gifted and talented. The discussion continues to highlight the nature of educational services while also examining both medical and social services. Definitions for each of the areas of exceptionality are presented, along with an overview of prevalence, characteristics, and causation.

WINDOW 3–3

*Shocked and
Scared Again*

My name is Kathleen, and I'm the parent of an adult who is much like a child. Tom is moderately retarded, but frankly he is doing quite well.

Sometimes it seems like I have spent the last twenty-two years being scared, shocked, numb, feeling helpless, angry, and all the other negative emotions that a person could possibly feel. It started while I was pregnant. During one of my regular checkups, my doctor became a bit worried about the baby. She talked with me a bit and indicated that things were not going well, even though I felt fine. Well, you can imagine how scared I felt; sort of a numbness went through me, starting with my feet and going all the way up. Anyway, she was right. When tests were run, we found that I was carrying a Down syndrome male child. I didn't know very much about it and neither did my husband, but we certainly have found out a lot since.

Giving only the *Reader's Digest* version, we had the typical problems that parents of handicapped children experience throughout childhood. We fought with the schools, it seemed like we fought with nearly every service agency one could think of; but in the end we got a pretty good assortment of services for Tom. Life could have been easier, but then it could have been a whole lot worse, too. I guess the last time that shock and frightened feeling came was when Tom was approaching the point where plans needed to be made for after he left school. By this time, my husband and I were no longer together and I was really on my own. I found out that Tom would lose many of the services that had made life tolerable while he was in school. I'd never thought about it much, but here was my child who no longer was a child but was still much like one and we needed help. Fortunately, we were in a good school district that offered Tom transition training and me transition counseling that would help when he was no longer in the public schools. Actual training for the process of leaving school saved us, and thank God it is becoming more widely available. Tom doesn't even live with me now; he is in a group home and is really doing fine. It hasn't been all that easy, but I'm doing fine, too.

Kathleen, *parent*

REVIEW

FOCUS 1: Why is it so important to provide early-intervention services to students at risk as early in the child's life as possible?

☐ The first years of life are important to the overall development of normal, at-risk, and disabled children.

☐ Early stimulation is critical to the later development of language, intelligence, personality, and a sense of self-worth.

☐ Interventions should begin as early as possible in an environment that is free of categorical labels.

☐ Early interventions have the potential of lessening the overall impact of disabilities as well as counteracting the negative effects of waiting to intervene.

FOCUS 2: Define early-childhood special education.

☐ Early-childhood special education is the process of carefully responding to a well-conceived individual education or treatment plan.

☐ The plan is based on the identified needs and strengths of the child.

☐ Early-childhood special education focuses on infants and children with all types and degrees of disabling and at-risk conditions.

FOCUS 3: What are some of the outcomes associated with early prevention and intervention for children at risk?

☐ Many infants who grow up to be disabled could clearly grow up to be normal if appropriate preventative steps were taken.

☐ Infants would be far less disabled if effective interventions were applied from birth.

FOCUS 4: What is the purpose of early-childhood special education services?

☐ Early-childhood special education addresses the needs of the whole child based on the Individualized Family Service Plan (IFSP).

☐ Intervention may include nutritional support, varied kinds of medical treatment (medication, surgery, physical therapy, etc.), speech and language therapy, parent and family training, and cognitive development.

☐ Early-childhood special education is designed to teach infants and very young children very specific skills (how to eat, in some cases, how to walk, how to talk, how to play successfully with other children, etc.); to lessen the impact of conditions that may worsen or become more severe without timely and adequate treatment; to provide specialized therapies for speech, language, and motor problems; to prevent children

from developing other, secondary disabling conditions; to prepare children as early as possible for meaningful experiences with their same-age peers; to teach children who exhibit troublesome behaviors (noncompliance, aggressiveness, etc.) that interfere with schooling more adaptive behaviors; and to provide children with the preacademic skills necessary for further learning.

FOCUS 5: What is meant by "adaptive fitting" for students with disabilities?

☐ The degree to which an individual is able to cope with the requirements of the school setting is described as the *adaptive fit*.

FOCUS 6: Distinguish between the consulting teacher, the resource-room program, the self-contained special class, and the special school for students with disabilities.

☐ Consulting teachers work directly with regular classroom teachers on the use of appropriate assessment techniques and intervention strategies.

☐ Students who work with consulting teachers are not removed from the regular classroom program, but remain with their nondisabled peers while receiving additional instructional assistance.

☐ Resource-room teachers provide specialized instruction to disabled students in a classroom that is separate from the regular education room.

☐ Under the resource-room program, the student still receives the majority of instruction in the regular education classroom, but is removed from the regular class for short periods to supplement his or her educational experience.

☐ Students who require intensive and specialized educational services that cannot be offered through the regular education classroom work with a teacher in a self-contained special education classroom or in a special school.

FOCUS 7: What is the role of the regular classroom teacher as a member of the multidisciplinary team?

☐ Regular classroom teachers must be aware of each disabled student's ability to acquire academic skills or cope socially within the school setting.

☐ Regular classroom teachers must be able and willing to recognize learning and behavior problems and work with the team to plan and implement an individualized program.

☐ When working with students with moderate and severe disabilities, the regular classroom teacher should assist the special education teacher in creating opportunities for interaction between disabled and nondisabled students.

FOCUS 8: Identify three curricular approaches that can be used in teaching students with learning and behavior disorders.

☐ The learning-of-basic-skills approach stresses that each student must learn a specified set of skills that are sequenced, each a prerequisite for the next step.

☐ The remediation approach identifies gaps in a student's skill development and then focuses on correcting the problems through the use of appropriate materials and instructional strategies.

☐ The functional life/compensatory approach teaches only those skills that would facilitate the student's successful adaptation to the environment.

FOCUS 9: Give four reasons why it is important to study the relationship between what is taught in school and the needs of an individual during the adult years.

☐ Disabled students leaving the public schools are not adequately prepared for life as adults in their local communities.

☐ Adult-service systems do not have the resources to meet the needs of disabled students following the school years.

☐ We have underestimated the capabilities of disabled adults.

☐ Definitions of *transition, adult, aging,* and *old* need to be clarified.

FOCUS 10: Give three factors involved in the definition of *transition.*

☐ Transition is a process that involves a series of choices about school experiences that will facilitate the disabled individual's adult life.

☐ Transition is the bridge between the security of the school and the reality of adult life in the community.

☐ The components of a transition system include an effective high school program, an array of adult services geared to the needs of each individual, and cooperative efforts across agencies for transition planning.

FOCUS 11: What are five aspects of the school's role in preparing a student for life during the adult years?

☐ High schools must attend to activities that facilitate success during the adult years.

☐ The needs of each high school student should be assessed across a variety of performance areas, including self-care, work, residential living, and recreation and leisure time.

☐ Schools must develop a formal transition-planning process that analyzes options during the adult years.

☐ Adult-service agencies must become involved in the student's high school program in order to target needed services during the adult years.

☐ Parents must be educated in the critical components of the adult-service system.

Debate Forum

Forgotten, Benign Neglect, or Priorities?

Adolescents and adults with handicaps have received relatively little attention over the years, in comparison to children and youth with similar conditions. This raises several questions. Have these people been literally forgotten in the process of focusing on childhood and the school years? Have they been the unfortunate victims of benign neglect because they do not need as much attention as handicapped children? Or does the relative lack of attention reflect conscious priority setting on the part of professionals and funding agencies? Choose a position and defend it.

Point With the exception of a rather small group (individuals with severe handicaps), most handicapped individuals who are beyond childhood can survive quite well without any attention from researchers or service providers. The historic focus on handicapped children during the school years is most appropriate because it is during the school years that most growth and development takes place. The school is also the environment in which people with handicapping conditions experience the most difficulty. Focusing our limited resources on older handicapped people is a waste of valuable tax dollars that are badly needed elsewhere. It makes more sense to use our funding to help children and youth who can benefit from it.

Counterpoint The historic lack of attention to adolescents and adults with handicaps represents nothing more than a generalized trend in education and psychology. Most professionals have focused on younger individuals generally, and handicapped people are no different. While it is true that many handicapped adults can fare rather well in the mainstream of society, it is very important to study and provide service to these people. From a pragmatic standpoint, such efforts are a very good investment of the tax dollar because the handicapped adult can become even more productive and thereby contribute to society as well as be a consumer of societal services. From a humanitarian perspective, neglect of these groups represents a neglect of social responsibility.

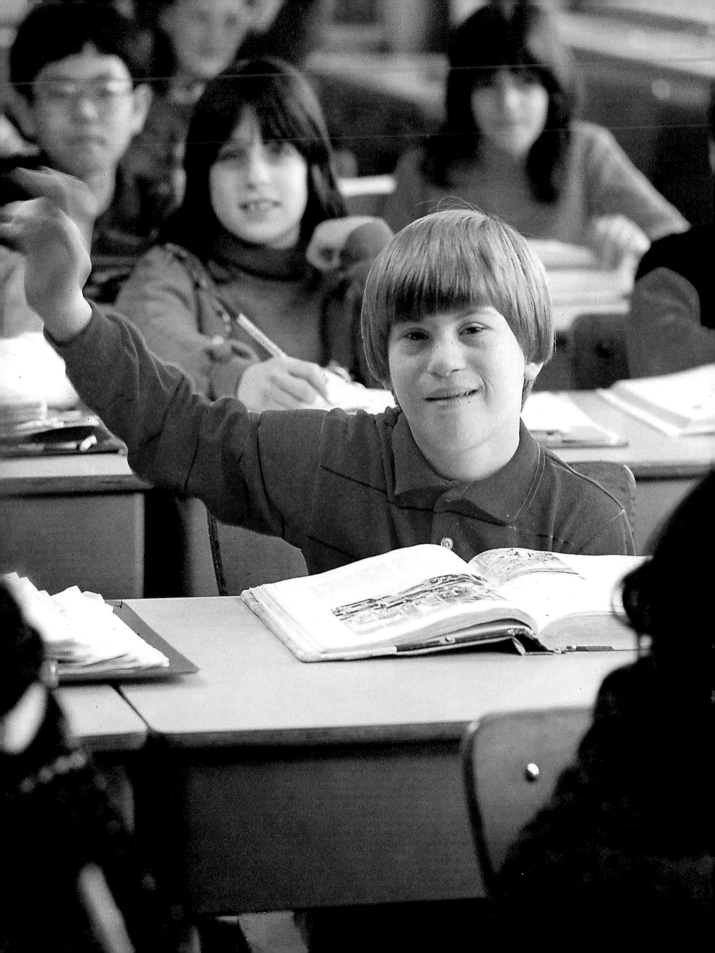

4 Mental Retardation

To Begin With...

■ Significantly more mentally ill persons are deinstitutionalized than are the mentally retarded (Blatt, 1987).

■ Older adults with mental retardation have little discretionary income. Many are poor. Most live in federally or state funded facilities (Stroud & Sutton, 1988).

■ In St. Louis, mothers who are mentally retarded can attend Parents Learning Together, a specially designed training program on child-care (Kantrowitz, King, & Witherspoon, 1986).

■ Persons with Down syndrome were referred to as "orangutans" in 1924, "nonpersons" in 1965 and "uneducable" as late as 1975. Today, such persons can attend Hope University, a private college for mentally retarded persons who are gifted in the fine arts (Turkington, 1987).

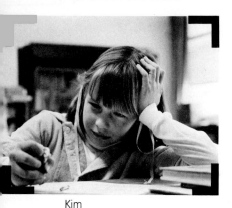

Kim

Kim developed much more slowly than her older brother, which caused some concern for her parents. Her family became concerned about Kim's hearing because of slow speech development, but this was judged to be normal when she was tested last year at the age of six. The **audiologist** referred the family to a psychologist for further evaluation. Although the audiologist said nothing specific, Kim's responses during the hearing test led her to suspect an overall developmental delay. The psychologist conducted a series of observations and administered a standardized intelligence test, along with tests to measure Kim's performance in reading and math. The test scores indicated that Kim's IQ was about 60, which placed her between two and three **standard deviations** below the average of 100. Her reading and math scores were also far behind those expected for a child of her age. Observations by her teacher suggested that Kim was delayed in the area of socialization skill development as well. Although she is now seven years old, Kim's functioning in many areas is much like that of a child three or four years younger. She does interact with other children her age in play activities, but if the game is complex or involves more than one or two children she tends to withdraw. Kim has learned the required self-help skills for her age level, including dressing, feeding, and personal hygiene. Kim is a child with mild **mental retardation.**

Roger is nineteen years old and lives at home with his parents. During the day he attends high school and works in a local toy company in a small work crew with five other disabled individuals. Roger and his working colleagues are closely supervised by a trained vocational specialist. Roger assembles small toys and is learning how to operate power tools for wood- and metal-cutting tasks. He earns wages, but not enough to be financially independent. It is likely that he will always be dependent on either his family or society for some financial assistance. Roger is capable of caring for his own physical needs. He has learned to dress and feed himself, and understands the importance of personal grooming and hygiene skills. He can communicate many of his needs and desires verbally, but is limited in his social language abilities. Roger has never learned to read, and his leisure hours are spent watching television, listening to the radio, and visiting with friends.

Becky is a six-year-old who has significant delays in her intellectual, language, and motor development. These problems have been evident from birth. Her mother experienced a long, unusually difficult labor, and Becky endured severe heart-rate dips; at times her heart rate was undetectable. During delivery, Becky suffered from birth asphyxiation and epileptic seizures. The attending physician described her as flaccid (soft and limp), with abnormal muscle reflexes. Becky has not yet learned to walk, is not toilet trained, and has no means of communication with others in her environment. She lives at home and attends a special class in a local elementary school during the day. Her educational program includes work with therapists to develop her gross motor abilities in order to improve her mobility. Speech and language specialists are examining the possibility of teaching her several alternative forms of communication (such as a language board or a manual communication system) because Becky has not developed any verbal skills. The special education staff is focusing on decreasing Becky's dependence on others by teaching some basic self-care skills such as feeding, toileting, and grooming. The medical and educational prognosis for Becky is unknown. The professional staff does not know what the ultimate long-term impact of their interventions will be, but they do know that although Becky is a child with severe mental retardation, she is learning.

INTRODUCTION

In this chapter we focus on people whose intellectual and social capabilities are significantly different from the norm. The growth and development of these individuals depends on the educational and social opportunities made available to them. Kim, who is mildly retarded, may be expected to achieve academically somewhere between second- and fifth-grade level if afforded an appropriate educational experience. As she grows older, she may achieve at least partial independence occupationally and socially within the community. Most likely, Kim will need some support from her family or other agencies to assist her in adjusting to adult life in the community.

Roger has completed school and is just beginning life as an adult in his local community. Roger is a person with moderate mental retardation. Although he will probably require on-going support on his job for a lifetime, he is earning wages which contribute to his successful adjustment in the community. Within a few years he will most likely move away from his family and into a group home or a supervised apartment of his own.

Becky has severe mental retardation. Although the long-term prognosis is unknown, she has many opportunities for learning and development that were not available until recently. Through a positive home environment and specialized educational services, Becky can reach a level of functioning that was once considered impossible.

Kim, Roger, and Becky are people with mental retardation, but they are not necessarily representative of the range of people who are characterized as mentally retarded. A six-year-old child described as mildly retarded may be no more than one or two years behind in the development of academic and social skills. Many mildly retarded children are not identified until they enter school at the age of five or six. This is because the child with mild mental retardation may not exhibit physical problems that are readily identifiable during the early childhood years. As this child enters school, these developmental lags become more apparent in the classroom environment. During early primary grades it is not uncommon for the child's intellectual and social difficulties to be attributed to immaturity. However, within a few years, school personnel generally recognize the need for specialized educational services beyond regular classroom instruction. Unfortunately, for many mildly retarded children, valuable time has been lost.

FOCUS 1
Describe the range of characteristics associated with mild to profound mental retardation.

Individuals with moderate to severe mental retardation have difficulties that transcend the classroom. Many are impaired in nearly every facet of life. Some have significant, multiple handicapping conditions, including sensory, physical, and emotional problems. Moderately retarded individuals are capable of developing skills that allow a degree of independence within their environment. These self-help skills include the ability to dress and feed themselves, to care for their personal health and grooming needs (such as toileting), and to develop safety habits that allow them to move safely wherever they go. These people have some means of communication. Most can develop verbal language skills, but some may be able to learn only manual communication. Their social-interaction skills are limited, however, making it difficult for them to relate spontaneously to others.

Contrast the above characteristics with those individuals who have severe to profound retardation and the diverse nature of these people becomes clear. Profoundly retarded individuals are dependent on others to maintain even their most basic life functions, including feeding, toileting, and dressing. They may not be capable of self-maintenance and often do not develop functional communication skills. The significance of their disorders may require a lifetime of complete supervision, whether it be in a special-care facility or at home. In terms of treatment or educational intervention, the only thing one can realistically say about this group is that the long-term prognosis for development is unknown. This does not mean that treatment beyond routine care and maintenance is not beneficial. The extreme nature of these handicaps is the primary reason such individuals were excluded from the public schools for so long. Drew, Logan, and Hardman (1988) indicate that exclusion was more for the protection of the schools rather than for the educational or social needs of the child with differences. Mori and Masters (1980) believe that exclusion could be justified "on the basis of lack of resources, lack of facilities, and lack of trained personnel to provide an adequate educational experience for this population" (p. 17). Given the present emphasis on research and alternative intervention approaches for people with mental retardation, the future may hold some answers and bring about a different outlook.

DEFINITIONS AND CLASSIFICATION

Definitions

FOCUS 2
Identify the three components of the definition of mental retardation.

People with mental retardation have been studied for centuries, by a variety of professional disciplines. The most widely accepted definition of mental retardation is that of the **American Association on Mental Retardation (AAMR)**, an organization of professionals from many backgrounds such as medicine, law, and education. The AAMR definition states that "mental retardation refers to significantly subaverage general intellectual functioning existing concurrently with deficits in **adaptive behavior,** and manifested during the **developmental period**" (Grossman, 1983). The essential features of this definition have also been adopted by the American Psychiatric Association (*Diagnostic and Statistical Manual of*

Mental Disorders, Third Edition Revised, 1987). The AAMR definition has three major components: intelligence, adaptive behavior, and the developmental period.

Intelligence. Significantly subaverage general intellectual functioning is assessed through the use of a standardized intelligence test. On an intelligence test a person's score is compared to the statistical average of age-mates who have taken the same test. The statistical average for an intelligence test is generally set at 100. We state this by saying that the person has an intelligence quotient (IQ) of 100. Psychologists use a mathematical procedure to determine the extent to which an individual's score deviates from this average of 100. This measurement is called a *standard deviation.* According to Best and Kahn (1989), standard deviations measure the dispersion of scores in a distribution. A score that deviates more than two standard deviations from the mean of 100 is considered to be significantly different. An individual who scores two standard deviations below the average on an intelligence test is in the range of mental retardation. Depending on the test, this means that individuals with IQs of approximately 70 to 75 and lower would be considered as having mental retardation. In the case of Kim from our opening vignettes, her IQ of 60 placed her in the range of persons with mental retardation, at least on the basis of an intelligence test.

Adaptive Behavior. Impairments in adaptive behavior are defined by AAMR as significant limitations in a person's ability to meet standards of maturation, learning, personal independence, and social responsibility that would be expected of another individual of comparable age level and cultural group (Grossman, 1983). Remember Becky from our opening vignette. She has significant impairments in her adaptive behavior skills. She is unable to walk and has a limited repertoire of self-help skills. At six years old, she still has no means of communicating with others.

As is true with intelligence, adaptive behavior can be measured by standardized tests. These tests are most often referred to as *adaptive behavior scales,* and generally use structured interviews or direct observations to obtain information. Adaptive behavior scales generally compare an individual to an established norm, and measure "the extent to which an individual takes care of personal needs, exhibits social competencies, and refrains from engaging in problem behaviors" (Bruininks & McGrew, 1987). Adaptive behavior may also be assessed through an informal appraisal, such as observations by people who are familiar with the individual or through anecdotal records of the individual's adaptive skills.

Developmental Period. In the AAMR definition, the developmental period is defined as "the period of time between birth and the eighteenth birthday" (p. 1). The reason for the inclusion of a developmental period within the definition is to clearly distinguish mental retardation from other conditions that may not originate until the adult years, such as head injuries or strokes.

The AAMR definition of mental retardation has evolved through years of effort to define the condition clearly. During the Middle Ages, retarded people were considered fools, demons, and witches. In the sixteenth century, terms such as *sot, simpleton,* and *idiot* were common names for those with mental retardation.

Reflect on This 4–1

How to Cure Mental Retardation

The current AAMR definition (Grossman, 1973, 1977, 1983) is a revision of an earlier one (Heber, 1961), which included a higher functioning group of people whose IQs were between 70 and 85. The definition we use today removes the label of retardation from all of these individuals. Burton Blatt commented that this change in definition

. . . has cured more mental retardation than all clinicians and scientists since the beginning of time! [It] reduced the incidence, or the theoretical incidence, or the psychometric incidence, from 16 percent to 3 percent. Just by changing the definition! Well, you can't do this with leprosy, you can't do this with syphilis, and you can't do this

with pregnancy. You can't do it with any objective disease. But you can do it with mental retardation (Jordan, 1973, pp. 223–24).

Throughout the nineteenth century, many individuals with mental retardation were identified according to their medical condition, such as cretinism, gargoylism, and mongolism. During this period the most common term to describe mentally retarded people was *feebleminded*. Feeblemindedness was broken down into three levels of retarded behavior: idiot (lowest level of functioning), imbecile, and **moron.**

Over the years, definitions of mental retardation have emphasized routine care and maintenance rather than treatment and education. However, recent legislation (including Public Law 94–142, The Education for All Handicapped Children Act, 1975; amended 1983, 1986) and litigation (such as *Homeward Bound* v. *The Hissom Memorial Center*, 1988) have opened new doors for mentally retarded people and put pressure on professionals to develop and use definitions aimed at assisting individuals in receiving appropriate services and improving their quality of life.

Classification

FOCUS 3
Identify the three methods of classifying people with mental retardation.

The purpose of developing classification systems is to provide a frame of reference for studying, understanding, and treating the many people labeled *mentally retarded*. People with mental retardation are often stereotyped as a homogeneous group of individuals, "the retarded", with similar physical characteristics and learning capabilities. Actually, mental retardation is a condition that results in a broad range of functioning levels and characteristics. In order to more clearly understand the diversity of people labeled *mentally retarded*, several classification systems have been developed. We discuss three methods of classifying individuals with mental retardation: by the severity of the condition, educability expectations, and medical descriptors.

Severity of the Condition. The extent to which a person's intellectual capabilities and adaptive behavior deviate from what is considered normal can be described by using such terms as *mild, moderate, severe,* and *profound.* Each of these four terms describes the significance of the intellectual deficit. *Mild* describes the highest level of performance for individuals classified as mentally retarded; *profound* describes the lowest level of performance for this population. The distinction between each of the severity levels associated with mental retardation is primarily determined through the use of scores on intelligence tests as well as indicators of maladaptive behavior. The AAMR uses four levels of intellectual functioning to group mentally retarded individuals according to the severity approach: (1) mild, IQ 55 to 70; (2) moderate, IQ 40 to 55; (3) severe, IQ 25 to 40; and (4) profound, IQ 25 or lower (IQ scores based on standard deviations of Wechsler Intelligence Scales). The American Psychiatric Association employs the same four severity classifications and uses basically the same IQ groupings.

A person's adaptive behavior, or the ability to adapt to or cope with environmental demands, can also be broken down into mild- through profound-severity descriptors. Grossman (1983) drew the distinction between intelligence and adaptive behavior: "Adaptive behavior refers to what people do to take care of themselves and to relate to others in daily living rather than the abstract potential implied by intelligence" (p. 42). As is true with intellectual functioning, adaptive behavior deficits may be described in terms of the degree to which an individual's performance differs from what is expected for his or her chronological age. For example, in the area of independent functioning, average three-year-olds are expected to feed themselves unassisted with the proper eating utensils, take care of their own personal hygiene, and be fully toilet-trained. A child with mild adaptive deficits may be able to use eating utensils, but with considerable spilling. This child can dress and take care of personal hygiene, but only with considerable help. The child may be partially toilet-trained; toileting accidents are common. The level of independence for each of the above skill areas decreases for individuals with moderate, severe, and profound adaptive behavior deficits. A three-year-old with profound adaptive behavior deficits generally must be fed by another individual, drinks from a cup with help, cannot take care of personal needs, and has no effective speech.

To better understand adaptive behavior let's return to our opening vignettes. Kim is an individual with mild mental retardation. As a twelve-year-old child, Kim has learned many of the required self-help skills for a child of her age, and although her socialization skills are below those expected, she is able to successfully interact with others in her environment. In contrast, Roger is an individual with moderate mental retardation. At nineteen, he has developed many skills that allow him to successfully live in his own community with supervision and assistance. It took longer for Roger to learn to dress and feed himself than it did for Kim, but he has learned these skills. His verbal communication skills are somewhat rudimentary, but nevertheless he is capable of communicating basic needs and desires. Becky is a child with severe to profound mental retardation. At age six, her development is significantly delayed in nearly every area of functioning. However, it is clear that with appropriate intervention, she is learning.

In the 1980s a new severity classification descriptor, **unspecified mental retardation,** was adopted by both AAMR and the American Psychiatric Association

Reflect on This 4–2

Moron, Imbecile, and Idiot

The terms *mild, moderate, severe,* and *profound* mental retardation have been used by professionals as classification descriptors for a relatively short period of time. Perhaps you are more familiar with such terms as *idiot, imbecile,* and *moron,* the forerunners of the current symptom severity descriptors. The use of *idiot* dates back to the late 18th century, when John Locke differentiated between idi-ocy and insanity by indicating that insane individuals put wrong ideas together and then reason from them, but idiots reason scarcely at all.

With the advent of the intelligence test in the beginning of the 20th century, the term *idiot* (IQ 0–25) along with *imbecile* (IQ 25–50), and *moron* (IQ 50–75) were used to identify three levels of retarded functioning. During the decades that followed these terms became part of our everyday language and took on very derogatory meanings. We have all used such phrases as "You idiot," "What an imbecile," and "He's a moron." It is obvious why professionals and parents have moved away from such labels in developing classification systems for people with mental retardation.

(DSM-III-R, 1987; Grossman, 1983). The term *unspecified* indicates that there are individuals with mental retardation whose condition has no known biological cause.

Educability Expectations. In response to the growing number of mentally retarded children entering the public schools during this century, the field of education has developed its own classification system. As the word *expectations* implies, retarded children are classified according to expected achievement in a classroom situation. The specific categories used vary greatly from state to state, depending on the locale and source consulted. Frequently this type of system specifies a label, an approximate IQ range, and a statement of predicted achievement.

☐ **Educable,** IQ 55 to about 70: Second- to fifth-grade achievement in school academic areas. Social adjustment will permit some degree of independence in the community. Occupational sufficiency will permit partial or total self-support.

☐ **Trainable,** IQ 40 to 55: Learning primarily in the area of self-help skills, some achievement in areas considered academic. Social adjustment is often limited to home and closely surrounding area. Vocational proficiencies include supported work in a community job or sheltered workshop.

☐ **Custodial,** IQ below 40: May be unable to achieve even sufficient skills to care for basic needs. Will usually require significant level of care and supervision during lifetime.

Table 4–1 compares the educability classification approach to the severity approach according to IQ level.

TABLE 4–1 Comparison of Educability and Severity Classification Approaches According to IQ Level

IQ Level	Approach	
	Educability expectation	*Severity of condition*
55–70	Educable	Mild
40–55	Trainable	Moderate
25–40	Custodial	Severe
Below 25	Custodial	Profound

The educability-expectation classification criterion was originally developed to determine for whom the schools would be responsible. As indicated by the terminology, *educable* implied that the child could cope with at least some of the academic demands of the classroom. *Educable* meant the child could learn basic reading, writing, and arithmetic skills. The term *trainable* indicated that the student was *noneducable* and only capable of being trained in noneducational settings. In fact, until the passage of Public Law 94–142, many children who were labeled *trainable* could not get a free public education. Public Law 94–142 redefined education to include the development of skills (e.g., self-help, motor, communication, etc.) that are not necessarily academic in nature.

The custodial category described children who were only capable of being maintained or cared for in a specialized setting. Any kind of learning experiences in a public school would be fruitless. We have learned that such an assumption was entirely false. Many of the children labeled as *custodial* only a few years ago are now receiving appropriate educational experiences that are decreasing their overall dependence on their families and society. *Custodial* is seldom used in today's public schools. In many states it has been replaced with the symptom-severity descriptors *severely* and *profoundly retarded*.

Medical Descriptors. Mental retardation may be classified on the basis of the origin of the condition rather than the severity or educational expectations associated with it. A classification system that uses the cause (etiology) of the condition to differentiate retarded individuals is often referred to as a *medical classification system* because it emerged primarily from the field of medicine. The most commonly used medical descriptor system is that proposed by AAMR (Grossman, 1983). This system uses the following ten categories:

☐ Infection and intoxication (e.g., syphilis, rubella)

☐ Trauma or a physical agent (e.g., injury during birth, prenatal injury)

☐ Nutritional or metabolic disorders (e.g., PKU, thyroid dysfunction)

☐ Gross postnatal brain disease (e.g., tuberous sclerosis)

☐ Diseases and conditions resulting from unknown prenatal influences (e.g., hydrocephalus)

☐ Chromosomal abnormality (e.g., Down syndrome)

☐ Gestational disorders (e.g., prematurity)

☐ Psychiatric disorders

☐ Environmental influences (e.g., sensory deprivation, social disadvantage)

☐ Other conditions (e.g., unknown causes or such known causes as blindness or deafness.

Each of these ten categories is discussed more thoroughly in the section entitled *Causation*.

PREVALENCE

FOCUS 4
What is the estimated prevalence of mental retardation?

It is generally estimated that from 1 to 3 percent of the total population has mental retardation (Grossman, 1983, Rantakallio & von Wendt, 1986). The U.S. Department of Education (1989), in the Eleventh Annual Report to Congress estimates that 15 percent of handicapped children in the public schools are considered mentally retarded. Mildly retarded individuals (IQs 55–70) comprise approximately 90 percent of this estimated prevalence. Based on a 3-percent prevalence estimate, approximately 2.5 percent of the general population would be classified as mildly retarded, or 5.5 million people in the United States.

Figure 4–1
Prevalence of Mental Retardation (U.S. Department of Education, 1989, Eleventh Annual Report to Congress)

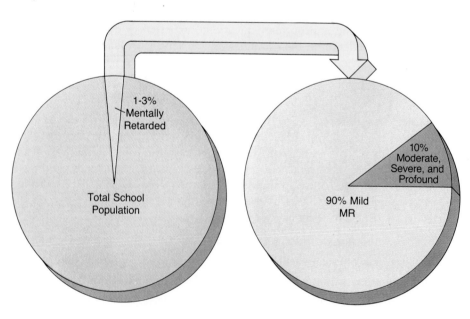

Individuals with moderate, severe, and profound retardation constitute a much smaller percentage of the general population. Even if we consider the multitude of conditions, prevalence estimates generally range from no more than 0.1 to 1 percent. Using an estimated prevalence of .5 percent, over 1 million people would fall into the range of moderate to profound mental retardation.

CHARACTERISTICS

Intellectual

The primary characteristic of mental retardation is an intellectual deficiency. There are, however, as many definitions of intelligence as there are people interested in defining the phenomenon. We will refer to intelligence as an ability to acquire, remember, and use information appropriately. People with mental retardation have, by definition, less capability in each of these areas when compared to intellectually normal individuals. They do not learn as effectively or efficiently as their nonhandicapped peers.

The learning and memory capabilities of people with mental retardation are deficient. Retarded children as a group are less able to grasp abstract, as opposed to concrete, concepts. They benefit from instruction that is meaningful and useful. The child with retardation learns more from contact with a real object than he or she does from a representation or symbol.

FOCUS 5
Identify four intellectual characteristics of individuals with mental retardation.

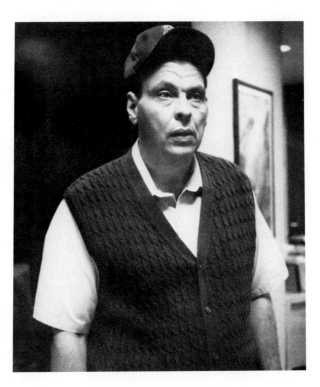

The media have only recently begun to portray people with mental retardation as active members of society. Larry Drake plays Benny Stulwicz, an office worker who is mentally retarded, on "L.A. Law." Drake won Emmys for Best Supporting Actor for the role in 1988 and 1989. (AP/Wide World Photos)

Intelligence is also associated with learning how to learn and the ability to apply what is learned to new experiences. This is known as establishing **learning sets.** Mentally retarded children and adults develop learning sets at a slower rate than nonretarded peers, and they are deficient in generalization of information to new situations (Agran, 1987; Payne, Polloway, Smith, & Payne, 1981).

These individuals also have difficulty in focusing on relevant stimuli in a learning situation (Borkowski & Day, 1987; Hallahan & Reeve, 1980); have inefficient **rehearsal strategies** that interfere with memory (Frank & Rabinovitch, 1974); and are unable to benefit from incidental learning cues in their environment (Hardman & Drew, 1975). In terms of overall control of memory processes (metacognition), mentally retarded children are generally characterized as unable to use appropriate task strategies. However, Borkowski, Peck, and Damberg (1983) suggest that they can be taught to change their control processes.

Adaptive Behavior

FOCUS 6
Identify seven in-school adaptive behavior deficiencies of students with mental retardation.

Adaptive behavior is the capability of individuals to take care of themselves and to relate to others around them. The adaptive functioning—social and personal competence—skills of individuals with mental retardation are deficient. Depending on the extent of the retardation, they may have difficulty coping with the demands placed on them in their daily lives. Table 4–2 describes the range of personal competence skills of individuals with moderate through profound mental retardation.

In the school setting, adaptive behavior is defined as the ability to apply the skills learned in a classroom to daily activities. The child must develop appropriate reasoning, judgment, and social skills that lead to positive interpersonal relationships with peers. The following are some examples of in-school adaptive behavior deficiencies that may be associated with mental retardation:

TABLE 4–2 Personal Competence Skills for Individuals with Moderate to Profound Mental Retardation

	Severity of Mental Retardation	
Moderate	*Severe*	*Profound*
Individuals may lack self-help skills but are capable of acquiring survival skills that enhance their independence within the environment; e.g., feeding, toilet-training, dressing, personal hygiene, and functional academics (reading, arithmetic).	Individuals lack basic self-help, survival skills. Habilitation is possible for very basic skills; e.g., feeding, toileting. However, many remain somewhat dependent on others for everyday needs. Individuals are generally not capable of learning functional academic skills.	Individuals generally do not profit from self-care training, except in very low-level skill areas; e.g., developmental skills for children under 6 months of age). Individuals require total care.

☐ Lack of school coping behaviors related to attention to learning tasks, organizational skills, questioning behavior, following directions, maintaining school supplies, and monitoring time use.

☐ Poor social skills related to working cooperatively with peers, social perceptions, response to social cues, use of socially acceptable language, and acceptable response to the teacher.

☐ Poor language skills related to the ability to understand directions, communicate needs, express ideas, listen attentively, and modulate the voice.

☐ Poor emotional development related to avoidance of work and social experiences as exemplified by tardiness, chronic complaints of illness, sustained or frequent idleness, aggressiveness under stress, classroom disruption, and social withdrawal.

☐ Poor self-care skills related to personal hygiene, dress, maintaining personal belongings, and mobility in and about the school.

☐ Limited success in applied cognitive skills related to initiating age-appropriate tasks, solving nonacademic problems, drawing conclusions from experience, and planning activities.

☐ Delayed academic development related to the ability to form letters, blend letter sounds, recall content from reading and listening, make mathematical computations, and repeat information in a logical sequence (State of Iowa Department of Public Instruction, 1981, pp. 15–16).

Some research has also suggested that individuals with mental retardation may have lower self-images (Westling, 1986) and a greater expectancy for failure (Zigler & Balla, 1981).

Academic Achievement

Research on the educational achievement of children with mild to moderate mental retardation has suggested that there are significant deficits in the areas of reading and mathematics. As early as 1940, Kirk indicated that children with IQs between two and three standard deviations below the mean would read anywhere from first- to fourth-grade level. Westling (1986), in a review of the literature on reading and mental retardation, suggests that "reading is generally

FOCUS 7
What are the expected reading and arithmetic deficiencies of students with mental retardation?

I like school because I have friends. I learn things that help me. Sometimes school is hard and I don't like school. My teacher says that school means that I have to work hard so I can learn. Walt [a brother] says he goes to school because Mom wants him to. I'm in a class with lots of friends. I don't think I'm as smart as some of the kids in my school, but I'm learning to do things that help me. When I grow up, I'm going to have my own apartment and not go to school anymore. I want to have a job and spend my own money. If I go to school, I'll get a job. I like school.

Ronald, *a student with mental retardation, in an elementary school*

WINDOW 4–1

I Like School

considered the weakest area of learning, especially reading comprehension. Comparatively, mildly retarded students tend to do better on reading words than on understanding what it is they have read" (p. 127). Most mentally retarded students read below their own mental-age level. Arithmetic skills are also deficient for these children, although their performance may be closer to their mental age. These children may be able to learn basic computations but be unable to apply concepts appropriately.

There is a growing body of research (Browder & Snell, 1987) indicating that children with moderate and severe mental retardation can be taught to read at least a protective or survival vocabulary. These children may be limited to recognizing their names and those of significant others in their life, as well as common survival words such as *men, women, danger,* and *stop*.

Speech and Language Characteristics

FOCUS 8
Identify three common speech problems and the most common language problem for individuals with mental retardation.

One of the most serious and obvious characteristics for individuals with mental retardation is delayed speech and language development. The most common speech problems are **articulation, voice,** and **stuttering problems.** Language problems are generally associated with delays in language development rather than the bizarre use of language (Cromer, 1974; Lenneberg, 1967). Kaiser, Alpert, and Warren (1987) emphasize that "the overriding goal of language intervention is to increase the individual's functional communication" (p. 248).

The severity of the speech and language problems is positively correlated with the severity of the mental retardation. Miller (1981) indicates that the mental age of the child is the single greatest predictor of language performance. Speech and language difficulties may range from minor speech defects, such as articulation problems, to the complete absence of **expressive language.** The relationship between language problems and mental retardation was postulated by Van Riper (1972). He suggests that children may appear to be or even become mentally retarded because they do not learn to speak. Mental retardation may cause speech problems, but speech problems may also directly contribute to the severity of the mental retardation. Table 4–3 describes the range of speech and language skills for individuals with moderate through profound mental retardation.

Physical Characteristics

FOCUS 9
Why are physical problems more evident in individuals with severe and profound mental retardation?

The physical appearance of most mentally retarded children does not differ from nonretarded children of the same age. However, there is a relationship between the severity of the mental retardation and the extent of physical problems for the individual (Hardman & Drew, 1977; Westling, 1986). For the person with severe mental retardation there is a significant probability of related physical problems. The mildly retarded individual may exhibit no physical problems whatsoever, because the retardation may be associated with environmental, not genetic, factors. Table 4–4 describes the range of physical characteristics associated with individuals who have moderate through profound mental retardation.

TABLE 4–3 Speech and Language Skills for Individuals with Moderate to Profound Mental Retardation

Severity of Mental Retardation		
Moderate	Severe	Profound
Most individuals are deficient in speech and language skills, but many develop language abilities that allow them some level of communication with others.	Without exception, individuals exhibit significant speech and language delays and deviations; e.g., lack of expressive and receptive language, poor articulation, and little, if any, spontaneous interaction.	Individuals do not exhibit spontaneous communication patterns. Bizzare speech may be evident; e.g., echolalic speech, speech out of context, purposeless speech. Language abilities are grossly inadequate.

Bruininks (1977) confirmed that physiological development is associated with severity of retardation. He found that nonretarded children were superior to both mildly and moderately retarded children on motor skill proficiency, and that the performance of mildly retarded children was superior to that of moderately retarded children.

Research studies have also suggested there is a higher prevalence of vision and hearing problems among retarded children (Bensberg & Siegelman, 1976; Fink, 1981; Lloyd, 1970). The vast majority of severely and profoundly retarded children have multiple handicaps and serious problems in nearly every aspect of intellectual and physical development.

TABLE 4–4 Physical Characteristics of Individuals with Moderate to Profound Mental Retardation

Severity of Mental Retardation		
Moderate	Severe	Profound
Gross and fine motor coordination are usually deficient. However, the individual is usually ambulatory and capable of independent mobility. Perceptual-motor skills do exist (e.g., body awareness, sense of touch, eye-hand coordination), but are often deficient in comparison to the norm.	As many as 80% have significant motor difficulties; i.e., poor or nonambulatory skills. Gross or fine motor skills may be present, but the individual may lack control, resulting in awkward or inept motor movement.	Some gross motor development is evident, but fine motor skills are inept. Individuals are usually nonambulatory and are not capable of independent mobility within the environment. Perceptual-motor skills are often nonexistent.

CAUSATION

FOCUS 10
What are the causes of mild mental retardation?

Mental retardation is the result of multiple causes, some known, many unknown. Possible causes of mental retardation include sociocultural differences, infection and intoxication, chromosomal abnormalities, gestation disorders, unknown prenatal influences, traumas or physical agents, metabolic and nutritional factors, and postnatal brain disease.

Sociocultural Influences

For mildly retarded individuals, such as Kim from our opening vignette, the cause of the problem is not generally apparent. There are a significant number of mildly retarded individuals who come from lower socioeconomic families and different cultural backgrounds. Individuals who are environmentally or culturally disadvantaged are often in home situations where there are fewer opportunities for learning, which only further contributes to their problems at school. Additionally, because these high-risk children are living in such adverse economic conditions, they are generally not receiving proper nutritional care. As stated by Westling (1986), "poor people have poor nutritional characteristics" (p. 100). MacMillan (1982) further explained that the highest prevalence of mental retardation occurs among—

> . . . people referred to as "culturally deprived," "culturally different," "culturally disadvantaged," or some other term that connotes adverse economic and living conditions. Children of high risk are those who live in slums and, frequently, who are members of certain ethnic minority groups. In these high-risk groups there is poor medical care for mother and child, a high rate of broken families, and little value for education or motivation to achieve (pp. 86–87).

An important question to be addressed in relationship to individuals who have grown up in adverse sociocultural situations is: How much of the person's ability is related to these sociocultural influences as opposed to genetic factors? This issue is referred to as the **nature-versus-nurture** controversy. There have been numerous studies over the years focusing on the degree to which both heredity and environment contribute to intelligence. What has been learned from these studies is that while there is a better understanding of the interactive effects of both heredity and environment, the exact contribution of each to intellectual growth remains unknown. The term to describe children whose retardation may be attributable to both sociocultural and genetic factors is **cultural-familial**. These individuals are often described as (1) being mildly retarded, (2) having no known biological cause for the condition, (3) having at least one parent or sibling who is also mildly retarded, and (4) growing up in a low socioeconomic-level home environment.

FOCUS 11
Identify seven causes of moderate to profound mental retardation.

For the majority of individuals with moderate, severe, and profound mental retardation, problems are evident at birth. The American Association on Mental Retardation has grouped the causes of mental retardation into several general categories (Grossman, 1983). In order to gain a greater understanding of the diversity of causes associated with mental retardation, we briefly review each of the categories.

Infection and Intoxication

Several types of **maternal infections** may result in difficulties for the unborn child. In some cases, the outcome is spontaneous abortion of the fetus, in others it may be severe birth defects. The probability of damage is particularly high if the infection occurs during the first three months of pregnancy. **Congenital rubella** (German measles) is the type of infection that is perhaps most widely known. Rubella is a viral infection that causes a variety of problems, including mental retardation, deafness, blindness, cerebral palsy, cardiac problems, seizures, and a variety of other neurological problems. Fortunately, a vaccine to prevent rubella infection has been developed. The widespread administration of this vaccine is one of the major reasons why mental retardation as an outcome of rubella has declined significantly in recent years.

Another infection associated with severe disorders is syphilis. Syphilis transmitted from the mother to the unborn child can result in severe birth defects. With syphilis, bacteria actually cross the placenta and infect the fetus. This results in damage to the tissue of the central nervous system as well as to the circulatory system. **Congenital syphilis** may result in spontaneous abortion or stillbirth. For the infant who survives, a variety of physical and cognitive problems result.

Several prenatal infections may result in other severe disorders. For example, **toxoplasmosis** is an infection carried by raw meat and fecal material. Evidence indicates that the damage of toxoplasmosis may be significant, with nearly 85 percent of surviving babies being mentally retarded and also having other problems such as blindness and convulsions (Sever, 1970). Toxoplasmosis is primarily a threat if the mother is exposed during pregnancy, whereas infection prior to conception seems to cause minimal danger to the unborn child.

Intoxication refers to disorders that occur when there is cerebral damage due to an excessive level of some toxic agent in the mother–fetus system. Excessive maternal use of alcohol or drugs, or exposure to certain environmental hazards such as x-rays or insecticides may cause damage to the child. Damage to the fetus that is caused by maternal alcohol consumption is known as **fetal alcohol syndrome.** This condition is characterized by facial abnormalities, heart problems, low birth weight, and mental retardation. Similarly, pregnant women who smoke are at greater risk of having a premature baby with complicating developmental problems such as mental retardation (Hetherington & Parke, 1986). The use of drugs during pregnancy has varying effects on the infant depending on frequency, amount taken, and drug type. According to Peterson (1987), drugs that are known to produce serious fetal damage include LSD, heroin, morphine, and cocaine. Prescription drugs, such as **anticonvulsants** and antibiotics have also been associated with infant malformations (Batshaw & Perret, 1986).

Another factor that can seriously affect the unborn baby is an incompatible blood type between the mother and the fetus. The most widely known form of this problem is when the mother's blood is Rh-negative while the fetus has Rh-positive blood. In this situation the mother's system may become sensitized to the incompatible blood type and produce defensive antibodies that damage the fetus. Medical technology can now prevent this condition through the use of a drug known as *Rhogam.*

Mental retardation may also occur after a baby is born, as a result of postnatal infections and toxic excesses. For example, **encephalitis** may damage the central nervous system following certain types of childhood infections (such as measles or mumps), as can certain toxic reactions such as lead poisoning, carbon-monoxide poisoning, or drugs.

Chromosomal Abnormalities

Chromosomes are threadlike bodies carrying the genes that play the critical role in determining inherited characteristics. Defects resulting from **chromosomal abnormalities** are typically dramatic, because the resulting damage is often severe and accompanied by visually evident abnormalities. Fortunately, genetically caused defects are relatively rare. The cell structure of the vast majority of humans is normal, and development proceeds without accident. Human body cells normally have forty-six chromosomes that are arranged in twenty-three pairs. Aberrations occurring in chromosomal arrangement, either before fertilization or during early cell division, may result in a variety of abnormal characteristics.

One of the most widely recognized types of mental retardation, **Down syndrome,** results from chromosomal abnormality. Down syndrome is a condition that results in facial and physical characteristics that are visibly distinctive. Facial features resemble those of Asians, which resulted in the term **mongoloid,** or *mongolism* (after the people of the Mongol empire, founded in the twelfth century by Genghis Khan). Facial features are marked by distinctive epicanthic eye folds, prominent cheekbones, and a small, somewhat flattened nose. There are three different types of Down syndrome, each resulting from a different chromosomal aberration.

The most common cause of Down syndrome is **nondisjunction,** when the chromosomal pairs do not separate properly as the sperm or egg cells are formed.

People with Down syndrome are no longer routinely institutionalized. They are successfully living in their own local communities. In school, they may be mainstreamed in regular education classes with their nonhandicapped peers. (Richard Hutchings/ Photo Researchers, Inc.)

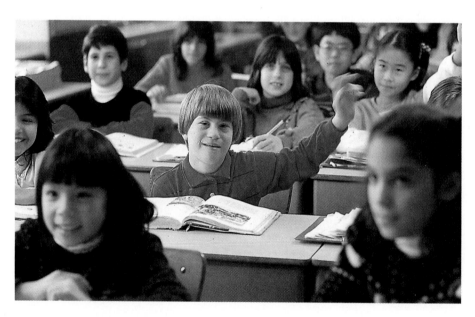

Down syndrome caused by nondisjunction is characterized by an extra chromosome at the twenty-first pair and thus is also known as **Trisomy 21.** The person then has forty-seven chromosomes instead of forty-six. The cell-division error occurs before fertilization, and the impact on the fetus is severe. Once the cell-division process is begun, all developing tissue carries the genetic makeup of those preceding cells.

Abnormal chromosome material in the twenty-first pair is also present in the second type of Down syndrome, known as **translocation.** Translocation occurs when a portion of the chromosome breaks off from the twenty-first pair and fuses with material of another pair. In this condition, the person has forty-five chromosomes instead of the normal forty-six.

Mosaicism, the third type of Down syndrome, is distinctly different from the other conditions because the chromosomal accident occurs after fertilization. Consequently the mosaic Down fetus develops normally for a period of time before the cell-division error appears. This individual thus has a mixed chromosomal configuration with some tissue being made up of normal cells and some made up of abnormal cells. Individuals with mosaicism are generally less retarded than those with Trisomy 21 or translocation.

Down syndrome has received widespread attention in the literature and has been a favored topic in both medical and special education textbooks for many years. Part of this attention has come because of the apparent ability to identify a cause with some degree of certainty. The cause of such genetic errors has become increasingly associated with the ages of both the mother and the father. MacMillan (1982) reported that for mothers between the ages of twenty and thirty the chances of having a child with Down syndrome is one in 1200. The probabilities increase significantly (1 in 20) for mothers older than forty-five years of age. Abroms and Bennett (1983) indicate that in about 25 percent of the cases associated with Trisomy 21, the age of the father (particularly those over fifty-five years old) is also a factor.

Gestation Disorders

The most typical gestation disorders involve **prematurity** and **low birth weight.** Prematurity refers to infants delivered before thirty-seven weeks from the first day of the last menstrual period. Low birth weight is viewed in terms of babies that weigh 2500 grams (five and one-half pounds) or less at birth. Prematurity and low birth rate significantly increase the risk of serious problems at birth, including mental retardation.

Unknown Prenatal Influences

There are several conditions associated with unknown **prenatal** influences, which can result in extremely severe disorders. One such condition involves malformations of cerebral tissue. The most dramatic of these malformations is known as **anencephaly.** Anencephaly is a condition in which the individual has a partial or even complete absence of cerebral tissue. In some cases, portions of the brain appear to develop and then degenerate. The prognosis for such individuals is not very promising, and most do not survive beyond a few hours or days.

Reflect on This 4–3

Information about People with Down Syndrome

- Down syndrome is universal and is not limited to race, nationality or social class.
- Approximately 4,000 individuals with Down syndrome are born each year in the United States.
- Women over 35 years of age give birth to more than 80% of individuals with Down syndrome.
- Paternal origin of the extra chromosomes has been verified in 20% of the cases.

- Compared with their "normal" peers, individuals with Down syndrome are usually smaller and their physical as well as intellectual development is slower.
- Approximately one-third of the individuals born with Down syndrome have heart defects. Most of these cardiac defects are now correctable by surgery.
- Some individuals with Down syndrome are born with problems in the gastrointestinal

tract. Surgery can correct these conditions.
- There is a wide variation in mental abilities, behavior and developmental progress in individuals with Down syndrome.
- Individuals with Down syndrome benefit from loving homes, early intervention, and special education.

Source: Information about Down Syndrome, 1984, Chicago, Ill.: National Down Syndrome Congress.

Hydrocephalus is another condition that results from unknown prenatal influence. In hydrocephalus an excess of cerebrospinal fluid accumulates in the skull and results in potentially damaging pressure on cerebral tissue. Hydrocephalus may or may not involve an enlarged head, depending on when the production or absorption imbalance occurs. If it is present at birth or shortly thereafter, the seams of the child's skull will not have grown closed and the pressure results in an enlarged head. Hydrocephaly may result in decreased intellectual functioning. If surgical intervention occurs early the damage may be slight, because the pressure has not been serious or prolonged. If such intervention does not occur or is not undertaken early, the degree of mental retardation may range from moderate to profound.

Traumas or Physical Agents

Traumas or physical accidents may occur either prior to birth (for example, excessive radiation), during delivery, or after the baby is born. Remember Becky from our chapter opening vignettes: The cause of her mental retardation is trauma during delivery. She suffered from birth asphyxiation as well as epileptic seizures. Our discussion here focuses on problems, such as those encountered by Becky, that are associated with a baby's delivery.

The continuing supply of oxygen and nutrients to the baby is a critical factor during delivery. One threat to these processes involves the position of the fetus. Normal fetal position places the baby with the head toward the cervix and the face toward the mother's back. Certain other positions may result in fetal damage as delivery proceeds. One of these is known as a **breech presentation,** in which the buttocks of the fetus, rather than the head, are positioned toward the cervix. Figure 4–2 illustrates a breech position. The breech delivery may result in several problems for the baby. The head exits last rather than first, and may be subjected to several types of stress that would not occur if the delivery were normal. The head is passing through the birth canal under stress, and the pressure of the contractions has a direct impact on the fetal skull rather than on the buttocks as in a normal position. In a breech presentation the umbilical cord may not be long enough to remain attached while the head is expelled, or it may become pinched between the baby's body and the pelvic girdle. In either case the baby's oxygen supply may be reduced for a period of time until the head is expelled and the lungs begin to function. The baby's lack of oxygen may result in damage to the brain. Such a condition is known as **anoxia** (oxygen deprivation).

Other abnormal positions can result in delivery problems and damage to the fetus. The fetus may lie across the birth canal in what is known as a **transverse position.** In such cases the baby may not be able to exit through the birth canal, or if the baby does exit, severe damage may occur. In other cases labor and delivery proceed so rapidly that the fetal skull does not have time to mold properly or in a sufficiently gentle fashion. Rapid births (generally less than two hours) are known as **precipitous births** and may result in mental retardation as well as other problems.

Metabolism and Nutrition

Metabolic problems are characterized by the body's inability to process (metabolize) certain substances that can then become poisonous and damage tissue in the central nervous system. **Phenylketonuria (PKU)** is one such inherited metabolic disorder. The baby is not able to process **phenylalanine,** a substance found in many foods, including the milk ingested by infants. The inability to process

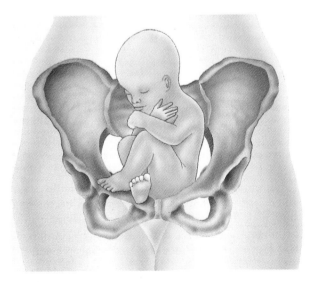

Figure 4–2
Example of a Breech Fetal Position

phenylalanine results in an accumulation of poisonous substances in the body. If it is untreated or not treated promptly (mostly through dietary restrictions), PKU causes varying degrees of mental retardation ranging from moderate to severe deficits. If treatment is promptly instituted, however, damage may be largely prevented or at least reduced. This is why most states now require mandatory screening for all infants in order to treat the condition as early as possible and prevent life-long problems.

Milk also presents a problem for infants affected by another metabolic disorder, **galactosemia.** In this case, the youngster is unable to properly process lactose, which is the primary sugar in milk and is also found in other foods. If galactosemia remains untreated serious damage results, such as cataracts, heightened susceptibility to infection, and reduced intellectual functioning. Dietary control by eliminating milk and other foods containing lactose must be undertaken.

Gross Postnatal Brain Disease

There are several disorders associated with gross postnatal brain disease. **Neurofibromatosis** is an inherited disorder that results in multiple tumors in the skin, peripheral nerve tissue, and other areas such as the brain. Mental retardation does not occur in all cases, although it may be evident in about 10 percent of the cases (Robinson & Robinson, 1976). The severity of mental retardation and other problems resulting from neurofibromatosis seems to relate to the location of tumors (e.g., in the cerebral tissue) and their size and growth. Severe disorders due to gross postnatal brain disease occur with a variety of other conditions, including **tuberous sclerosis,** which also involves tumors in the central nervous system tissue, and degeneration of cerebral white matter.

Although we have presented a number of possible causal factors associated with mental retardation, it is important to remember that the cause is unknown and undeterminable in many cases. Additionally, many conditions associated with mental retardation are due to the interaction of both hereditary and environmental factors. While we are unable to always identify the causes of mental retardation, there are measures that can be taken to prevent its occurrence.

PREVENTION

FOCUS 12
Identify four measures that may prevent mental retardation.

Preventing mental retardation is a laudable goal, and has for many years been the focus of professionals in the field of medicine. Over the years prevention has taken many forms, including the sterilization of people with mental retardation. More recently, preventive measures have focused on immunization against disease, maternal nutritional habits during pregnancy, appropriate prenatal care, and screening for genetic disorders prior to and at birth.

Immunization can protect family members from contracting serious illness and in addition guard against the mother becoming ill during pregnancy. Diseases such as rubella, which may result in severe mental retardation, heart disease, or blindness, can be controlled through routine immunization programs.

Improper nutritional habits during pregnancy may also contribute to fetal

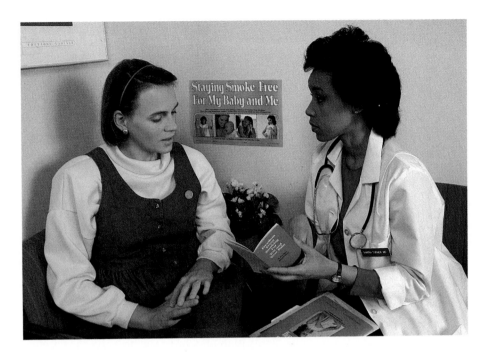

The prevention of mental retardation is a central goal of prenatal care. (© Andrew Brilliant/The Picture Cube)

problems. Drew, Logan, and Hardman (1988) report that "**maternal malnutrition, which frequently is part of the mother's life-long state of nutritional inadequacy, has been implicated as exerting possible damaging influence on the fetus, particularly on the developing central nervous system**" (p. 181).

Poor nutritional habits are part of a much larger social problem: the lack of appropriate prenatal care during pregnancy. In 1983 the President's Commission for the Study of Ethical Problems in Medicine and Biomedical and Behavior Research indicated that delays in prenatal care can have "significant health consequences, as many conditions that are amenable to timely medical treatment can develop serious complications if neglected" (p. 111). The Commission documented several case studies of pregnant women who were unable to obtain prenatal care in their local communities. These women were already in labor when they entered the hospital, and were considered to be at high risk for complications at delivery (President's Commission, 1983a).

A medical history can alert the attending physician to any potential dangers for the mother or the unborn infant that may result from family genetics, prior trauma, or illness. The physician is able to monitor the health of the fetus, including heart rate, physical size, and position in the uterus. At the time of birth, several factors relevant to the infant's health can be assessed. A procedure known as **Apgar Scoring** evaluates the infant on heart rate, respiratory condition, muscle tone, reflex irritability, and color. This screening procedure alerts the medical staff to infants who may warrant closer monitoring and more in-depth assessments. Other screening procedures conducted in the medical laboratory within the first few days of life can detect anomalies that, if not treated, will eventually lead to mental retardation, psychological disorders, physical disabilities, or even death. The effects of disorders such as phenylketonuria and Rh incompatibility can be substantially diminished if assessed at birth and treated immediately.

Other methods of prevention are more involved with issues of morality and ethics. These include genetic screening and counseling, and therapeutic abortion. **Genetic screening** is defined as "a search in a population for persons possessing certain genotypes that (1) are already associated with disease or predisposed to disease, (2) may lead to disease in their descendants, or (3) produce other variations not known to be associated with disease" (National Academy of Sciences, 1975, p. 9). Genetic screening may be conducted at various times in the family planning process or during pregnancy (President's Commission, 1983b). When screening is conducted prior to conception, the purpose is to determine whether the parents are predisposed to genetic anomalies that could be inherited by their offspring. If screening takes place after conception, the purpose is to determine if the fetus has any genetic abnormalities. This can be accomplished through one of several medical procedures, including **amniocentesis, fetoscopy,** and **ultrasound.**

Once genetic screening has been completed, it is the responsibility of a counselor to inform parents of the results. Parents are then made fully aware of potential outcomes and options. While the genetic counselor does not make decisions *for* the parents regarding family planning, he or she prepares the parents to exercise their rights: "The information-giving function is at the heart of genetic counseling. . . . The primary emphasis on information-giving is based on an ideal of 'nondirectiveness,' a goal that attempts to recognize the person counseled as an autonomous decision-maker" (President's Commission, 1983b, p. 37).

The primary outcome of **genetic counseling** can be viewed as informing parents concerning decisions they have to make about whether to (1) have children based on the probability of a genetic anomaly occurring, or (2) abort a pregnancy if prenatal assessment indicates that the developing fetus has a genetic anomaly. The decision of whether or not to abort involves a moral controversy that society has been attempting to deal with for years. For example, if a Down syndrome fetus is detected, what are the intervention options? Certainly, one option involves continuing the pregnancy and making mental, physical, and financial preparations for the additional care that may be required by such an individual, both as a child and in the years beyond childhood. The other option is to terminate the pregnancy. Often termed a **therapeutic abortion,** it is an abortion nonetheless and presents ethical dilemmas for many people. These issues have begun to emerge in the literature on mental retardation (see, e.g., Drew et al., 1984; Hardman & Drew, 1978, 1980; Hardman, 1984), but they have long been a concern in the literature of other fields such as religion, medicine, and philosophy (e.g., Fletcher, 1975; Ramsey, 1973; Williams, 1966). In certain cases, the time immediately following birth, known as the **neonatal period,** presents some of the most difficult ethical dilemmas for parents and professionals (Burt, 1976; Diamond, 1977; Duff & Campbell, 1973; Fletcher, 1968; Horan & Mall, 1977; President's Commission, 1983b; Robertson, 1975; Shaw, 1977). During the neonatal period, the issue is usually whether to withhold medical treatment from a defective newborn. This raises such ethical and moral questions as who makes these decisions; what the circumstances are under which the decisions are made; and what criterion is used to determine whether treatment is to be withheld.

EDUCATIONAL ASSESSMENT

FOCUS 13
What is the role of the multi-disciplinary team in regard to the educational assessment of the mentally retarded student?

Just as a physician assesses an individual with mental retardation to determine the extent of medical intervention, so do professionals from several disciplines assess the need for special education services. This group of professionals join with the child's parents to assess needs and plan for intervention, and are often referred to as the **multidisciplinary team.** The professionals on this team usually include the school psychologist, the classroom teacher, and a school administrator. Depending on the needs of the child, other professionals may be involved as well, including a social worker, speech or language specialist, occupational or physical therapist, **adaptive physical education teacher,** school counselor, and school nurse.

The multidisciplinary team has two critical functions with regard to assessment of a child. First, they must determine whether the child in question meets the criteria of mental retardation before placing the child in a special education program. Second, it is the responsibility of the team to assess the educational needs of the child so that an appropriate educational program can be implemented.

An intelligence test and a measure of adaptive behavior deficits must be completed to determine whether the child meets criteria to be labeled mentally retarded. The most commonly used scales for measuring intelligence in school-age children are the **Wechsler Intelligence Scales** and the Stanford-Binet Intelligence Scale.

Adaptive behavior may be measured by both formal and informal appraisals. Informal appraisals include direct observations as well as asking people who are in regular contact with the child (such as parents and classroom teachers) about his or her ability to cope with the demands of the environment. Formal appraisals include the use of standardized adaptive behavior scales such as the **Vineland Social Maturity Scale,** the **Scales of Independent Behavior,** and the **AAMR Adaptive Behavior Scale.**

Once it has been determined that the child meets the criteria for mental retardation, the team sets in place specific assessment procedures that will determine the nature of an appropriate educational experience for this particular child. The team members contribute information from their areas of expertise to build a broad base for determining the child's needs. The psychologist and the classroom teacher select, administer, and interpret appropriate psychological, educational, and behavioral assessment instruments. In addition, they observe the child's performance in an educational setting and consult with parents and other team members regarding the child's overall development. Parents provide the team with information regarding the child's performance outside of the school setting. They must provide written consent for testing the child in order to change his or her educational placement. Physical therapists, occupational therapists, and adaptive physical education specialists assess the motor development of the child. The speech or language specialist assesses the child's communication abilities. The social worker may collect pertinent information from the home setting as well as other background data relevant to the student's needs. The school nurse assists in the interpretation of information regarding the student's health, including hearing and vision screenings, conferences with physicians, and monitoring medication).

Although each team member has specific responsibilities in assessing the educational needs of the child, it is important for the members to work together as a unit. Each member of the team has the responsibility to maintain on-going communication with other members, actively participate in problem-solving situations, and follow through with assigned tasks.

EDUCATIONAL INTERVENTIONS

Education is a relatively new concept as it relates to children with mental retardation, particularly the more severely and profoundly retarded ones. Historically, many of these children were defined as noneducable by the public schools because they did not fit the programs offered by general education. Educational programs have been built on a foundation of academic learning that emphasizes reading, writing, and arithmetic. Thus children with mental retardation could not meet the academic standards set by the schools and, as such, were excluded from public education. Schools were not expected to adapt to the needs of the retarded individual, the individual was expected to adapt to the system.

Through both state and federal mandates (P.L. 94–142), the schools, which excluded these children for so long, are now faced with a new challenge: appropriate education for all children and youths with mental retardation. Based on a new set of values, education has been redefined. No longer do the schools dictate a general curriculum emphasizing only academic learning. Instead, education is defined as advancing an individual to the next higher level of functioning, regardless of how developmentally delayed he or she may be. For those who are severely and profoundly retarded, the differences are substantial and require services far beyond the scope of a single profession. Although educators have traditionally been autonomous in their classrooms, this practice cannot continue if the needs of these individuals are to be met. When working in harmony, the fields of medicine, the social services, and education form a network of professionals that provide the best means available to meet the needs of the mentally retarded individual. To gain a more in-depth perspective on intervention strategies, we will analyze both childhood and adolescent programs for individuals with mental retardation.

Early Childhood Education

FOCUS 14
Why is there such a critical need for early-intervention services for children with mental retardation?

Education and training for people with mental retardation, particularly individuals such as Becky, who is severely mentally retarded, may be a lifetime process. For people who are severely retarded, intervention should begin at birth and continue through to the adult years. The importance of early intervention cannot be overstated. Gentry and Olson (1985) report that significant advances have been made in the area of early intervention, including (1) improved assessment, curricular, and instructional technologies, (2) increasing numbers of children receiving services, and (3) appreciation of the need to individualize services for families as well as children. McDonnell and Hardman (1988), in a review of the literature in early intervention, suggest that "best practice" indicators include programs that are integrated with nonhandicapped students, comprehensive, normalized, adaptable, peer- and family-referenced, and **outcome-based.**

Early-intervention techniques, such as **infant stimulation** programs, focus on the acquisition of sensorimotor functions and intellectual development. This involves learning simple reflex activity and equilibrium reactions. Subsequent intervention then expands into all areas of human growth and development. Intervention based on normal patterns of growth is often referred to as the developmental milestones approach (Bailey & Wolery, 1989) because it seeks to develop, remedy, or adapt learner skills based on the retarded child's variation from what is considered normal. This progression of skills continues as the child ages chronologically, and the child's rate of progress depends on the severity of the condition. Some profoundly retarded children may never exceed a developmental age of six months. Some moderately or severely retarded children develop to a functioning level that later enables them to live as adults with varying levels of societal support and supervision.

The preschool-age, mildly retarded child may exhibit subtle developmental discrepancies in comparison to age-mates, but parents may not identify these discrepancies as significant enough to seek intervention. Even if parents are concerned and seek help for their child prior to school age, they are often confronted with professionals who are apathetic toward early childhood education. Some professionals believe that early-childhood services may actually create rather than remedy problems, since the child may not be mature enough to cope

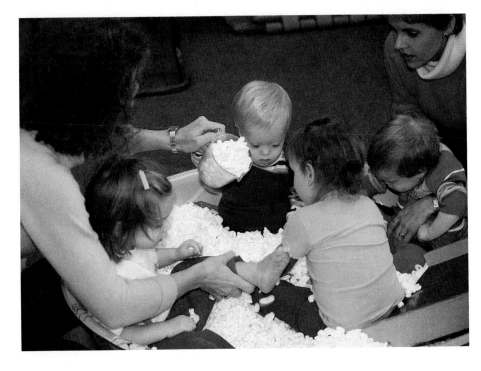

Infant stimulation programs focus on the acquisition of sensorimotor functions and intellectual development. (The Institute for the Study of Developmental Disabilities at Indiana University)

with the pressures of structured learning in an educational environment. This **maturation philosophy** has been ingrained in educators and parents. Simply stated, it means to wait for the child to reach a point of maturation where he or she is ready to learn certain skills. Unfortunately, this philosophy has kept many children out of the public schools for years while waiting for them to mature. The antithesis of the maturation philosophy is the prevention of further learning and behavior problems through intervention. **Project Head Start,** initially funded as a federal preschool program for disadvantaged students, is a prevention program that attempts to identify and instruct high-risk children prior to their entering public school. Although Head Start programs did not generate the results that were initially anticipated (the virtual elimination of school-adjustment problems for the disadvantaged student), it did represent a beginning. The rationale for early education is widely accepted in the field of special education and is part of the mandate of the Education of the Handicapped Act under the 1986 amendments (P.L. 99–457).

Education for Elementary School–Age Children

FOCUS 15
Identify five skill areas for elementary-age mentally retarded children.

Educational programming for elementary school–age children with mental retardation is concerned with decreasing dependence on others while concurrently teaching adaptation to the environment. Therefore the educational curriculum must concentrate on those skills that facilitate the child's interaction with others and emphasize independence in the community. Programs for mentally retarded children generally include skill areas such as motor development, self-care, social skills, communication, and functional academics.

Motor Skills. The acquisition of motor skills is a fundamental component of the developmental process and a prerequisite to successful learning in other content areas, including self-care and social skills. Moon and Bunker (1987) suggest that:

> Both fine and gross motor skills are involved in the accomplishment of almost all activities within every domain. . . . A general rule of thumb should be to train fine and gross motor skills within the context of functional activities. . . . Walking can be instructed during community activities such as learning to use the neighborhood grocery store or traveling independently to school or work (p. 232).

Gross motor development involves general mobility, including the interaction of the body with the environment. Gross motor skills are developed in a sequence ranging from movements that make balance possible, to higher order locomotor patterns. Locomotor patterns are intended to move the person freely through the environment. Gross motor movements include head and neck control, rolling, body righting, sitting, creeping, crawling, standing, walking, running, jumping, and skipping. **Fine motor development** requires more precision and steadiness than the skills developed in the gross motor area. Fine motor skills include reaching, grasping, and manipulation of objects. The development of fine motor skills is initially dependent on the ability of the child to "visually fix" on an object and "visually track" a moving target (Mori & Masters, 1980). Coordination of the eye and hand is an integral factor in many skill areas as well as in fine motor development. Eye–hand coordination is the basis of social- and leisure-time activities and is essential to the development of the object-control skills required in vocational situations.

Self-Care Skills. The development of self-care skills is another important content area related to independence. Self-care areas include feeding, dressing, and personal-hygiene skills. Feeding skills range from finger-feeding, drinking from a cup, and proper table behaviors such as the use of utensils and napkins, to serving food and etiquette. Dressing skills include buttoning, zipping, buckling, lacing, and tying. Personal-hygiene skills also range on a continuum from rather basic developmental skills to high-level skills relevant to adult behavior. Basic skills include toileting, face- and hand-washing, bathing, toothbrushing, hair-combing, and shampooing. Skills associated with adolescent and adult years include skin care, shaving, hair-setting, use of deodorants and cosmetics, and menstrual hygiene.

Social Skills. Social-skills training is closely aligned with the self-care area in that it relates many of the self-care concepts to the development of good interpersonal relationships. Social-skills training emphasizes the importance of physical appearance, proper manners, appropriate use of leisure time, and sexual behavior. The area of social skills may also focus on the development of personality characteristics conducive to successful integration into society.

Communication Skills. The ability to communicate with others is also essential to growth and development. Without communication there is no interaction.

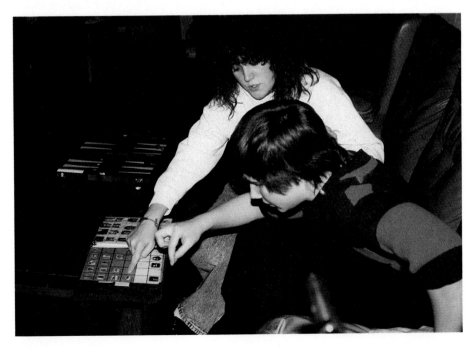

Communication boards are used by nonverbal people to express requests and answer simple questions. (The Institute for the Study of Developmental Disabilities at Indiana University)

Communication systems for children with mental retardation take three general forms: (1) verbal language, (2) **manual communication,** such as sign language or language boards, or (3) a combination of the verbal and manual approaches. The approach employed depends on the child's capability. If he or she is able to develop the requisite skills for spoken language, everyday interactive skills will be greatly enhanced. Manual communication must be considered when a child is unable to develop verbal skills as an effective means of communication. What is important is that the individual develop some form of communication.

Functional Academic Skills.   A **functional academic curriculum** is intended to expand the child's knowledge in daily living, recreation, and vocational areas. Functional academics are taught only when a child has acquired the prerequisite skills. When teaching functional academic skills, the classroom teacher uses instructional materials that are realistic and part of the context of the child's environment. Browder and Snell (1987), reviewing the literature related to learning functional reading skills, reported that students with mental retardation, including those with moderate to severe problems, can learn to read sight words and acquire reading comprehension or decoding skills (p. 437). A functional reading program contains words that are frequently encountered in the environment, such as labels or signs in public places; words that warn readers of possible risks; and symbols such as the skull and crossbones on poisonous substances. A functional math program involves such activities as learning to use a checkbook, shop in a grocery store, or operate a vending machine.

FOCUS 16
What are related services for students with mental retardation?

Related Services.   In order to provide an appropriate education for children with mental retardation, many different professionals must be involved in the instructional process. In fact, federal legislation mandates that a team consisting of professionals from several disciplines assess the educational needs of exceptional children. The law also provides that services not usually defined as educational in nature must be made available if they assist a student in benefiting from a special education program. They are defined by law as related services.

> Related services means transportation and such developmental, corrective, and other supportive services (including speech pathology and audiology, psychological services, physical and occupational therapy, recreation, and medical and counseling services) . . . as may be required to assist a handicapped child to benefit from special education, and includes the early identification and assessment of handicapping conditions in children (U.S. Congress, Education for All Handicapped Children Act, Public Law 94–142, 1975).

Education for Adolescents

FOCUS 17
Identify four educational goals for adolescents with mental retardation.

The goals of an educational program for adolescents with mental retardation are to (1) increase personal independence, (2) enhance opportunities for participation in the local community, (3) prepare for employment, and (4) facilitate a successful transition to the adult years.

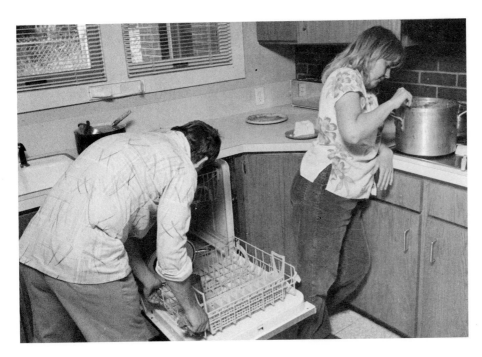

The development of independent-living skills allows an individual to become more self-sufficient. (John Telford)

Independence refers to the development and application of skills that lead to greater self-sufficiency in one's daily personal life. These skills include personal hygiene, self-care, and appropriate leisure activities. Participation in the community includes access to those community programs, facilities, and services that non-handicapped people often take for granted—grocery stores, shopping malls, restaurants, theaters, parks, and so forth. Adolescents with mental retardation should have opportunities for contact with nonhandicapped individuals other than care-givers, access to community events, sustained social relationships with other people, and involvement in the choices that affect their lives. Work is a critical measure of any person's success during the adult years. Work provides mentally retarded adults with their primary opportunities for social interaction, a basis for personal identity and status, and a chance to contribute to the community.

Vocational training for mentally retarded adolescents has been fraught with problems because of a pessimistic attitude that professionals and the general public have about its effectiveness. Today the negative philosophy about vocational training has largely been replaced by a commitment to the development of relevant vocational programs for this population, particularly in competitive employment settings (Bellamy & Wilcox, 1981; Brickey, Campbell, & Browning, 1985; Gold, 1975; Peck, Apolloni, & Cooke, 1981; Pomerantz & Marholin, 1977; Wehman & Hill, 1985). As a content area, vocational preparation is essentially a composite of basic skills taught in other areas. These include communication, motor development, recreation, and self-care. Vocational training for mentally retarded adolescents focuses on perseverance, sustained performance,

Reflect on This 4–4

Circles of Friends in Schools

Toronto, Ontario—Marsha Forest came away from her Joshua Committee experiences as if she had put on a better pair of glasses. Her position as a well-ensconced professor of special education at York University suddenly seemed less important to her. She spent long hours on the road helping school boards, principals, and teachers to see how everybody can experience richness when someone with a severe disability is placed in a regular classroom and the so-called regular students are encouraged to form a circle of friends around that person.

Forest always believed in getting teachers down to meticulous detail when it came to educating persons with disabilities. Now, however, she saw that some of the most valuable educational steps can come naturally from regular classmates, if the right conditions exist in the classroom. She saw how peer-group concerns can become a fountainhead of power.

She also knew that parents and teachers fear peer-group pressure. After all, when kids get together these days, they can give themselves quite an education—one that often shapes lives more powerfully than adults can shape them. But peer-group education doesn't always lead to belligerence and destruction and drugs. It can lead to caring and nurturing and helping others do healthy things they had never done before.

This twist, however, generated fears in some teachers when it dawned on them that a circle of friends might foster better growth and development in a student than they were capable of teaching.

And so Marsha moved into regular schools and worked hard at:

- helping boards and principals understand the circles of friends process
- finding a teacher and class willing to include a person with a severe disability
- helping the regular teacher handle any initial fears about the venture
- letting the teacher and class call the shots as much as possible
- providing strong support persons—integration facilitators—who would assist only when they really were needed

response to motivation and rewards, and work-adjustment skills such as punctuality, task correction, responsibility, socialization, independence on the job, initiative, and safety.

Educational Placement Considerations

FOCUS 18
Why is the integration of mentally retarded students with their nonhandicapped peers an important part of an appropriate educational experience?

The educational placement of students with mental retardation has been a critical concern for school personnel and parents for many years. Prior to the late 1960s, special education for mentally retarded children and youth meant segregated education. Since then much of the focus on educational placement has been concerned with mainstreaming retarded children with their nonretarded age-mates (Polloway, 1984). *Mainstreaming* may be defined as the placement of mentally retarded students in regular education classrooms with nonhandicapped peers, consistent with an established educational plan for each individual. Some mentally retarded students may be mainstreamed for a small part of the school day and attend only those regular education classes that are consistent with their needs and functioning level (e.g., physical education, industrial arts, or home

■ then finding a handful of kids willing to work at being friends with their classmate with the disability

"The first placement in a school is the toughest," she said. "After that, it's usually easy to include others."

Forest sees the building of a circle of friends as a person-by-person process, not an all-encompassing program. And so she focuses on students with disabilities one at a time, setting up a framework that enables a circle to surround that person.

Because no two settings are alike, she watches as the circle, the regular teacher, and the rest of the students develop and coordinate their own routines for helping. Then, never predicting an outcome, she waits. And when new learning takes place in the person with the disability, Forest

moves in and makes all the students, the teacher, the principal—even the board members—feel simply great.

According to her, the average school can handle up to twelve of these arrangements. After that, the efficiency of the process may diminish.

She doubts that circles of friends will work in every school. "If a school is all screwed up," she said, "and if it has lost its zest and commitment for really helping kids learn—forget it. On the other hand, I'm sure that circles of friends can help make a good school—especially the kids—better. Then coming to school takes on fresh values and meaning. Some enjoy coming to school as they never did before."

According to Forest. . . .

"Circles of friends are not an alternative to learning. They are a precondition.

"They move us beyond integration—into community.

"I hate labels. I just see people who challenge the school system.

"Wait for schools to be ready for people with challenging behaviors, and you can wait until hell freezes over.

"The term *gifted* is an insult. All people have gifts. Sometimes those with challenging behaviors have the greatest gifts.

"You can't learn to like kids with disabilities by watching puppets. Puppets don't smell or drool. They aren't real. Kids learn to accept people with differences by really living with them."

Source: From *Circles of Friends* by Robert & Martha Perske. Copyright © 1988 by Robert & Martha Perske. Used by permission of the publisher, Abingdon Press.

economics). The majority of their school day is spent in a self-contained classroom for mentally retarded students. Other students with mental retardation may attend regular education classes for the majority of the school day. For these students, special education consists mostly of support services to facilitate their opportunities for success in the regular education classroom.

Segregated educational facilities (often referred to as **special schools**) have been a placement option for moderately, severely, and profoundly retarded children for several years. Proponents of the special school argue that they provide for (1) greater homogeneity in grouping and programming, (2) teacher specialization in such areas as art, language, physical education, and music, and (3) centralization of teaching materials, which results in a more efficient use of available programs. In addition, some parents of severely retarded individuals believe that their children will be happier in a segregated environment that "protects" the child.

However, the research on the efficacy of segregated educational environments does not support these premises (McDonnell & Hardman, 1989). On the contrary, investigations over the past twenty years strongly indicate that mentally retarded students, regardless of the severity of the condition, benefit from placement in a regular education facility where opportunities for integration with nonhandicapped peers are systematically planned and implemented (Brinker, 1984; Schutz, Williams, Iverson, & Duncan, 1984; Stainback & Stainback, 1985; Wehman & Hill, 1982; Voeltz, 1982; Wilcox & Bellamy, 1982). Integration does not necessarily mean mainstreaming moderately and severely retarded students in the regular education classroom, but includes a variety of opportunities within the total school environment. These opportunities may include, but not be limited, to:

> Homeroom, art, music, recess, Thanksgiving and birthday parties, show-and-tell times, and rest periods. Nonhandicapped students could be encouraged to visit the special education classroom to work as tutors or simply spend a little time with a severely retarded friend. In addition, teachers can facilitate interactions between nonhandicapped and severely retarded students in the school cafeteria, at assembly programs, in the hallways, and at the bus loading and unloading zones (Stainback & Stainback, 1982).

Stainback and Stainback also report that regular education teachers who have the opportunity for interaction with severely retarded children are not fearful of or intimidated by their presence in the school building. Segregated schools generally offer little, if any, opportunity for interaction with normal peers and deprive the mentally retarded child of valuable learning and socialization experiences. McDonnell and Hardman (1989) argue that segregated facilities cannot be financially or ideologically justified. Public school administrators must now plan to include these children in existing regular education facilities.

OTHER INTERVENTION STRATEGIES

Medicine

FOCUS 19
What is the role of medicine in meeting the diverse needs of people with mental retardation?

In order to meet the diverse needs of people with mental retardation, several professionals must be involved in intervention. Most individuals with moderate to profound mental retardation exhibit problems that are evident at birth. Consequently, a physician is usually the first professional to come in contact with these children. In a survey of physicians in the state of Texas, more than 85 percent indicated they were the initial informants to parents regarding their child's handicapping condition (McDonald, Carson, Palmer, & Slay, 1982). The physician's primary roles are as diagnostician, counselor, and care-giver. As a diagnostician, the physician analyzes the nature and cause of the child's condition and then, based on the medical information available, counsels the family concerning the medical prognosis. The physician's role as a family counselor has been challenged by some professionals in the behavioral sciences and by parents, because such counseling often exceeds the medical domain (Hardman & Drew, 1980). This concern reflects the opinion that medical personnel should counsel families only on medical matters and recommend other resources such as educators, psychologists, social workers, clergy, or parent groups when dealing with issues that do not relate to issues other than the child's medical needs.

Social Services

The appropriate social services for people with mental retardation extend into many aspects of the individual's life, such as the primary family unit, the extended family, the neighborhood, the educational environment, and the community at large. Necessary social services may be put into five general categories: (1) community support services, (2) family support services, (3) alternative living arrangements, (4) vocational services, and (5) leisure-time services. Figure 4–3 illustrates some of the services included within each of these general categories.

The availability of services provides for mentally retarded individuals a greater opportunity to achieve what is commonly referred to as **normalization.** This principle emphasizes the need to make available to the individual "the patterns and conditions of every day life which are as close to the norms and patterns of mainstream society as possible" (Nirje, 1970, p. 181). The principle of normalization goes far beyond the mere physical integration of the retarded individual in a community. It promotes the availability of needed support services, such as training and supervision, without which the retarded individual may not be prepared to cope with the demands of community life.

FOCUS 20
Identify five social services necessary for people with mental retardation.

Figure 4–3
Classification of Community Service Needs

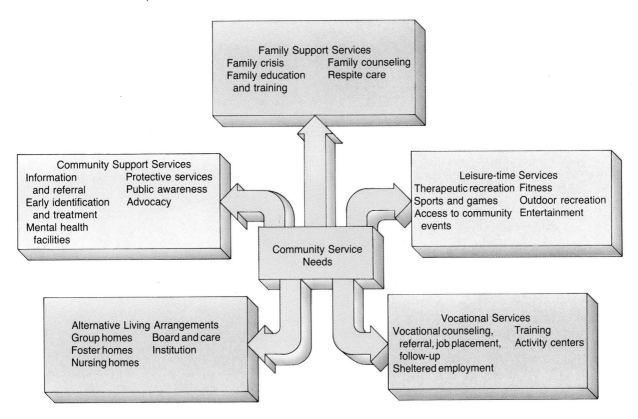

REVIEW

FOCUS 1: Describe the range of characteristics associated with mild to profound mental retardation.

☐ Mildly retarded children have learning difficulties that are usually school-related.

☐ Children with moderate to severe mental retardation have difficulties that transcend the classroom, and they may be impaired in nearly every facet of life.

☐ Severely retarded individuals are capable of developing skills that allow a degree of independence within their environment.

☐ Profoundly retarded individuals generally are dependent on others to maintain even their most basic life functions.

FOCUS 2: Identify the three components of the definition of mental retardation.

☐ Significantly subaverage general intellectual functioning is defined as two standard deviations below the mean on an individual test of intelligence.

☐ Adaptive behavior deficits are defined as significant limitations in a person's ability to meet standards of maturation, learning, personal independence, and social responsibility.

☐ Developmental period is defined as birth to eighteen years of age.

FOCUS 3: Identify the three methods of classifying people with mental retardation.

☐ The severity of the condition may be described in terms of mild, moderate, severe, and profound mental retardation.

☐ Educability expectations are discussed in terms of children who are educable, trainable, and custodial.

☐ Medical descriptors classify mental retardation on the basis of the origin of the condition (e.g., infection, intoxication, trauma, or chromosomal abnormality).

FOCUS 4: What is the estimated prevalence of mental retardation?

☐ It is generally estimated that from 1 to 3 percent of the general population have mental retardation.

FOCUS 5: Identify four intellectual characteristics of individuals with mental retardation.

☐ Intellectual deficiencies include learning and memory deficiencies, difficulties in establishing learning sets, inefficient rehearsal strategies, and incidental learning problems.

FOCUS 6: Identify seven in-school adaptive behavior deficiencies of students with mental retardation.

☐ School adaptive behavior problems include (1) lack of school coping behaviors, (2) poor social skills, (3) poor language skills, (4) poor emotional development, (5) poor self-care skills, (6) limited success in applying cognitive skills, and (7) delayed academic development.

FOCUS 7: What are the expected reading and arithmetic deficiencies of students with mental retardation?

☐ Students with mental retardation exhibit significant deficits in the areas of reading and mathematics.

☐ School-age students with mild mental retardation have poor reading mechanics and comprehension compared to their age-mates.

☐ Children with moderate and severe mental retardation can be taught to read at least a protective or survival vocabulary.

FOCUS 8: Identify three common speech problems and the most common language problem for individuals with mental retardation.

☐ The most common speech problems are articulation, voice, and stuttering problems.

☐ Language problems are generally associated with delays in language development rather than the bizarre use of language.

FOCUS 9: Why are physical problems more evident in individuals with severe and profound mental retardation?

☐ Physical problems generally are not evident for individuals with mild mental retardation because the retardation is usually not associated with genetic factors.

☐ The more severe the mental retardation, the greater the probability of compounding physiological problems.

FOCUS 10: What are the causes of mild mental retardation?

☐ The cause of mental retardation is generally not known for mildly retarded individuals.

FOCUS 11: Identify seven causes of moderate to profound mental retardation.

☐ Causes associated with moderate to profound mental retardation include infection and intoxication, chromosomal abnormalities, gestation disorders, unknown prenatal influences, traumas or physical agents, metabolism or nutrition problems, and gross postnatal brain disease.

FOCUS 12: Identify four measures that may prevent mental retardation.

☐ Widely accepted preventive measures include immunizations against disease, appropriate nutrition for the mother during pregnancy, appropriate prenatal care, and screening for genetic disorders at birth.

FOCUS 13: What is the role of the multidisciplinary team in regard to the educational assessment of the mentally retarded student?

☐ The multidisciplinary team joins together to assess each individual's needs, and to plan for intervention based on identified problem areas.

FOCUS 14: Why is there such a critical need for early-intervention services for children with mental retardation?

☐ Early-intervention services are needed to provide the child with a stimulating environment to enhance growth and development.

☐ Early-intervention programs focus on the development of communication skills, social interaction, and readiness for formal instruction.

FOCUS 15: Identify five skill areas for elementary-age mentally retarded children.

☐ Programs for elementary-age mentally retarded children include instruction in the areas of motor development, self-care, social skills, communication, and functional academics.

FOCUS 16: What are related services for students with mental retardation?

☐ Related services include transportation and such development, corrective, and other support services as may be required to assist a handicapped student to benefit from special education.

FOCUS 17: Identify four educational goals for adolescents with mental retardation.

☐ Educational goals for adolescents are to (1) increase the individual's personal independence, (2) enhance opportunities for participation in the local community, (3) prepare for employment, and (4) facilitate a successful transition to the adult years.

FOCUS 18: Why is the integration of mentally retarded students with their nonhandicapped peers an important part of an appropriate educational experience?

☐ Regardless of the severity of the condition, students with mental retardation benefit from placement in regular education environments where opportunities for integration with nonhandicapped peers are systematically planned and implemented.

FOCUS 19: What is the role of medicine in meeting the diverse needs of people with mental retardation?

☐ The physician's roles are diagnostician, counselor, and care-giver.

FOCUS 20: Identify five social services necessary for people with mental retardation.

☐ Appropriate social services include community support services, family support services, alternative living arrangements, vocational services, and leisure-time services.

Debate Forum

Social Integration or Social Separation of Children with Mental Retardation

The principle of normalization and the least-restrictive-environment clause in Public Law 94–142 state that individuals with mental retardation should have available to them conditions and opportunities in every day life that are as close as possible to those available to nonhandicapped people. The following are two different viewpoints on the applications of these principles to children with mental retardation in an educational setting. One point of view is from the vantage of professionals working in a special school (separate educational facility for handicapped students); the

counterpoint is from the position of social integration for students in a regular education building or classroom.

Special School Programs as the Least Restrictive Environment

Point Oftentimes it is a special school program that can provide the least restrictive environment for a handicapped student. It is here where a greater variety of opportunities in which the student can attain full participation is offered. These settings provide the necessary adaptive instruction in a noncompetitive environment, which leads to the mastery of skills and growth of self-esteem that cannot be duplicated in many of our neighborhood schools. Special school programs can concentrate on adaptive and functional instruction and therapy, leisure activities, social skills, community participation, and vocational preparation.

For many students, special school programs are the least restrictive environment because of the appropriate delivery of services and the "philosophical" commitment to severely handicapped students. . . . Although mainstreaming may provide the most appropriate environment for the majority of handicapped students, let's not assume that this is the least restrictive environment for all students at all times. There will always be a need for special school programs as long as there are students with unique, special needs.*

The Movement to Social Integration

Counterpoint For the preschool-age child, the world is defined primarily through family and a small same-age peer group. As the child progresses chronologically the world expands to the neighborhood, the school, and eventually to a larger heterogeneous group we call the community. As educators we must then ask, How do we structure a student's educational program to effectively foster full partici-

pation as the life space of the individual is expanded? What are the barriers to full participation, and how do we work to break them down?

One critical barrier is the separation or segregation of students with severe disabilities from the people with whom they will participate in the heterogeneous world, whether it be at school, where they live, at work or play. Such segregation promotes dependence and isolation, and limits opportunities for students to learn skills that enhance independent living and social participation. . . . Students with severe disabilities are to be educated to the maximum extent possible with their nondisabled peers, which includes attending a regular school unless extenuating individual circumstances preclude this as an appropriate placement decision.

Recent research on social, educational, and financial outcomes is also supportive of the social integration of students with severe disabilities. Appropriately implemented integration efforts include planned, sustained interactions between students with severe disabilities and their nondisabled peers. In fact, such interactions yield improved attitudes and interaction patterns, while exposing the student to socially appropriate role models.†

Sources: *J. Curtis & M. Riding, 1989, Special School Programs as the Least Restrictive Environment, *The Special Educator*, 9(5), 6. †M. L. Hardman, 1988, Educational Services for Students with Severe Disabilities: The Movement toward Social Integration, *The Special Educator*, 9(1), 9–10.

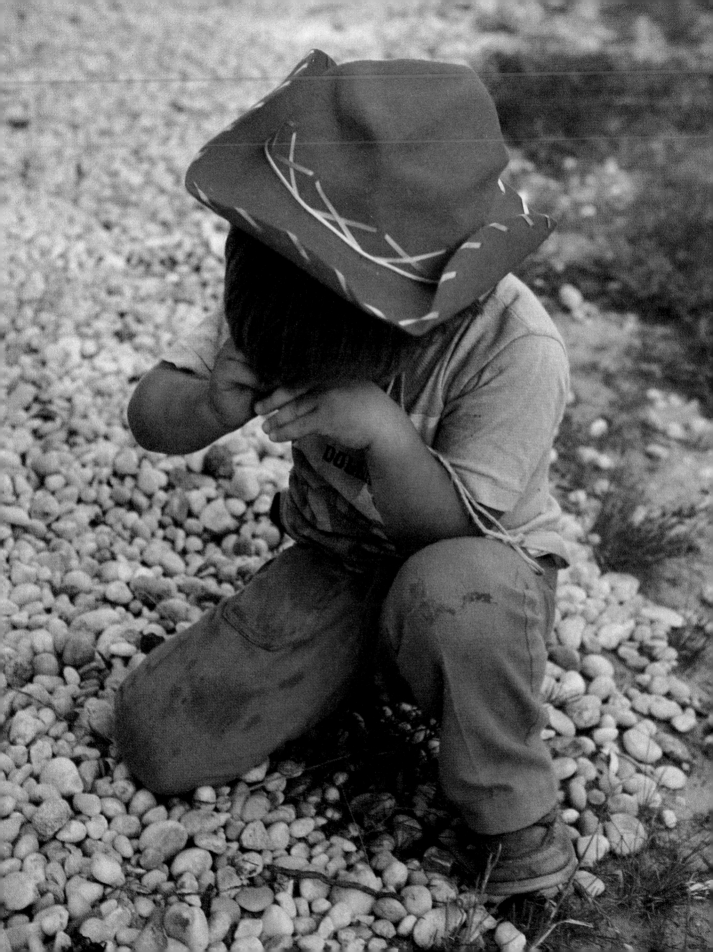

5 Behavior Disorders

To Begin With...

- One Day in the Lives of American Children, 1987: 1,293 teenagers will give birth; 6 teens will commit suicide; 1,849 children will be abused; 3,288 children will choose to run away from home; 1,629 children will be incarcerated in adult jails; 2,989 children will see their parents divorce (Children's Defense Fund, 1989).

- The therapeutic benefits of pets are being studied as more than 1,100 programs in hospitals and other institutions use animals to help youths and adults develop social relationships (Associated Press News Service, 1989).

- Referring to a 1989 report released by the Institute of Medicine, Yale University, Dr. Frederick Solomon, director of the Mental Health Division, noted that for seriously emotionally disturbed children, "the evidence is that less than 30 and maybe less than 20 percent are served."

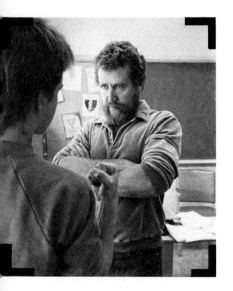

Steve's overall appearance and demeanor were something to behold. I have worked with several hundred very difficult boys, but Steve in many ways represented the most difficult of the difficult. It was as if he had become a belligerent vagrant at the early age of twelve. His clothing was dirty, or should I say filthy. His countenance, clothing, and conduct said, "Stay away from me or you'll be very, very sorry!"

I thought I was prepared for almost anything after teaching disturbed children for ten years, but Steve drew off all the patience and skill that was in me during the first two months in my class. His refusal and outright opposition to almost any request made of him was incredibly frustrating to me and his house parents. Moreover, he was exceptionally skilled in what I refer to as teacher torture techniques. These included various forms of pencil tapping, quiet but distinguishable junglelike vocalizations, and careful applications of mucus applied to reading and math assignments. His other school assignments were rarely submitted without some grotesque or sexually explicit drawing. Assignments replete with numerous erasures and erasure-induced holes and purposeful errors were commonplace.

His feelings of disdain for himself, other students, and his situation were expressed in numerous ways. Spitting was a constant threat to anyone who sat near him or chose to interact with him, particularly when he was upset. He was a time bomb of sorts. The treatment staff, including myself, could rarely predict what it was that set him off, nor could we reliably predict when he would explode. The unpredictability of his behavior kept us continually on our toes. He excelled in irritation and outright intimidation of adults and fellow students. Teasing, bullying, harassing, bothering, and fighting were his specialty. He was continually hassling the younger, more demure students in the class. His manipulative skills and capacity to talk one out of an assignment or talk one into a preferred activity of his choosing were well-developed behaviors. Even in fairly informal settings that were recreational in nature and devoid of demands of adults and other authority figures, he seemed to be unhappy and unfulfilled.

Cherie was an attractive, bright sixth grader. Her work was always completed punctually and accurately. She was, in fact, unusually conscientious, conforming, and eager to please. She seemed to enjoy school a great deal and liked being a part of all our classroom activities. The school year came to an end and delightful Cherie left my classroom to enjoy the summer.

The next school year was an altogether different story. She began her junior high school year with her peers and with much anticipation. Seven teachers per day, lockers and locker partners, and a host of other new school variables were only a few of the features of junior high school life that captured her attention. She did well during the first week of school. Then suddenly, without any real warning signs, Cherie complained about not feeling very well and asked if she could stay home. Her actual request to stay home was preceded by episodes of nausea and vomiting. She also said that she felt dizzy and faint during the afternoon of the previous day. Her mother was prompt in responding to her symptoms of illness and allowed her to stay home that day. This was the beginning of a consistent pattern of refusal to go to school.

The precipitating events appeared to be two low scores that she had received the previous day in two of her classes, history and advanced math. She was also perplexed with the challenges that were an integral part of her P.E. class. Undressing, dressing, and showering with so many peers present was highly stressful for her. She felt as if everyone was watching her. School became socially and psychologically aversive.

Many attempts were made to persuade Cherie to attend school following these events, but they were unsuccessful. Her anxiety actually bordered on what many would describe as sheer panic at times. Sometimes she would have chest pains. Other times she would feel very dizzy. She fought attempts by her parents to forcibly take her to school. She often locked herself in her room, or she just took off if she felt her parents were going to force her to go to school. Just thinking about school was anxiety provoking for her.

Jan, our daughter, was very close to completing her junior year in high school. With the exception of the last six months, her behavior had been normal. She didn't have a lot of friends as she was fairly shy and enjoyed doing things by herself. She didn't like or dislike school. Occasionally she would participate in extracurricular school activities if her friends went out of their way to invite her. Her interests, concerns, loves, and fears were like those of any teenager. But after Christmas break her behavior began to change, not in an abrupt fashion but very slowly. One of the first signs was the deterioration of her relationship with her friends. They stopped calling her and she had no interest in talking to them.

One morning during this post-Christmas period after I awakened her for school and began making breakfast, she entered the room still attired in her pajamas and told me that she did not need to go to school that day. When I asked her why she wasn't going to school, she told me that a voice had told her not to go. These voices began to impact her life in many ways. Gradually I watched as my once-competent daughter became another person, and I was powerless to do anything about it. Her face was at times immobile. The normal emotional intensity that was so much a part of her earlier junior high and high school days had practically vanished.

Her thoughts, as expressed in conversations with family members and others, were often disconnected. She rapidly shifted from one topic to another, completely unrelated topic of discussion without realizing that she was not making sense.

Another behavior that really concerned us during this time was her loss of self-initiated, goal-directed activity. Her behavior became very random both in school and at home. At times she appeared to know what she was doing and other times she seemed to be totally unaware of her behavior and its impact on others.

With the presence of these and other behaviors we knew that something was definitely wrong with Jan. We consulted with our family physician and he referred us to Dr. Holmes, a psychiatrist in our area. After a number of preliminary visits, we were told that Jan has schizophrenia.

INTRODUCTION

Individuals with behavior disorders, such as Steve, Cherie, and Jan, experience great difficulties in relating appropriately to peers, siblings, parents, and teachers. They also have difficulty responding to academic and social tasks that are essential parts of their schooling. In some cases they may exhibit too much behavior. For example, Steve's placement in a specialized treatment facility was a function of his excessive aggressive or oppositional behaviors. In other cases, individuals with behavior or emotional problems may not have learned the coping behaviors necessary for successful participation in school settings, as demonstrated by Cherie. She, for a variety of reasons, was unable to respond to the demands of her new junior high school environment. Jan, as described by her mother in the last vignette, gradually lost her capacity to engage in meaningful relationships and goal-directed behaviors. Her inability to communicate and relate effectively to her family members, teachers, and peers had a profound impact on her achievement educationally, socially, and occupationally.

STUDYING BEHAVIOR DISORDERS

FOCUS 1
What five factors influence the ways in which we view others' behaviors?

Many factors influence the ways in which we view the behaviors of others. Our perceptions of others and their behaviors are significantly influenced by our personal beliefs, standards, and values about what constitutes normal behavior. If we were to observe Jan hearing voices in our classroom, we would probably become very concerned about her behavior. Also, imagine how her peers might react to her hearing voices in a classroom. Our range of tolerance for various behaviors varies greatly. Steve's aggressive and oppositional behaviors were not tolerated at school, nor were they well liked by his brothers and sisters, or his mother, who was often manipulated by his aggressive behaviors. Now he is receiving his education in a more restrictive setting. When he learns to control his behaviors and act more appropriately, he can return to the normal school environment.

What may be viewed as normal by some of us may be viewed by others as abnormal. Steve's toughness and willingness to continually oppose authority was viewed as normal by his father. Others, including his teachers, viewed it as totally inappropriate and abnormal.

The context in which behaviors occur dramatically influences our views of their appropriateness or inappropriateness. For example, if Jan were to hear voices in a church setting or as a part of a religious service, fellow worshippers might view her as being very spiritual. Similarly, Steve's toughness may be highly valued by a little league football coach who observes his zealousness in pursuing and attacking his fellow teammates during practice.

Sometimes it is the intensity or sheer frequency with which a given behavior or cluster of behaviors occurs that leads us to suspect the presence of behavior or emotional problems. Jan's parents observed a gradual change in her behavior. Initially they were uncertain about the significance of her symptoms. However, with the passage of time and the increase in frequency of certain behaviors (conversation devoid of meaning, hallucinations, and withdrawal from social activities), her parents realized that she needed psychiatric help.

VARIABLES IN BEHAVIOR DISORDERS

Many variables influence the types of behaviors that are exhibited or suppressed by individuals with behavior disorders. These include the parents' and teachers' management styles; the school or home environment; the social and cultural values of the family; the social and economic climate of the community; the responses of peers and siblings; and the academic, intellectual, and social-emotional characteristics of the individuals with the disorders.

FOCUS 2
What five variables influence the types of behaviors that are exhibited or suppressed by individuals with behavior disorders?

The vignettes of Steve, Cherie, and Jan help us to partially understand the severity of various behavior disorders. Jan and her family will have to deal with the challenges of schizophrenia throughout her lifetime. Steve's aggressive and oppositional behaviors were extremely difficult to treat, but the staff were successful in helping him learn other, more functional ways of successfully dealing with problems than by acting aggressively. Cherie's refusal to go to school was a major challenge for her parents and therapist, but she eventually returned to her junior high, completed her high school preparation, and went on to graduate from college as a certified teacher. Some behavior disorders are very severe and require the services of many trained individuals working together cooperatively. Other disorders may be treated in a relatively short time, with fewer personnel and at less expense.

TERMINOLOGY: EXTERNALIZING AND INTERNALIZING DISORDERS

At this juncture, it is important to note that a number of terms have been used to describe individuals with emotional, social, and behavioral problems. These terms include *behavior disorders, social maladjustment, emotional disturbance,* and others. Childhood, adolescent, and adult behavior problems can frequently be grouped into two broad but overlapping categories: externalizing and internalizing disorders. The latter category refers to behaviors that seem to be directed more at the self than at others. Depressions and phobias are examples of behaviors that we would include in the internalizing category. Some clinicians would describe individuals with these conditions as being emotionally disturbed.

FOCUS 3
What differentiates externalizing disorders from internalizing disorders?

Youngsters exhibiting externalizing disorders may be described as engaging in behaviors that are directed more at others than at themselves. Furthermore, these behaviors may have greater observable impact on parents, siblings, and teachers. The juvenile offender who chronically engages in crimes involving property damage or injury to others might be identified as being socially maladjusted. The distinction between the two categories is not clear-cut. For example, adolescents who are severely depressed certainly have an impact on their families and others. However, the primary locus of the distress for these youths is internal or emotional.

Throughout this chapter we use the term *behavior disorders* to describe persons with both external and internal problems. Our use of the term *behavior disorders* reflects our interest in observable behaviors. Our observations and those of others help to determine whether a child is depressed, aggressive, suicidal, anxious, delinquent, hyperactive, socially withdrawn, or extremely shy. So as we proceed, please keep in mind that behavior disorders as we perceive them may be internal (emotional) and/or external (social) in nature. Our knowledge of their presence is a function of our ability to carefully observe and measure them.

The behavior of children who exhibit externalizing disorders is often directed more at others than at themselves. (D & I MacDonald/The Picture Cube)

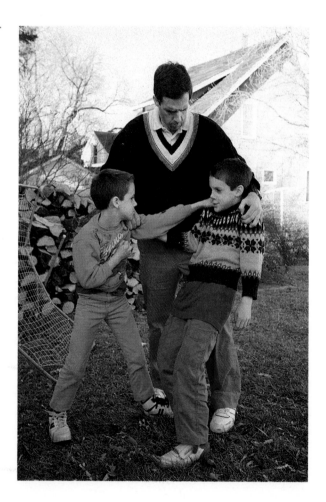

DEFINITIONS AND CLASSIFICATIONS

Definitions

A variety of definitions have been created to describe children and youth with behavior disorders. The current definition, used in conjunction with the rules and regulations governing the implementation of Public Law 94–142, is as follows:

"Seriously emotionally disturbed" is defined as . . . :

(i) The term means a condition exhibiting one or more of the following characteristics over a long period of time and to a marked degree, which adversely affects educational performance:

(A) An inability to learn which cannot be explained by intellectual, sensory or health factors;

(B) An inability to build or maintain satisfactory relationships with peers and teachers;

(C) Inappropriate types of behavior or feelings under normal circumstances;

(D) A general pervasive mood of unhappiness or depression; or

(E) A tendency to develop physical symptoms or fears associated with personal or school problems.

(ii) The term includes children who are schizophrenic [or autistic]. The term does not include children who are socially maladjusted, unless it is determined that they are seriously disturbed. (U.S. Department of Health, Education and Welfare, *Federal Register*, 1977, 42, No. 163, p. 42478)

This description of severe emotional disturbance or behavior disorders is a derivation of an earlier definition created by Bower (1959). This definition has been criticized because of its vagueness (Kauffman, 1982) and exclusion of individuals described as socially maladjusted (Benson, Edwards, Roseel, & White, 1986; Position Paper on Definition, 1987).

Each of the five characteristic behaviors identified by Bower in the federal definition helps us to see more clearly the ways in which behavior disorders may be exhibited. For example, the learning difficulties that young students with behavior disorders demonstrate are not attributable to intellectual retardation, sensory impairments, or health factors. Children or youths with behavior disorders have difficulties in initiating and maintaining relationships, exhibiting appropriate behaviors in various settings, expressing emotions appropriately, dealing with fears successfully, and maintaining dispositions that reflect satisfaction or achievement. We observed many of these difficulties in our vignettes of Steve, Cherie, and Jan. It is important to note that autism has been recently removed from the P.L. 94–142 definition of "seriously emotionally disturbed." **Autism** has now been placed in the "other health-impaired" category. However, we discuss aspects of this disorder very briefly in the classification section below.

An Alternate Definition.   Another definition has been developed by Kauffman (1977). He defined behavior disorders according to three levels of severity and identified the settings in which such children might receive special assistance.

Furthermore, he provided an optimistic perspective regarding the capacity of these children for positive growth.

> Children with behavior disorders are those who chronically and markedly respond to their environment in socially unacceptable and/or personally unsatisfactory ways, but who can be taught more socially acceptable and personally gratifying behavior. Children with mild and moderate behavior disorders can be taught effectively with their normal peers (if their teachers receive appropriate consultive help) or in a special resource or self-contained class with reasonable hope of quick reintegration with their normal peers. Children with severe and profound behavior disorders require intensive and prolonged intervention and must be taught at home, in a special class, special school, or residential institution (p. 23).

Behavior disorders are defined and classified in the context of normal behavior. A precise notion of normality is not simple to derive. Clarizio and McCoy (1976) indicated that although there is no acceptable definition of normality, there are specific components every definition must include. They suggested that the following must be taken into account:

1. The child's developmental level, since what is viewed as normal at one age might well be viewed as abnormal at another
2. The child's culture or subculture
3. Allowances for individuality
4. A multidimensional approach; that is, the definition must take into account how the child functions in various representative areas of development.

Later in this chapter, we review some of the procedures that are used to identify children and adolescents with behavior disorders. Although there are many screening and assessment devices that have been designed to aid clinicians in identifying children with behavior problems, the judgments are greatly influenced by the viewer's conception of **normality.**

Classifications

FOCUS 5
List three reasons why classification systems are important to professionals who diagnose, treat, and educate individuals with behavior disorders.

Classification systems serve several purposes for human services professionals. First, they provide a means for describing various types of behavior problems in children. Second, they provide a common set of terms for communicating with others. For example, children who are identified as having Down syndrome, a type of mental retardation, share some rather distinct characteristics. Physicians and other health care specialists use these characteristics and other information as a basis for diagnosing and treating these children. Unfortunately, there is no consistent use of a standardized set of criteria for determining the nature and severity of behavior disorders (Forness, 1988; Kavale, Forness, & Alper, 1986; Swartz, Mosley, & Koenig-Jerz, 1987). If valid eligibility and classification systems did exist, they would provide educational or psychiatric clinicians with extremely valuable information about the nature of various conditions, effective treatments, and associated complications.

The area of behavior disorders is broad and includes many different types of problems. Thus it is not surprising that many approaches have been used to classify them. Some classification systems describe individuals according to statistically derived categories. Patterns of behavior that are strongly related to each other are identified through sophisticated statistical techniques. Other classification systems are clinically oriented. They are derived from the experiences of physicians and other social scientists who work directly with children and adults with behavior disorders. Still other classification systems help us understand behavior disorders in terms of their relative severity.

Statistically Derived Classification Systems.　For a number of years researchers have collected information about children with behavior disorders (Ackerson, 1942; Hewitt & Jenkins, 1946; Peterson, 1961; Quay, 1972, 1975). Data collected from parent and teacher questionnaires, interviews, and behavior rating scales have been analyzed using a variety of advanced statistical techniques. Certain clusters or patterns of related behaviors have emerged from these studies. For example, Peterson found that the behavior problems exhibited by elementary school children could be accounted for by two dimensions—withdrawal and aggression. Similarly, several researchers have intensively studied child psychiatric patients to develop a valid classification system (Achenbach, 1966; Achenbach & Edelbrock, 1981). Statistical analysis of data generated from these studies revealed two broad clusters of behaviors: externalizing symptoms and internalizing symptoms. Externalizing clusters of behaviors included stealing, lying, disobedience, and fighting. Internalizing clusters of behaviors included physical complaints (such as stomachaches), phobias, fearfulness, social withdrawal, and worrying.

Other researchers (Quay, 1975, 1979; Von Isser, Quay, & Love, 1980), using similar methodologies, have reliably identified four distinct categories of behavior disorders in children and adolescents:

1. **Conduct disorders** involve such characteristics as overt aggression, both verbal and physical; disruptiveness; negativism; irresponsibility; and defiance of authority—all of which are at variance with the behavioral expectations of the school and other social institutions.

2. **Anxiety-withdrawal** stands in considerable contrast to conduct disorders, involving, as it does, overanxiety, social withdrawal, seclusiveness, shyness, sensitivity, and other behaviors implying a retreat from the environment rather than a hostile response to it.

3. **Immaturity** characteristically involves preoccupation, short attention span, passivity, daydreaming, sluggishness, and other behavior not in accord with developmental expectations.

4. **Socialized aggression** typically involves gang activities, cooperative stealing, truancy, and other manifestations of participation in a delinquent subculture (Von Isser, Quay, & Love, 1980, pp. 272–73).

Behaviors related to each of these categories may be very severe to very mild in nature. In thinking about these categories, recall for a moment the vignettes of Steve, Cherie, and Jan. How would they be classified according to these categories? Did Steve have a conduct disorder? Was Cherie's refusal to go to school and her other related behaviors an anxiety-withdrawal disorder? And what about Jan's behavior? Does she qualify for placement in any of these categories?

Clinically Derived Classification Systems. Several clinically derived classification systems have been developed; however, the major system used by medical and psychological personnel is the *American Psychiatric Association Diagnostic and Statistical Manual of Mental Disorders, Third Edition, Revised* (DSM-III-R). It was developed and tested for its usefulness by groups and committees of psychiatric, psychological, and health care professionals. Participants on each of these teams were persons who served or worked closely with children, youths, and adults with behavior disorders. The categories and subcategories of the DSM-III (American Psychiatric Association, 1980) were developed after years of investigation and field testing. The DSM-III was preceded by earlier publications of the DSM-I in 1952 and DSM-II in 1968. The current manual, DSM-III-R (American Psychiatric Association, 1987), identifies nine major groups of disorders that may be exhibited by infants, children, or adolescents. They include:

I. Developmental Disorders
  A. Mental Retardation
    1. Mild Mental Retardation
    2. Moderate Mental Retardation
    3. Severe Mental Retardation
    4. Profound Mental Retardation
    5. Unspecified Mental Retardation
  B. Pervasive Developmental Disorders
    1. Autistic Disorder
    2. Pervasive Developmental Disorder Not Otherwise Specified
  C. Specific Developmental Disorders
    1. Academic Skill Disorders
    2. Language and Speech Disorders
    3. Motor Skills Disorder
II. Disruptive Behavior Disorders
  A. Attention-Deficit Hyperactivity Disorder
  B. Conduct Disorder
  C. Oppositional-Defiant Disorder
III. Anxiety Disorders of Childhood or Adolescence
  A. Separation Anxiety Disorder
  B. Avoidant Disorder of Childhood or Adolescence
  C. Overanxious Disorder
IV. Eating Disorders
  A. Anorexia Nervosa
  B. Bulimia Nervosa
  C. Pica
  D. Rumination Disorder of Infancy

Reflect on This 5–1

Internal Suffering: Shyness

We have talked about external versus internal disorders. One of the conditions associated with internal disorders is extreme shyness. What does it feel like to be extremely shy? How does shyness affect an individual? Shirley Radl shares with us what it is like to feel shy even as a mother.

Having personally suffered from shyness in varying degrees nearly all of my life, I know full well how it got started—skinny, homely little girl, skinnier and homelier teenager—and know all too well that neither the shyness researchers nor those I've interviewed exaggerated how really awful and crazy it feels. I have known what it is to, no matter what the circumstance, feel self-conscious of my every gesture, have trouble swallowing and talking, see my hands tremble for no apparent reason, feel as if I were freezing to death while perspiring profusely, be confused about issues I am thoroughly familiar with, and imagine all sorts of terrible things that might happen to me—the least of which being that I would lose my job for being a public disgrace.

I have experienced dizzy spells and twitching when in the company of absolutely nonthreatening men, women, and children. I've known what it is to avoid going to the grocery store because I couldn't face the checker, to become excessively nervous while chatting with the man who delivers the milk, or to be unable to tolerate the watchful gaze of my children's friends while making popcorn for them. I have known what it is like to have the feeling that I was stumbling naked through life with the whole thing being broadcast internationally. . . . (Radl, 1976, as cited by Zimbardo, 1978, p. 24)

V. Gender Identity Disorders
 A. Gender Identity Disorder of Childhood
 B. Transsexualism
 C. Gender Identity Disorder of Adolescence or Adulthood, Nontranssexual Type

VI. Tic Disorders
 A. Tourette's Disorder
 B. Chronic Motor or Vocal Tic Disorder
 C. Transient Tic Disorder

VII. Elimination Disorders
 A. Functional Encopresis
 B. Functional Enuresis

VIII. Speech Disorders Not Elsewhere Classified
 A. Cluttering
 B. Stuttering

IX. Other Disorders of Infancy, Childhood, or Adolescence
 A. Elective Mutism
 B. Identity Disorder

C. Reactive Attachment Disorder of Infancy or Early Childhood

D. Stereotypy/Habit Disorder

E. Undifferentiated Attention-Deficit Disorder

Some of the DSM-III-R categorical groups for infants, children, and adolescents overlap with other exceptionalities. For example, children and youth who exhibit Developmental Disorders may also be identified as retarded, autistic, and learning disabled. We now explore some of the more prevalent disorders that have been identified in the DSM-III-R.

Developmental Disorders. For a moment let us examine one of the conditions identified as a developmental disorder. Autism has received increased attention during the past several years, by both researchers and the media, with movies such as 1988's "Rain Man," which starred Dustin Hoffman as an adult with autism. One of the essential features of autism is a lack of social responsiveness to others. Imagine being the parent of a young infant who is completely non-responsive to your nurturing. When you pick up your new baby son, he tells

Dustin Hoffman won an Academy Award for his performance as Raymond, a man with autism, in 1988's *Rain Man.* (Wide World Photos)

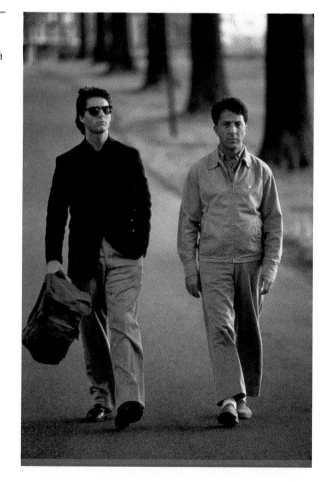

you in no uncertain physical terms that he does not enjoy being held. He arches his back, turns his head away from you and says, in effect, "Put me down! Get away from me! I don't want to look at you! I don't want you to talk to me!" Infants with autism do not enjoy the holding, cuddling, and nurturing behaviors that are so readily received by most normal infants. Inconsolable or unexplained crying, fascination with spinning objects, complete lack of language or very limited language, repetitive hand movements, and bizarre responses to certain stimuli are only a few of the characteristic behaviors of children with autism.

Disruptive Behavior Disorders. Classifications identified in the Disruptive Behavior Disorders category correspond to some of the clusters of behavior identified earlier in the statistically derived classification system. The first condition is **Attention-Deficit Hyperactivity Disorder,** or ADHD. It is closely related to the Immaturity category of the statistically derived classification system. Children with this disorder have difficulty attending to and completing tasks, responding carefully and reflectively to academic and social tasks, and controlling or restricting their level of physical activity. In fact, often their activity appears to be very random or purposeless in nature. These behaviors are also characteristic of some children with learning disabilities.

Now let us examine the second condition found within the Disruptive Behavior Disorders category, conduct disorders. Does Steve, the young boy described in our first vignette, meet the prerequisites for this condition as defined by the DSM-III-R?

Diagnostic Criteria for Conduct Disorder

A. A disturbance of conduct lasting at least six months, during which at least three of the following have been present:
   (1) has stolen without confrontation of a victim on more than one occasion (including forgery)
   (2) has run away from home overnight at least twice while living in parental or parental-surrogate home (or once without returning)
   (3) often lies (other than to avoid physical or sexual abuse)
   (4) has deliberately engaged in fire-setting
   (5) is often truant from school (for older person, absent from work)
   (6) has broken into someone else's house, building, or car
   (7) has deliberately destroyed other's property (other than by fire-setting)
   (8) has been physically cruel to animals
   (9) has forced someone into sexual activity with him or her
   (10) has used a weapon in more than one fight
   (11) often initiates physical fights
   (12) has stolen with confrontation of a victim (e.g., mugging, purse-snatching, extortion, armed robbery)
   (13) has been physically cruel to people
   Note: The above items are listed in descending order of discriminating power based on data from a national field trial of the DSM-III-R criteria for Disruptive Behavior Disorders.
B. If 18 or older, does not meet criteria for Antisocial Personality Disorder.

Criteria for Severity of Conduct Disorder:

Mild: Few if any conduct problems in excess of those required to make the diagnosis, and conduct problems cause only minor harm to others.

Reflect on This 5-2

What's It Like?

Siblings of autistic children experience a variety of challenges in growing up with a sister or brother who is severely disturbed. Following are a number of excerpts that have been written by siblings of autistic children and teenagers (Sullivan, 1979):

My Brother, Eddie

As soon as we got to her house, Eddie insisted that he be allowed to walk around outside. We didn't think that would be too good an idea, so we said no. Eddie didn't think that was a good idea, so he ran out anyway. My father and I spent the next thirty-five minutes chasing him all over the scenic routes of Brentwood. We finally caught him with the help of local police and had him back in our station wagon. I sat with him so that he would not hit my dad while he was driving. During the whole ride back, he went through a series of emotional straits—first violently upset, then sobbing, then screaming and swinging at dad, then crying again. (p. 289)

For the Sake of Others

My parents were very helpful in assisting us to readjust our "normal" expectations. It was a good meal if Chris ate half of his strained bananas without screaming and spitting. I remember the day that Chris finally held his bottle by himself. The pride I took in his accomplishment could not be dampened by the fact that at his age other children had long been weaned from bottles and were drinking from cups. Living with Chris made us aware of the little things one hardly ever notices. "Chris put his chair up to the sink today to climb and play in the water!" "Mom, he's watching me change the rec-

---

Moderate: Number of conduct problems and effect on others intermediate between "mild" and "severe."

Severe: Many conduct problems in excess of those required to make the diagnosis, or conduct problems cause considerable harm to others, e.g., serious physical injury to victims, extensive vandalism or theft, prolonged absence from home. (*American Psychiatric Association: Diagnostic and Statistical Manual of Mental Disorders*, Third Edition, Revised, 1987, p. 55)

Actually, we probably have not provided you with sufficient information about Steve for you to make an informed choice about his classification; however, if you had access to all the information in Steve's file, the choice would be very clear. He would be identified as conduct disordered.

Anxiety Disorders. The Anxiety Disorders of Childhood or Adolescence category is very similar to the Anxiety-Withdrawal category of the statistically derived classification system. Children with Anxiety Disorders have problems dealing with anxiety-provoking situations. They also may have problems separating themselves from parents or other attachment figures (e.g., close friends, teachers, coaches, etc.). Unrealistic worries about future events, overconcern about achievement, excessive need for reassurance, and somatic complaints are characteristic of young people who have anxiety disorders. Cherie, our junior high student, suffered from an anxiety disorder.

ord!" "Today when I put his coat on, he helped put one arm in!" "He raised his arms so I could pick him up today!" We quickly learned the meaning and value of individual differences. (p. 292)

Ben

We were walking home from school, she and I, and the discussion was focused on my unusual little brother. Unusual, that is, to everyone else. To me, he was just my little brother. Since I only had one, he was unique, regardless of his other qualities. Anyhow, my friend asked me why my

brother did not talk yet, as he was almost five years old. I thought for a moment and said, very seriously, "Well, he only speaks French and none of us can speak or understand French, so it presents a terrible problem." She nodded with a vague comprehension of the "problem." I chuckled all the way home. We were in the fourth grade. (p. 293)

Sibling of a Handicapped Child

I have often wished that my brother were normal. Since we are the only two children that my parents have, I really can't imagine what it would be like

to have a true brother—one that you could talk to about special things or share secrets with, as most siblings do. I guess that is why all during my school years, and even now, I tend to be closer to guys, platonically of course, than to girls. They provide me with a brother or a reasonable facsimile. (p. 295)

Source: From Ruth Christ Sullivan, Ph.D., Editor, "Parents Speak" column, *Journal of Autism and Developmental Disorders*, 9(3), 1979, pp. 287–297.

Eating Disorders. The fourth category, Eating Disorders, provides information about **anorexia nervosa** and **bulimia nervosa**. These conditions are evidenced by gross disturbances in eating behavior. In the case of anorexia nervosa, the most distinguishing feature is body weight that is 15 percent below that which is expected. Bulimia is characterized by repeated episodes of binging, followed by self-induced vomiting or other extreme measures to prevent weight gain.

Gender Identity Disorders. Gender identity disorders were not a part of the previous DSM classification system for infants, children, and youth. At the heart of these disorders is an incongruence between the youth's perception of his or her biologically assigned sex and his or her gender identity.

Tic Disorders. Tic Disorders, the sixth category, involve stereotyped movements or vocalizations that are involuntary, rapid, and recurrent over time. Tics may take the form of eye-blinking, facial gestures, sniffing, snorting, repeating certain words or phrases, and grunting. Stress often exacerbates the nature and frequency of tics.

Elimination Disorders. Elimination disorders deal with soiling and wetting behaviors in older children. Children who continue to have consistent problems with bowel and bladder control past their fourth or fifth birthdays may be diagnosed as having an elimination disorder, particularly if the condition is not a function of any physical disorder.

Speech and Other Disorders. The remaining categories in the DSM-III-R refer to speech and other disorders that are not easily placed in other categorical areas. We briefly review two conditions identified in these categories. **Elective mutism** is a persistent refusal to talk in typical social and school environments. This disorder is really quite rare, occurring less than 1 percent of the time in psychiatric referrals. Identity disorders are characterized by severe stress and uncertainty about one's goals, values, social relationships, sexual orientation, and religious preference. This condition generally surfaces in late adolescence or young adulthood, when individuals are moving away from their families and forming relationships with others.

The older DSM-III classification system has been criticized by a number of professionals and researchers (McLeMore & Benjamin, 1979; Schacht & Nathan,

TABLE 5–1 Characteristics of Children Who Exhibit Maladaptive Behavior

Definition	Mildly Disturbed	Severely Disturbed	Comment
Intellectual or cognitive ability: as measured by a standardized intelligence test.	Average IQ score in low-normal or dull-normal range.	Average IQ in mentally retarded range.	Actual range for both groups is from retarded to gifted.
Achievement: as measured by achievement test scores predominantly in reading and arithmetic.	Generally achieve at a lower level than their IQ level would imply. Children classified as conduct disordered or delinquents further behind than other categories.	Markedly deficient in academic areas. Generally function at basic levels in language, toileting, eating, rudimentary reading, and math.	Both levels range the spectrum, but most are generally below average. Any seriously disturbed high achievers are usually erratic in responding.
Underselectivity: difficulty focusing on relevant stimuli and screening out irrelevant stimuli. *Overselectivity:* attention to limited aspects of a task, lacks ability to zero out.	Difficulty focusing on task at hand. Tend to be underselective.	Tend to be overselective. Often exhibit "gaze aversion," will not make or maintain eye contact.	Both levels as a group have attending problems; however, research indicates that the type of attending problem may be different depending on the seriousness of the emotional disturbance.
Hyperactivity: inability to modulate motor behavior in accordance with the demands of a situation. *Impulsivity:* quick, almost instantaneous response to stimulation.	Frequently exhibit hyperactivity and impulsivity.	Frequently exhibit hyperactivity and impulsivity.	Reflectivity, the tendency to look, think, and consider alternatives, is the reverse of impulsivity.

1979; Harris, 1979; Harris & Achenbach, 1980), but it is a vast improvement over the previous systems (DSM-I and DSM-II) developed earlier by the American Psychiatric Association. The DSM-III-R reflects a new emphasis on the importance of data gathered from field trials in constructing valid and reliable criteria for mental disorders.

Classification According to Severity of Behaviors. Various researchers have attempted to differentiate mild-to-moderate behavior disorders from severe problems. As you might expect, the behavioral characteristics of individuals with severe disorders are identified more easily than those associated with mild disorders. Stainback and Stainback (1980) contrasted the characteristics of individuals with mild and severe disturbances. As illustrated in Table 5–1, severely disordered children differ significantly from those with mild disorders in a variety of intellectual, social, academic, and behavioral domains.

Persons who exhibit severe behavior disorders are often described as psychotic, crazy, or insane. **Psychosis** is a general term. The DSM-III-R uses such terms as pervasive developmental disorders, schizophrenia, and others to refer to infants, children, youths, and adults that are psychotic or very seriously disturbed. The

Definition	Mildly Disturbed	Severely Disturbed	Comment
Withdrawal: includes withdrawal from human contact and/or general overall withdrawal of interest in the environment.	May consistently refrain from initiating conversation, refrain from play with others, or exhibit lack of concern or interest in the environment— shy, immature, wallflower, but not oblivious to surroundings.	May lack contact with reality and subsequently develop own world— often called autistic, schizophrenic, psychotic.	Depression is sometimes associated with withdrawal.
Physical aggression: destructive actions against self and other people and things. *Verbal aggression:* includes yelling, cursing, abusive language, threats and self-destructive statements.	May be obnoxious, negative, oppositional, and/or generally nasty. Generally *not* violent, brutal, destructive, assaultive, or physically damaging to others and self.	May frequently, consistently over a long period of time, display aggressive behaviors of a serious nature.	"Normal" children also display aggressive behaviors, but usually less onerous and at a lower rate.
Helplessness: does not appear to be interested in trying to do anything, does not set goals for self, often does not respond to assigned tasks.	May exhibit lack of joy and interest in life, fail to perform tasks previously exhibited, unwillingness to try, tends to give up quickly.	May be highly dependent, pessimistic, and suicidal; may be unable to perform basic life skills.	Teacher's task is to provide appropriate training that is based on the level the child is actually functioning.

Source: Reprinted, by permission of the authors and the publisher, from S. Stainback and W. Stainback, *Educating Children with Severe Maladaptive Behaviors* (New York: Grune & Stratton, 1980), pp. 26–27.

following statements reflect the views of teachers of children with severe behavior disorders about severely disturbed children:

1. A residential center is the best placement for most of these children.
2. These children are often classified as autistic or schizophrenic.
3. These children usually show no social interest in relating to others.
4. These children are most often multihandicapped.
5. The problems of this group of children are more likely to be genetically or organically based (Olson, Algozzine, & Schmid, 1980; p. 100).

Work completed by Newcomer (1980) also helps us understand other important features of severe behavior disorders (see Table 5–2). One of these parameters is an insight index, which relates to the child's awareness or understanding of his or her behavior problems. Is the child aware of the behavioral deviance, and does he or she understand the reasons for the behavior and its impact on self, family, and others? Another parameter of similar importance is the conscious-control dimension, which relates to whether the child makes an attempt to control the behavior problem and the degree to which such attempts are successful. These parameters and others are particularly helpful to professionals and parents who are responsible for referring a student for further evaluation. In the next section, we examine the prevalence of behavior disorders.

TABLE 5–2 Criteria for Determining Degree of Disturbance

	Degree of Disturbance		
Criteria	**Mild**	**Moderate**	**Severe**
Precipitating events	Highly stressful	Moderately stressful	Not stressful
Destructiveness	Not destructive	Occasionally destructive	Usually destructive
Maturational appropriateness	Behavior typical for age	Some behavior typical for age	Behavior too young or too old
Personal functioning	Cares for own needs	Usually cares for own needs	Unable to care for own needs
Social functioning	Usually able to relate to others	Usually unable to relate to others	Not able to relate to others
Reality Index	Usually sees events as they are	Occasionally sees events as they are	Little contact with reality
Insight Index	Aware of behavior	Usually aware of behavior	Usually not aware of behavior
Conscious control	Usually can control behavior	Occasionally can control behavior	Little control over behavior
Social responsiveness	Usually acts appropriately	Occasionally acts appropriately	Rarely acts appropriately

Source: From Phyllis L. Newcomer, *Understanding and Teaching Emotionally Disturbed Children*, p. 111. Copyright © 1980 by Allyn and Bacon. Reprinted with permission.

Steven was two and a half years old when our daughter, Katherine, was born. This is the time when I seriously began to search for help. I knew something was wrong shortly after Steve's birth. But when I tried to describe the problem, no one seemed to understand what I was saying. In spite of chronic ear infections, Steve looked very healthy, and his coordination was good. He was slow in developing language, but that could easily be attributed to his ear trouble. Since he was our first baby, I thought that maybe we just weren't very good parents.

Katherine's infancy was like a revelation to me. Everything she did made some kind of sense. I could pretty much tell what she wanted when she cried. When she was happy, she smiled and cooed at me. She put up her arms to be picked up. She understood a lot of what I said even before she could speak.

This was in sharp contrast to Steve's behavior. He screamed most of the time from birth until four years of age. He was virtually inconsolable. He didn't seem to understand when we spoke to him, and he couldn't tell us what he wanted.

We determined that Steven was afraid of certain sounds, such as those made by bathroom ventilating fans. This fear seriously affected our ability to take him anywhere. Often, when we would enter a public restroom, Steve would immediately resist because of the fan noise. We would then turn off the fan by turning off the light switch. This only made things worse, for he wouldn't enter a dark bathroom. Tantrums were often a part of the restroom experience. Rarely were these rooms truly *rest*rooms. Yes, Steven had a need to use the restrooms, but there was no way that he would dare enter many of them. Dilemmas like these are commonplace in my life with Steven.

Steven is now fourteen years old. He has had counseling and therapy for many years. He achieves above grade level in academics, but he still lacks the ability to relate meaningfully with others. Because of this inability, Steve has severe and chronic social problems that may limit his life as an adult.

Sheri, *Steve's Mother*

WINDOW 5–1

Comment from a Mother Regarding Her Son, Steve

PREVALENCE

Estimates of the **prevalence** of behavior disorders vary greatly from one source to the next, ranging from 0.05 to 15.0 percent. The U.S. Office of Education estimated that 2 percent of the children in the country have behavior disorders. However, Bower (1982) indicated that "approximately 10% of children in school have moderate to severe emotional problems" (p. 60). Approximately two to four out of every 10,000 children exhibit some form of severe behavior disorder.

Kelly, Bullock, and Dykes (1977) provided some prevalence figures from an educational perspective, which were also cast according to the severity of the condition. They employed three classifications: mild, moderate, and severe. Approximately 20 percent of the students in this study were identified by their teachers as exhibiting behavior disorders. Among these youngsters, 12.6 percent were judged to be mildly disordered, 5.6 percent were classified in the moderate category, and 2.2 percent were put in the severe category.

Kauffman (1985) suggested that 6 to 10 percent of the school-age population need specialized services because of behavior disorders. Other specialists would suggest that as many as 33 percent of school-age children experience behavior problems during any given year (Cullinan & Epstein, 1986). Of this number, about a third need the assistance provided by personnel outside the typical classroom. Another third of this number need special education and related services.

Behavior disorders are not a randomly distributed phenomenon. Referral rates for very young children (preschool through the primary grades) are quite low (Redick, 1973). By contrast, the rate increases dramatically during the preadolescent and adolescent years (Morse, Cutler, & Fink, 1964). Clarizio and McCoy (1976) suggested that these differences in rates between young and older children may be a function of referral policies rather than age itself.

Behavior disorders are not equally distributed between the sexes either. Males outnumber females at least two to one (Kelly, Bullock, & Dykes, 1977). In addition, researchers have found that boys, particularly during the school years, are at far greater risk for developing behavior disorders than are girls (Schultz, Salvia, & Feinn, 1974). However, the ratio of males and females becomes more nearly equal as they reach the young adult years. During the 1987–1988 school year, about 9 percent of all the special education students in the United States were identified and served in the behavior disorders category (U.S. Department of Education, 1989). From 1987 to 1988, the number of behavior disordered students served in special education settings grew by a mere .7 percent (U.S. Department of Education, 1989).

As we can readily see, the growth of programs for youth with behavior disorders has occurred rapidly during the past several years. However, there are still many children and youth who need specialized services but are not yet receiving them (Kauffman, 1987). This is particularly true in rural and remote areas throughout the United States.

CHARACTERISTICS

Intelligence

FOCUS 6
What are five general characteristics (intellectual, adaptive, and achievement) of children and adolescents with behavior disorders?

Researchers from a variety of disciplines have studied the intellectual capacity of individuals with behavior disorders. In an early national study of disturbed children enrolled in public school programs, the majority of these students exhibited above-average intelligence (Morse, Cutler, & Fink, 1964). However, other research, conducted more recently, reveals a different picture. Rubin and Balow (1978) studied three groups of disturbed children. The first group was composed of students who had been referred and identified as disturbed by medical or psychological personnel but not by their teachers. Their average IQs on two separate intelligence tests were 109 and 107. The second group of students, who were consistently referred and identified by teachers, had IQs of 96 and 92 on the same measures. The last group, who were sporadically identified as having difficulties by teachers, had average IQs of 102 on both tests of intelligence. Bower (1982) compared the IQs of disturbed children to those of normal children. He found that disturbed children had average IQs of 92, whereas the normal children had average IQs of 103.

Studies dealing with children who have been identified as psychotic reveal still another picture of intellectual functioning. Researchers have found that the majority of these children have IQs in the retarded range of functioning (Kauffman, 1985; Freeman & Ritvo, 1984). Of course, some of these children do have average or above-average IQs but they are in the minority.

The preponderance of evidence leads us to the conclusion that disturbed children tend to have average to lower-than-average IQs compared to their normal peers (Coleman, 1986). Additionally, children with severe behavior disorders tend to have IQs that fall within the retarded range of functioning. These inferences closely parallel the conclusions reached by Kauffman (1985).

What impact does intelligence have on the educational and social-adaptive performance of children with behavior disorders? What do you think? Is a disturbed child's intellectual capacity a good predictor of other types of achievement and social behavior? The answer is yes. Kauffman (1985) believes that "the IQs of disturbed children appear to be the best single predictor of academic and future social achievement" (p. 143). The below-average IQs of many disturbed children contribute significantly to the challenges that they experience in mastering academic and social tasks in school and other environments. In the next section, we examine the adaptive behavior of children and youth with behavior disorders.

Adaptive Behavior

Individuals with behavior disorders exhibit a variety of problems in adapting to their homes, schools, and community environments. Furthermore, they have difficulties in relating socially and responsibly to persons such as peers, parents, teachers, and other authority figures.

Listening, asking for teacher assistance, bringing materials to class, following directions, completing assignments, and ignoring distractions are some of the school-related, adaptive behaviors that do not come naturally to disturbed children. In addition, these behaviors may not have been successfully taught to these children. Socially, they may have difficulty introducing themselves, beginning and ending conversations, sharing, playing typical age-appropriate games, and apologizing. They may be unable to deal appropriately with situations that produce strong feelings such as anger and frustration. Recall Cherie's difficulty in dealing with fears and frustrations, which profoundly influenced her desire to stay out of school.

Social problem solving, accepting consequences of misbehavior, negotiating, expressing affection, and reacting appropriately to failure are behaviors that are not generally part of a disturbed child's repertoire. Because children with behavior disorders have deficits in these adaptive-social behaviors, they frequently experience difficulties in meeting the demands of the classroom or other environments in which they must participate. Steve, the aggressive boy described in our first vignette, experienced many difficulties in accepting the consequences of behavior, dealing with strong feelings, and expressing affection. Cherie's refusal to go to school was directly related to her deficits in coping with her first week of junior high school. Jan's problems surfaced much later in her school career. It was a deterioration of her adaptive skills that caused her significant problems in completing her schooling and maintaining her relationships with friends and others.

Earlier in the classification section, we talked about statistically derived categories of behaviors that were common to children and adolescents with behavior disorders. You may recall the categories: conduct disorder, anxiety-withdrawal, immaturity, and socialized aggression. Conduct disordered children engage in verbal and physical aggression, are disruptive, negative and irresponsible, and defy authority. Children who are characterized as being anxious and withdrawn exhibit behaviors such as anxiety, social withdrawal, seclusiveness, and shyness. Children who exhibit the behaviors associated with the immaturity dimension have difficulty attending to tasks, particularly academic ones, tend to daydream, and respond to learning tasks in a very lethargic fashion. Gang activities, drug abuse, cooperative stealing, truancy, and other delinquent acts characterize youths who are identified as socialized aggressives. They relate well with each other, but engage in antisocial acts that are offensive to the communities in which they take place. It is easy to see how the behaviors associated with these categories are maladaptive and how they interfere with school and family success. Moreover, we can see how gang activities and cooperative stealing on the part of youths would antagonize and agitate community members who are affected by these behaviors.

A number of researchers (Safer & Heaton, 1982; Whalen, 1983) have found that children who frequently display behaviors associated with hyperactivity, distractibility, and impulsiveness have problems in developing friendships and achieving satisfactorily in school. Swift and Spivack (1973) investigated overt classroom behaviors of high school students and their relationship to academic achievement. They found that low achievers had difficulties in managing stress related to tests, were quiet and withdrawn in class, and rarely interacted with peers. Furthermore, they exhibited poor work habits, were inflexible and unreceptive to other's opinions, verbally negative with teachers and peers, unable to sit still, often involved in disturbing others, had to be controlled or reproved by the teacher, and expressed negative beliefs about themselves and the work load. Statements such as, "I can't do this stuff!" and "Why do you give us so much to do?" are representative of these negative beliefs. Although the researchers did not investigate the behavior of disturbed children per se, they clearly identified the behaviors that many disturbed children are likely to exhibit in normal classroom settings.

Severely and profoundly disturbed children (schizophrenic and psychotic) exhibit social and adaptive patterns of behaviors that closely parallel children who are moderately to severely retarded. They may need extensive assistance in developing self-help skills (such as toileting, grooming, dressing, and caring for themselves), language competency, and social skills that permit them to interact adequately with others in their home environments and elsewhere.

Academic Achievement

A variety of studies have been conducted to assess the academic characteristics of children with behavior disorders. Tamkin (1960) evaluated the achievement of children who had recently been institutionalized for behavior disorders. He found that 41 percent of the sample were academically advanced in comparison to their actual grade level, 27 percent were performing at grade level, and 32 percent were performing below grade level. Reading achievement for the disturbed children as a whole was significantly higher than their math performance. In a more recent study, Coutinho (1986) found a significant relationship between early reading achievement problems and eventual classification as behavior disordered, as well as continued subaverage performance in reading at the secondary level.

Other researchers have collected data that provide a different perspective of the academic characteristics of children with behavior disorders. Stone and Rowley (1964) evaluated children referred for psychiatric services on the basis of their chronological age. Of the 116 children tested, 20 percent were academically above average for their grade level, 21 percent were at grade level, and 59 percent were below grade level. Graubard (1964) investigated the achievement of institutionalized children in conjunction with their mental age, that is, their intellectual capacity as measured in years and months on an IQ test. In reading and math, these children were found to be severely disabled in relation to their mental ages.

Similar observations have been made by other researchers. Motto and Wilkins (1968) determined that forty-two out of the forty-eight children they assessed in a state mental hospital were severely behind in math and reading performance. More recent, large-scale studies (Bower, 1981) of disturbed and normal children revealed that disturbed students are significantly behind their peers in reading and math achievement. As a rule, the academic achievement of disturbed children is not on a par with their expected achievement as indicated by mental age. In fact, many disturbed students could be identified as **learning disabled** if the selection were based primarily on discrepancy scores (i.e., the difference between one's ability as represented by IQ scores and one's actual academic performance as represented by achievement test scores) (O'Donnell, 1980). This is particularly true for children who have mild to moderate disorders.

The picture is quite different, however, for children who are identified as schizophrenic or psychotic. Very few of them compare favorably to their peers in achievement. Severely disturbed youngsters are generally retarded, and as such their performance in areas such as math and reading is significantly substandard compared to normal children (Coleman, 1986; Kauffman, 1985). Next we examine the causes of behavior disorders and the theories that undergird them.

CAUSATION

Theoretical Perspective

Throughout history, philosophers, physicians, theologians, and others have attempted to explain why people behave as they do. Historically, the mentally disturbed were described as being possessed by evil spirits. It was presumed that the presence of evil spirits within these individuals made them behave the way they did. The treatment of choice at that time was religious in nature. Later, Sigmund Freud and others promoted the notion that behavior could be explained in terms of subconscious phenomena or early traumatic experiences. More recently, some theorists have attributed disordered behaviors to inappropriate learning

FOCUS 7
What can we accurately say about the causes of behavior disorders?

or complex interactions that take place between individuals and their environments. From a biological perspective, others have suggested that aberrant behaviors are caused by certain biochemical substances, brain abnormalities or injuries, or chromosomal irregularities.

With such a wealth of etiological explanations, it is easy to see why practitioners might choose different approaches to treating and preventing the various disorders. However, the variety of theoretical frameworks and perspectives provides clinicians with a number of choices for explaining the presence of certain behaviors. Kauffman (1977) stated, "The first or ultimate cause of behavior disorders almost always remains unknown. . . . The focus of the special educators' concern should be on those contributing factors that can be altered by the teacher" (p. 263). We believe that this statement also holds true for other professionals such as physicians, psychologists, social workers, and community planners. Table 5–3 provides an overview of etiologies and causal factors associated with various theoretical frameworks.

The Biological Approach.   The biological framework explains behavior disorders as a function of inherited or abnormal biological conditions within the body or injury to the central nervous system. Behavior problems presumably surface as a result of some physiological, biochemical, or genetic abnormality or disease.

TABLE 5–3   Etiologies and Causal Factors Associated with Behavior Disorders

Theoretical Framework	Etiologies/Causal Factors
Biological	Genetic inheritance Biochemical abnormalities Neurological abnormalities Injury to the central nervous system
Psychoanalytical	Psychological processes Functioning of the mind: id, ego, and superego Inherited predispositions (instinctual processes) Traumatic early-childhood experiences
Behavioral	Environmental events 1. Failure to learn adaptive behaviors 2. Learning of maladaptive behaviors 3. Developing maladaptive behaviors as a result of stressful environmental circumstances
Phenomenological	Faulty learning about oneself Misuse of defense mechanisms Feelings, thoughts, and events emanating from the self
Sociological/ecological	Role assignment (labeling) Cultural transmission Social disorganization Distorted communication Differential association Negative interactions and transactions with others

The Psychoanalytical Approach.   Subconscious processes, predispositions or instincts, and early traumatic experiences explain the presence of behavior disorders from a psychoanalytic perspective. The internal processes are unobservable events that occur in the mind among the well-known psychic constructs of the **id** (the drives component), **ego** (the reality component), and **superego** (the conscience component). As we gain insight into psychic conflicts by means of psychotherapy, we may be able to eliminate or to solve the problem behaviors. The return to normalcy may also be aided by a caring therapist or teacher. For children, this process theoretically occurs through play therapy, in which inner conflicts are revealed and subsequently resolved through family therapy and therapeutic play experiences with understanding adults.

The Behavioral Approach.   The behavioral approach focuses on aspects of the environment that produce, reward, diminish, or punish certain behaviors. Through treatment, adults and children are given opportunities to learn new adaptive behaviors by identifying realistic goals and receiving **reinforcement** for attaining these goals. Gradually, aberrant behaviors are eliminated or replaced by more appropriate ones.

The Phenomenological Approach.   From a phenomenological point of view, abnormal behaviors arise from feelings, thoughts, and past events tied to a person's self-perceptions or self-concepts. Faulty perceptions or feelings are thought to cause individuals to behave in ways that are counterproductive to self-fulfillment. Therapy using this approach is centered on helping people develop satisfactory perceptions and behaviors that are in agreement with self-selected values.

The Sociological-Ecological Approach.   The sociological-ecological model is by far the most encompassing explanation of behavior disorders. Aberrant behaviors are presumed to be caused by a variety of interactions and transactions with other people (Patterson & Bank, 1986; Ramsey & Walker, 1988). For some, the deviant behaviors are taught as a part of one's culture. For others, the behaviors are a function of labeling. Individuals labeled as juvenile delinquents, according to this perspective, gradually adopt the patterns of behavior that are associated with the assigned label. In addition, others who are aware of the label begin to treat the labeled individuals as if they were truly delinquent. Such treatment theoretically promotes the delinquent behavior. Another source of aberrant behavior associated with this model is differential association. This source of deviance is closely related to the cultural-transmission explanation of deviance: People exhibit behavior problems in an attempt to conform to the wishes and expectations of a group with which they wish to join or maintain affiliation. Finally, the sociological-ecological perspective views the presence of aberrant behavior as a function of a variety of interactions and transactions that are derived from a broad array of environmental settings.

Each of these models contributes different explanations for the causes of behavior disorders. Unfortunately, we are rarely able to isolate the exact cause of a child's behavior disorders, but we do have an understanding of many conditions and factors that contribute to disordered behavior. We concur with Wicks-Nelson and Israel (1984), who wrote: "With few if any exceptions, behavior can be explained only by multiple influences and their continuous interaction. A vast array of variables—biological structure and function, inheritance, cognition, social/emotional status, family, social class—can usually be expected to come into play" (p. xvii).

Family and home environments play a critical role in the emergence of behavior disorders. Poverty, malnutrition, increased homelessness, family discord, divorce, child-rearing practices, and child abuse have an impact on the behaviors we observe in youngsters (Gelfand, Jenson, & Drew, 1988). Young mothers who are malnourished during pregnancy are likely to give birth to low birth-weight babies. Babies weighing less than 4 pounds are at risk for developing a variety of handicapping conditions (attention deficit disorders, epilepsy, and other neurological disorders). Young mothers in impoverished environments are often single and inexperienced in child care. Others are experienced in child care but are frequently burdened with the survival tasks of providing food, clothing, and housing for themselves and their children. Little time may be available for stimulating and interacting with their young infants. Moreover, these mothers may have little energy at the end of the day to play and talk with their children. Lacking appropriate stimulation these children suffer intellectually, cognitively, socially, and emotionally (Perterson, 1987).

Family discord and divorce also play a role in the development of behavior disorders in some children. The impact of divorce on children is influenced by a variety of factors (age of the child, financial status of the family, gender of the child, amount of acrimony between the partners, etc.). Therefore, it is difficult to predict with great precision who will be severely affected by divorce. As a rule, boys appear to be more negatively influenced by divorce than are girls (Emery, Hetherington, & DiLalla, 1984). Girls who are affected often exhibit behaviors associated with anxiety and withdrawal. Boys, in contrast, exhibit aggressive and hyperactive behaviors (Guidubaldi, Perry, & Cleminshaw, 1984).

Child management and discipline procedures also play important roles in the development of behavior disorders. Children whose parents are extremely permissive, overly restrictive, and/or aggressive often produce children who are conduct disordered (Kazdin, 1985). Home environments that are devoid of consistent rules and consequences for child behavior; that are lacking in parental supervision; that reinforce aggressive behavior; and that have parents who model aggression and use aggressive child-management practices produce children who are very much at-risk for developing disruptive behavior disorders. Also, marital discord, family separation, and divorce are found more frequently in families of children and youths identified as having conduct disorders.

Child abuse, too, plays a major role in the development of aggression and other problematic behaviors in children and youths. Rogeness (1986) found that serious abuse during later childhood and adolescence was often accompanied by destructive, noncompliant, and aggressive behaviors. MacFarlane (1978) referred to sexual abuse as the "psychological time bomb." The bomb's impact is a function of several factors. These factors include the age at which the child or youth was abused, the degree of violence involved, the relationship of the abuser to the child or youth, the duration of the abuse, the response of parents and professionals to the abuse, and the degree of guilt or discomfort expressed by

WINDOW 5-2

*Comment from a
Parent of a
Severely Disturbed
Child Regarding
Causation*

When Steven was a baby, I attributed his problems to constant ear infections. When his speech did not develop normally, I thought he might have a hearing loss. But after he had tubes put in his ears, the infections cleared up and his hearing was normal.

When he was two and a half, we enrolled him in a diagnostic nursery school. He did not seem to understand us when we spoke. I wondered if he was retarded or had some other developmental problem. The nursery school gave us their opinion when he was four. They said he seemed to have normal intelligence, but he perseverated, was behind socially, and did not seem to process verbs. They said he had some signs of autism and some signs of a learning disability.

When Steve was four and a half, he did some amazing things. He began to talk, read, write, and play the piano. I was taking beginning adult piano lessons at the time. He could play everything I did. In fact, he could play any song he heard and he added chords with his left hand. Relatives and friends began to tell us that he was a genius and that accounted for his odd behavior. I really wanted to believe this genius theory, but it didn't fit with what I knew about gifted children.

I enrolled him in a public kindergarten at age five. The teacher had a theory about his strange behavior. She believed that we were not firm enough with him. She also sent the social worker to our home to see what we were doing with him.

I often wondered if we were just very poor parents. I certainly had enough people tell us so. Whenever I went to anyone for help, I was likely to begin crying. Then the doctor, or whoever, would start to watch my behavior closely. I could just see them forming a theory in their minds: the child is okay but the mother is a mess. I wondered if I was a very cold mother. Maybe I was subtly rejecting my son. Then again, maybe it was his father. My mother always said he didn't spend enough time with Steve. After all, she never saw them play ball together.

I didn't understand when the psychiatrist told me Steve had a pervasive developmental disorder. I began to get the picture when the words *psychotic* and *schizoidal* were mentioned. Something was terribly wrong, but it had a physical basis. It was not my fault at all. This was a relief and a tremendous blow. If I was doing something wrong, then I could possibly change and cure the problem. He was trying to tell me that Steve had a mental illness and there wasn't any cure.

It really helps to have a name for the problem. We used to wonder if Steve was lying awake nights dreaming up new ways to get our attention. We lived from crisis to crisis. We would just handle one problem to have a new one develop in its place. Steve still does bizarre things, but it doesn't send us into a panic. We just address the problem behavior with him and add it to his behavior chart. Sometimes we just adjust his medication.

Sheri, *Steve's Mother*

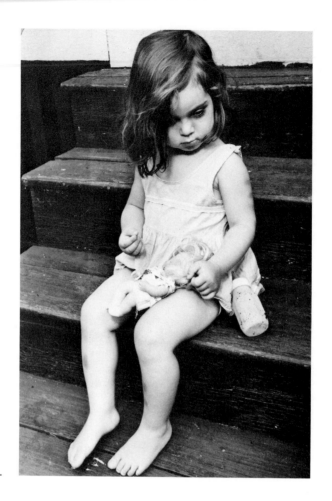

What long-term effects will abuse and neglect have on this child? (© Andrew Brilliant/The Picture Cube)

the affected child or youth. Most victims of sexual abuse are girls between the ages of 11 and 14. Very little research has been devoted to sexual abuse of males or its impact (Browne & Finkelhor, 1986).

ASSESSMENT

Screening and Referral

The first step in the assessment process is screening. The major purpose of **screening** is to identify infants, children, and youths who are most in need of treatment. Screening is also based on the belief that early identification leads to early treatment, which may lessen the overall impact of the behavior disorders on the individual and family. However, very few school systems or social agencies engage in any kind of grand-scale screening for behavior disorders. First, such a task is generally very expensive and time consuming. Most school systems and state social service agencies do not have sufficient financial or human resources to conduct systematic screening programs for behavior disorders. Furthermore, it is possible that many more children would be identified than could be adequately handled by a school system or social agency. However, research conducted in one statewide screening program has not confirmed this outcome (Smith, 1985).

In most school environments, children are considered for screening only after concerned or perplexed teachers have initiated referrals for them. For example, an experienced kindergarten teacher became very concerned about a boy named John. He was continually involved in a variety of behaviors atypical for his age. These included taking off his clothes, prolonged periods of crying without any apparent reason, and physically attacking children for no obvious reason. These behaviors and others prompted John's kindergarten teacher to take some action, not only with his parents but also with the principal.

The actual submission of a referral for a student is generally preceded by a number of parent–teacher conferences. The conferences help the teacher and parents determine what action ought to be taken. For example, the problems may be a symptom of family problems such as an extended parental illness, marital difficulties, or severe financial challenges. If the parents and teacher continue to be perplexed by a child's behavior, a referral may be initiated. Referrals are generally processed by principals, who review them, consult with parents, and then pass them on to a psychologist or assessment team leader.

Gropper and his colleagues (1968) have developed a means of helping teachers and others evaluate the seriousness of problematic behaviors of children. Using questions such as, "Is the behavior a reasonable response to the situation?," "How long does the behavior episode last?," and "How often does the behavior occur?" teachers are able to determine whether the challenging behaviors exhibited by children in their classrooms and other locations are basically normal, problematic, or referable (see Table 5–4). Think about a child whose behaviors have been a concern to you. Respond to the questions listed in Table 5–4 and determine whether you would refer the child based on your responses.

Once a referral has been appropriately processed and parental or guardian permission for testing and evaluation has been obtained, assessment team members proceed with the tasks of carefully observing and assessing a child's strengths and weaknesses. Their task is to determine whether the child has a behavior disorder and whether he or she qualifies for special education services. Furthermore, the team is responsible for identifying treatment strategies that may be helpful to the parents and teacher.

Factors in Assessment

The severity of behaviors such as those exhibited by the kindergartner, John, may be examined from several perspectives. First, it is necessary to determine whether any discrepancy exists between his chronological age and the behaviors he consistently displays. This is important in determining John's status in relationship to various norms. In addition to determining whether John's behaviors are age-appropriate, assessment team members must analyze the frequency of

FOCUS 8
What are four factors that need to be carefully assessed in determining whether or not a child has a behavior disorder?

TABLE 5–4   Criteria for Classifying Problem Behaviors

Description of Criteria	Normal	Problem	Referable
Intensity How disruptive of the child's other activities is the problem behavior?	*NONDISRUPTIVE* Behavior does not interfere with the child's other activities.	*DISRUPTIVE* Behavior interferes with the child's other activities.	*EXTREMELY DISRUPTIVE* Behavior completely disrupts child's other activities.
Appropriateness Is the behavior a reasonable response to the situation?	*REASONABLE* Response is acceptable or expected for the situation.	*INAPPROPRIATE* Response is undesirable for the situation.	*EXCESSIVE* Response is out of proportion to the situation.
Duration How long does the behavior episode last?	*SHORT-LIVED* Episode lasts only a short time (short time within a class period).	*MODERATELY LONG* Episode extends over a longer period (some carryover from one class to the next).	*LONG-LASTING* Episodes are long-lasting (greater part of a day).
Frequency How often does the behavior occur?	*INFREQUENT* Behavior usually is not repeated (rarely repeated in a day; rarely repeated on other days).	*FREQUENT* Behavior is repeated (may be repeated several times a day; may be repeated on several days).	*HABITUAL* Behavior happens all the time (repeated often during day; repeated on many days).
Specificity/generality In how many types of situations does the behavior occur?	*OCCURS IN SPECIFIC SITUATION* Behavior occurs in specific type of situation.	*OCCURS IN SEVERAL SITUATIONS* Behavior occurs in more than one type of situation.	*OCCURS IN MANY SITUATIONS* Behavior occurs in many types of situations.

problematic behaviors. They must assess how often his peculiar behaviors occur and under what circumstances. They must also determine if his inappropriate behaviors are related to specific activities or individuals, and whether his problems continue even after someone intervenes.

Assessment team members have the responsibility for evaluating the influence of his behaviors on classmates, teachers, and the family unit. Additionally, team members have an obligation to assess the teacher's contribution to the present problems (Slate & Saudargas, 1986). John's interactions with individuals in his school setting and his responses to his home environment significantly influence the recommendations that team members make regarding his classification, placement, and eventual treatment.

Techniques Used in Assessment

A variety of techniques are used to identify children with behavior disorders. These techniques closely parallel the theoretical framework or philosophical perspective of the evaluator. Usually an actual diagnosis of the behavioral problems is preceded by a set of screening procedures. Screening is done using behavior checklists or a variety of sociometric devices (such as peer ratings) and teacher

Description of Criteria	Normal	Problem	Referable
Manageability How easily does the behavior respond to management efforts?	EASILY MANAGED Responds readily to management efforts.	DIFFICULT TO MANAGE Inconsistent or slow response to management efforts.	CANNOT BE MANAGED Does not respond to management efforts.
Assessability of circumstances How easily can the circumstances that produced the behavior be identified?	EASILY ASSESSED Easy to identify situation or condition producing behavior.	DIFFICULT TO ASSESS Situation or condition producing behavior difficult to identify.	CANNOT BE ASSESSED Cannot identify situation or condition producing behavior.
Comparison with maturity level of class How close to the norm of the class is the problem behavior?	NO DEVIATION FROM LEVEL OF CLASS Behavior is par for the group.	BELOW LEVEL OF CLASS Behavior is below the group level.	CONSIDERABLY BELOW LEVEL OF CLASS Behavior is considerably below the group level.
Number of problem behaviors exhibited	Rarely more than one.	Usually more than one.	Usually many and varied.
Acceptance by peers Does the child have difficulty being accepted by peers?	ACCEPTED Is accepted by peers.	HAS DIFFICULTY GETTING ALONG May have difficulty with particular individuals.	NOT ACCEPTED Unaccepted by group.

Source: Reprinted, by permission, from G. Gropper, G. Kress, R. Hughes, and J. Pekich, "Training Teachers to Recognize and Manage Social and Emotional Problems in the Classroom," *Journal of Teacher Education,* 1968, *19,* 481.

rating scales. Information is collected about children's intellectual abilities as well as their academic achievement.

Bower and Lambert (1962) developed an extensive process for conducting in-school screening. Others have also developed rating scales for use in screening children with suspected behavior disorders (e.g., Achenbach, 1980, 1981; Burks, 1977; Long, Fagan, & Stevens, 1971; Spivack & Spotts, 1966; Spivack, Spotts, & Haimes, 1967; Spivack & Swift, 1967; Walker, 1983). Some of these rating scales provide measures of standard deviation that allow the clinician to compare the child's ratings to nonhandicapped students. For example, the Walker Problem Behavior Identification Checklist (Walker, 1983) provides five scales that describe various types of problem behavior: acting out, withdrawal, distractibility, disturbed peer relations, and immaturity. Each of these scales can be tabulated to represent a student's deviation from the mean (T-Score of 50) on a Profile Analysis Chart (see Figure 5–1). Students whose scores fall above a T-Score of 60 are considered to have serious behavior disorders. For instance, a female student who receives a rating of 3 on the acting-out scale would be considered average or normal in terms of aggressive behavior. In contrast, a female student with a rating of 16 on this scale would be considered for referral and further assessment, since such a score would fall well beyond two standard deviations from the mean on this measure.

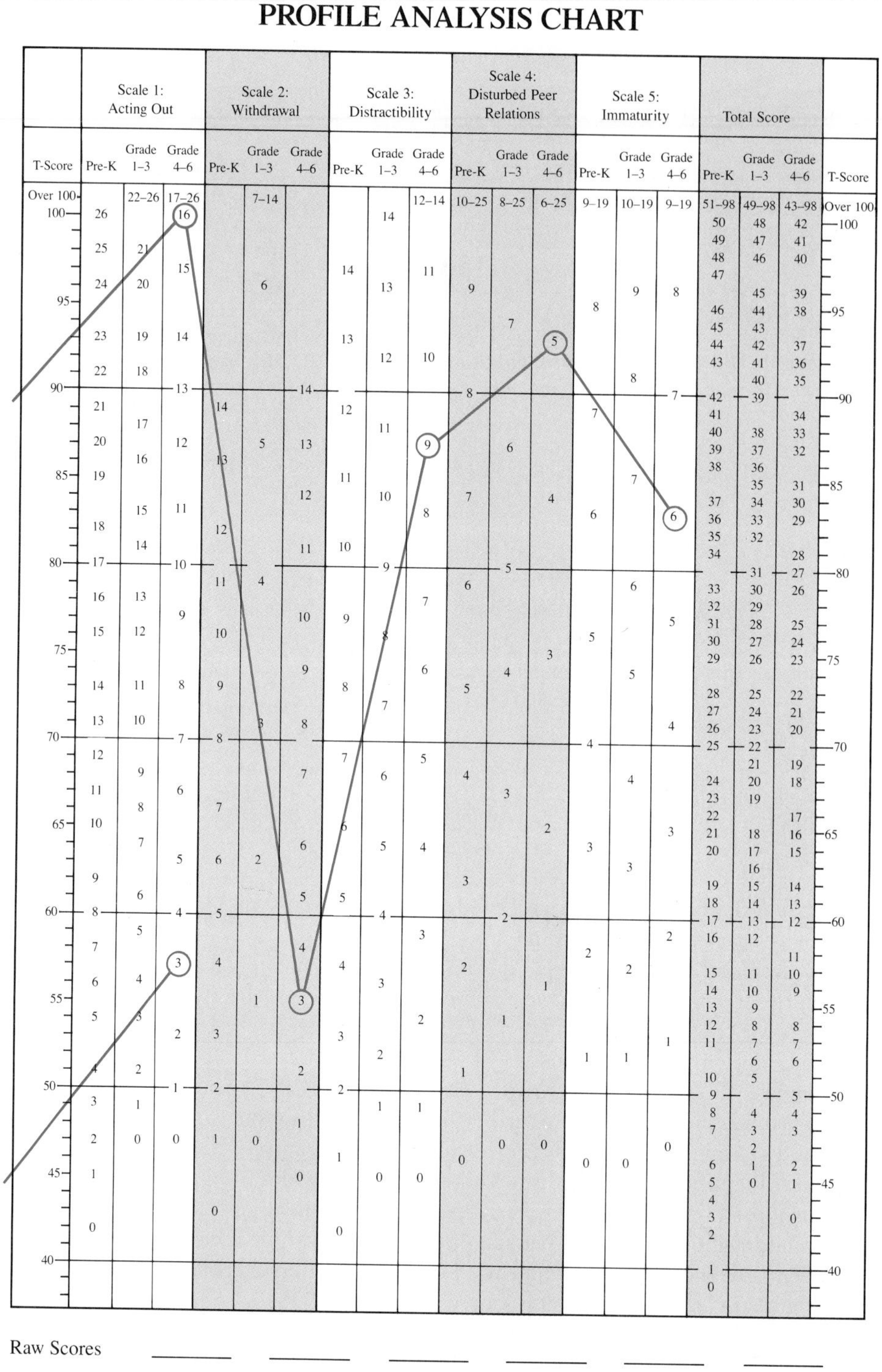

PROFILE ANALYSIS CHART

T-Score	Scale 1: Acting Out			Scale 2: Withdrawal			Scale 3: Distractibility			Scale 4: Disturbed Peer Relations			Scale 5: Immaturity			Total Score			T-Score
	Pre-K	Grade 1–3	Grade 4–6	Pre-K	Grade 1–3	Grade 4–6	Pre-K	Grade 1–3	Grade 4–6	Pre-K	Grade 1–3	Grade 4–6	Pre-K	Grade 1–3	Grade 4–6	Pre-K	Grade 1–3	Grade 4–6	
Over 100	26	22–26	17–26	7–14					12–14	10–25	8–25	6–25	9–19	10–19	9–19	51–98	49–98	43–98	Over 100
100	26		16					14								50	48	42	100
	25	21														49	47	41	
	24	20	15	6			14	13	11	9				9	8	48	46	40	
95											7		8			47	45	39	95
	23	19	14				13									46	44	38	
	22	18						12	10							45	43	37	
																44	42		
															5	43	41	36	
90	21		13	14		14	12			8				8		42	40	35	90
	20	17	12	13	5	13		11			6		7		7	41	39	34	
		16														40	38	33	
85	19		11	12		12	11	10		7		4		7		39	37	32	85
	18	15				11	10		8				6			38	36	31	
		14	10		4			9								37	35	30	
80	17			11					7	5			5	6	5	36	34	29	80
	16	13	9	10		10	9			6		3				35	33	28	
	15	12				9		7	6		4			5		34	32		
75	14	11	8	9	3		8	6		5					4	33	31	27	75
	13	10	7	8		8	7	5	5	4	3	2	4		3	32	30	26	
70	12	9		7		7			4					4		31	29	25	70
	11	8	6			6	6	4		3			3			30	28	24	
65	10	7	5	6	2	5	5	3	4		2	1		3	3	29	27	23	65
	9	6		5					3	2			2	2	2	28	26	22	
60	8	5	4	4	1	4	4	2			1					27	25	21	60
	7	4		3		3	3	1	2	1			1	1	1	26	24	20	
55	6	3	2		0	2			1		0					25	23	19	55
	5	2	1	2		1	2	0	0	0		0	0	0	0	24	22	18	
50	4	1	0	1		0	1									23	21	17	50
	3	0		0	0		0									...	...	...	
45	2																		45
	1																		
40	0																		40

Raw Scores _____ _____ _____ _____ _____ _____

Figure 5–1

Profile Analysis Chart (PAC) (*Source:* H. M. Walker, *Walker Problem Behavior Identification Checklist, revised 1983.* Copyright © 1970, 1976, 1983 by Western Psychological Services. Reprinted by permission of the publisher, Western Psychological Services, 12031 Wilshire Blvd., Los Angeles, Calif. 90025.)

Spivack et al. (1966; 1967) also developed a number of rating scales for evaluating the behaviors of children and youths, which can be summarized using profiles. An example drawn from the Devereaux Child Behavior (DCB) Rating Scale (Spivack & Spotts, 1966) illustrates their approach to reporting scores in deviation units. Ratings on this instrument are accomplished in a straight-forward fashion. The rater is given a listing of various descriptive statements such as the following:

Compared to normal children, *how often does the child*

Item 8:   Have a fixed facial expression that lacks feeling?

Item 16: Appear completely inactive and lethargic?

Item 32: Have a blank stare or faraway look in the eyes?

Item 34: Daydream?

Item 35: Look unhappy, sad, and unsmiling?

Item 53: Look happy, smiling, and cheerful?

The score obtained on this rating scale provides a measure of the degree of deviation between the rated child and normal children. As such, these measures and attendant scores are helpful to teachers, parents, or child-care workers in quantifying their perceptions of a child's overall behavior.

Behavioral-analysis techniques are also used to make comparisons between children and youths suspected of exhibiting serious behavioral problems. One such technique is direct observation. Using this method, a well-trained observer can count and record a variety of behaviors that may be of concern to a teacher or parent while at the same time monitoring these behaviors in a number of other students. Comparisons drawn from these types of observations can be very helpful in accurately assessing the behavior pattern of a student in contrast to his or her peers.

Once the screening process has been concluded, specialists and/or consultants, including psychologists, special educators, social workers, and psychiatrists complete in-depth assessments of the child's academic and social-emotional strengths and weaknesses in various environmental settings such as the classroom, home, and playground. The assessment team may analyze classroom and playground interactions with peers and teachers using behavioral-analysis techniques (i.e., observations with frequency counts of various types of behaviors or interactions); administer various tests to evaluate personality, achievement, and intellectual factors; and interview the parents and the child. Additionally, they may observe the child at home and apply an array of other assessment procedures.

Unfortunately, many assessment devices, particularly the projective and personality inventories, do not provide information that reliably differentiates disordered individuals from nondisordered ones (Gelfand, Jenson, & Drew, 1988). Likewise, information gained from these devices cannot be readily translated into specific programming for individuals with behavior disorders. Of greatest promise at this point are behavioral analysis measurement techniques, which provide a concrete means for evaluating problem behaviors, selecting appropriate IEP goals, and assessing intervention effects. Unfortunately, the agreement between diagnostic or assessment data and students' IEP goals and associated interventions is poor (Fiedler & Knight, 1986).

INTERVENTIONS

FOCUS 9
What six major treatment approaches generally are used in treating children and adolescents with behavior disorders?

Approaches to Treatment

Interventions for individuals with mild, moderate, or severe behavior disorders include a variety of approaches (Center, 1986). Major approaches to treatment include insight-oriented therapies, play therapy, group psychotherapy, behavior therapy, marital and family therapy, and drug therapy (see Table 5–5). Each of these approaches is discussed very briefly.

Insight-Oriented Therapies.   Insight-oriented therapies include psychoanalytic, nondirective, and client-centered therapy. These approaches assume that children who feel rage, rejection, and guilt can be helped by an understanding and caring therapist. The therapist endeavors to establish a relationship with the child or

TABLE 5–5   Summary of Intervention Approaches

General Goals	Intervention Approaches					
	Insight-oriented therapy	Play therapy	Group psychotherapy	Behavior therapy	Marital and family therapy	Drug therapy
Relieve symptoms	•					•
Treat causes of behavior	•		•		•	
Develop a therapeutic relationship	•	•	•		•	
Play out emotional problems		•				
Develop positive peer relationships		•	•			
Teach language skills				•		
Teach self-help skills				•		
Teach academic skills				•		
Reduce and/or eliminate behaviors				•		
Teach adaptive behavior				•		
Teach social skills		•		•		
Develop problem-solving skills		•	•		•	
Understand unconscious causes of behavior	•		•			
Control disordered or unusual behavior				•		•
Control aggression				•		•
Control behavior				•		•

adolescent by creating an atmosphere that is conducive to the sharing and expression of feelings. The goal of therapy is to help the child or youth develop insight or self-understanding. Insight provides the basis for the relief of symptoms and the development of new, more adaptive behaviors.

Play Therapy. Play therapy for young children serves several purposes. It is designed to help them become aware of their own unconscious thoughts and the behaviors that emanate from these thoughts. For children who have been emotionally abused or neglected, another purpose is to provide them with an opportunity to interact with a caring, sensitive adult. The vehicle for communication between the therapist and children is free play and other, related small-group activities. Through play therapy children may reveal information about themselves that they cannot talk about, such as sexual abuse, sibling rivalry, and damaging discipline practices. Play therapy can be a valuable source of information for therapists.

Group Psychotherapy. Group psychotherapy and other group-oriented treatment approaches are occasionally used with children; however, they are used more frequently with adolescents and young adults. Slavson's **activity group therapy** for children is operated much like a club (Slavson & Shiffer, 1975). A mix of aggressive and withdrawn boys meet together weekly for club (therapy) meetings. The therapist's role in the group setting is primarily one of modeling appropriate, healthy behaviors, helping aggressive children become more co-operative, and promoting and developing outgoing behaviors in children who are shy and withdrawn. Group-treatment approaches for older youth are varied and often quite similar to the procedures used with adults. The major difference lies in the concerns and issues that are the focus of therapy sessions. Vorrath's Positive Peer Culture has been used with a variety of youth-related problems, including disruptive classroom behaviors, delinquency, and substance abuse (Sandler, Arnold, Gable, & Strain, 1987; Vorrath & Brendtro, 1974). This treatment approach capitalizes on the power inherent in peer approval and peer-selected rules, contingencies, and solutions. It requires the skill of an experienced therapist, group leader, or teacher.

Behavior Therapy. Behavioral interventions for children and youth focus on developing or improving various self-help, social, language, and academic behaviors. Increasing the rates of desirable behavior is achieved in a variety of ways. Teachers and special education personnel make extensive use of the principles of behavior modification in this approach. Rule-review procedures (Rosenberg, 1986), rewards, **token reinforcement systems, contingency contracting,** and other motivational systems are used to encourage children to engage in normal, adaptive behaviors.

Another focus of behavioral interventions is the reduction or elimination of maladaptive behaviors. Reductions in certain behaviors may be achieved through a variety of means. For instance, a young boy's fighting behavior may be reduced by rewarding his cooperative and problem-solving behaviors and punishing his fighting behaviors. For engaging in fighting, he may lose accumulated tokens (response cost) or be placed in a time-out area where he cannot earn tokens or participate in the on-going, reinforcing activities of the classroom. In extreme cases and when other strategies have failed, a severely disturbed child who engages in self-injurious behavior may receive physical **punishment** that is aversive yet brief. For example, consider a young child with infantile autism who engages in self-injurious behavior such as head banging or eye gouging. These behaviors are not only physically harmful to the child but they occur frequently enough to interfere with important learning that should be taking place. Also, many of the children who engage in these behaviors may use them to evade interaction with others or to avoid taking part in various instructional activities.

Marital and Family Therapy. Marital therapy and family therapy are designed to help married individuals and their families enjoy greater success in dealing with problems and relating more effectively with one another. Several types of family therapy have been developed. Some therapists are psychodynamically oriented; that is, they are interested in helping family members understand the unconscious dynamics and other factors that may be influencing their interactions. Family therapists (Haley, 1963; Satir, 1967) who adhere to the systems orientation direct their efforts at helping family members understand the roles and functions they play in the family systems. They may determine that a child's disturbance serves some specific family function and is thereby supported by the other family members. Structural family therapy (Minuchin, 1974) emphasizes the assessment of family functioning. The ways in which family members solve problems and interact with each other are assessed. Coalitions within the family are isolated. The views that family members have of themselves and others are evaluated. Therapists using this approach become actively involved with families by assigning homework between sessions and giving participants other family-related tasks to complete.

Children with severe behavior disorders may be treated with medication to control disorganized or highly erratic behavior. (John Telford)

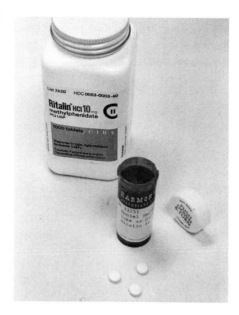

Drug Therapy.   Drug therapies for children are frequently used to treat a variety of conditions and related behaviors (Epstein & Olinger, 1987). Hyperactive, inattentive, and impulsive children are often treated with stimulant drugs. Children with severe behavior disorders may be treated with medications to control disorganized or highly erratic behavior. In other cases medications may be prescribed for children who have chronic problems with bed wetting or involuntary urination. Older teenagers or young adults may be prescribed drugs that are ordinarily taken by adults for depression and other psychiatric conditions.

A number of service delivery systems are used to make these and other treatments available to children, youths, and their families. The type of service delivery and the emphasis of the approach taken depends on the age of the student, the severity of the disorder, the type of disorder, and the theoretical orientation of the providers. Moreover, the effectiveness of past interventions and input from the family must be considered. For example, a young preschooler who is out of control will need an altogether different treatment than an adolescent who is severely depressed. We now review briefly some of the service delivery systems and treatment approaches that may be used with children of varying ages.

Early Childhood Interventions

Service delivery systems for young disturbed children are many and varied. However, there are four systems generally used to provide disturbed children with necessary services (Karnes & Zehrbach, 1979). These include the home-based system, the home-based system followed by involvement with a specialized center, the home-and-center-based system, and the center-based system. Personnel in these service delivery systems may use a variety of intervention approaches to assist children and families with whom they work (see Table 5–6).

The home-based program approach provides disturbed children with specialized services through a home teacher. These teachers train parents to use

TABLE 5–6   Childhood Service Delivery Systems and Intervention Approaches

Early-Childhood Service Delivery Systems	Intervention Approaches					
	Insight-oriented therapy	Play therapy	Group psychotherapy	Behavior therapy	Marital and family therapy	Drug therapy
Home-based program				•		•
Home-based program followed by specialized center	•	•		•	•	•
Home- and center-based system	•	•	•	•	•	•
Center-based program	•	•	•	•	•	•

behavior modification and other therapeutic procedures. The parents then employ these techniques to assist their handicapped children in learning and mastering new, developmentally appropriate skills. Home-based behavioral interventions seem to produce better results for young children with conduct disorders than do other service delivery systems (Scruggs, Mastropieri, Cook, & Escobar, 1986). Referrals for a home-based service program come from physicians, local guidance clinics, public school personnel, and county health nurses. Home teachers assist parents in selecting appropriate goals for their children, which are based on actual performance data of the child as observed first hand by the parents and the home teacher. Using these data the home teacher and the parents develop a program that is consistent with the child's needs. The program consists of training related to self-help, language, socialization, and motor skills. On a weekly basis the family is visited by the home teacher, and the child is observed relative to weekly goals that have been established. The parent is also observed, to be sure that he or she is encouraging the behaviors associated with the weekly goal; and the home teacher discusses any problems that may be occurring in the training process. The home teacher also provides demonstrations and instructions that are relevant to the goals that the parents and child are presently pursuing.

Home-based programs may be followed by a specialized center program. The intent of these programs is to provide a carefully conceived, sequential program in which objectives for the home and center programs are interrelated. In general, children served in this manner receive home-based instruction from birth to approximately three years of age. When a child is about two and one-half to three and one-half years old, he or she is moved into a center-based program that builds on the skills developed in the home program.

Center-based programs for young children with severe emotional problems provide treatments drawn from a variety of perspectives and orientations. For example, a center may emphasize both behavioral and psychodynamic principles. Teachers and therapists in such a center would attempt to determine all of the dynamics that may play a role in the children's present behaviors. Feelings, thoughts, past negative and positive experiences, relationships with parents and siblings, and family values would all be considered in the treatment process and daily education of young children. Various forms of play therapy may be used to encourage children to play out their conflicts and to develop trusting relationships with adults. Teacher-child relationships are very important to the teachers and other persons who work directly with children in centers.

Teachers and therapists are also free to use the techniques associated with the behavior therapy. Rewards for positive behavior, use of task analysis (breaking down behaviors into their most elementary parts for teaching), behavior shaping (gradually helping a child develop a behavior that has not yet been exhibited or mastered), and other behavioral techniques may be used.

Interventions for Elementary-Age Children

Elementary children with behavior disorders are likely to exhibit below-average performance in reading and math as well as other areas within the typical school curriculum. In addition to their academic problems, they may have difficulties relating to others, observing class rules, and handling emotional situations. The academic problems may be addressed through specialized instruction and materials provided by a consulting teacher. How and when the special materials are used depends on the staffing patterns and resources available in each school. Young children with behavior disorders may be tutored by an older, academically capable student. Some children are assisted by an aide or the regular class teacher, with follow-up provided by a consultant or special education resource room teacher.

The behavioral difficulties may be addressed in a variety of ways. Sometimes misbehavior is a function of a lack of satisfactory rules, routines, and structures within the regular classroom. If this is the case, a consulting teacher may assist the regular class teacher in developing a classroom management system that not only benefits the disturbed child but other children in the classroom as well.

Small training groups may be formed by a teacher to assist a youngster in developing social and problem-solving skills (Amish, Gesten, Smith, Clark, & Stark, 1988). Structured Learning (McGinnis, Goldstein, Sprafkin, & Gershaw, 1984) is a program that uses (1) **modeling,** (2) **role playing,** (3) **performance feedback,** and (4) **transfer of training.** Prior to the initiation of training, a careful assessment is completed to determine the skills that need to be taught through the structured learning sequences. The first phase of the training consists of modeling activities in which the students are given an opportunity to carefully observe various types of prosocial behaviors. For example, a trained peer may model some healthy and effective ways to respond to teasing. Observational learning or modeling activities are followed by role playing. During role playing, students rehearse and practice the behaviors that have been modeled. Students are then given performance feedback directly related to the success with which they have adequately performed the targeted social behavior. After children have demonstrated a solid level of performance in the small group setting, they are given many opportunities to try their newly learned skills in regular classrooms, during recess periods, and at home.

Research regarding the effectiveness of programs like Structured Learning are beginning to emerge. These interventions have been effective in teaching specific social skills to students with behavior disorders in well-controlled environments, but the transfer of these skills over time to the home, neighborhood, and employment settings appears to be negligible (Schloss, Schloss, Wood, & Kiehl, 1986; Simpson, 1987).

Children with Moderate to Severe Behavior Disorders.   Children who exhibit moderate to severe behavior disorders are primarily served in special classes. These classes may be housed in a number of different types of facilities. In some school systems the special classes are found within the elementary school itself. In fact, there may be a small cluster of two to three classes in selected buildings. Other special classes may be found within a hospital unit, a special school, a residential program, or a specialized treatment facility.

Special classes for children with moderate to severe disorders are characterized by a number of significant features (Morgan & Jenson, 1988). The first is a high degree of structure; that is, rules are clear and consistently enforced. The second feature is teacher monitoring of student performance; students are frequently

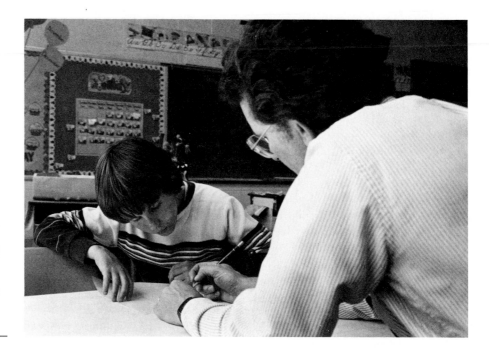

Children with moderate to severe behavior disorders are often served in special self-contained classrooms. What are the advantages and disadvantages of such an arrangement? (John Telford)

provided with feedback and reinforcement based on their academic and social behaviors. Furthermore, expectations for student behavior are well known by all class participants.

In addition to behaviorally oriented interventions, students may also receive individual counseling or group and family therapy. Many children with behavior disorders may be on some form of medication as well. In these cases, teachers are encouraged to carefully monitor the effectiveness (or ineffectiveness) of the medications that have been prescribed. Signs of negative side effects are immediately reported to parents or guardians.

One of the most comprehensive and successful programs developed for disturbed elementary children is Project Re-Ed (Hobbs, 1965; Weinstein, 1969), which has an ecological focus. Interventions are directed not only at the children but also at their families, schools, and communities. Initially the program was a residential one: Children attended school at a residential site and went home on weekends. Through teacher-counselors, enrolled children received relevant educational and therapeutic support in special class environments. At the same time, the parents of these children and regular school personnel were kept informed of the children's progress by liaison teachers. The liaison teachers were also responsible, in conjunction with other personnel, for helping families and school personnel ready themselves for the reentry of the children into regular classrooms. A variety of treatment approaches were used in helping these children and their families develop the behaviors necessary for successful individual and family living; however, the distinguishing characteristic of this program was its ecological focus. Not only were the children treated, but the major social and education environments of the children were also treated and prepared for their return.

Programs for seriously disturbed children who may be described as autistic, schizophrenic, or exhibiting pervasive developmental disorders are similar in nature to those previously discussed. However, they may involve a variety of other specialized medical, speech or language, and social services personnel. For young autistic children, the continued thrust of their training is language development. For children with pervasive developmental delays, the thrust may be training in the self-help skills of toileting, feeding, dressing, bathing, and grooming.

Intervention for Adolescents

Secondary-age school programs for disturbed youth are in a state of emergence (Whelan, 1981). Progress has been made in the amount and kind of literature available to educators who are interested in programs and strategies for youth with behavior disorders (Brown, McDowell, & Smith, 1981; D'Alonzo, 1983; Jones, 1980; Rizzo & Zabel, 1988; Shea & Bauer, 1987; Towns, 1981); however, the total percentage of youths with behavior disorders who are actually served through special programs remains relatively small (44.1 percent) in comparison to the number who may need the service but are not yet identified (Miller, Sabatino, & Larsen, 1980).

Service delivery systems for adolescents with behavior disorders closely parallel those for elementary-age students. The major differences lie in the types of intervention strategies that are applied, the roles educational specialists fulfill, and the types of problems that become the focus of the invention efforts. The various parts of a program for disturbed youth vary according to the severity and nature of the individual's social and academic problems. For example, a youngster who is chronically delinquent and has been found guilty of a number of felony offenses (physical assaults, armed robbery, etc.) is treated differently than one who is schizophrenic or school-phobic. Similarly, a student who has great difficulty in dealing with the academic and social demands of the regular high school academic and social environment would not receive the same placement or interventions as one who is autistic and still unable to communicate effectively.

Special educators, vocational specialists, rehabilitation personnel, social workers, probation counselors, psychologists, psychiatrists, and other professionals use a variety of intervention techniques to prepare behavior-disordered youth for the next appropriate transition. Interventions may include preparing youths to leave a secure facility for delinquents in order to reenter their homes and communities, or to move from a residential facility to their own homes. Some special educators may prepare students to move from a self-contained class within a special school to a regular secondary school, or equip the older adolescent with the skills necessary for the transition from secondary school education to full-time work in the community. Other support personnel may prepare the adolescent to handle personal challenges such as school disappointments, peer challenges, and parental control without intensive therapeutic assistance.

The support personnel may use various forms of individual and group therapy coupled with appropriate medications to assist a disordered teenager. Special educators, vocational, and career development specialists may collaborate to identify the type of vocational or professional training that may be most helpful to disturbed students, given their abilities and interests (Phelps & Clark, 1977; Dick, 1987). Special educators may also provide instruction that is related to specific job-related behaviors that may be social or academic in nature. They may also give instruction that is directly related to adult survival skills in the areas of emergency care, accident prevention, and consumerism. For example, D'Alonso (1983) contended that secondary special educators should not attempt to continue teaching elementary developmental skills and their remediation per se, but "teach the academic, vocational, social, and personal skills needed for work, future education, and maintenance of successful, sound relationships and harmonious interpersonal adjustment" (p. 10). Rather than adhering to the traditional high school curriculum or remedial work, special educators are encouraged to focus their instruction on a "life oriented program that offers alternatives to social conflict" (Miller, 1978, p. 72).

The probation counselor may use a probation agreement or contract with a delinquent youth and his or her family to formalize goals and determine the conditions for coming off court probation (Polsgrove, 1977). Positive peer-group procedures may be used in a residential or group treatment center to establish appropriate patterns of behavior (Vorrath & Brendtro, 1974). The recreational therapist may use a variety of camping and other leisure activities to give disturbed youth a new perspective about themselves, their peers, and immediate surroundings.

One of the greatest challenges is the coordination of all of these services. This is particularly true for disturbed teenagers who are about to leave the public school system and enter the adult world and employment market. Fortunately, considerable effort is now being exerted to develop training systems and approaches that prepare disturbed and other handicapped youth to enter the post–public school period prepared to contribute and live as independently as their skills allow (Greenan, 1985).

REVIEW

FOCUS 1: What five factors influence the ways in which we view others' behaviors?

□ Our personal beliefs, standards, and values influence our perceptions of others and their behaviors.

□ Our tolerance for certain behaviors varies, again because of our standards, values, and level of emotional fitness at the time the behaviors are exhibited.

□ Perceptions of normality are frequently in the "eye of the beholder" rather than some objective standard of normality as established by consensus or research.

□ The context in which a behavior takes place has a profound effect on our view of its appropriateness or inappropriateness.

□ The frequency with which the behavior occurs or its intensity strongly affects our interpretation of its suitability or appropriateness.

FOCUS 2: What five variables influence the types of

behaviors that are exhibited or suppressed by individuals with behavior disorders?

□ The variables that influence types of behaviors that are exhibited by children and adolescents with behavior disorders include the parents' and/or teachers' management styles; the school or home environment; the social and the cultural values of the family; the social and economic climate of the community; the responses of peers and siblings; and the academic, intellectual, and social-emotional characteristics of the individuals with behavior disorders.

FOCUS 3: What differentiates externalizing disorders from internalizing disorders?

□ Externalizing disorders involve behaviors that are directed at others (fighting, assaulting, stealing, vandalizing, and so on).

□ Internalizing disorders involve behaviors that are directed inwardly or at oneself more than at others (fears, phobias, depressions, and so on).

FOCUS 4: What are six essential features of definitions describing serious emotional disturbances or behavior disorders?

□ The behaviors in question must be exhibited to a marked extent.

□ Learning problems that are not attributable to intellectual, sensory, or health deficits are common.

□ Satisfactory relationships with parents, teachers, siblings, and others are few.

□ Behaviors exhibited by these children occur in many settings, and under normal circumstances are inappropriate.

□ A pervasive mood of unhappiness or depression is frequently displayed by children with behavior disorders.

□ Physical symptoms or fears associated with the demands of school are common in some children and adolescents.

FOCUS 5: List three reasons why classification systems are important to professionals who diagnose, treat, and educate individuals with behavior disorders.

□ Classification systems provide professionals with a common language for communicating about various types and subtypes of behavior disorders.

□ Classification systems provide professionals with a means of describing and identifying various behavior disorders.

□ Classification systems sometimes provide a basis for treating a disorder and making predictions about treatment outcomes.

FOCUS 6: What are five general characteristics (intellectual, adaptive, and achievement) of children and adolescents with behavior disorders?

□ Disturbed children and adolescents tend to have average to lower-than-average IQs compared to their normal peers.

□ Children and youths with severe behavior disorders tend to have IQs that fall within the retarded range of functioning.

□ Disturbed children and adolescents have great difficulty relating socially and responsibly to peers, parents, teachers, and other authority figures.

□ Disturbed students perform less well than their ability would predict, as measured by intellectual instruments.

□ Seriously disturbed students, particularly those with IQs in the retarded range, are substantially substandard in their academic achievement.

FOCUS 7: What can we accurately say about the causes of behavior disorders?

□ Behavior disorders are caused by sets of continuously interacting biological, genetic, cognitive, social, emotional, and cultural variables.

FOCUS 8: What are four factors that need to be carefully assessed in determining whether or not a child has a behavior disorder?

□ The discrepancy between the child or adolescent's behavior and expected performance, given his or her age, culture, temperament, and intellectual endowment, should be assessed.

□ The frequency, intensity, and location of the various problematic behaviors must be assessed.

□ The relationship of the behaviors to various events and people should be assessed.

□ The influence of family and cultural factors should be evaluated and analyzed.

FOCUS 9: What six major treatment approaches generally are used in treating children and adolescents with behavior disorders?

□ Major approaches to treating behavior disorders include insight-oriented therapies, play therapy of various types, group psychotherapy, behavior therapy, marital and family therapy, and drug therapy.

□ The therapies are used in conjunction with various types of service delivery systems, including home-based and center-based programs, school-based programs (consulting teacher, resource rooms, self-contained programs, specialized schools), residential programs, hospitals (outpatient and inpatient programs), and one-to-one or family therapy provided by a private practitioner.

Debate Forum

Drugs: Is There Adequate Support for Their Continued Use with Great Numbers of Children?

There is considerable disagreement regarding the practice of prescribing stimulant drugs for "disturbing" children, and children who have been identified as inattentive, hyperactive, impulsive, or difficult to manage. Consider for a moment the following:

1. Stimulant drugs do improve school children's short-term academic performance in some language areas and arithmetic skills (Douglas et al., 1986).

2. IQ scores, grades, and basic learning abilities are not improved with stimulant medication (Ross & Ross, 1982).

3. Researchers report that stimulant medication enhances children's classroom performance and makes them less impulsive, easier to control, and more attentive (Barkley, 1985).

4. Parent-child and teacher-child interactions appear to improve with stimulant medication (Whalen, Henker, & Dotemoto, 1981; Whalen, Henker, & Finck, 1980).

5. Reduced aggression, more goal-directed activity, enhanced short-term memory, reduced impulsiveness, and improved performance on rote learning and fine motor tasks seem to be the major positive outcomes of stimulant medication for children (Weiss, 1979).

6. Long-term academic achievement does not appear to be significantly affected by stimulant medication (Ross & Ross, 1982).

7. Drug therapy may be a poor substitute for effective teaching and parenting, or nothing more than a form of control that makes children more manageable for adults (Stroufe, 1975).

8. Research regarding the effectiveness of stimulant medication compared to behaviorally oriented treatment strategies has produced mixed results (Brown, Wynne, & Medenis, 1985; Pollard, Ward, & Barkley, 1984).

9. Behavioral procedures seem to produce more positive results. Targeted behaviors are increased or reduced. Changes in the child's environment are brought about through the use of behavioral procedures. The child may attribute the changes in behavior to his or her actions rather than to medication (Gelfand, Jenson, & Drew, 1988).

10. Stimulant medication may temporarily suppress normal growth and weight gains in children, but rapid recuperation occurs during drug holidays (Gualtieri et al., 1982).

11. However, several studies suggest that small but significant decreases in height and weight occur with certain individuals with chronic treatment (Mattes & Gittelman, 1983; Greenhill et al., 1984).

12. State-dependent learning may be one of the outcomes of consistent use of medication in that the child is only able to learn and demonstrate learning when he or she is medicated (Gelfand, Jenson, & Drew, 1982).

13. Medication appears to decrease activity in structured classroom settings and significantly increase activity during physical recreation periods (Porrino et al., 1983).

14. There is no reliable method for predicting who will respond or benefit from medication (Klein et al., 1980).

15. Follow-up studies of youngsters who have used medication extensively over a long period of time to control their behavior may develop problems associated with substance abuse (Hectman, Weiss, & Perlman, 1984).

Point The administration of stimulant drugs improves children's functioning in a variety of school-related behaviors. They enhance general classroom performance as observed by teachers; improve children's on-task behaviors; reduce aggression; increase goal-directed activity; and reduce behaviors associated with impulsiveness. They should be prescribed for children who need help in these areas.

Counterpoint The administration of stimulant drugs does not improve children's basic learning abilities or academic achievement over time. It appears that other interventions are equally effective in changing children's behaviors, and these other procedures do not appear to produce any negative side effects. Furthermore, researchers are uncertain as to the long-term effects of continual use of stimulant drugs by children. The continued use of stimulant drugs to change children's behaviors should be stopped.

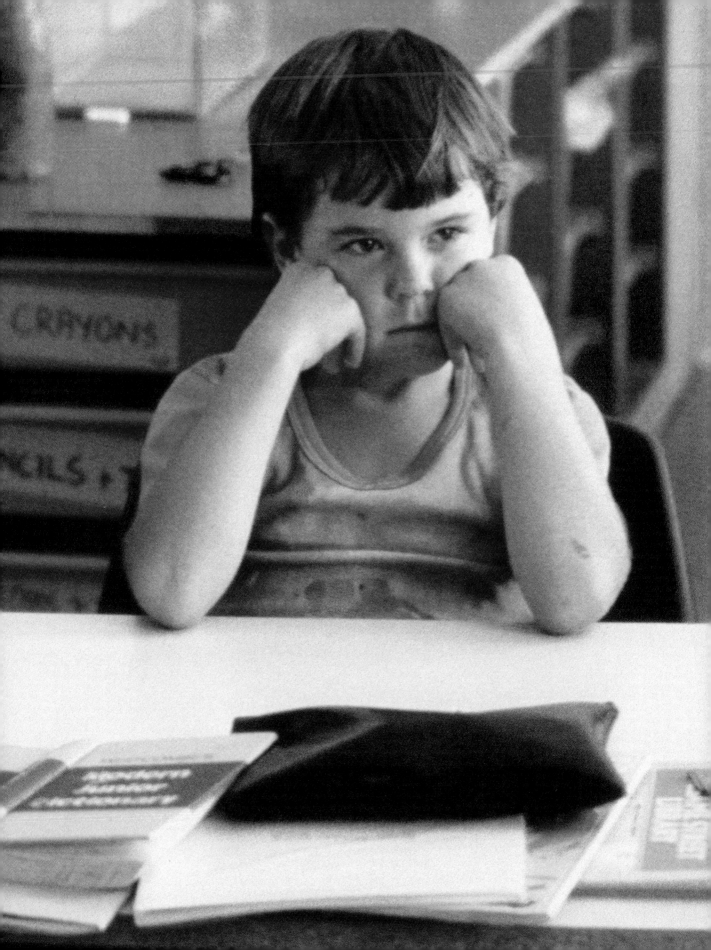

6 Learning Disabilities

To Begin With...

- In the period from 1978–79 to 1986–87, the number of special education students increased from 3.9 to 4.4 million, largely due to the rise in the number of students who were classified as learning disabled. The growth of this category exceeded all other handicapping conditions combined (National Center for Education Statistics, 1988).

- A college student, in an interview with the author, describing her young sister who has a learning disability: "It just gets me, the same child who forgets her own telephone number remembers word-for-word almost any commercial you see on TV. You want the Pepsi jingle? Just ask Sarah."

- Show-business entertainer Cher, in discussing her learning disability: "Numbers and I have absolutely no relationship" (Kelman, 1983).

- By the early 1990s, it is estimated that over one million children will be receiving stimulant medication (Associated Press News Service, 1989).

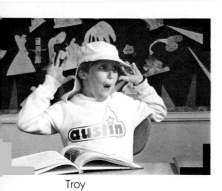

Troy

Troy is now in the fourth grade at Valley View Elementary School. He experienced minor learning difficulties as a young child, which did not receive adequate attention. When he entered elementary school, matters became much more difficult. He now reads at about the second grade level, and for two years he has been on medication to control hyperactivity. Troy's teacher describes him as a bright boy but one who "raises a lot of hell," particularly when he comes to school without taking his medication. Troy has been diagnosed by the district child study team as learning disabled. His academic problems are fairly mild and mostly involve reading and social adaptation. Troy's interaction with his peers is characterized by frequent episodes of bullying and aggression, and he seldom allows others to choose play activities or lead the way. Troy now lives with his mother and her boyfriend in a small apartment. He expresses a lot of affection for both of these people but seems troubled about school. He has been recommended for the resource room on a part-time basis, to work primarily on reading skills but also on the development of appropriate social behavior.

Michelle's difficulties in learning academic skills have been evident from the time she entered school. Although her intelligence score is well within the normal range, she has been unable to master the foundation skills in reading, spelling, and handwriting and has deficits in gross motor development. Each year her teachers report that she is capable of doing the work required but that her problems with visual perception interfere with her performance. Michelle is unable to align words on a page, she reverses numbers and letters, she writes words from the bottom to the top of the page, and she reads from right to left. Now, at the age of fourteen, Michelle is facing high school with reading skills that are more than four years behind grade level. Her reading vocabulary is comparable to that of a third- or fourth-grader, but she has great difficulty using reading as a tool for learning. A tape recorder is one of her most valued possessions. In addition to providing a constant source of rock music (much to her parents' consternation), it allows her to sit comfortably through lectures, knowing she does not have to fumble with taking notes. She can play back the discussion over and over to obtain the necessary information. Michelle performs much better in the area of math, especially when she is required to do computations in which little reading is involved. Most of Michelle's early school experiences have been in a regular classroom with resource room assistance. As she moved into the middle grades, however, her school educational team recommended she receive a more extensive special education program in a self-contained classroom. This recommendation was based on her substantial withdrawal from peer relationships and interactions, and her inconsistent performance in academic subjects.

INTRODUCTION

Compared with other handicaps, **learning disabilities** are a recently identified and defined area of exceptionality. They have often been viewed as mild handicapping conditions because most individuals with learning disabilities have normal or near normal intelligence but experience problems in academic areas such as reading and mathematics. However, recent thinking suggests that the term *learning disabilities* is a generic label representing a very heterogeneous group of handicaps, ranging from mild to severe. In many cases, learning disabled people have been described as having "poor **neurological** wiring" and other such maladies that are somewhat mystical in terms of explaining their problems. Our vignettes describe "typical" children with learning disabilities: They have normal intelligence but experience academic difficulties and perhaps social ones as well. They represent a substantial challenge to both school and family settings. They present a highly variable and complex set of characteristics and needs.

DEFINITIONS AND CLASSIFICATIONS

Learning disabilities have generated more controversy, confusion, and polarization among contemporary professionals than any other exceptionality. Educational services for learning disabled children were virtually nonexistent prior to the 1960s. In the past, many children now identified as having specific learning disabilities would have been labeled **remedial readers,** remedial learners, emotionally handicapped, or even mentally retarded—if they received any special or additional instructional support at all. Today learning disabilities command the largest single program for exceptional children in the United States. Although relatively new, its growth rate has been unparalleled by any other area in special education (U.S. Department of Education, 1989).

Definitions

Definitions of learning disabilities reflect great variation. This may be because of the field's unique evolution, highly accelerated growth pattern, and strong interdisciplinary nature. Several disciplines (including medicine, psychology, speech-language, and education) have contributed to the confusion associated with inconsistent terminology. For example, education coined the phrase *specific learning disabilities;* psychology uses such terms as **perceptual disorders** and **hyperkinetic behavior;** speech and language employ the terms **aphasia** and **dyslexia;** and medicine uses labels of *brain damage, minimal brain dysfunction, brain injury,* and *impairment. Brain injury, minimal brain dysfunction,* and *learning disabilities* are among the more commonly used terms, although all appear in various segments of the literature.

A brain-injured child is described as having an organic impairment resulting in perceptual problems, thinking disorders, and emotional instability. A child with minimal brain dysfunction manifests similar problems, but there is often evidence of language, memory, motor, and impulse-control difficulties. Individuals

FOCUS 1
What are four reasons why definitions of learning disabilities have varied?

with minimal brain dysfunction are often characterized as average or above average in intelligence, distinguishing the disorder from mental retardation.

Specific Learning Disabilities. Kirk (1963) introduced the phrase *specific learning disabilities,* and his original concept remains largely intact today. The concept is presently defined by delays, deviations, and performance discrepancies in basic academic subjects (such as arithmetic, reading, spelling, or writing), as well as speech and language problems. Additionally, these disabilities cannot be attributed to mental retardation, sensory deficits, or emotional disturbance. It has become common practice in education to describe learning-disabled individuals on the basis of *what they are not.* For example, although they have a number of problems, they are not mentally retarded, emotionally disturbed, or deaf. *Learning disabilities* is a general educational term—an umbrella label—that includes a variety of different conditions and behavioral and performance deficits (Gelfand, Jenson, & Drew, 1988).

Until recently, educational literature virtually ignored the notion of severity in definitions and concepts of learning disabilities. However, current research and writing in learning disabilities is focusing more on problem severity (see McLoughlin & Nettick, 1983; Weller, Strawser, & Buchanan, 1985; Wilson, 1985). Learning disabilities have probably been defined in more different ways than any other type of handicap. In fact, Cruickshank (1972) noted that over forty different terms were being used to describe essentially the same behaviors.

Other Theories. The wide variety of terminology and definitions in learning disabilities has emerged partly because of the different theoretical views of the problem. For example, **perceptual-motor theories** emphasize an interaction between various channels of perception and motor activity. Perceptual-motor theories of learning disabilities focus on normal sequential development of motor patterns and compare it with the motor development of children with learning disabilities. Children with learning disabilities are seen as having perceptual-motor abilities that are unreliable and unstable, which presents problems when they encounter activities involving time and spatial orientation. In contrast, *language disability theories* concentrate on the child's reception or production of language. Because language is so important in learning, these theories emphasize the relationship between learning disabilities and language deficiencies. On the basis of only these two theories, it is clear we are examining very different viewpoints. Learning disabilities is a field with many theoretical perspectives regarding the nature of problems as well as causation and treatment.

Recent literature has taken a different view of learning disabilities than was evident earlier. Instead of focusing on differing terminology, some researchers suggest that many different, specific disorders are being grouped under one term. "*Learning disabilities* is a general educational term. . . . The term can be used only as a generalized referent in that it encompasses a variety of specific types of problems" (Gelfand, Jenson, & Drew, 1988, p. 224). Benton and Pearl (1978) also support this notion by suggesting that even specific *types* of learning disabilities, specifically dyslexia, represent a collection of different disorders. In one sense, this thinking is not surprising. It has long been acknowledged that people with learning disabilities are a very heterogeneous group. However, professionals

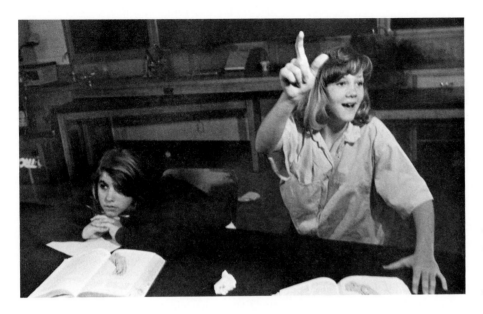

The category of learning disabilities includes widely divergent behaviors and skills. (John Telford)

continue to characterize people with learning disabilities as though they were uniform. Such characterizations typically reflect the theoretical or disciplinary perspective of the professional rather than an objective behavioral description of the individual being evaluated. Thus there has been a tendency to characterize the disorder rather than to describe the characteristics of an individual with problems. Such characterizations will inevitably be in error in a population representing a wide variety of disorders.

The problems with defining learning disabilities are evident in research on learning disabilities. The wide range of characteristics associated with children who have learning disabilities and myriad methodological problems (such as poor **research designs** and measurement error) have caused difficulties in conducting research on learning disabilities (Swanson, 1988). Generalizing research results is questionable, and replication of studies is very difficult. Consequently efforts to standardize and clarify definitions are important, both for research and intervention purposes.

Public Law 94–142.   One widely used definition of learning disabilities was presented by the National Advisory Committee on Handicapped Children (1968) of the U.S. Office of Education. This definition is similar to Kirk's (1963) early concept and was initially incorporated into Public Law 91–320, the Learning Disabilities Act of 1969. It was also used in Public Law 94–142, the Education of All Handicapped Children Act of 1975. The definition in P.L. 94–142 reads as follows:

"Specific learning disability" means a disorder in one or more of the basic psychological processes involved in understanding or in using language, spoken or written, which may manifest itself in an imperfect ability to listen, think, speak, read, write, spell, or to do mathematical calculations. The term includes such conditions as perceptual handicaps, brain injury, minimal brain dysfunction, dyslexia, and developmental aphasia. The term does not include children who have learning problems which are primarily the result of visual, hearing, or motor handicaps, of mental retardation, of emotional disturbance, or of environmental, cultural, or economic disadvantage (U.S. Education of All Handicapped Children Act, 1975, Section 5(b) (4).

Many thought P.L. 94–142's definition was exclusionary (i.e., a definition of conditions that are *not* learning disabilities rather than explaining substantively what learning disabilities *are*) and ambiguous because of a lack of measurement specification. Consequently the National Joint Committee for Learning Disabilities proposed a new definition in 1981:

> *Learning disabilities* is a generic term that refers to a heterogeneous group of disorders manifested by significant difficulties in the acquisition and use of listening, speaking, reading, writing, reasoning, or mathematical abilities. These disorders are intrinsic to the individual and presumed to be due to central nervous system dysfunction. Even though a learning disability may occur concomitantly with other handicapping conditions (for example, sensory impairment, mental retardation, social and emotional disturbance) or environmental influences (such as cultural differences, insufficient/inappropriate instruction, psychogenic factors), it is not the direct result of those conditions or influences (Hammill, Leigh, McNutt, & Larsen, 1981, p. 336).

Hammill et al. (1981) also point out that "the purpose of the definition was to establish learning disabilities theoretically—not to set up specific operational criteria for identifying individual cases" (p. 339). This definition is important to the present discussion for two reasons. First, it describes *learning disabilities* as a generic term that refers to a heterogeneous group of disorders. Second, a person with learning disabilities must manifest *significant* difficulties. The use of the word *significant* is an obvious attempt to remove the connotation of a mild problem.

In our examination of learning disabilities, we describe behavioral characteristics from different theoretical viewpoints. This is a field with an insufficient research base to allow us to select *one* perspective to explain learning disabilities. It is important to provide examples of how a person might be classified as having a learning disability using different perspectives. Hallahan and Kauffman suggested that five general areas are usually present in definitions of learning disabilities. They are "(1) academic retardation, (2) uneven development between different areas of functioning, (3) central nervous system dysfunction may or may not be present, (4) the learning problems are not due to environmental disadvantage, and (5) learning problems are not due to mental retardation or emotional disturbance" (1976, p. 20). Combinations of these and other behavioral characteristics have periodically appeared in the many theoretical views of learning disabilities. For example, uneven development of skill areas (**intraindividual** discrepancies) has been increasingly prominent in the literature since 1968.

Classification

FOCUS 2
What are four different ways in which people with learning disabilities can be classified?

Individuals who are labeled *learning disabled* represent a complex constellation of behaviors and conditions. However, people with learning disabilities have seldom been formally classified into differing severity categories. As noted earlier,

Reflect on This 6–1

Defining and Labeling

You are now in the fourth grade. School has been pretty frustrating for you, even though you have survived this far. The reading seems to be most difficult. When the teacher talks about passages from assignments, it isn't clear what exactly is going on. It is very hard to find the same information from reading assignments that others seem to find so easily. It takes a long time to read. For example, last night you were doing your studies and reading this paragraph: "Mary pelieveb than things would get detter. What they hab left Missouri they hab enough foob dut now there was darely enough for one meal a bay. Surely the wagon-master woulb finb a wet to solve the broblem." It didn't make much sense, but maybe history is not supposed to make sense. The other students seemed to understand quite well.

Today there will be some tests to take, but they are just for you. You are supposed to go down the hall to meet Mr. Jacobsen. This makes you a bit nervous, since everyone that goes to see him is called a "retard." The teacher had said something about "learning disabilities," but you didn't understand what that meant—the kids just called students who went to Mr. Jacobsen "retards." But the teacher said that you would get extra help that would make school better.

Consider the label of *learning disabilities*. Does the gain offset the loss for you? Do you want to be labeled *learning disabled* to obtain the extra help? What would it mean for you personally?

---

learning disabilities have generally been seen as mild disorders, despite the fact that clinicians have observed a range of symptoms, from mild to severe, for years. Instead of a severity scheme, learning-disabled individuals have been described relative to the classification parameters discussed earlier. For example, the DSM-III-R (1987) uses the labels of Undifferentiated **Attention-Deficit Disorder** and **Attention-Deficit Hyperactive Disorder.** Here, a generic label, *learning disabilities*, connoting academic deficits is combined with adaptive behavior problems, hyperactivity. DSM-III-R also discusses (1) age-specific features, (2) associated features, (3) age at onset, (4) course (how the problems develop or diminish), (5) complications, and (6) family patterns, among other things. Attention-deficit disorder is emerging more frequently in current literature as a term for learning disabilities. *In some cases,* however, this has been *only* a general terminology substitution without more precise behavioral use, despite the additional specificity provided in DSM-III-R.

Children with learning disabilities have also been viewed from other perspectives. For example, the federal rules and regulations published to clarify P.L. 94–142 provided additional information. According to these rules and regulations, any criterion for classifying a child as learning disabled must be based on an already existing *severe* discrepancy between capacity and achievement. The determination for placement was related to:

1. Whether a child achieves commensurate with his or her age and ability when provided with appropriate educational experiences

2. Whether the child has a *severe* discrepancy between achievement and intellectual ability in one or more of seven areas relating to communication skills and mathematical abilities (U.S. Department of Health, Education, and Welfare, 1977, p. 65082).

The person's learning disability must be determined on an individual basis, and the severe discrepancy between achievement and intellectual ability must be in one or more of the following areas: (1) oral expression, (2) listening comprehension, (3) written expression, (4) basic reading skill, (5) reading comprehension, (6) mathematical calculation, and/or (7) mathematical reasoning (U.S. Department of Health, Education, and Welfare, 1977, p. 65083).

The intended meaning of the term *severe discrepancy* is open to debate among professionals. This concept coincides with severity as a classification parameter, although it is not specified in terms of measurement. What is an acceptable discrepancy between a child's achievement and expected grade level— 25 percent? 35 percent? 50 percent? Bateman (1965) first introduced the discrepancy concept as an added dimension to the definition of learning disabilities. She defined learning-disabled children as "those who manifest an educationally significant discrepancy between their estimated intellectual potential and actual level of performance related to basic [learning processes]" (p. 220). Here, we see intelligence and academic achievement parameters involved in the area of learning disabilities.

A review of the literature on definitions and classifications of learning disabilities, either historical or current, presents a confusing and conflicting array of ideas. There is no precise set of concepts one can identify that *most* researchers totally agree to. This causes a number of difficulties with respect to both research and treatment. However, the people with learning-disabilities characteristics present some of the most interesting challenges in behavioral science today.

PREVALENCE

FOCUS 3
What are two estimate ranges for the prevalence of learning disabilities?

Determining prevalence (the total number of existing cases) is always a difficult task because actually counting on a large scale is time consuming and expensive. Problems of determining accurate figures are magnified by the differing definitions, theoretical views, and assessment procedures employed. Wallace and McLoughlin (1988) cite estimates that range from 1 to 28 percent.

A relative scarcity of empirical evidence is a problem that further compounds the difficulties in determining the prevalence of learning disabilities. Studies collecting such information have not been conducted in learning disabilities to the degree that they have in other areas. However, some data have been collected with larger samples than are typical. For example, Meier (1971) studied over 3,000 second-grade children in the Rocky Mountain area and derived an estimated 15 percent prevalence figure. Myklebust and Boshes (1969) also conducted an investigation in which 2,767 schoolchildren were screened to identify underachievers. Their data indicated that 15 percent of this population would be considered *underachievers*, based on a learning quotient of 89 or below. However, when exclusionary criteria were applied (i.e., no serious deficits in emotional

Reflect on This 6–2

Prevalence Distribution by Handicapping Condition

Despite the definition and classification difficulties involved with the learning disabilities area, it has become one of the largest groups served in special education. Since this term emerged in 1963, the number of people served has grown more rapidly for this group than for any other exceptional population typically considered a special education population; a number of other categories have shown a decrease during the same time period. Hallahan and Cruickshank (1973) noted that the label *learning disabilities* was accepted "in some cases . . . with religious fervor" (p. 7). This use of the *learning disabilities* label for service still continues to grow, as illustrated in the table. The growth and high level of service for learning disabilities have come under some criticism by federal support agencies as well as others. With definitional problems and uncertain research evidence, does it make much sense to have this group of exceptional individuals representing such a high proportion of those served? Does the

Changes between 1986–87 and 1987–88 in Number and Percentages of Children Ages 6 through 21 Served under Education of All Handicapped Act, by Handicapping Condition

Handicapping Condition	Changes (1986–87 to 1987–88)	
	Number	*Percentage*
Learning disabled	37,264	+2.0
Speech impaired	17,221	+1.9
Mentally retarded	−16,875	−3.0
Emotionally disturbed	2,407	+.7
Hard of hearing and deaf	441	+1.1
Multihandicapped	1,696	+2.8
Orthopedically impaired	1,851	+4.7
Other health impaired	2,365	+5.8
Visually handicapped	−484	−2.8
Deaf-blind	40	+5.4
All conditions	45,926	+1.2

Source: U.S. Department of Education (1989). Eleventh Annual Report to Congress on the Implementation of The Education of All Handicapped Act. Washington, D.C.: Division of Educational Services, Special Education Programs.

learning-disabled population really represent such a high proportion of exceptional populations, or has this label become a dumping ground for those in special education as mild mental retardation did a few years ago? Examine the table, as well as other information, to determine your answer.

adjustment, vision, hearing, intelligence, or motor ability were included) half the group could not be classified as learning disabled (Myklebust, Bannochie, & Killen, 1971). Thus the result was 7.5 percent of the original sample being identified as learning disabled. These data clearly suffer from being quite old, which raises the question of how relevant they are for the 1990s. Briefing papers presented in hearings before the National Council on the Handicapped on June 8, 1989, indicate that 5 to 10 percent is a reasonable estimate of the persons affected by learning disabilities (Stanford Research Institute, 1989). (See Figure 6–1.) These figures are remarkably similar to the earlier levels noted.

The learning disabilities population has had a high prevalence figure, when compared with other exceptionalities, since the term was first conceived, a source of controversy for many years. It has been difficult to focus on one figure that is agreed on by all involved in the field. The 1989 Report to Congress indicates somewhat over 4.1 million exceptional children being served in the schools during 1987–88, of which there were over 1.9 million classified as learning disabled. This represents 44 percent of the exceptional population being served. Needless to say, professionals and others with vested interests in a particular group view this as somewhat problematic. In some cases, their apprehension is due to competition for limited funds between different exceptionalities. In other cases, there are concerns that the learning disabilities label is being overused to avoid the stigma associated with other labels or because of misdiagnosis, which may not result in the most appropriate treatment.

Discrepancies in prevalence occur in all fields of exceptionality, although the area of learning disabilities seems more variable than most. Part of this diversity can be attributed to different procedures used between agencies, states, or researchers who are doing the counting and estimating. Another source of discrepancy may be found when definitions differ or are vague. Prevalence figures are unlikely to be the same when different definitions of what is being counted are used. This situation is not at all uncommon in the field of learning disabilities, where various definitions are evident, the definitions are often ambiguous, and therefore different characteristics may be used by those conducting prevalence studies.

CHARACTERISTICS

FOCUS 4
What are seven characteristics attributed to the learning disabled, and why is it difficult to characterize this group?

Although specific learning disabilities has been characterized by many professionals as a mild disorder (Idol-Maestas, Lloyd, & Lilly, 1981; Gelfand, Jenson, & Drew, 1988), there has been little attempt to empirically validate this premise. Identification of subgroups and severity levels in this heterogeneous population have been largely ignored in the past. However, there have been some attempts to attend to the issue of severity during the last decade (Deloach, Earl, Brown, Poplin, & Warner, 1981; Larsen, 1978; Torgesen & Dice, 1980; Weller et al., 1985). For example, Weller et al. (1985) used model-consolidating criteria from several sources as a means of identifying severity level. This model uses functional/adaptive ability criteria to differentiate students with mild disorders from those with more severe problems. It focuses on a variety of skill areas, including the effect of the problem on other abilities (such as social skills) and the need to alter the person's future life.

Deloach et al. (1981) suggest that the differences between mildly and severely disabled populations may be determined through the perceptions of teachers in the field. Results of this study indicate that teachers view students with learning disabilities as a heterogeneous group functioning at differing levels of severity. These levels range from non–learning disabled to severe disabilities. Approximately 20 percent of the students in classes for the learning disabled are functioning at a level that warrants classification as severely learning disabled. The authors

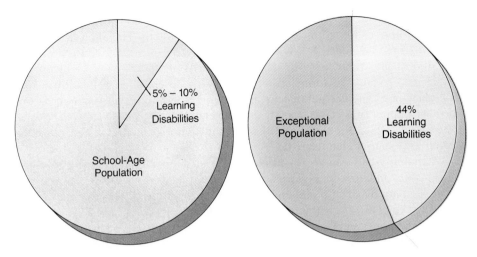

Figure 6–1
Prevalence of Learning Disabilities (Stanford Research Institute, 1989; Eleventh Annual Report to Congress, 1989.)

report that the most significant factors in distinguishing mild from severe problems are the needs of students with severe learning disabilities for individualized instruction, a necessity for alternative curricular approaches for severely disabled students, and a significant discrepancy between a student's scores on intelligence scales and grade-level as measured by achievement tests.

Teachers in the study by Deloach et al. (1981) indicated that approximately 30 percent of the students in their classrooms had learning problems that they did *not* attribute to learning disabilities. This finding is consistent with the belief that many students currently being served as learning disabled have been inappropriately referred. Larsen (1978) commented on this phenomenon:

> It is . . . likely that the large number of students who are referred for mild to moderate underachievement are simply unmotivated, poorly taught, come from home environments where scholastic success is not highly valued, or are dull-normal in intelligence. For all intents and purposes, these students should not automatically be considered as learning-disabled, since there is little evidence that placement in special education will improve their academic functioning (p. 7).

Intelligence

When comparing mild behavior-disordered and learning-disabled populations, intelligence is considered a common attribute. By definition, both categories involve people thought to be average or near average in intelligence. Differences between mild behavior disorders and specific learning disabilities have focused primarily on social-adjustment differences and learner characteristics. However, learning-disabled individuals may also exhibit secondary behavioral disorders, and mild behavior-disordered populations may also have learning difficulties similar to those exhibited by learning-disabled individuals (Hallahan, Kauffman, & Lloyd, 1985; Wallace & McLoughlin, 1988).

Student classroom performance also suggests that behavior problems are not specific to any one intellectual functioning level. It is well known that individuals with intellectual deficits and learning disabilities also exhibit a considerable amount of social and interpersonal behavior that is maladaptive (deHaas, 1986; Reid, 1988; Richardson, 1978). Problems in social adjustment must be viewed as a shared characteristic.

Variability between areas of functioning (such as measured intelligence and performance) and between performance areas has long been viewed as characteristic of the learning-disabled population. General descriptions of learning disabilities have often emphasized great intraindividual differences between skill areas (Gelfand et al., 1988). For example, a youngster may have a disability (very low performance) in reading but not in arithmetic. Frequently this variability in aptitude patterns has been used as a distinguishing characteristic between learning-disabled and mentally retarded populations. Typically, individuals thought to be retarded are expected to exhibit a rather flat or consistent profile of abilities (i.e., somewhat even, low performance levels in all areas), as contrasted to the pronounced intraindividual variability associated with learning disabilities. As with other attributes, however, intraindividual variability is not limited to students with learning disabilities. Intraindividual variability is definitely evident in students with mental retardation and behavior disorders (Hallahan, Kauffman, & Lloyd, 1985; Hammill, Leigh, McNutt, & Larsen, 1981).

Hyperactivity

Hyperactivity is a behavioral characteristic commonly associated with children labeled as learning disabled. Hyperactivity, also termed **hyperkinesis,** is typically thought of as a general excess of activity. Professionals working in the area of learning disabilities, particularly teachers, often mention hyperactivity first in describing their students. Such children are frequently depicted as fidgeting a great deal and being unable to sit still for even a short time. Most descriptions involve the characterization of an overly active child.

Certain points need to be considered as we discuss hyperactivity in learning-disabled children. First, not all learning-disabled children are hyperactive nor vice versa. Rosenthal and Allen (1978) highlighted these facts when they sought to differentiate learning disabilities, hyperkinesis, and minimal brain dysfunction. They noted, "There is probably such a degree of overlap between these categories that perhaps half of the subjects in a learning disability study might also be labeled either minimally brain dysfunctional or hyperkinetic" (p. 693). This should not be interpreted to mean that *half* the learning disabled are hyperactive. More correctly, this statement emphasizes the confusion regarding learning disabilities and how they relate to or are distinguishable from hyperkinesis.

A second point to consider involves the view that hyperkinesis is characterized as a *general* excess of activity. This idea may be more a function of stereotyped expectations than descriptions based on accurate observations. Some research

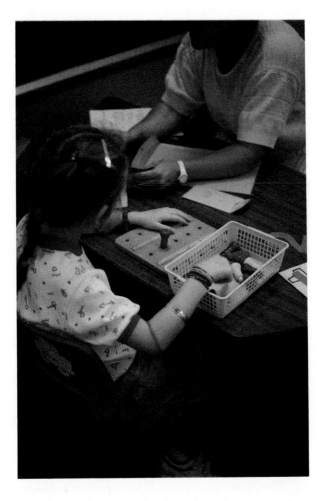

Most people with learning disabilities are thought to be of average or near average intelligence. (The Institute for the Study of Developmental Disabilities at Indiana University)

suggests that it may be more helpful to consider the *appropriateness* of a child's activity *in particular settings;* it may be incorrect to view hyperkinesis as a general excess of activity. Evidence does indicate that hyperactive children have a higher level of activity than their normal peers in structured settings (which may be descriptive of certain classroom circumstances). However, relatively unstructured settings (such as play periods) seem to result in no differences between hyperactive children and other children (Baxley & LeBlanc, 1976; Whalen & Henker, 1976).

Learning Modalities

Learning disabilities have also been associated with perceptual abnormalities. Such problems have been conspicuous in the historical development of the field of learning disabilities. Interest in this perspective has declined over the years, although some researchers have continued to view perception difficulties prominently with respect to behavior and causation of learning disabilities.

Perception. Perception difficulties in learning-disabled persons represent a constellation of behavioral abnormalities, rather than a single characteristic. Descriptions of these problems have included the visual, auditory, and haptic sensory systems. (**Haptic** refers to touch sensation and information transmitted to the individual through body movement and/or position.) Visual-perception difficulty has been closely associated with learning disabilities. It is important to remember that the definitions of learning disabilities exclude impaired vision in the traditional sense. Visual-perception problems in learning-disabled persons refers to something distinctly different. This type of abnormality is evident when a child sees a visual stimulus as unrelated parts rather than as an integrated pattern. In such cases, the youngster may not be able to identify a letter in the alphabet because he or she perceives only unrelated lines rather than the letter as a meaningful whole. Clearly such perception causes severe performance problems in school.

Visual perception problems may also emerge in **figure–ground discrimination**, the process of distinguishing an object from its background. Most of us have little difficulty with figure–ground discrimination. However, certain children labeled as learning disabled are unable to accomplish such a task. Children with this type of problem may have difficulty focusing on a word or sentence on the page of a textbook, which of course results in school difficulties. This example also presents an illustration of the theoretical problems in learning disabilities. A given behavior may be interpreted quite differently, depending on the research, theory, or disciplinary perspective being employed. The example above *may* be a figure–ground discrimination disorder, but it may also represent an attention deficit or memory problem—these have also been associated with the difficulties of learning-disabled children. Thus the same abnormal behavior can be accounted for by several theories.

Discrimination. Other discrimination problems have also appeared in descriptions of learning-disabled persons. Difficulties in **visual discrimination** have often been associated with learning disabilities. Individuals with such problems may be unable to distinguish one visual stimulus from another (e.g., between words such as *sit* and *sat* or letters such as *V* and *W*). This may result in the reversal of such letters as *b* and *d*, which has often been noted in learning-disabled children. This type of error is common among young children and often causes great concern for parents. However, most youngsters develop normally and show few reversal or rotation errors on visual images by about seven or eight years of age. The child who "continues to have difficulty and who makes frequent errors on easily discriminable letters" should be viewed as being a potential problem and perhaps given extra help (Hallahan, Kauffman, & Lloyd, 1985, p. 33).

We mentioned that auditory perception problems have also been associated with learning disabilities. Some children have been characterized as unable to distinguish between the sounds of different words or syllables, or even to identify certain environmental sounds (such as a ringing telephone) and differentiate those from others. Such problems have been termed **auditory discrimination**

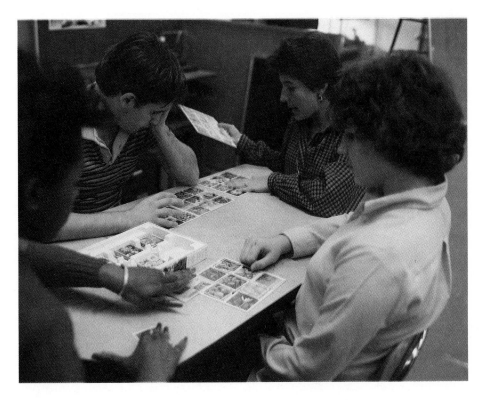

Visual-perception difficulty has been closely associated with learning disabilities. (The Institute for the Study of Developmental Disabilities at Indiana University)

deficits. Learning-disabled persons have also been described as having difficulties in **auditory blending, auditory memory,** and **auditory association.** Those with blending problems may not be able to blend word parts into an integrated whole as they pronounce it. Auditory-memory difficulties may result in an inability to recall information presented verbally. An auditory-association deficiency may cause the person to be unable to associate ideas or information presented verbally. Difficulties in these areas naturally create school performance problems for a child (Nix & Shapiro, 1986).

Haptic perception (touch, body movement, and position sensation) problems have also been associated with learning disabilities. Such difficulties are thought to be relatively uncommon, but may be important in some areas of school performance. For example, handwriting requires haptic perception because tactile information about the grasp of a pen or pencil must be transmitted to the brain. In addition, **kinesthetic** information is transmitted regarding hand and arm movements as one writes. Learning-disabled children have often been described by teachers as having poor handwriting, with difficulties in spacing letters and staying on the lines of a piece of paper. However, such problems could also be due to visual-perception abnormalities. Precisely attributing some behaviors to a single factor is difficult. Figure 6–2 presents an example of writing by a college freshman with learning disabilities. There are two samples in this figure, which were written on two consecutive days, each in a *forty-minute period.* The note provides a translation of what was written.

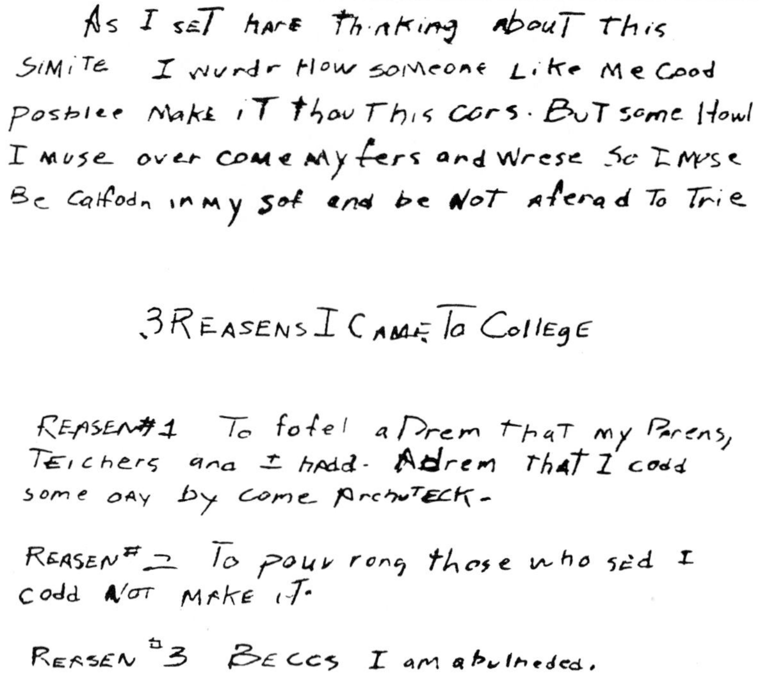

The text of these samples reads as follows:

> As I sit here thinking about this semester, I wonder how someone like me could possibly make it through this course. But somehow I must overcome my fears and worries. So I must be confident in myself and not be afraid to try.

Three Reasons I Came To College

Reason #1.   To fulfill a dream that my parents, teachers, and I had — a dream that I could some day become an architect.
Reason #2.   To prove wrong those who said I could not make it.
Reason #3.   Because I am bullheaded.

Figure 6–2
Writing Samples of a College Freshman with Learning Disabilities

Not all individuals labeled as having learning disabilities exhibit behaviors that suggest perceptual problems. Widely varying patterns of deficiencies are evident. We should also mention the relative lack of empirical evidence regarding perceptual problems in those labeled as learning disabled. In many cases, the notion of perceptual dysfunction is represented more by clinical impressions than by rigorous research. However, such clinical lore is widespread enough that it should be discussed in the learning disabilities area.

Cognition/Information Processing

Many other characteristics have been attributed to those with learning disabilities, some of which are in the area of **cognition** or **information processing** (Reid, 1988). Information processing has long been used in psychology as a model for studying cognition. This approach essentially relates the way a person acquires, retains, and manipulates information. Each of these areas has periodically emerged as problematic for learning-disabled individuals. For example, teachers have long complained about poor memory in such children. In many cases, the youngsters seem to learn material one day but cannot recall it the next. Research on the memory of learning-disabled children has been relatively scanty although such study is central to understanding how information is acquired, stored, selected, and recalled. Certain evidence suggests that the learning disabled do not perform as well as normal children on some memory tasks (Agrawal & Kaushal, 1987; August, 1987; Swanson, 1987), whereas other results indicate no differences (Griffith, Ripich, & Dastoli, 1986; Swanson, 1979, 1987). Research in this area needs increased effort to confirm, refute, or clarify clinical impressions.

Research also suggests that such children have different rather than deficient cognitive abilities (Hall, 1980). This type of finding has led to the development of specific, highly focused instruction for individuals with learning disabilities, instead of a generic curriculum that assumes their cognitive skills are *generally* poor (Finch & Spirito, 1980; McKinney & Haskins, 1980).

Attention problems have also been associated with learning disabilities. Such problems have often been clinically characterized as a **short attention span.** Parents and teachers often note that their learning-disabled children cannot sustain attention for more than a very short time. Some evidence has supported observations of a short attention span in these children (Aman & Turbott, 1986), but other research has indicated that learning-disabled children have difficulty in certain *types* of attention problems and attending *selectively* (Cotungo, 1987; Draeger, Prior, & Sanson, 1986; Pelham & Ross, 1977; Tarver, Hallahan, Kauffman, & Ball, 1976; Zentall & Kruczek, 1988). **Selective-attention** problems cause difficulty in focusing on centrally important tasks or information rather than peripheral or less relevant stimuli (Loper, 1980). Such problems might emerge when children with learning disabilities are asked to compute simple math problems that are on the chalkboard (which also means they must copy from the board). They may focus their attention on the copying task rather than on the math problems. This example presents a situation where the teacher can easily modify the task (e.g., by using worksheets rather than copying from the board) as a means of facilitating completion of the important lesson.

Academic Achievement

One of the primary areas that resulted in the development of learning disabilities as an identified exceptionality is academic achievement. These individuals, while

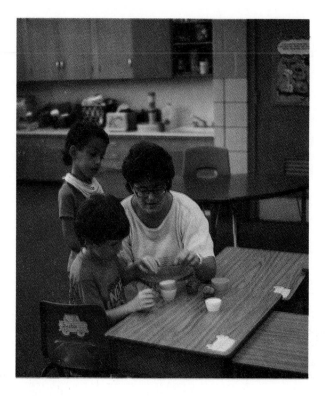

Some research suggests that children with learning disabilities do not perform as well as normal children on some memory tasks. (The Institute for the Study of Developmental Disabilities at Indiana University)

generally of normal or above average intelligence, seem to have many academic problems.

Reading.   Children with learning disabilities often have reading problems. In fact, learning disabilities grew out of what was once known as *remedial reading*. Some estimates suggest that over 85 percent of all learning-disabled students have reading disabilities (Kaluger & Kolson, 1978). The specific reading problems that students with learning disabilities have are as varied as the many elements involved in the reading process.

Word knowledge and word recognition are important parts of reading that cause difficulty for people with learning disabilities. When we encounter a word that we know, it needs only to be recalled from our mental dictionary to determine the meaning (Samuels & Kamil, 1984). Other words, however, are not a part of our mental dictionary and so we must sound the letters out and pronounce them based on our knowledge of typical rules regarding spelling patterns and pronunciation. Skill in this latter process is particularly important, since there are too many words for a person to memorize, especially when one is constantly encountering and learning new material. This dimension of word knowledge presents particular problems for students with learning disabilities. To recognize novel words, students must know the rules, be able to generalize letter patterns, and draw analogies with considerable flexibility to attain word recognition. Good readers usually accomplish this rather easily, fairly quickly, and almost auto-

I am LD—I learn differently. Rather than read a textbook like you're doing, I follow along as I listen to a recording of the text. When a recording of the text is unavailable, I rely on a reader. Rather than take notes, I photocopy another student's notes or tape the lecture, or sometimes both. Rather than write the complete answer to an essay question, I write a rough outline and from that I present my answer to the instructor (or record my answer on a cassette tape) so the instructor can assess my knowledge of the subject.

Educators say that background knowledge is extremely important to facilitate learning. To help develop my background knowledge (as well as for my enjoyment), I have a home library somewhat different from that of many people. It consists of illustrated books, books on many subjects that are primarily photographs, children's books (these really helped to begin building background knowledge), and educational books and tapes that go with them. I also have novels and short stories on tapes read by professional artists (these can be purchased at many bookstores). Another important source of both information and enjoyment are videotapes of movies made from books, documentaries, lectures, and classic and more recent movies. I have a specially designed radio that broadcasts the local newspaper, current magazine articles, books or chapters from books, and old-time radio shows. In addition to these, I receive a weekly world newspaper with larger print, less cluttered format, and less difficult reading level than papers available at the newsstand. The last item that I will mention here (I could go on much longer) is a consumer news digest that is extremely important. It covers a wide variety of topics, but the articles are short (*really* short) and therefore easy for me to read. This is a great source of consumer awareness and protection. I use it constantly for background information, and it helps a great deal in social conversation as well.

Learning differently is not without difficulty but I choose to focus on my strengths. It is my strengths that I need to spend time developing. It is by developing and using my strengths that I can compensate for my deficits. It is through utilizing my strengths that I'm successful. By focusing on my strengths and allowing myself to be different, to be creative, to accept that there are many alternatives by which I can get from A to B allows me to accept who I am—helps me to be my own best friend. I am a human being—I am *not* a learning disability, I am *not* an Attention Deficit Disorder, I am *not* a *label!* I am a person who learns differently, a person who approaches learning and living differently. If you let me I will share with you from my world, sensitivity, adventure, and discovery. You may even find new personal options, more creative approaches, and a new way of looking at people and life.

Deborah, *graduate student*

matically. Students with reading disabilities experience great difficulty with this process and when they can do it, they do so only slowly and laboriously. They can, however, be taught through specific training in the process (Anderson, Hiebert, Scott, & Wilkinson, 1985; Englert & Palincsar, 1988; Patberg, Dewitz, & Samuels, 1981).

Another important element in reading is the use of context to determine meaning. Good readers tend to be very adept at inferring the general meaning of an unknown word from the contextual information surrounding it. Poor readers have difficulty using context to aid in word recognition and reading (Bransford, Stein, Nye, Franks, Auble, Mezynski, & Perfetto, 1982; Patberg, Dewitz, & Samuels, 1981). However, specific instruction on using context improves the reading performance of students with learning disabilities (Wong & Sawatsky, 1984).

Good and poor readers are also different in the degree to which they have and use background knowledge (Bransford et al., 1982). Failure to use background information is likewise a problem for students with learning disabilities (Wong, 1980). Similarly, students with learning disabilities do not seem to perceive or use the organization of important ideas in text material, often focusing on details and factors that are less relevant (Bos & Filip, 1984; Englert & Thomas, 1987).

Reading is a complex process, involving many skills that are also found, in one form or another, in other areas (such as the ability to focus on the important rather than irrelevant aspects of a task). Thus some of the difficulties experienced by people with learning disabilities emerge in more than one facet of behavior, as we will see in discussing other academic characteristics. Depending on the severity of the problem, specific instruction may improve performance, although there may not be significant generalization beyond the limited focus of the training. In some cases, if the disability is quite severe (as in dyslexia), a person must be taught to compensate for the difficulty through alternative means of accessing information, and even then use reading sparingly.

Writing and Spelling.   Children labeled as learning disabled also often have markedly different writing performance than their nondisabled peers, which affects their academic achievement. These difficulties include areas such as handwriting (slow writing, spacing problems, poor formation of letters), poor spelling skills, and immature composition (Hallahan, Kauffman, & Lloyd, 1985). Several such problems were illustrated in Figure 6–2 presented earlier.

Some children are poor at handwriting because they have not mastered the basic developmental skills required for the process. Earlier we discussed theories regarding haptic perception problems in children with learning disabilities. Such deficits contribute to the very fundamental processes of grasping a pen or pencil and moving it in a fashion that results in legible writing on the page. In some cases, the fine motor development seems delayed in children with learning disabilities, which can contribute to the inability to physically use handwriting materials well. Handwriting also involves an understanding of spatial concepts such as up, down, top, and bottom. These are abilities that frequently are less well developed in youngsters with learning disabilities than in their nondisabled age-mates. The physical acts involved in using writing tools (such as a pencil or pen) as well as problems in spatial relationships can contribute to difficulty in forming letters and spacing letters, words, and lines. Some youngsters with rather mild handwriting problems may be exhibiting a slowness in development, which will improve as they grow older, receive instruction, and practice. However, there are also more severe examples (such as the young adult whose writing sample appeared in Figure 6–2) where age and practice have not resulted in writing-skill mastery.

Some researchers view the handwriting abilities of youngsters with learning disabilities as being closely related to their reading ability. For example, research does not clearly indicate that children with learning disabilities write more poorly than their normally achieving peers who are reading on a similar level (Grinnell, 1988; Tansley & Panckhurst, 1981). Letter reversals and, in severe cases, **mirror writing,** have often been used as illustrations of poor handwriting. However, it is also questionable whether children with learning disabilities commit these types of errors more often than their nondisabled peers *at the same reading level* (Nelson, 1980). The logic connecting handwriting and reading abilities has certain intuitive appeal. Most youngsters write to some degree on their own prior to receiving instruction in school (Harste, Burke, & Woodward, 1981). In general, children who write spontaneously also seem to read spontaneously and tend to have considerable practice at both before they enter school. Their homes (thereby implicating their parents) tend to have writing materials readily available for experimentation and practice. Likewise, writing is an activity they often observe their parents doing and may be one that the parents and child do together. Further research concerning the relationship between reading and handwriting is definitely in order. Instruction in writing for children with learning disabilities has historically been somewhat isolated from the act of reading, focusing instead primarily on the technical skills (Grinnell, 1988).

Poor spelling is often a problem among students with learning disabilities (also evident in Figure 6–2). These youngsters frequently omit letters or add unnecessary ones. Their spelling also shows evidence of letter-order confusion and reflects developmentally immature mispronunciation (Polloway & Smith, 1982). Interestingly, there has been relatively little research conducted on these spelling difficulties, and teaching has been based primarily on opinion (Grinnell, 1988). Recent studies suggest that spelling skills of students with learning disabilities seem to follow similar developmental patterns to those of their nondisabled peers, but they are delayed (Gerber, 1985, 1986). Characteristics such as visual and auditory memory problems, deficiencies in auditory discrimination, and **phonic generalizations** have also been implicated in the spelling difficulties with learning disabilities (Polloway & Smith, 1982). Further research on spelling is needed to more clearly understand this area.

Mathematics. Arithmetic is another academic achievement area where in-dividuals with learning disabilities have considerable difficulty (Ackerman et al., 1986). They often have problems with counting, writing numbers, and mastering other simple math concepts.

Counting objects is perhaps the most fundamental mathematics skill and provides a foundation for the development of the more advanced, yet basic, skills of addition and subtraction. Counting is also an area where students with learning disabilities encounter problems. Some of these youngsters omit numbers when counting sequences aloud (such as, "1, 2, 3, 5, 7, 9"), whereas others can count correctly but do not understand what the numbers mean with respect to relative value. Students with arithmetic learning disabilities also have additional

In the News 6–1

Dyslexia

■ At first glance, Tom Cruise, one of the hottest young actors in Hollywood, seems to lead a charmed life. His rise to stardom in only eight years (with movie credits that include *Risky Business, Top Gun, The Color of Money,* and *Rainman*), his good looks, charming manner, and air of self-confidence are in contrast to a childhood that was less than idyllic.

Cruise suffers from severe dyslexia. "For me, it began in kindergarten," he recalls. "I was forced to write with my right hand when I wanted to use my left. I began to reverse letters, and reading became so difficult I was always put in remedial classes, and I felt ashamed, like we were the dummies."

Cruise's family moved often and by the time he was eighteen, he had attended fifteen different schools. As a result, his dyslexia was never officially diagnosed or properly treated. He says, "With my reading difficulties, I'd never catch up. But people would excuse me: 'He's the new kid. We'll just help him through this year.'"

Fortunately, Cruise's mother had studied special education and she recognized the signs of dyslexia in her young son. She spent hours tutoring him in his studies and devising methods to help him overcome his disability. "I had to train myself to focus my attention," he explains. "I became very visual and learned how to create mental images in order to comprehend what I read."

When Cruise was sixteen, the family moved once again, to Glen Ridge, N.J. It was there that Cruise discovered his passion for acting when he played the lead in the senior class play, *Guys and Dolls.* "I could express myself in a way I'd never experienced before," he says. "I felt I needed to act the way I needed air to breathe." He asked his mother and stepfather to give him ten years to either succeed or fail as an actor. Tom Cruise's acting career took off, and today he is a top box office attraction.

■ Landmark College, founded in 1985 in Putney, Vermont, is the first post-secondary school devoted exclusively to teaching people with dyslexia.

counting difficulties when they are asked to proceed beyond nine, where more than one digit is used. This is a somewhat more advanced skill than single-digit counting and involves knowledge about place value.

Place value involves even more of a conceptual skill than the simple counting of objects and is fundamental to the arithmetic functions of adding and subtracting. Many students with learning disabilities in math have problems understanding place values and particular difficulty with the idea that the same digit (for example 6) represents different magnitudes when placed in various number positions (such as 16, 61, 632). Place value concepts are central to addition and subtraction since they are important to the processes of carrying and borrowing. Grinnell (1988) states that the four problems students with learning disabilities encounter include "(1) understanding the grouping process, (2) understanding that each position to the left represents another multiple of ten, (3) understanding the placement of one digit per position, and (4) understanding the relationship between the order of the digits and the value of the numeral" (p. 349).

Basic arithmetic difficulties such as those mentioned place major problems in the paths of students with learning disabilities. Those listed above are the

Developing students' self-esteem is a critical goal at Landmark College. Most people with dyslexia have experienced years of failure in the public school system. Some believe that they are stupid and destined to be failures. In reality, most people with dyslexia have average or above average intelligence, and many have overcome their difficulties to become highly successful. Some notable examples include Agatha Christie, Thomas Edison, Woodrow Wilson, Nelson Rockefeller, Cher, and Greg Louganis, Olympic diver.

The curriculum at Landmark College is grueling: intensive tutoring in all academic areas, with special attention given to reading and writing. Currently, there are 160 students enrolled at the school, which has an impressive student-teacher ratio of 4:1. But this special schooling does not come cheaply: for the 1989–90 school year, tuition, room and board will come to $22,900.

■ In 1986, Karen Morse sued her New Hampshire high school on the grounds that it failed in its duty to teach her to read and write. It wasn't until her junior year that the school diagnosed Karen with dyslexia. "I was smart enough to work around the system," she says. Karen was student-council president, editor of the school newspaper, and a member of the National Honor Society.

Specialized treatment for students with dyslexia is expensive, especially for public schools that must balance tight budgets. Consequently, many students don't get the help they need, and scores, like Karen, go undiagnosed. Often such students are assigned to remedial classes and grouped with other learners who have a variety of unrelated learning problems.

Sources: Ellen Hawkes, "'I Had to Grow Up Fast,'" *Parade*, January 8, 1989, pp. 10–12.

Ezra Bowen, "Good Timers Need Not Apply," *Time Magazine*, April 21, 1986, pp. 70–71.

"A Dyslexic Sues to Read 'n' Write," *Newsweek*, August 11, 1986.

very beginning quantitative concepts and are vital to learning further, more abstract, and complex mathematics. Students with learning disabilities are increasingly seeking to complete high school and attend colleges or universities. For these young adults, it is essential to achieve a certain level of mathematics mastery, including work in algebra and geometry during their years in secondary education. These topics have traditionally received minimal or no attention in curriculum design because of an emphasis on computation (Fair, 1988). Further research on mathematics difficulties and effective instruction for students encountering such problems is more important as the goals and achievements of such young people change.

Achievement Discrepancy. Youngsters with learning disabilities frequently find the fundamental and basic areas of academic achievement problematic, as indicated above. These students tend to be below their age-mates in achievement, but they also perform below what would be expected based on their measured potential. This has led to the discrepancy notion, which basically involves a discrepancy between academic achievement and what one would expect given the student's assessed ability and age. Attempts to quantify the academic achievement/potential discrepancy in learning disabilities have appeared in the literature for some time (Kaluger & Kolson, 1978; Myklebust, 1968). However, the field remains without an agreed-on formula. School-age youngsters may be two to four, or more, years behind their peers in academic achievement. Frequently a student falls progressively behind as he or she continues in the educational system. This often results in students dropping out of high school (Gartner & Lipsky, 1989; Stanford Research Institute, 1989), or graduating even though they are not proficient in basic reading, writing, or math skills.

Comments

We have described several behavioral characteristics that have been attributed to individuals labeled as learning disabled. It is increasingly evident that learning disabilities represent a very heterogeneous set of problems and that many different specific problems are involved under this general label. It is important to repeat that *learning disabilities* is a generalized educational term representing many different disorders. In many cases, solid empirical evidence for certain characteristics of the learning disabled is scanty or even absent. A substantial amount of what is known about people with learning disabilities can be considered simply clinical lore. This is also evident as we discuss the causes of learning disabilities.

CAUSATION

FOCUS 5
What are four causes thought to be involved in learning disabilities?

The behaviors of learning-disabled individuals have been explained in a number of ways, with a number of causes implicated. In some segments of the special education profession, determining causation (and classification) in learning disabilities is viewed from a rather pessimistic standpoint. For example, Lynn, Gluckin, and Kripke (1979) note that, "In fact, the causes of learning disabilities are unknown. If we knew what caused a learning disability, we would call it by another name" (p. 139). These authors further state that, "No *honest* classification of learning disabilities can be based on causes, because the causes are unknown" (p. 158, emphasis ours). This view, however, is not held by all professional groups working in learning disabilities. Interest and research on the causes of learning disabilities have been substantial over the years. In learning disabilities, as in many other areas, determining precise causation *is* difficult. This does not detract from the importance of such efforts; it merely limits the information available at any given time.

Neurological Causation

Over the years, learning disabilities have often been viewed as caused by structural neurological damage or, if not structural, some type of neurological-activation abnormality. A number of the professionals within the field support this contention (Gaddes, 1985; Reid, 1988; Rourke, 1987). Neurological involvement has even been specified as an identification criterion in some studies of learning disabilities (Kavale & Nye, 1981).

A variety of factors may result in the neurological damage such as that associated with learning disabilities. Part of what was discussed in relation to mental retardation (Chapter 4) is relevant here as well. To repeat, damage may be inflicted on the neurological system at birth, in several ways (e.g., abnormal fetal positioning during delivery, or anoxia, a lack of oxygen). Infections may also result in neurological damage and learning disabilities. Specific injury or infection has also long been implicated as a causal factor in brain damage and learning disabilities (Houck, 1984). However, neurological damage as a cause must be largely inferred, since direct evidence is usually not available.

Maturational Delay

Somewhat related to neurological causation is that of maturational delay. There have been some theories advanced that suggest a maturational delay of the neurological system results in the difficulties experienced by some individuals with learning disabilities (Goldstein & Myers, 1980). In many ways, the behavior and performance of children with learning disabilities resembles that of much younger individuals (Reid, 1988). They often exhibit delays in skills maturation, such as slower development of language skills, and problems in the visual-motor area and several academic areas, as noted above. Maturational delay is most likely not a causative factor in all types of learning disabilities but it has received considerable support as one of many.

Genetic Causation

Genetic causation has also been implicated in learning disabilities. Genetic abnormalities, which are inherited, are thought to cause or contribute to one or more of the problems categorized learning disabilities. This is always a concern for parents with regard to all types of learning and behavior disorders. Some evidence is available that would suggest genetic influences. Most likely we are examining many different specific problems with multiple causes. Over the years some research has obtained results suggesting an inheritance linkage (Hallgren, 1950; Healy & Aram, 1986), including studies of both **identical** and **fraternal twins** (Hermann, 1959; Matheny, Dolan, & Wilson, 1979). These findings must be viewed cautiously, because of the well-known problems in separating the influences of heredity and environment (Gelfand, Jenson, & Drew, 1988), but evidence lends a certain degree of support to the inherited causation of some learning disabilities (Houck, 1984).

Environmental Causation

Environmental influences are often mentioned as a possible cause of learning disabilities. Such factors as diet inadequacies, food additives, radiation stress, fluorescent lighting, unshielded television tubes, smoking, drinking, and drug consumption are now only beginning to be investigated. In some cases, these influences appear to be primarily prenatal concerns, whereas in others, the problems seem limited to the postnatal environment or both. Research on environmental causes remains inconclusive but it is the focus of continuing study.

Comments

Learning disabilities have many different causes, and in some cases a given type of learning disability may have multiple causes. We cannot always determine the origins of these problems, although considerable research has been conducted over the years with this aim. In many cases, it is more practical to direct attention to assessment issues in order to determine who can be helped with specialized instruction and what the nature of that instruction should be.

ASSESSMENT

FOCUS 6
What four questions are being addressed by screening assessment for learning disabilities?

Assessment for learning disabilities has several purposes. The ultimate goal is appropriate screening, identification, and placement of individuals who require services beyond those needed by most people. This may mean additional help academically, socially, or in various combinations, including nearly all aspects of life and nearly all human service disciplines. Decisions of such a varied nature require differing types of information from a variety of assessment procedures (Achenbach, 1986; Connors, 1986; Gordon, 1986). We examine here the assessment for learning disabilities in terms of purpose and domain of assessment; and focus on the areas of intelligence, adaptive behavior, and academic achievement.

Preliminary Concepts

As we begin discussing the assessment of learning-disabled individuals, certain preliminary concepts need to be mentioned. These concepts play an important role with respect to both the purpose and method of assessment. An individual's status in performance, skills, and ability may be evaluated in a number of ways. They may be assessed by either formal or informal means. The notions of formal and informal have grown to mean standardized versus teacher-made tests or techniques. Standardized instruments are those that are published and distributed widely on a commercial basis, such as intelligence tests and achievement tests. Teacher-made (or those devised by any professional) generally refer to techniques or instruments that are not commercially available. These may be constructed for specific assessment purposes and are often quite "formal" in the sense that great care is taken in the evaluation process. Both formal and informal assessment techniques are effective ways of evaluating learning-disabled students, and other students as well. Both are used for various evaluation purposes and in a number of performance or behavior areas.

Two other background concepts are also important, norm- and criterion-referenced assessment. **Norm-referenced assessment** compares an individual's skills or performance with that of others, such as age-mates or national average scores. Thus a student's counting performance might be compared with that of his or her classmates, others in the school district of the same age, or state or national average scores. In contrast, **criterion-referenced assessment** does not compare an individual's skills with some norm. Instead, his or her performance is compared with a desired level (criterion) that is a goal. The goal may involve counting to 100 with no errors by the end of the school year or some other criterion, depending on the purpose.

Both norm- and criterion-referenced assessment are useful with learning-disabled students. The two types tend to be used for different purposes, however. Norm-referenced assessment tends to be used more often for administrative purposes such as census data on how many students are achieving at the state or national average. Criterion-referenced assessment is helpful for specific instructional purposes and ongoing intervention planning.

It is very important to note that we are using these two terms as *concepts*, with no implied reference to specific instruments or procedures. Depending on how a technique, instrument, or procedure is employed, it may be used in a norm-referenced or criterion-referenced manner. Some areas of assessment, such as intelligence, are more typically evaluated using norm-referenced procedures. However, even a standardized intelligence test can be scored and used in a criterion-referenced fashion (although then it would become no more than a source of test items, and a student's performance could not be viewed exactly as the test developer intended). Assessment should *always* be undertaken with careful attention to the purpose and use of evaluation (Fuchs & Fuchs, 1986; Gronlund, 1985).

Screening

Screening and identification have always been important in assessment. For these purposes, assessment of youngsters occurs *prior* to any labeling or treatment. There are, however, usually suspicions of a problem by the clinicians or others (often parents) who come into contact with the child. This may occur at a rather young age for some individuals and involve assessment to compare the child with others of a similar age. Screening has the purpose of "throwing up a red flag," suggesting that more investigation is needed for one or more of several reasons. The questions to ask at this point of the assessment process are:

1. Is there a reason to more fully investigate the abilities of this child?
2. Is there a reason to suspect that this child is handicapped in any way?
3. If the child appears handicapped, what are the relevant characteristics and how should we move to intervention?
4. How should we plan for the future of this individual?

Answers to all of the above screening questions might well involve classification, placement for services, psychological or educational treatment, and evaluation of progress for the person. It is important to emphasize that assessment is not a simple, isolated event resulting in a diagnosis and is then completed. It is complex, involving many different steps. Assessment includes diagnosis, but it must be an ongoing process that provides the basis for a progression of decisions throughout the time an individual is receiving services (Drew, Logan, & Hardman, 1988; Houck, 1984). Approaches to assessment, for our purposes, come back to the three basic foci of intelligence, adaptive behavior, and academic achievement.

Intelligence.   Learning-disabled individuals have long been described as having average or near-average intelligence while experiencing problems in school more often found with students having lower intelligence. In many cases, the measured intelligence may not be accurate because of specific visual, auditory, or other limitations that might make it inaccurate. However, intelligence assessment remains an important matter with learning-disabled individuals (Swanson & Watson, 1982) and is typically evaluated with a standardized instrument such as an IQ test.

Adaptive Behavior.   The learning disabled have frequently been described as exhibiting behaviors that are not appropriate or adaptive in their environment. This has primarily appeared in clinical reports and has not historically been a routine part of the assessment to the degree it has in other areas of exceptionality such as mental retardation. However, some work has been undertaken to address adaptive-behavior assessment for learning-disabled individuals. Such efforts have been based on the assumption that an ability/academic discrepancy alone is insufficient to fully assess and describe learning disabilities (Weller et al., 1985). Adaptive behavior has contributed to concepts of subtypes and severity levels in learning disabilities (Weller et al., 1985; Weller & Strawser, 1987).

Academic Achievement.   Academic achievement has always been a major problem for learning-disabled youngsters. Achievement assessment is used to determine if there is a discrepancy between a student's ability and his or her academic achievement. Assessment of academic achievement is also of central importance to help evaluate the student's level of functioning in one or more areas. Instruments have been developed and used in an attempt to diagnose specific academic problems. For example, a number of reading tests are used to determine the nature of reading problems, including the Woodcock Reading Mastery Tests, the Diagnostic Reading Scales, and the Stanford Diagnostic Reading Test. Likewise, mathematics assessment has received attention, resulting in instruments such as the Key Math Diagnostic Arithmetic Test and the Stanford Diagnostic Mathematics Test (Swanson & Watson, 1982).

Academic assessment for learning-disabled students is very important. For the most part, assessment techniques are the same as those used in other areas of exceptionality. This is because deficits in academic achievement are a common problem among students with disabilities. However, specific skill-deficit diagnosis is more prominent in learning disabilities and has prompted focused skill-oriented academic achievement assessment in other disability areas as well.

INTERVENTIONS

FOCUS 7
What are three types of intervention or treatment employed with those diagnosed as having learning disabilities?

Intervention strategies for learning-disabled individuals have changed as professionals have come to view learning disabilities as a constellation of specific problems rather than a generic category. Much of the current literature addresses the area in terms of specific disabilities such as perceptual, cognitive, attention and hyperactivity, social and emotional, spoken language, reading, writing, and mathematics (Dudley-Marling & Searle, 1988; Hallahan, Kauffman, & Lloyd,

1985; Reid, 1988). A consequence of this current view is intervention aimed at specific problems, rather than general treatment of a problem that includes many different discrete disabilities.

Interventions used for adolescents or adults with learning disabilities may be different than those for children. In some cases, changes in treatment are due to different intervention goals emerging as individuals grow older (e.g., the acquisition of basic counting skills versus math instruction in preparation for college). Various professions are involved in the interventions for persons with learning disabilities. Although the different professionals often function as a team, each makes a unique contribution to the overall treatment program.

Childhood

There are several approaches to treatment and education of young children with learning disabilities. Many such children are first diagnosed as having learning disabilities when they enter school and begin to encounter academic difficulties. In these circumstances, it is often the educator and related school personnel that are involved in interventions. Other children with learning disabilities are first evaluated and treated by medical professionals.

Medical Interventions. Physicians often diagnose childhood abnormal or delayed development in the areas of language and behavior as well as motor functions. Pediatricians often participate in diagnosing physical handicaps that may significantly affect learning and behavior, and interpret medical findings to the family and other professionals. Physicians may be involved with a learning-disabled child early because of the nature of the problem, such as serious de-

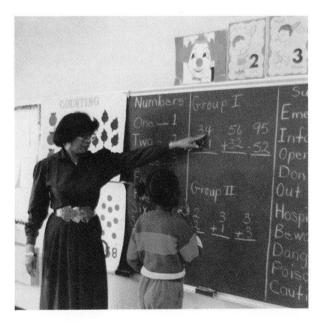

Instructional intervention should pinpoint specific problem areas. (The Institute for the Study of Developmental Disabilities at Indiana University)

velopmental delay or hyperactivity. Often, however, a medical professional sees the young child first because he or she has not entered school yet, and the family physician is the primary advisor for parents. When other professional expertise is needed the physician may refer the family to other specialists and then function as a team member in meeting a child's needs (Johnston, 1987).

Hyperactivity and the Use of Medication. One example of therapeutic intervention is in the area of hyperactivity. On the surface, hyperactivity may lead one to believe that such children are overly aroused; that is, suffering from greater-than-normal physiological arousal. Such notions led many researchers to recommend environments with few distracting stimuli, known as low-stimulus or stimulus-free settings. However, one treatment often employed with hyperactive children has called into question the overarousal theory. The medication often used to control hyperactivity is from the amphetamine family and is known as Ritalin. Although amphetamines increase activity in most people, they decrease activity in hyperactive children.

Other theories regarding hyperactivity may make sense of the paradoxical reactions to amphetamines. Some researchers have suggested that hyperactive individuals may be plagued by abnormally *low* physiological arousal; they are not functioning at an *optimal* arousal level, rather than being generally overly aroused (Zentall & Kruczek, 1988). It has been hypothesized that the apparent high level of motor activity in hyperkinetic individuals may be the result of the person trying to increase stimulation, much as a person who yawns is trying to stay alert. Such a notion would explain the higher level of activity in certain circumstances, plus the apparent quieting effect of amphetamines. Hyperactive children may receive adequate stimulation on the playground but not in a structured instructional setting. If amphetamines actually raise arousal in hyperactive individuals, as they do with most of us, then these children might not require an extraordinary level of activity to maintain an adequate level of stimulation. More research is crucial in this area because much remains unknown about medication and learning disabilities. For example, exactly which drug will be effective is seldom known until after treatment has begun. Adding to the disconcerting confusion is a problem with dosage level. Pelham (1983) stated:

> One of the problems with previous studies of drug effects on learning is the dosages of psychostimulants that have been administered in the great majority of studies (and in *all* long-term studies) have been considerably higher than the doses shown to maximize cognitive improvement. . . . Teacher ratings show greatest improvement with high doses of medication, with the result that the children in these studies have received mean doses of stimulants that improve *social behavior* but are 50% to 400% higher than the dose . . . recommended as the maximum to improve *cognitive abilities* (pp. 15–6).

Some professionals have seriously questioned the use of medication in light of the available evidence on its effectiveness (Pelham, 1986; Rosenberg, 1987). There has also been concern about side effects of the medication as well as possible abuse (Weiss & Hechtman, 1986). The physical side effects of using stimulant medication include insomnia, irritability, decreased appetite, and headaches. These side effects seem to be relatively minor and mostly temporary, although they vary greatly among individuals. Current thinking indicates that the successful treatment of hyperactivity requires multiple interventions, often differing greatly among individuals, and may be a lifelong undertaking (Whalen, 1987).

Instructional Interventions.   Instructional interventions include a variety of programs such as perceptual, cognitive, attention, spoken language, reading, writing and mathematics treatment (Choate & Rakes, 1989; Enright, 1989; Rakes & Choate, 1989). Even within these areas there have been an array of instructional procedures aimed at pinpointing specific problems. For example, as part of cognitive training, attention has focused on such instructional areas as problem-solving (Hamlett, Pellegrini, & Conners, 1987), problem attack–strategy training (Lloyd, 1980), and social competence (la Greca, 1987; Osman, 1987). Learning disabilities involve a very heterogeneous population, as our discussions thus far has indicated. Likewise, cognitive interventions also vary; they are tailored to address specific problems and often include combinations of approaches (Whelan & Henker, 1986).

Multiple intervention approaches and programs have been developed for the specific subtypes of learning disabilities noted above, and it is not surprising that controversies have emerged in some (see, for example, Hallahan, Kauffman, & Lloyd, 1985). For example, two general approaches to intervention for perceptual disabilities are process-training programs and the behavioral approach. Each has a number of specific procedures that have variously been called *programs, techniques,* or other labels. In all cases, with children the main purpose is to build skills that seem to be deficient so the students have a more promising potential in later school programs.

One example of building a foundation of skills for later learning is in the area of mathematics. Earlier we noted that children with arithmetic learning difficulties may have problems with basic counting and place values. For these students, counting may be most effectively taught with manipulative objects. Repetitive experience counting buttons, marbles, or any such objects helps the student to practice counting as well as learn the basic concepts of magnitude associated with numbers. Counting more than nine objects can help children begin to grasp rudimentary place-value concepts. In these cases, each ten objects that are counted are placed separately in a group, with those remaining being then counted and grouped separately. For students with learning disabilities these activities must be quite structured.

The illustration above involves counting, as a beginning math concept, using commonly available objects. However, there are also commercially available programs involving instruction in basic math concepts. Cuisenaire Rods (Davidson, 1969) are a set of 291 color-coded rods for manipulative learning experiences. These rods differ in length, with the color and size systematically associated with numbers. They may be used to teach basic arithmetic processes, either with individual students or groups.

Basic computational skills (addition, subtraction, multiplication, and division) may also be taught using the Computational Arithmetic Program (Smith &

Lovitt, 1982). This program was developed on the basis of the authors' research on students with learning disabilities. It also may be used with either individuals or groups. The manual includes methods for pupil placement, student-performance charting and analysis, and procedures for evaluating progress.

The programs mentioned above are selected from several available that can be used effectively for students with arithmetic learning disabilities. Others include DISTAR Arithmetic (Engelmann & Carnine, 1972), KeyMath Teach and Practice (Connolly, 1985), and Corrective Mathematics Program (Engelmann & Carnine, 1982). (The Corrective Mathematics Program is mentioned here although it is designed for use with students in the third grade through adulthood.)

Our rapid advances in computer technology have also found their way into the teaching of math skills to students with learning disabilities. Kirk and Chalfant (1984) suggest that microcomputers are particularly appealing for teaching math to these students because the fundamental structure of the content can be sequenced and programmed to present systematic instruction. Computers also have an advantage in that they provide a great deal of drill and practice on an individualized basis, something that is often difficult for teaching staff to accomplish with several children present, each adding to instructional responsibilities in different ways. Kirk and Chalfant (1984) point out that "the computer capability to present forms, objects, number problems, and word problems and to reinforce the student visually in a highly prescriptive, systematic fashion may replace many of the instructional methods used today" (p. 253). These points are well taken and do provide an effective means of instruction for some students with learning disabilities. One limitation, however, that cannot be addressed through the use of microcomputers is the manipulation of objects for students who find this helpful. Long-term research is needed regarding the effectiveness of computer instruction to determine its most useful application for these children.

Reading has been recognized for many years as a serious problem for students with learning disabilities, as indicated earlier. Consequently, this area of instruction has had a great deal of attention, and many different procedures have been used. Each has had some success with certain children but not with all, emphasizing the current belief that many different disabilities are involved even in students experiencing problems in the same area. Instructionally oriented research on specific types of problems, such as the inability to use context to determine meaning, has resulted in significant improvements for students with learning disabilities (e.g., Wong & Sawatsky, 1984). Information based on research like this is being incorporated into instructional programs more than ever before. Combined with the realization that we face many specific disabilities requiring focused instruction—that is, one approach does *not* fit all students—the instructional picture for students with learning disabilities appears promising.

Developmental reading instruction programs are often successful for students with learning disabilities (Lerner, 1985) and typically use the approach of introducing controlled sight vocabulary with an analytic phonics emphasis. Perhaps the most widely used developmental approaches involve basal readers such as the Holt Basic Reading; Ginn 720 Series; Scott, Foresman Reading; and Macmillan Series E. Basal readers are most useful for group instruction (often designed for three levels), are well sequenced developmentally, and most have sufficient detail for use by relatively inexperienced teachers. They tend to be oriented toward group instruction and therefore may present some limitations for students with learning disabilities who need heavy doses of individual, specific attention.

Individualized reading instruction is often required for a student with serious reading disabilities. Such individualization may be accomplished with many different materials (such as trade books), which are typically selected for reading levels and topics of high interest to the students. The basis for individualization falls on the shoulders of the teacher, who needs to have considerable knowledge of reading skills and procedures for specific, individually tailored instruction. Effective individualized instruction also requires a high level of progress evaluation, ongoing monitoring, and detailed record keeping. Individualized reading instruction seldom comes in a package (even when a publisher claims it), although most materials can be used in an individualized manner. The teacher's training, skills, and knowledge for effective individualized teaching must be applied in a flexible manner based on student needs.

Specific skill-oriented reading instruction may also be found in several diagnostic-prescriptive programs that are commercially available, such as the Fountain Valley Reading Support System available from Zweig and Associates and the Ransom Program from Addison-Wesley. There are also diagnostic-prescriptive reading programs that use computer-assisted instruction, such as the Harcourt Brace CAI Remedial Reading Program and the Stanford University CAI Project. Diagnostic-prescriptive reading programs provide for individualization in that the students work at their own pace. However, because they are packaged, commercially available materials, the skills that can be taught are only those that lend themselves to the format used. This reduces, to a degree, the level of individualization, but these programs do not require the high level of teacher knowledge and skill described above for the totally individualized reading instruction. Diagnostic-prescriptive programs generally provide ongoing assessment and feedback, and developmental skills are usually well sequenced.

There are many approaches and programs available for reading instruction beyond those mentioned above, each with strengths and limitations for students with learning disabilities. Other approaches that are developmentally based include synthetic phonics basals, linguistic phonemic programs, and language experience approaches. In addition, there are procedures that use multisensory techniques such as Fernald's method, developed initially in 1943 and recently revised by Idol (1988). Selection of an appropriate method and proper application of instructional technique is most effective when a student's particular disability and needs are addressed.

Computer software for use in reading instruction presents some potential assistance for students with learning disabilities and will likely be more commonly seen in the future. For these students, computer-presented reading instruction offers some particular advantages. Individual instruction can be provided to a student, and the computer provides for never-ending drill and practice. Programs can also provide feedback combined with corrective instruction. As we gain experience in writing computer programs, reading instruction software will improve (currently, word recognition programs seem to be of a higher quality than is comprehension software) and become more widely available (Lindsey, 1987).

As children progress into the upper elementary grades, they may also need to be taught some compensatory skills or methods to circumvent deficit areas that have not been remedied. These interventions may involve tutoring by an outside agency or individual specializing in the problem, or they may mean placement in a resource room or even a self-contained class for learning disabilities. Each approach reflects the severity of the difficulty, area of deficiency, and, unfortunately, the resources and attitudes of those involved (such as families and school districts).

Behavioral Interventions. Distinctions between behavioral and instructional interventions are not always sharp and definitive. Both involve the person's learning of skills and changing the ways they behave. Behavioral treatments, however, generally use the most basic principles of learning, the pointed use of stimuli, or stimulus conditions, and manipulation of the consequences of behavior, such as reinforcement. Behavioral interventions such as the structured presentation of stimuli (e.g., letters or words) and reinforcement for correct responses (e.g., specific praise) are used in many instructional interventions including several mentioned earlier. In this section we briefly discuss some behavioral treatments that are used outside of traditional academic areas.

With certain children, treatment may include social skills that are causing difficulty. Some students with learning disabilities who experience repeated academic failure become frustrated and depressed despite trying so hard. They may not understand why their nondisabled classmates seem to do little more than they do yet achieve more success. These students may show extreme withdrawal or express frustration and anxiety by acting out or becoming aggressive. When this type of behavior emerges, it may be difficult to distinguish these students with learning difficulties from those with behavior disorders as a primary disability. In fact, at this point there is an overlap between them with regard to many behaviors. Social and behavioral difficulties of students with learning disabilities are receiving increasing attention in the literature (e.g., Deshler & Schumaker, 1983).

One type of intervention often used to change undesirable behavior is the **behavioral contract.** Using this approach, a teacher or behavioral therapist establishes a contract with the child that provides him or her with reinforcement if appropriate behavior is exhibited. Such contracts may be either written or verbal, usually focus on some specific behavior (such as remaining in his or her seat for a given period of time), and rewards the child with something that he or she really likes and therefore considers reinforcing (such as going to the library or using the class computer). It is important that the pupil understand clearly what is expected and that the event or consequence be appealing to *that child* so that it really does reinforce the appropriate behavior. Behavioral contracts have considerable appeal because they give the youngsters a certain amount of responsibility for their own behavior (Brown, 1986), and they can also be used effectively outside of school settings, including by parents, at home. Contracts also have applications in various forms, at widely different ages.

Another behavioral intervention involves what is known as a **token economy.** Token-economy systems arrange conditions in a manner where the students can earn tokens for appropriate behavior, which can then be exchanged for something that is of value *to them* (i.e., something rewarding, as noted above). Token economies resemble the work-for-pay lives that most of us have as adults, and so the approximation of that life can also teach the child skills that are generalizable later. Token economies require considerable time and effort to plan and implement (Morris, 1985), but they can be used effectively to improve behavior.

Behavioral interventions are based on the fundamental principles of learning and largely developed from the early work of experimental psychologists such as Skinner (1953; 1957; 1971). These principles have been widely applied, in many settings, for students with learning disabilities as well as other exceptionalities. One of their significant strengths is that, given knowledge of the basic theory, they can be modified to suit a wide variety of needs and circumstances.

One factor that must be considered for all interventions is the age of the person being treated. In this section we have discussed interventions that may be used during childhood. Obviously childhood covers a broad age span. The *exact* elements (content or specific approach) of an appropriate intervention for a child of six are not likely to be useful for one who is twelve years old. Age-appropriate modifications are essential to the effectiveness of any treatment and most often must be made by the professional involved in the intervention.

Adolescence

Medical Interventions. Intervention with learning-disabled adolescents is somewhat different than with children. If they are receiving medication to control hyperactivity or other problems, it is likely that they have been taking it for a number of years, since many physician assessments and prescriptions are made during childhood. There are, however, a number of cases in which learning-disabled adolescents and adults have struggled through the earlier years and have not received medication until after childhood. In many cases, the medication to assist with behavior and attentional problems is again one in the amphetamine family (Coons, Klorman, & Borgstedt, 1987). Adolescents with learning disabilities may have social-behavior deficits somewhat similar to those exhibited by juvenile delinquents (Fleener, 1987; Perlmutter, 1987).

FOCUS 8
How are the interventions used for adolescents with learning disabilities different from those employed during childhood?

Instructional Interventions. Instructional/academic interventions are also different at this age than with younger individuals. Research suggests that the instructional system fails adolescents with learning disabilities. Forty-seven percent drop out of school by the age of sixteen (Gartner & Lipsky, 1989) and do not receive diplomas. If the goal of secondary education is to prepare individuals for postschool life and careers, there is serious doubt that this goal is being accomplished for adolescents with learning disabilities. Not only do these young people still need to achieve at least minimal survival-level skills academically (for some, preparation for college), but they are also often deficient socially, without comfortable interpersonal relationships. Clearly, a comprehensive model, with a variety of components, needs to be developed to address a broad spectrum of needs for learning-disabled adolescents. Deshler, Schumaker, and Lenz (1984) discussed such a model and suggested seven components that specifically emphasize (1) motivation, (2) detailed, specific instruction targeting academic and cognitive skills, (3) generalization of mastered skills to other content areas and settings, (4) content to be mastered, (5) communication enabling a coordinated service to the student from various professionals, (6) transition from secondary school to postschool life, and (7) evaluation to obtain intervention feedback (p. 109). Such a comprehensive model program, however, rests primarily in the literature as a recommendation; it remains to be developed or implemented on a widespread basis. To this list we would add instruction and experiences in socially related areas that are relevant to young people just entering adulthood—information seldom taught but essential to a successful and happy adult life.

One of the continual difficulties facing teachers of adolescents with learning disabilities is *time*. There is a limited amount of time for instruction for these young people, progress for them is often slow, and determining what to focus on during this time is difficult (Deshler, Schumaker, Lenz, & Ellis, 1984). These adolescents and their teachers face a difficult task. In some areas, the students may not have progressed beyond the fifth grade academically (Warner, Schumaker, Alley, & Deshler, 1980). And they may have only a rudimentary grasp of some academic topics, yet they are reaching an age where life after secondary school must be addressed. This may mean college plans, which is happening with increasing frequency, vocational goals, and preparations for social and interpersonal life beyond childhood. Thus at a time when they need to be building and expanding on a firm foundation of knowledge, many students with learning disabilities are operating on a rather beginning to intermediate level.

Secondary-school instruction for students with learning disabilities may also involve compensatory skills to circumvent those not acquired earlier. These compensations are often focused on specific deficits such as writing, listening, and social behaviors. For example, tape recorders may be used in class, to offset difficulties in taking notes during lectures, which would compensate for a listening (auditory-input) problem.

For some individuals, there are residual or accompanying personal problems related to their disabilities, requiring counseling or other mental-health assistance. Adolescents with learning disabilities tend to have low social status among nearly all the people around them including peers, teachers, and even their parents (Dudley-Marling & Edmiaston, 1985). Certain learning-disabled youth may also become involved in criminal activities at this time in their lives (Fleener, 1987; Perlmutter, 1987). Despite this fact, which is mentioned periodically in the literature, the empirical link between learning disabilities and juvenile delinquency is inconclusive (Wallander, 1988), and evidence suggests that arrests or jail terms for them do not occur at substantially higher rates than for their nondisabled peers (McLoughlin, Clark, Mauck, & Petrosko, 1987; White, Deshler, Schumaker, Warner, Alley, & Clark, 1983).

Transition Interventions. In many cases, the adaptations of adolescents (as well as adults) identified as learning disabled have been accomplished by themselves over the years (Lynn et al., 1979). However, the difficulties that youngsters with learning disabilities experience do not disappear (Kramer, 1986; McCue et al., 1986), and specialized services are often needed through adolescence, perhaps into adulthood. Unfortunately, transition services remain rather sparse for this population on a widespread basis, but they are beginning to receive increased emphasis as interest in adolescence becomes greater. Both research and personnel preparation efforts are now being undertaken on a level that would not have been predicted a few years ago.

Transition programs for adolescents with learning disabilities must basically consider similar life goals as would be relevant for nondisabled young people. Some students view their postsecondary-school years as involving employment that does not require further education in a college setting. A portion of these pupils continue their schooling in vocational and trade schools (Stanford Research Institute, 1989). However, there are growing numbers of young people with learning disabilities who have definite college or university plans. There is little question that they will encounter difficulties (Vogel, 1982). However, with as much academic mastery as possible, compensatory skills where needed, and perseverance, college education is certainly possible.

College-bound students with learning disabilities find that many of their specific deficit areas are basic survival skills in higher education. Matters such as taking notes during lectures, absorbing lecture information auditorially, written language skills, reading, and study habits are all assumed in normal college classrooms. Transition programs preparing these students must elevate their abilities in these areas as much as possible and show the students how to compensate as well. Tape recorders may circumvent difficulties in lectures because the student need not receive all the information from notes or auditorially, at least not quickly, *during* the lecture. Taped lectures can be played and replayed many times to understand the information. Students with reading disabilities often obtain the help of readers, who tape textbooks for their use in much the same manner as others tape lectures.

Perhaps the most helpful survival skill that can be taught to a youngster with learning disabilities is actually more than a specific skill—it is a way of thinking about survival. Recall Deborah, the graduate student in Window 6–1. Deborah describes an amazing array of techniques that she uses to acquire knowledge while circumventing her specific deficit areas. No list of detailed suggestions like those in the last paragraph can cover all possible situations when a college student with learning disabilities will need special assistance. Transition programs preparing these students for college are most effective if, in addition to suggestions, they can teach a survival attitude, or way of thinking about how to compensate for their severe deficit areas.

As part of survival skills, these students should also be taught how to establish an interpersonal network of helpers and advocates. In many cases, a faculty-member advocate is more successful than the student in asking a colleague to allow for special testing arrangements or other consideration (at least for the first time). Faculty in higher education are bombarded with student complaints and requests, most of which are not based on extreme needs. They are therefore wary of students' requests for considerations like extra time. Additionally, many faculty in higher education are uninformed about learning disabilities, and thus to receive the initial overtures from a faculty colleague carries more credibility.

Students with learning disabilities can lead productive, even distinguished, adult lives. Some research suggests that even after they complete a college education, adults with learning disabilities have limited career choices (Gottfredson, Finucci, & Childs, 1984). A more complete research base is needed in this area. However, we do know that learning disabilities are reported to have plagued notable people like Thomas Edison (scientist and inventor), Woodrow Wilson (President of the United States), Albert Einstein (scientist), and Nelson Rockefeller (Governor of New York and Vice President of the United States). We also know that Deborah graduated with her Masters degree, and that the young man whose writing we saw in Figure 6–2 did become a successful architect. Such achievements are not accomplished without considerable work, but the outlook for students with learning disabilities can be very promising.

REVIEW

FOCUS 1: What are four reasons why definitions of learning disabilities have varied?

- *Learning disabilities* is a broad, generic term that involves many different specific types of problems.
- The study of learning disabilities has been undertaken by a variety of different disciplines.
- The field of learning disabilities per se has existed for only a relatively short period of time and is therefore relatively "immature" with respect to conceptual development and terminology.
- The field of learning disabilities has grown at a very rapid pace.

FOCUS 2: What are four different ways in which people with learning disabilities can be classified?

- By the type of atypical behavior exhibited.
- Historically, as a mild disorder but with increasing attention to varying severity.
- By theorized causation.
- By the type of academic deficit exhibited.

FOCUS 3: What are two estimate ranges for the prevalence of learning disabilities?

- From 1 to 28 percent, depending on the source.
- From 5 to 10 percent is a reasonable current estimate.

FOCUS 4: What are seven characteristics attributed to the learning disabled, and why is it difficult to characterize this group?

- Typically, average or near-average intelligence.
- Uneven skill levels in various areas.
- Hyperactivity.
- Perceptual problems.
- Visual- and auditory-discrimination problems.
- Cognition deficits, such as memory.
- Attention problems.

- In other words, the group of individuals included under the umbrella term *learning disabled* is so varied that it defies simple characterization with a single concept or term.

FOCUS 5: What are four causes thought to be involved in learning disabilities?

- Neurological damage or malfunction.
- Maturational delay of the neurological system.
- Genetic abnormality.
- Environmental factors.

FOCUS 6: What four questions are being addressed by screening assessment in learning disabilities?

- Is there a reason to investigate the abilities of this child more fully?
- Is there a reason to suspect that this child is handicapped in any way?
- If the child appears handicapped, what are the characteristics and how should we move to intervention?
- How should we plan for the future of this individual?

FOCUS 7: What are three types of intervention or treatment employed with those diagnosed as having learning disabilities?

- Medical interventions, in some circumstances involving medication to control hyperactivity.
- Academic interventions in a wide variety of areas that are specifically aimed at building particular skill areas.
- Behavioral interventions aimed at improving social skills or remediating problems in this area. Behavioral procedures may also be a part of academic instruction.

FOCUS 8: How are the interventions used for adolescents with learning disabilities different from those employed during childhood?

☐ Interventions with younger children focus primarily on building the most basic skills.

☐ Interventions during adolescence may include skill building but also involve assistance in compensatory skills that permit the circumvention of deficit areas.

☐ Interventions during adolescence should include instruction and assistance in transition skills that will prepare students for adulthood, employment, and further education, based on their own goals.

Debate *Forum*

Is *Learning Disabilities* Too Broad a Category?

Some have argued that *learning disabilities* is too broad a category to be practically useful and that the label should be dropped in favor of the more specific subtype labels that are included under this broad term. Others contend that this would be a mistake, since there is a trend toward eliminating categories anyway.

Point *Learning disabilities* is a general category of exceptionality that includes many different specific problems that are extremely diverse. These conditions vary greatly from perceptual problems to hyperactivity and poor academic performance in specific areas. Both research and interventions must be pinpointed at the specific area of difficulty to be effective. The general label *learning disabilities* has promoted the notion that there is a single unitary problem that can be treated with a general intervention useful for all individuals that are so diagnosed. This is clearly not the case. The term *learning disabilities* should be eliminated and replaced with multiple labels that more accurately describe the specific problems. This approach would communicate more clearly to all involved (e.g., parents, professionals) that a specific disability exists and requires intervention that is pinpointed at the particular problem.

Counterpoint There are already too many different categories of exceptionality. Adding more by employing more specific terminology for those involved in learning disabilities would only cause problems. Such a move would create an administrative nightmare and further confuse professionals and laypeople alike. It runs counter to the conceptual trends currently gaining momentum in special education that suggest minimizing or eliminating categories. In fact, the field of learning disabilities is ahead of the game and leading the way with regard to minimizing categories. Educators and other professionals can use the term *learning disabilities* very easily and simply keep in mind that varying types exist.

There are good points to each of these arguments and also certain limitations. Take a position and argue for that position using information provided in the book plus other sources you might find.

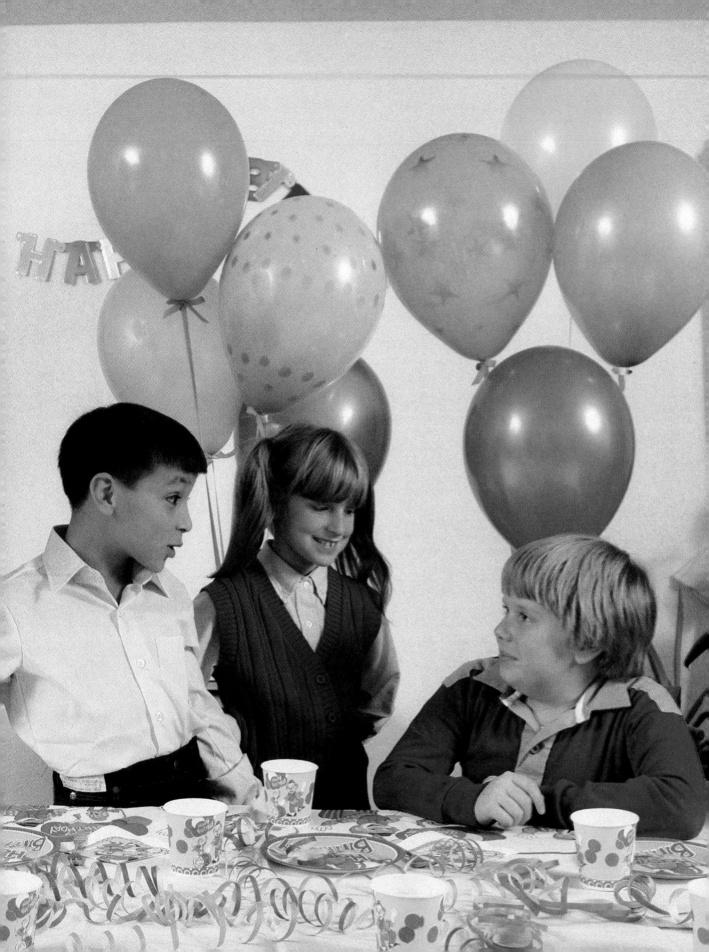

7 Cross-categorical Perspectives

To Begin With...

- The classification of children into specific categories, such as learning disabled, mentally retarded, or emotionally disturbed, may not be justified. There does not appear to be a relationship between these categories and the instructional needs of each individual student. An example of this is the classification of learning disabilities, described by some professionals as ill-defined and poorly conceptualized. Yet the term is used to describe a vast number of children who are unsuccessful in school (Goldman & Gardner, 1989).

- Approximately 80% of the entire student populaton in our nation's schools could be classified as learning disabled by one or more of the definitions presently in use (Ysseldyke, 1987).

- Procedures for classifying students with disabilities are often unreliable, invalid, time consuming, and costly. These classifications result in stereotyping students and isolating them from their nondisabled peers. It is also true that once a label is found, it is seldom lost (Wang, 1989).

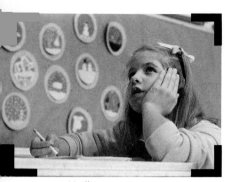

Marilyn

Marilyn is nine years old and in her second month of fourth grade at Willowbrook Elementary School. Her classroom teacher describes her as a slow learner and a poorly motivated student. Marilyn is unable to cope with the behavioral or academic requirements of the classroom without assistance beyond that required by the other students. She has a reading vocabulary that is beginning third-grade level and consistently struggles with reading-comprehension activities. In math she is still attempting to master basic subtraction facts but is proficient in number identification and single-digit addition.

Marilyn has communicated to her parents and teacher the frustrations she encounters at school. She sees school as a negative aspect of her life. Her teacher confirms this negative attitude and reports that Marilyn has difficulty completing assigned tasks and is often reprimanded for daydreaming or visiting with classmates at inappropriate times. Marilyn was recently referred to the school psychologist for an analysis of her educational skills. A standardized test battery indicates that Marilyn is functioning below average on an individual test of intelligence (IQ 83); achievement-test scores range from the end of second-grade level in reading to second grade, first month, in math; and language expression and reception are below the average for students in her classroom.

Jared was a very disruptive student who had been referred numerous times to a variety of public school and community agencies. From the time he was in the second grade until he reached fifth grade, he had been in constant trouble, not only with his parents but also with his teachers and neighbors. A review of his school history showed that he had been described as obnoxious, a holy terror, and downright sneaky. In terms of his academic performance he had not done well either. He was considerably below the level of his classmates in all subjects except for art and physical education. In creative activities, particularly artwork, he did extremely well.

His most obvious problem was his behavior. He was extremely noncompliant. He did things when he felt like doing them, regardless of setting or rules. He had few if any close friends. He was regularly involved in fights and teasing. The regular classroom teacher used all available resources and personnel to assist Jared and his family in dealing with their problem, but these efforts were to no avail. His misbehavior was not limited solely to school environments. Children in his neighborhood avoided him, and his family had a difficult time relating to him. During the middle of Jared's elementary-school years his mother and father were divorced. Jared's father maintained custody of the children (two younger sisters and Jared). Within a year, Jared's father remarried. His new mother made sincere attempts to become Jared's friend, but that friendship never materialized to any significant degree. Over time, Jared and his stepmother became bitter enemies. With the demise of his family relationships and lack of any substantive success in school, his already dismal school record became worse. He was eventually referred at the beginning of the fifth grade for placement in a self-contained class for students with behavior disorders. The placement was finalized during the seventh week of school. Jared now regularly attends this class.

Kevin is 14 years old and attends school at Eastmont Junior High. Kevin does not speak, walk, hear, or see. Throughout the day, his classroom support team works diligently to meet Kevin's most basic needs, including feeding and toileting. In spite of his profound and multiple handicapping conditions, Kevin has learned to make his wants known through a communication board, is able to maneuver through his environment in a wheelchair, and is learning to feed himself independently. Kevin lives at home with his family. He participates in all family activities, including shopping at the local mall, eating at a fast-food restaurant, relaxing on the lawn in the neighborhood park, and playing miniature golf at the community recreation center.

INTRODUCTION

Marilyn is a student with a **mild learning and behavior disorder.** She has remained in the regular classroom environment, with no additional educational services, since she was six years old. While Marilyn's academic and behavioral performance in the classroom deviates enough to require some additional instruction programming beyond that given to her classmates, it is anticipated that once these services are available she can remain in the regular classroom. The problems of children with mild learning and behavior disorders are most evident in school; they have less difficulty adjusting to life outside the classroom setting. Consequently, as these individuals move into adulthood the learning and behavior disordered classification is usually no longer applicable if adequate special services have been provided during the school years.

Jared is a student with a **moderate learning and behavior disorder.** His behavior problems occur not only in a school setting, but at home and within his neighborhood. He and his family need additional help, beyond educational services, including ongoing counseling provided by the local mental health agency. With considerable effort on the part of teachers, support services, and family, Jared may be back in the regular class in the next school year.

Kevin is an individual with **profound/multiple disorders.** In one way or another, he will be dependent on others throughout his life. Marilyn, Jared, and Kevin are certainly not representative of all individuals with learning and behavior disorders, but they are representative of the range of problems experienced by this population. The previous three chapters discussed learning and behavior disorders using the traditional **categorical descriptors** of mental retardation, behavior disorders, and learning disabilities. In this chapter we view individuals with learning and behavior disorders from the perspective of **crosscategorical definitions** and intervention strategies. Our purpose is to familiarize you with an alternative approach to traditional categorical labels. The crosscategorical approach used in this chapter groups individuals with learning and behavior disorders on the basis of severity—mild, moderate, and severe learning and behavior disorders. The labels *mental retardation, behavior disorders,* and *learning disabilities* are not used in the description of the individuals.

CATEGORICAL VERSUS CROSSCATEGORICAL APPROACHES

FOCUS 1
Why is the *crosscategorical approach* considered an alternative way of defining and classifying individuals with learning and behavior disorders?

Categorical and crosscategorical approaches represent alternative ways of defining and classifying individuals with learning and behavior disorders. While both approaches are useful in certain instances, neither alone can serve the broad range of learning and behavior disorders adequately. The issue regarding categorical and crosscategorical approaches to defining and classifying learning and behavior disorders has gained considerable attention in the field of education in recent years (Dickie, 1982; Gartner & Lipsky, 1989; Gartner & Lipsky, 1987; Lilly, 1987; Marston, 1987; Reynolds, Wang, & Walberg, 1987). Some professionals have maintained that the traditional categories of mental retardation, behavior disorders, and learning disabilities do not clearly define nor adequately differentiate the needs of exceptional students in the classroom (Eysenck, Wakefield, & Friedman, 1983; Jenkins, Pious, & Peterson, 1988; Hardman, 1981; Laycock, 1980; Lilly, 1987; Reynolds & Birch, 1988). Jenkins et al. (1988) summarized this view: "We can see no justification for separating students by categorical labels" (p. 157). Granger and Granger (1986) indicate that "every time a child is called mentally defective and sent off to the special education class for some trivial defect, the children who are left in the regular classroom receive a message: no one is above suspicion; everyone is being watched by the authorities; nonconformity is dangerous" (p. xii).

An alternative viewpoint is that crosscategorical labels are nonfunctional, and that the individual categories are more relevant to educational programming (Becker, 1978; Braaten, Kauffman, Braaten, Polsgrove, & Nelson, 1988; Keogh, Becker, Kukic, & Kukic, 1972). As suggested by Braaten et al., "To argue that BD [behavior disordered] students' stigma derives from their label misses that point that these students become social outcasts before they are referred for special education" (1988, p. 23).

Many psychologists and educators have attempted to break away from the traditional categories. In large part, efforts to date have been unsuccessful. Some approaches have represented little more than semantic exercises that used different terms but maintained the same categorical framework. Others have been dramatically different, but have accomplished little except to fuel a polarized debate between advocates of crosscategorical and categorical classification systems. Little serious effort has been given to a careful examination of the bases or parameters employed for classification and to the circumstances under which they may be functional or nonfunctional.

Our discussion now focuses on learning and behavior disorders using a crosscategorical approach. The learning and behavioral characteristics of the individual are broken down into mild, moderate, and severe and profound/multiple conditions. A mild learning and behavior disorder is representative of the highest level of performance; severe and profound/multiple is the lowest level of performance.

MILD LEARNING AND BEHAVIOR DISORDERS

Every educator has been confronted with students who exhibit mild learning and behavior problems. As is true of Marilyn in the opening vignette, the significance of such problems depends on a number of factors. First, what is the discrepancy between how the student is performing on school-related tasks and what is expected? For Marilyn, reading performance is about a year behind her classmates. In math, she is about two years behind peers. Her classroom teacher also describes her as a poorly motivated student. From the school's standpoint, the problem is often viewed in terms of its effect on the student's academic achievement and social adjustment, as well as any negative effect on the student's classmates, which may be evident (or anticipated).

Definition

The framework for our discussion of mild learning and behavior disorders is the following definition:

> *Individuals with mild learning and behavior disorders exhibit academic and/or social-interpersonal performance deficits that range from one to two **standard deviations** below average on **normative** and **criterion-referenced assessments**. These deficits generally become evident in a school-related setting. The cause of the performance deficits is generally unknown. A student with a mild disorder remains in the regular classroom setting for the majority, if not all, of the school day. Additional support services beyond those typically offered in a regular education setting should be made available as necessary.*

FOCUS 2
Identify the four components of the definition of mild learning and behavior disorders.

This definition emphasizes the breadth of this population and allows for considerable flexibility in identifying and providing educational support services. This crosscategorical definition stresses that the primary reason for identifying this population is to enhance the opportunity for success in the regular education classroom. In order to deal with the variety of characteristics exhibited by these students, the definition purposely does not limit the areas for assessment. Depending on the problem that has resulted in a referral, assessment may include several measures, such as **adaptive behavior, academic achievement,** and **cognitive functioning.** This provides the professional with the flexibility of using whatever assessment tools are necessary to determine the extent of the academic or behavioral deficits and to make recommendations for educational intervention. The definition is meant to emphasize *present* functional deficits that may well be corrected or improved through educational intervention. In the crosscategorical approach, educators must focus directly on functional descriptions of the specific problem behavior, rather than on a label that may have no specific relevance for instruction.

There are four major components in the definition of mild learning and behavior disorders: (1) academic and/or social-interpersonal deficits are one to

Everything You Ever Wanted to Know About a Standard Deviation

The definitions of learning and behavior disorders introduced in this chapter include a term that may not be familiar to you. Standard deviation is merely a *measure* of the amount that an individual score differs from the average. Put another way, standard deviation gives us a way to measure the percentage of difference between what is the average score of a group of people and how well a given individual performed in comparison to that average. Let's take, for example, an intelligence test. Questions are put together by a group of researchers that, for the sake of our discussion, measure the construct known as *intelligence*. Once the questions are developed, this test is administered to a group of people to see how well they do on each of the questions. When all the scores are added up and divided by the number of people who have taken the exam, the average score turns out to be 100. This certainly doesn't mean that everyone scored 100, it is merely an arithmetical way of establishing what is average.

When we look at individual scores on the intelligence test, we find that some people actually do score 100, whereas others are either higher or lower than our average score. Johnny, for example, has a score of 85. So just what does the score of 85 mean in comparison to the rest of the people who have taken this test? We can now use a mathematical procedure to determine the extent to which Johnny's score differs from the average score of 100. This measurement is called a **standard deviation** from the average. Again

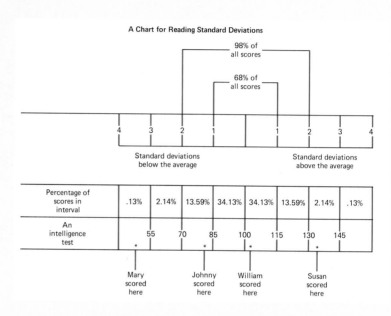

for the sake of discussion, we find that on this intelligence test each standard deviation is about 15 points. Now, looking at the chart for reading standard deviations we can see that because Johnny scored 85 he is one standard deviation *below* the average score on the test. Mary, on the other hand, scored 50. Looking at the chart, we see that she is more than three standard deviations below the average. William scored 104 on the test, so he is less than one standard deviation *above* the average. Susan scored 134, so she is more than two standard deviations above the average. We now know how many standard deviations each of these individuals is away from the average, but the information is still not very meaningful. Let's convert these standard deviations into percentages. The mathematical procedure used to determine a standard deviation also

reveals the *percentage* of people taking the test who score at each of the standard deviation levels. The chart reveals that Johnny's score of 85 means he is better than only 16 percent of all the people who took the test. In other words, 84 percent of the people taking the test had a better score than Johnny. Mary's score of 50 is better than less than 1 percent of everyone taking the test. William's score is close to the average, so he did better than 50 percent of those taking the test. Susan's score of 134 is better than about 98 percent of all the scores.

Remember, the standard deviation is simply a means to measure percentages. Whether a test is a measure of intelligence, academic achievement, behavior, weight, height, age, or some other characteristic, the idea is the same.

two standard deviations below the average on normative and criterion-referenced assessments, (2) problems are primarily evident in school settings, (3) the cause is generally unknown, and (4) the student remains in the regular class, with support services. (See Figure 7–1.)

The phrase *academic and/or social-interpersonal performance deficits* is necessary because such deficits are generally shared attributes of these students. It is not uncommon to find a student with a mild disorder who is lower in academic ability than his nondisabled classmates and exhibits social adjustment problems. The definition allows for the independent occurrence of an academic deficit or behavior problem, but it also suggests that if both disorders occur in a parallel fashion they are included within the single definition. For example, Marilyn is unable to cope with either the academic or behavioral requirements of the classroom. We can assume that an individual functioning at this level is generally able to adapt to the social environment outside the classroom setting. Problems that do emerge are not likely to be serious enough to cause a referral on behavior alone.

The phrase *one to two standard deviations below the average* specifies severity level. For example, Marilyn's IQ is 83, which is between one and two standard deviations below the mean of 100. This IQ level differs somewhat from certain trends in more traditional categories. For example, in 1973 the AAMR moved to two standard deviations as the upper limit on IQ in defining mental retardation, and essentially declassified as mentally retarded all individuals functioning between that level and the average. (Review Reflect on This! 4–1 in Chapter 4, How to Cure Mental Retardation.)

The crosscategorical approach permits individuals with a mild disorder to receive specialized services in a *regular education classroom,* but it avoids using the label *retardation,* which has such a negative connotation. Even though the AAMR has ceased viewing mental retardation as unchangeable, the general connotation of the label is one of permanence and social stigma. The crosscategorical definition emphasizes a person's functional performance, which may well be changed by specific intervention techniques.

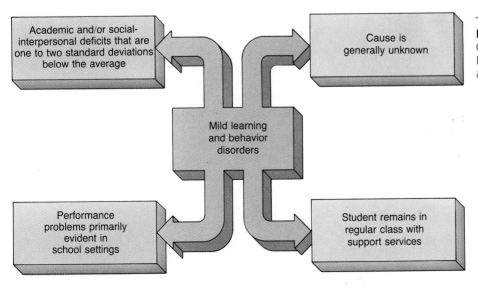

Figure 7–1
Components of the Definition of Mild Learning and Behavior Disorders

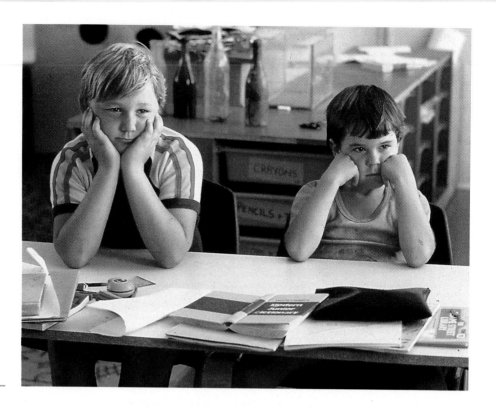

Interindividual differences occur in all children. (Photo Researchers © Ulrike Welsch)

It is our contention that the term *mild learning and behavior disorders* is broad enough that it is unlikely to become a diagnostic term, but it can be used in a number of ways that are functional for intervention purposes. Educators would therefore be required to focus more directly on a functional description of the problem behavior than has historically been the case (labels became diagnostic entities). For example, Marilyn is a fourth-grade student with a reading vocabulary that is beginning third-grade level. The deficit in reading vocabulary is a functional description of Marilyn's problem that indicates the discrepancy between actual performance and what is expected for a child of her age. The categorical label placed on Marilyn might be a *learning disability*, which provides no specific information regarding her specific academic problems.

An individual's performance may be described statistically by comparing him or her with others of the same chronological age (**interindividual differences**), or the person may be described in terms of an analysis of his or her individual strengths and weaknesses (**intraindividual differences**).

An interindividual assessment is often referred to as a *norm-referenced* or **standardized** measure of student abilities, because the individual is compared to a larger group where a mean or average score has been determined. Intraindividual assessment, often referred to as *criterion-referenced* measurement, does not compare the student to other students, but analyzes the student's individual strengths and weaknesses. As with interindividual assessment, a mean or average is determined. However, the average is calculated on several of the *individual's* performance areas (e.g., giving letter sounds, recognizing common word parts, or sound blending). Then each area of performance is compared to the individual's average, in addition to an assessment of differences between performance areas. Depending on the nature of the problem, one may need to view the child on an interindividual basis, an intraindividual basis, or both. The use of average performance (means) does not restrict this definition to standardized tests in which means have been established through norms. Such an anchor point can be determined using **behavior checklists** and **precision-teaching** techniques on both inter- and intraindividual bases. The basic premise of this part of the definition is that a functional analysis of the individual's performance areas is made.

The phrase *on normative or criterion-referenced assessments* is necessarily broad because of the variety of specific attributes required for assessment. Depending on the problem that resulted in the referral, the attributes may include one or more of several measures, such as adaptive behavior, academic achievement, and intellectual functioning. This provides the flexibility to use normative referenced (interindividual) instruments, criterion-referenced (intraindividual) assessments, observations, interviews, and so forth, as well as systems of assessment that combine several types of measures.

In large part, the performance deficits of mildly disordered individuals "become evident in school-related settings where the cause of the problem is generally unknown." Problems may well occur in other settings, such as the home, but the most pronounced difficulties clearly relate to the structured environment of formal schooling. This has led to certain characterizations such as the **"six-hour retardate"** (MacMillan, Meyers, & Morrison, 1980). This notion arose from observations that certain youngsters appeared retarded only during the six hours a day they were in school. These children, often from low socioeconomic backgrounds, are labeled *retarded* in the school setting, but the label is not transferred to their home and community lives. The retardation label also disappears once the student transitions out of school into the adult years. Given that the occurrence of mild learning and behavior disorders is associated primarily with the student's educational experience, the estimated prevalence of the condition is based on services provided during the school years.

Prevalence

Whether a student is labeled *handicapped* (as defined by federal or state regulation) depends on the level of educational intervention required. This decision is best handled by a **multidisciplinary** team responsible for determining the most appropriate educational program and environment for the student. Depending on federal and state funding patterns, this team must generally work within the parameters of the 12-percent prevalence figure established for services to handicapped children under P.L. 94–142 (see Chapter 2).

Approximately 13 percent of all school-age children perform between one and two standard deviations below the mean and are thus considered to have a mild learning and behavior disorder according to the definition presented in this chapter. Obviously, not all mildly learning and behavior disordered students qualify for special education services or are labeled *handicapped* under P.L. 94–142. Given the 12-percent ceiling, we estimate that about 6 percent of the school-age population qualifies for funds under the description "mild learning and

FOCUS 3
What is the estimated prevalence of mild learning and behavior disorders?

behavior disorders." An additional 7 percent of school-age students needs educational support services and are considered mild learning and behavior disordered, but do not qualify for federal money targeted for students who are handicapped.

Characteristics

FOCUS 4
Identify the discrepancies between definitions of mental retardation, behavior disorders, and learning disabilities and the actual performance of children in each category.

Individuals with mild learning and behavior disorders share a variety of characteristics that cut across the more traditional categorical definitions. Although many special educators have attempted to preserve categorical purity, some professionals indicate that when the child's actual performance in the classroom is examined, there is considerable overlap, particularly at the mild severity level (Gartner & Lipsky, 1987; Gartner & Lipsky, 1989; Jenkins, Pious, & Peterson, 1988; Laycock, 1980; Lilly, 1987; Reynolds & Birch, 1988; Wang, 1981; Wang & Walberg, 1988).

Many educators have begun to focus on the relationship between learning environment, material content, and individual learner and teacher styles, rather than the differences between categorical labels. This approach directs attention to specific instructional approaches rather than centering on a label. Hardman (1981) indicates that educational programming has been based more on definitional expectations according to categorical labels than on the individual student's actual task performance. This educational phenomenon is illustrated in Table 7–1 (see page 224), which compares expectations according to traditional categorical definitions with the actual performance of students in a given categorical area.

There is real danger in adhering strictly to the categorical approach at the mild severity level, because it implies that each category is homogeneous. An examination of individuals with mild learning and behavior disorders reveals that this is not the case.

> The term *mental retardation*, for example, is currently applied to hundreds of different syndromes. Likewise, *learning disabilities* and *emotional disturbance* are generic or global terms covering a variety of specific problems. It is misleading to use the labels as though all children within the category exhibit common attributes. . . . In addition to variance within categories, there is also overlap between categories. Human beings cannot be pigeon-holed as neatly as definitions would lead us to believe (Laycock, 1980, p. 53).

Students with mild learning and behavior disorders are often defined and categorized primarily by exclusion—by what they are not. For example, the learning-disabled child is usually defined as one who is *not* intellectually inferior, even though children of varying intellectual functioning levels may exhibit specific learning disabilities (Hammill, 1976). Additionally, learning-disabled students do not demonstrate distinct and reliable differences from other low achievers in the educational system (Ysseldyke, Algozzine, Shinn, McGue, 1982).

When comparing mild behavior-disordered and learning-disabled students, intelligence is considered a common attribute: By definition, these two categories involve individuals who are normal in intelligence. The differences between mild behavior disorders and specific learning disabilities have been explained more in terms of social-adjustment differences and learner characteristics. However, learning-disabled individuals may also exhibit secondary behavioral disorders. In addition, mild behavior-disordered populations may also have learning difficulties comparable to those exhibited by individuals defined as learning disabled (Hallahan & Kauffman, 1976). The performance of students in the classroom also suggests that behavior problems are not specific to any one intellectual functioning level. It is well known, both clinically and from the scientific literature, that individuals with mental retardation also exhibit a considerable amount of behavior that is socially and interpersonally maladaptive (Drew, Logan, & Hardman, 1988). Problems in social adjustment must therefore be viewed as a characteristic that is shared by learning-disabled, behavior-disordered, and mentally retarded students to a considerable degree.

One factor that has long been viewed as characteristic of learning-disabled individuals is variability between areas of functioning. General descriptions of learning disabilities have often emphasized great intraindividual differences between skill areas. For example, Marilyn is a fourth grader reading at about a third-grade level, with some difficulties in comprehension. However, her skills in math are at least a full grade below her reading level, and two grades below the expectancy for her age. Frequently this variability in aptitude patterns has been used to distinguish between learning-disabled and mentally retarded students. Typically, individuals thought to be retarded are expected to exhibit a rather flat or consistent profile of abilities, in contrast to the pronounced intraindividual variability associated with learning disabilities. It is expected that a child with mild mental retardation would achieve at about the same level across all academic areas, reading, writing, and arithmetic. As with other attributes, however, intraindividual variability does not seem to be the sole domain of students with learning disabilities. Intraindividual variability can occur for students with mental retardation and behavior disorders as well.

Our discussion has emphasized the considerable similarities of behavioral attributes within traditional categories at the mild level. This does not negate the fact that differences do exist between the traditional categories, especially in terms of overall ability, rate of learning, and attention to task. It does, however, stress that the categorical labels are not useful in the development of an educational program for students with mild learning and behavior disorders. As summarized by Reynolds and Birch (1988),

> In view of the major problems of reliability in the classification of children, it can be fairly concluded that for the present, instruction for exceptional children ought to proceed mainly on the basis of highly individualized evaluations of both children and their situations, disregarding the classification criteria as educational mentally retarded, learning disabled, and emotionally disturbed (p. 56).

Our effort to conceptualize mild disorders in a crosscategorical fashion requires that the traditional categories be viewed within an "umbrella model" of symptom severity. It also requires that accommodation be made for the shared and discrepant behavioral characteristics of students with mild learning and behavior disorders.

Causation

The cause (or causes) of mild learning and behavior disorders is largely unknown. Because so many factors can interact and contribute to these learning and behavior differences, it may not be possible to ever determine cause. However, we do

FOCUS 5
Identify five possible causes of mild learning and behavior disorders.

TABLE 7–1   Capacity, Achievement, and Social Performance by Special Education Categorical Area

	Definitional Expectation	Actual Performance
Capacity (Intelligence)	*Mild Behavior Disorders:* Average or above-average performance on intelligence tests.	*Mild Behavior Disorders:* Behavior problems occur in all ranges of intelligence, e.g., mentally retarded range.
	Learning Disabilities: Average or above-average performance on intelligence tests.	*Learning Disabilities:* Specific learning disabilities occur in all ranges of intelligence, e.g., mentally retarded range.
	Mild Mental Retardation: Low potential—significantly subaverage (two standard deviations below the mean) performance on intelligence tests.	*Mild Mental Retardation:* Mental retardation is limited by definition to IQ below 70. Definition excludes children whose IQ is *between* one and two standard deviations below the mean (IQ 70–85).
Achievement (Academic Learning)	*Mild Behavior Disorders:* Definitions do not generally include low achievement as a criterion.	*Mild Behavior Disorders:* Low achievement can be secondary effect of behavior disorders (behavior problems interfere with academic learning).

know that individuals exhibiting mild learning and behavior disorders are not usually characterized by physical or sensory deficits. These are individuals whose problems are primarily educationally related. They are not easily identified as disordered once they are outside the educational environment. It may not be until the child enters school, often at the age of five, that a handicapping condition is actually recognized.

Numerous causal factors have been associated with mild learning and behavior disorders; for example, diverse cultural backgrounds, socioeconomic differences, and poor teaching. Mercer and Lewis (1979) confirm that students whose cultural backgrounds are different from the dominant core culture, and whose socioeconomic status is on the lower end of the continuum, are more likely to be identified and labeled as having a disability by the public education system. These authors also indicate that the same population is not viewed by the community as deviant outside the school setting.

Effective teaching practices are critical to the success of mildly handicapped students in an educational environment (Larrivee, 1986; Lovitt, 1977). Poor teaching may be a primary reason for many of the school-related problems exhibited by students with mild learning and behavior disorders: "Perhaps 90 percent or more of the children who are labeled 'learning disabled' exhibit a

	Definitional Expectation	Actual Performance
	Learning Disabilities: Low achievement is an integral part of the learning disabilities (LD) definitional concept. Child will perform at least one or two years below grade level.	*Learning Disabilities:* Child performs at least one or two years below grade level.
	Mental Retardation: Low intelligence indicates poor academic potential.	*Mental Retardation:* Mildly retarded child performs at least one or two years below grade level.
Social Skills (Adaptive Behavior)	*Behavior Disorders:* Child will be deficient in socialization and classroom adaptation skills.	*Behavior Disorders:* Child is deficient in socialization and classroom adaptation skills.
	Learning Disabilities: Social deficits are not included in LD definitional structure.	*Learning Disabilities:* Poor performance in social and adaptive behavior may be secondary effect of learning problems.
	Mental Retardation: Adaptive behavior skills are an integral part of mental retardation definition.	*Mental Retardation:* IQ continues to be *major* factor for categorization. Social deficits are not necessarily correlated with poor performance on intelligence tests.

Source: Reprinted, by permission of the publisher, from M. L. Hardman, "Learner Characteristics of Students with Mild Learning and Behavior Differences," in M. L. Hardman, M. W. Egan, and E. D. Landau, *The Exceptional Student in the Regular Classroom* (Dubuque, Iowa: William C. Brown Co., 1981), p. 60.

disability not because of anything wrong with their perception, **synapses,** or memory, but because they have been seriously mistaught. Learning disabilities are made, not born" (Engelmann, 1977, pp. 46–47). There is a need to examine more closely the way teachers are educated in university-preparation programs and their effectiveness in applying what they have been taught (Marston, 1987). Are teachers utilizing the appropriate procedures, methods, and materials necessary to ensure maximum growth and development in their students?

Several other factors are associated with mild learning and behavior disorders, including high absenteeism during the early school years and differing value systems within the home concerning the importance of school. Poor motivation or inadequate memory and retention skills have also been linked to school-related problems. The list goes on, but the issues of causality remain unresolved.

MODERATE LEARNING AND BEHAVIOR DISORDERS

Our discussion of mild learning and behavior disorders emphasized the shared characteristics of individuals at this severity level. Individuals with mild learning and behavior disorders are the most likely candidates for a crosscategorical approach to services (Forness & Kavale, 1984). As we move to individuals at the moderate severity level, traditional categories become more distinct, and individuals with various characteristics are more different from one another than before. However, certain behavioral characteristics remain shared by individuals with different primary diagnoses. The identification of a primary disabling condition is more easily accomplished at this severity level.

Definition

FOCUS 6
Identify the four components of the definition of *moderate learning and behavior disorders.*

Despite greater reliance on the traditional categories, the notion of a crosscategorical approach for individuals with moderate learning and behavior disorders is still a viable alternative. In this context, the definition of moderate learning and behavior disorders is as follows:

> *An individual with moderate learning or behavior disorders exhibits intellectual, academic, and/or social-interpersonal performance deficits that range between two and three standard deviations below the average on normative and criterion-referenced assessments. These performance deficits are not limited to the school setting but are typically evident in the broad spectrum of environmental settings. The cause(s) of the problem(s) may be identified in some cases but typically cannot be precisely determined. Individuals with functional disorders at this level require substantially altered patterns of service and treatment and may need modified environmental accommodations.*

This definition presents a crosscategorical framework that is consistent with our approach to mild learning and behavior differences. The four major components of the definition of moderate learning and behavior disorders are (1) intellectual, academic, and/or social-interpersonal deficits that range from two to three standard deviations below the average, (2) performance problems beyond the school setting, (3) identifiable causes in some cases, and (4) the necessity for substantially altered patterns of service and treatment. (See Figure 7–2.)

The phrase *intellectual, academic, and/or social-interpersonal performance deficits* focuses on problems that require a more intense level of service than that provided to students with mild disorders. The term *intellectual* has been added to the definition because at the moderate severity level when an intellectual deficit is involved it is far more evident and pronounced than at the mild severity level. (Some individuals with mild learning and behavior disorders may exhibit learning or achievement difficulties that suggest intellectual deficits, but the deviations in measured intelligence are not sufficient to be considered a primary problem.) The terms *academic and social-interpersonal performance* were also used in the definition of mild disorders, but differ in the areas of severity and the environment in which a performance problem may be apparent—difficulties are evident in a broader range of environments than in the case of mild disorders. Performance problems may be exhibited in more than one area of functioning. Individuals with moderate disorders exhibit multiple performance deficits that are more frequent and serious than at the mild severity level. However, the primary disabling condition is more easily identified than with a mild disorder. Additionally, causes for some of the conditions may be identifiable at this level of severity.

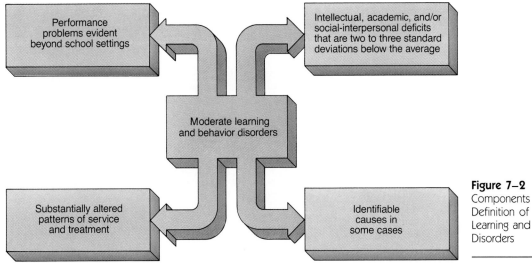

Figure 7–2
Components of the Definition of Moderate Learning and Behavior Disorders

Prevalence

Approximately 2 percent of all school-age individuals exhibit moderate learning and behavior disorders. This figure is based on our definition of moderate disorders, which requires that the performance deficits for these individuals range between two and three standard deviations below interindividual or intraindividual means on any given assessment.

FOCUS 7
What is the estimated prevalence of moderate learning and behavior disorders?

Characteristics

The primary distinguishing characteristics associated with the traditional categories of mental retardation, behavior disorders, and learning disabilities become more distinct at the moderate level of severity. It is true that many people with moderate learning disorders also manifest behavior problems and vice versa, but in many cases of moderate disorders one can assess which is the primary difficulty and which is the secondary one. This is not as easily accomplished with those who are described as having a mild learning and behavior disorder.

FOCUS 8
Why are many children with moderate learning and behavior disorders not identified until they reach school age?

Many children with moderate learning and behavior disorders are not identified until they enter school at the age of five or six. This is because these children may not exhibit severe physical anomalies that are readily identifiable during the early-childhood years. Nevertheless, the preschool child with a moderate disorder exhibits one- or two-year delays, particularly in the development of socialization skills and academic readiness. As the child enters school, these developmental lags become more apparent in the classroom environment. During the first one or two years in school, the child's intellectual, academic, and/or social differences may be attributed to immaturity. However, school professionals eventually realize the need for specialized intervention beyond the regular class. Unfortunately, valuable instruction time may be lost by not intervening when the problem is first suspected. (For a more in-depth discussion of the characteristics

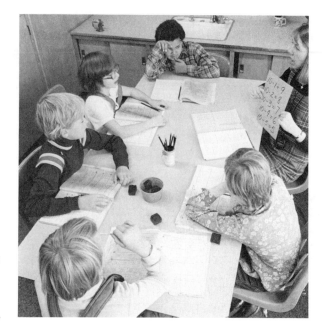

Children with moderate disorders may go undetected until they enter school and their developmental lags become more apparent in the classroom environment. (John Telford)

of these individuals according to the traditional categorical areas of mental retardation, behavior disorders, and learning disabilities, see the Characteristics sections of Chapters 4, 5, and 6.)

Causation

FOCUS 9
Identify five possible causes of moderate learning and behavior disorders.

The causes of moderate learning and behavior disorders run the same gamut as the causal factors associated with mental retardation, behavior disorders, and learning disabilities. Causal factors may range from socioeconomic differences, poor motivation or achievement orientation, and inadequate memory and retention, to identifiable neurological dysfunction, genetic or **metabolic errors,** drug or alcohol abuse, poor maternal nutrition, or infectious diseases. The cause of the disorder is often unknown or unidentifiable.

SEVERE AND PROFOUND/MULTIPLE DISORDERS

Individuals with severe and profound/multiple disorders may be impaired in nearly every facet of life. Some of these people have severe intellectual, learning, and behavior disorders; others are physically disabled or sensory impaired. Most have disorders that transcend our ideas of single-handicap categories; they have significant, multiple problems. Recall that Kevin, from our opening vignette, cannot speak, walk, hear, or see.

The needs of these people cannot be met by one profession. The nature of these disorders extends equally into the fields of medicine, psychology, and social services. Since these individuals present such diverse characteristics and need several professional perspectives, it is not surprising that numerous definitions and intervention strategies have been employed to describe and treat them.

Definition

Our crosscategorical definition of severe and profound/multiple disorders is as follows:

> *Individuals with severe and profound/multiple disorders exhibit physical, sensory, intellectual, and/or social-interpersonal performance deficits that range beyond three standard deviations below the average on normative and criterion-referenced assessments. These deficits are not limited to any given setting but are evident in all environmental settings and often involve deficits in several areas of performance. Cause(s) is more likely to be identifiable at this level of functioning, but exact cause(s) may be unknown in a large number of cases. Individuals with functional disorders at this level require both substantially altered patterns of service and treatment and modified environmental accommodations.*

The four major components of this definition are (1) physical, sensory, intellectual, and/or social-interpersonal deficits more than three standard deviations below the average, (2) deficits evident in all environmental settings and across several areas of performance, (3) identifiable causes in some cases, and (4) substantially altered patterns of service and treatment. (See Figure 7–3.)

The severity of the condition has increased in this definition, moving *beyond three standard deviations below the average on the measure(s) being recorded*. This statement is self-explanatory, although a point regarding the handicap impact needs reemphasizing here. You may note that we have focused on the term *disorder* and carefully avoided *handicap* in most of this discussion. The reason for this is that the two notions are not synonymous. For example, a person may have a severe visual disorder (i.e., be blind) but not be severely *handicapped*, because of accommodations in the environment, special mobility

FOCUS 10
Identify the four components of the definition of severe and profound/multiple disorders.

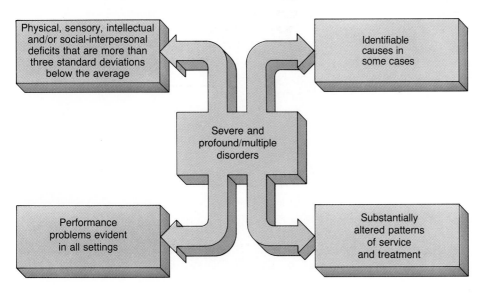

Figure 7–3
Components of the Definition of Severe and Profound/Multiple Disorders

training, and special instructional technology. Kevin has multiple disorders, including the inability to communicate verbally. However, through the technology of a communication board, he is able to make his wants known to others. Thus, in certain circumstances a disorder may be severe while the handicap impact is less pronounced.

The term *multiple* disorders is used because the vast majority of persons with severe and profound disorders exhibit multiple problems. The nature of these problems may include a combination of any one or more of the several categories of exceptionality. However, mental retardation is a primary symptom in the greatest number of cases. Persons with profound retardation invariably suffer from significant physical and psychological disorders in addition to subaverage intellectual functioning. Severely and profoundly retarded persons have a higher incidence of congenital heart disease, epilepsy, respiratory problems, diabetes, and metabolic disorders. They exhibit poor muscle tone and are often plagued with such conditions as **spasticity, athetosis,** and **hypotonia** (Mori & Masters, 1980). These people may also have sensory impairments, including vision and hearing disorders.

The relationship between severe retardation and emotional disturbance has not been understood as clearly as that between retardation and physical disorders. In fact, there has been a great deal of confusion concerning the overlapping characteristics of these supposedly different populations. Characteristics of severely emotionally disturbed persons appear to be closely related to those of individuals with severe and profound retardation, but by definition severely disturbed individuals are not truly retarded.

There are also multiple disorders in which mental retardation is not a primary symptom. One such disorder is **deaf-blindness.** The concomitant vision

In addition to mental retardation, people with severe and profound disorders may also exhibit problems such as poor muscle tone, epilepsy, and vision and hearing disorders. (Photo Researchers, Inc./Will & Deni McIntyre)

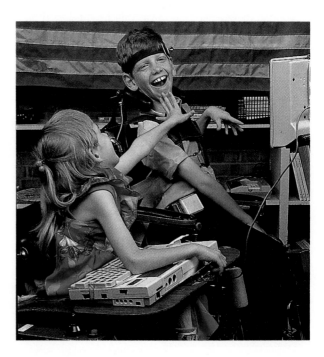

and hearing disorders exhibited by deaf-blind people result in severe communication deficits as well as developmental and educational difficulties. These multiple problems preclude placement in single-category programs for either the deaf or the blind and necessitate highly specialized services.

There are many terms used to describe individuals with severe and profound/multiple disorders. These include **severely handicapped, profoundly handicapped,** or **severely multiply handicapped.** Note, however, that few crosscategorical definitions distinguish between severe and profound conditions. There is little consensus on the distinction between the two. Thus these conditions are often treated as a single category within the educational system.

Prevalence

Individuals with severe and profound/multiple disorders constitute a very small percentage of the general population. Even if we consider the multitude of conditions, prevalence estimates generally range from no more than 0.1 to 1.0 percent. Approximately 4 out of every 1000 persons are severely and profoundly handicapped where the primary symptom is mental retardation. An additional 2 to 4 out of every 10,000 children exhibit some other form of severe mental disorder.

FOCUS 11
What is the estimated prevalence of severe and profound/multiple disorders?

Characteristics

Individuals with severe and profound/multiple disorders can exhibit any combination of physical, psychological, intellectual, or sensory problems. Some combinations are more prevalent than others, but there is an incidence of all combinations. Bellamy (1985) defined individuals with severe and profound/multiple handicaps as individuals "who require ongoing support in several major life areas in order to participate in the mainstream of community life" (p. 6).

FOCUS 12
Identify seven behavioral and physical characteristics associated with severe and profound/multiple disorders.

Individuals with severe handicaps can also be characterized according to their instructional needs. Snell (1987) suggests that professionals working with these students concentrate on instructional need and less on general, often stereotyped, population characteristics. For Kevin, this would mean focusing on educational outcomes that can decrease his dependence on others in his environment, and can create opportunities to enhance his participation at home, school, and in the community. Instruction is developed with these outcomes in mind, rather than with a set of general characteristics associated with the label *severe handicaps.* As proposed by Snell, "Such appropriate methods for these difficult-to-teach students include those that reduce errors, and facilitate **generalization** of skills learned under one set of conditions to other conditions. Further, teachers need to collect accurate student performance data so that progress can be monitored" (1987, p. 3).

Other authors (Falvey, 1986; Wilcox, 1979) have also supported a stronger emphasis on instructional need and suggest that definitions of severe handicapping conditions refer directly to the individual's level of functioning. "Definitions which reference absolute functioning levels, though admittedly arbitrary, do carry reasonable information regarding the probable content of instruction and do allow for the removal of the label 'severely handicapped' based on demonstrated student progress: As students acquire more skills, they lose the label" (Wilcox, 1979, p. 139).

The multitude of characteristics exhibited by people with severe and profound disorders is mirrored by the numerous definitions associated with these individuals. A close analysis of these definitions reveals a great deal of repetition from one to another; all describe people whose life needs cannot be met without substantial assistance from society. These people have been, and are likely to continue to be, dependent in some fashion on social support systems for a lifetime.

Causation

FOCUS 13
Identify five possible causes of severe and profound/multiple disorders.

Multiple problems result from multiple causes. For the vast majority of this population, the problems are evident at birth. Birth defects may be the result of genetic or metabolic disorders, including **chromosomal abnormalities, phenylketonuria, or Rh incompatibility.** Birth defects may also be caused by drugs, smoking, or alcohol-related problems; poor maternal nutrition; infectious diseases (such as rubella); exposure to radiation; venereal disease; or advanced maternal age. Severe and profound disorders can also be the result of factors that occur later in life, such as poisoning, accidents, malnutrition, physical and emotional neglect, and disease.

This chapter has focused on learning and behavior disorders using a crosscategorical approach. The learning and behavioral characteristics of the individual have been broken down into mild, moderate, and severe and profound/multiple conditions. Success in the educational setting for these students depends on the **adaptive fit** between the demands of the school and the needs and ability of each student, regardless of severity level (see Chapter 3). Several factors must be considered in this adaptive process, including the development of appropriate goals and objectives, modification of the instructional program (such as basic skills, remediation, functional life skills), and an analysis of the time available to meet these objectives.

REVIEW

FOCUS 1: Why is the crosscategorical approach considered an alternative way of defining and classifying individuals with learning and behavior disorders?

- ☐ The crosscategorical approach does not use the traditional categories of mental retardation, behavior disorders, or learning disabilities in defining or classifying students with learning and behavior disorders.
- ☐ Some professionals have suggested that the traditional categories of mental retardation, behavior disorders, and learning disabilities do not clearly define or adequately differentiate the needs of each student.
- ☐ The crosscategorical approach characterizes students with learning and behavior disorders on the basis of the severity of the problem: mild, moderate, and severe and profound/multiple disorders.

FOCUS 2: Identify the four components of the definition of mild learning and behavior disorders.

- ☐ The four major components in the definition of mild learning and behavior disorders are (1) academic and behavioral deficits that are two standard deviations below the average, (2) school-related problems, (3) cause is generally unknown, and (4) student remains in regular class.

FOCUS 3: What is the estimated prevalence of mild learning and behavior disorders?

- ☐ Approximately 13 percent of all school-age children perform between one and two standard deviations below the average.
- ☐ Only 6 percent of school-age children functioning be-

tween one and two standard deviations below the average receive special education services.

FOCUS 4: Identify the discrepancies between definitions of mental retardation, behavior disorders, and learning disabilities and the actual performance of children in each category.

□ Behavior problems may be evident in children with mental retardation and learning disabilities as well as those with behavior disorders.

□ Learning disabilities occur in all ranges of intelligence.

□ Low academic achievement is evident in children with behavior disorders as well as in those with learning disabilities and mental retardation.

FOCUS 5: Identify five possible causes of mild learning and behavior disorders.

□ The causes associated with mild learning and behavior disorders are largely unknown.

□ Factors such as diverse cultural backgrounds, low socioeconomic status, poor teaching, and high absenteeism in school have all been associated with mild learning and behavior problems.

FOCUS 6: Identify the four components of the definition of moderate learning and behavior disorders.

□ An individual with moderate learning or behavior disorders exhibits intellectual, academic, and/or social-interpersonal deficits that are two to three standard deviations below the average.

□ Problems are evident in a broad spectrum of environmental settings.

□ Causes are identifiable in some cases.

□ Individuals with moderate learning and behavior disorders require substantially altered patterns of service and treatment in comparison to nonhandicapped peers.

FOCUS 7: What is the estimated prevalence of moderate learning and behavior disorders?

□ It is estimated that approximately 2 percent of all school-age children exhibit moderate learning and behavior disorders.

FOCUS 8: Why are many children with moderate learning and behavior disorders not identified until they reach school age?

□ Children with moderate learning and behavior disorders are generally not identified prior to school age because they may not exhibit physical or learning problems that are readily identifiable during the early-childhood years.

FOCUS 9: Identify five possible causes of moderate learning and behavior disorders.

□ Possible causes associated with moderate learning and behavior disorders include socioeconomic differences, low motivation or achievement orientation, inadequate memory and retention, genetic or metabolic errors, and poor maternal nutrition.

□ The cause may also be unknown.

FOCUS 10: Identify the four components of the definition of severe and profound/multiple disorders.

□ Individuals with severe and profound/multiple disorders have physical, sensory, intellectual, and/or social-interpersonal deficits that range beyond three standard deviations below the average.

□ These deficits are evident in all environmental settings.

□ Causes are identifiable in some cases.

□ Individuals with severe and profound/multiple disorders require significantly altered environments with regard to care, treatment, and accommodation.

FOCUS 11: What is the estimated prevalence of severe and profound/multiple disorders?

□ Prevalence estimates generally range from no more than .1 percent to 1 percent of the general population.

FOCUS 12: Identify seven behavioral and physical characteristics associated with severe and profound/multiple disorders.

□ These individuals may exhibit a range of characteristics, including not being able to walk, speak, hear, or see.

□ They may have severe language or perceptual problems.

□ Some individuals with severe and profound/multiple disorders cannot attend to even the most pronounced stimuli, and self-mutilate, self-stimulate, and have intense temper tantrums.

□ An extremely fragile physiological condition may also be evident.

FOCUS 13: Identify five possible causes of severe and profound/multiple disorders.

□ Problems are generally evident at birth.

□ Birth defects may be the result of genetic or metabolic problems.

□ Factors associated with poisoning, accidents, malnutrition, physical and emotional neglect, and disease are also known causes.

Debate Forum

Categorical and Crosscategorical Programs

The merits of categorical versus crosscategorical programs for students with learning and behavior problems have been a topic of discussion for several years. In Chapters 4, 5, 6, and 7 of this text, you had the opportunity to review such material as definitions, characteristics, and intervention strategies from both a categorical (mental retardation, behavior disorders, learning disabilities) and a crosscategorical perspective. The following discussion focuses on some of the issues in the debate on the merits of each approach.

Point The traditional categories of mental retardation, behavior disorders, and learning disabilities are essentially nonfunctional in an instructional situation. They are *not* necessary, because they do not adequately differentiate the needs of exceptional students in the classroom setting.

Counterpoint It is the crosscategorical approach to instruction that is nonfunctional. The crosscategorical approach forces the teacher to deal with children who have a wide variety of educational and behavioral problems. How can individualized programs be implemented when the teacher has to work every day with such a wide range of individual problems and needs?

Point The crosscategorical approach stresses that the reason you identify and label children is to ensure that they receive adequate and appropriate services based on individual need. On the other hand, the categorical approach often forces children into neat and tidy boxes that describe the individual according to a set of characteristics associated with the label. This can result in the realization of a self-fulfilling prophecy. "Johnny cannot be expected to read because Johnny is mentally retarded." Using the crosscategorical approach, the professional assesses the individual to determine the range of academic and behavioral deficits and to make recommendations for educational intervention. On the other hand, the primary purpose of assessment under the categorical approach is to make sure the child fits into one of the boxes (categories) known as mental retardation, behavior disorders, or learning disabilities.

Counterpoint Your assumption that the crosscategorical approach results in more clearly defined groups of individuals and, consequently, adequate programming based on individual need is certainly questionable. Let's look at the effect of the crosscategorical approach on research studies concerned with educational programming for these children. Researchers must have clearly defined groups of subjects in order to determine the efficacy of instructional approaches for this population. The crosscategorical approach makes research very difficult to conduct, because the groups from which subjects are selected are very broad and not well defined.

What are some other issues that need to be discussed as we assess the merits of categorical and crosscategorical approaches to working with students who have learning and behavior disorders?

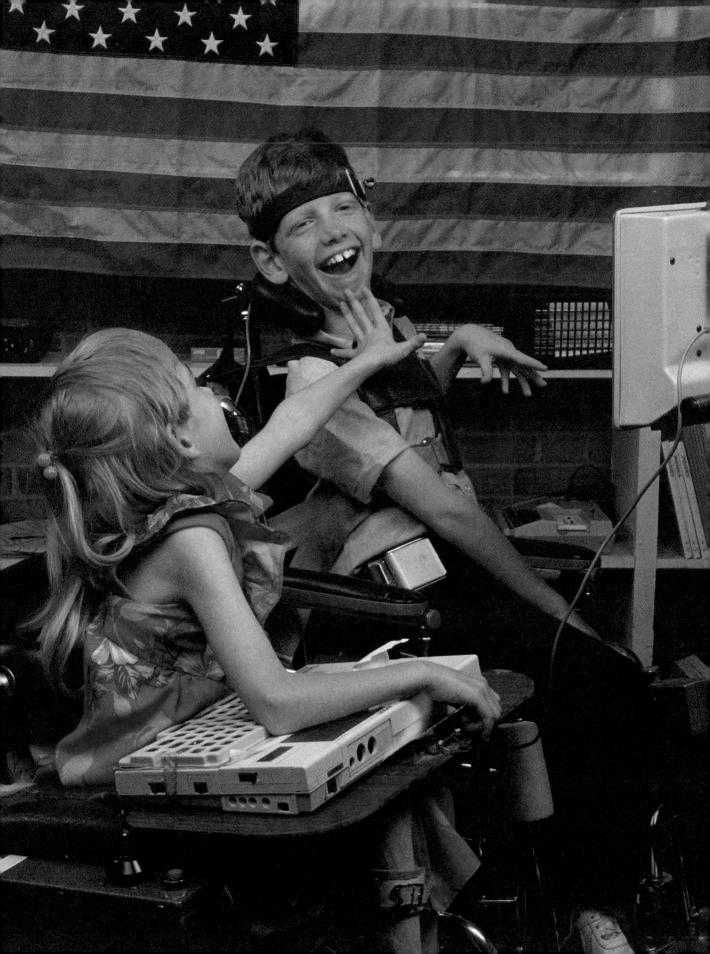

8 Speech and Language Disorders

To Begin With...

- Nearly half of the American population identified as disabled experience difficulty in speaking, reading or writing (Burrough, 1986).

- John Eulenberg, head of Michigan State University's Artificial Language Laboratory, programmed computers to produce traditional Hebrew chanting for a Bar Mitzvah ceremony. He says, "As long as there are going to be talking refrigerators and talking automobiles, let there be talking people first" (*Education Daily*, 1983).

- Welcome to Wendy's! Using the Fast Food Passport™, a customer with limited language or speech that is difficult to understand can flip to cards that have pictures of food items available at these restaurants. The disabled person simply points to the desired items (Crestwood Company, 1987–88).

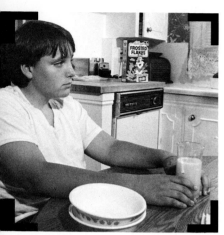

Doug

The first years of Doug's life were basically normal. He was an active and intelligent child. His father and mother were both well educated—his father, a chemistry professor; his mother, a nurse. Doug exhibited all the normal behaviors of a young child. There was no evidence of serious abnormality in his initial speech development, but at the age of four his parents began to observe an unusual lack of fluency in his speech. Doug's father was the first to label the problem as **stuttering,** and he began to work with Doug to correct it. Doug's mother was concerned about attempting to solve the problem in this manner. She was inclined to seek professional assistance, but was not successful in convincing Doug and his father to agree. The results of the corrective program provided by his father were not great. We now find Doug at age thirteen. In his diary, Doug recounts part of a day in his life:

> The best time of day is before I get out of bed because I don't have to talk. The only problem during this time is that I dread the rest of the day. I have to see my Mom and Dad at breakfast and say something—which will always end up in me stuttering; Dad trying to correct or help me; and Mom trying to anticipate what I am struggling to say. Since I have to go to breakfast, I try to wait until Dad has left for the office so that the number of people I have to deal with is reduced. This morning I was successful in avoiding Dad, but Mom was still there—trying to please and asking what I wanted for breakfast. God, I wish that she would just put something in front of me. Even if it wasn't great it would be better than having to talk, and stutter. I asked for a hot roll this morning. I really wanted cereal but I knew that I would block on that, plus Mom would have asked why I didn't want something hot.

Millie was fifty-two years old when the accident happened. She was a successful real estate broker and developer, owning her own agency and working on commercial projects between her office in Lubbock and Brownsville. That basically covered the State of Texas from north to south and involved a lot of opportunity, responsibility, and travel. Millie was driving home late one evening when she fell asleep at the wheel. The Texas State Trooper found her car lodged against a rock at the bottom of a gulley. Millie had pulled herself out of the wreck and made it about fifty yards up the rock-strewn gulley. She was diagnosed in the rehabilitation unit of the hospital as **aphasic.** One year after the accident, Millie still has great difficulty speaking and she communicates mostly through notes. She seems to understand most of what is said to her, although there are times when she shakes her head indicating that she does not comprehend what the speaker is trying to say. She can no longer personally show property to potential investors and can only make suggestions by writing notes to her Associate Broker, who has worked in her agency for several years. Her rehabilitation program is focusing on relearning language and adjusting to the vocational limitations that might well exist for the rest of her life.

We communicate with others many times a day, to order food in a restaurant, thank a friend for doing us a favor, ask a question in class, call for help in an emergency, or give directions to someone who is lost. **Communication** is one of the most complicated and vital processes people undertake, yet we seldom think much about it unless there is a problem. **Speech** and **language** are two components of communication. They are highly interrelated, and problems in either can significantly affect a person's daily life. Because of their complexity, determining the cause of a problem is often perplexing.

Communication is the interchange of ideas, opinions, or facts between senders and receivers. It requires that a sender (an individual or group) compose and transmit a message, and that a receiver decipher and understand the message (Bernstein, 1985). In this manner, the sender and receiver are partners in the communication process. Communication is an extremely important tool that "helps us adapt to and change our environment" (Hurt, Scott, & McCrosky, 1978, p. 9). Part of this tool involves the use of speech and language.

Although related, speech and language are not synonymous. Kretschmer and Kretschmer (1978) stated:

> *Language may be expressed through speech, but not in all cases.* Speech is the audible production of language, the result of manipulation of the vocal tract and oral musculature. Language, on the other hand, denotes the intended messages contained in the speaker's utterances. It is possible to have speech without language, as with parrots . . . , or language without speech, as with deaf persons who express language in a manual mode (p. 1, emphasis in the original).

Communication is the broader concept. Language is a part of communication. Speech is often thought of as a part of language, although language may exist without speech. Figure 8–1 illustrates the interrelationship of speech, language, and communication.

The Structure of Language

Language, whether English, Russian, or Arabic, is generally viewed as including several major components: phonology, syntax, morphology, semantics, and pragmatics. **Phonology** represents the system of speech sounds that an individual utters; that is, rules regarding how sounds can be used and combined. For example, the word *cat* has three phonemes. **Syntax** involves the rules governing sentence structure—the "order and the way in which words and sequences of words are combined into phrases, clauses, and sentences" (Cole & Cole, 1981, p. 4). For example, the sentence "Will you help Linda?" suggests a question that changes in meaning when the order of words is changed to "You will help Linda." **Morphology** is concerned with the form and internal structure of words; that is, the transformations of words in terms of such areas as tense and number—like present to past tense, or singular to plural. When we add an *s* to *cat* we have produced the plural form, *cats,* with two morphemes or meaning units—the concept of cat and the concept of plural. Such transformations involve

FOCUS 1
What are four ways speech, language, and communication are interrelated?

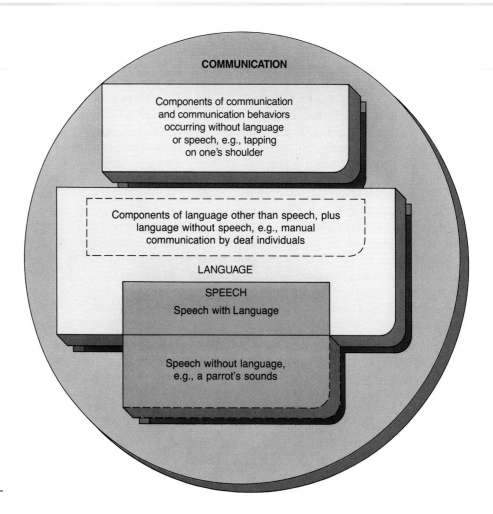

Figure 8–1
Conceptual Model of
Communication, Language,
and Speech

prefixes, suffixes, and inflections. Syntax and morphology combine to form what we know as grammar. **Semantics** represents the "component of language most concerned with the meaning or understanding of language" (Cole & Cole, 1981, p. 8). It involves the meaning of a word to an individual, which may be unique in one's personal mental dictionary (e.g., the meaning of the adjective *nice* in the phrase "nice house"). **Pragmatics,** as a component of language, has received increased attention in recent language literature. It is concerned with "the use of language in social contexts, including rules that govern language functions (the reason for communicating) and rules that govern the choice of codes (alternate message forms) to be used when communicating" (Bernstein, 1985, p. 4). An example of pragmatics can be found in the different ways a professor talks when lecturing to a class versus chatting at a party.

Language Development

The development of language is a complex process, and one that is fascinating to observe firsthand, as parents of infants know well. Young children normally progress through several stages in developing language, from a preverbal stage, to the use of words together in sentences. At first a baby's verbal communication is limited primarily to crying, which is usually associated with discomfort (from hunger, pain, or being soiled or wet). Before long (around two months), babies begin to coo as well as cry, verbally expressing reactions to pleasure as well as discomfort. They begin to babble at about three to six months of age, which involves making some consonant and vowel sounds. At this point, babies often make sounds repeatedly when they are alone, seemingly experimenting with their sound making and not necessarily trying to communicate with anyone. They may also babble when their parents or others are with them, playing or otherwise handling them.

The baby's first word is always a momentous event, and parents often attach words to sounds that stretch the imagination of more objective observers and likely have no meaning to the child. What usually happens is that the baby begins to string sounds together that resemble words. To the delight of the parents, these sounds frequently include such sounds as "da-da" and "ma-ma" which, of course, are echoed, repeated, and reinforced greatly by Father and Mother. As a baby begins to actually listen to the speech of adults, exchanges or "conversations" seem to occur, where the youngster responds by saying "da-da" when a parent says that sound. While this type of interchange sounds like a conversation, the child's vocal productions may only be understood by those close to him or her (such as parents or siblings); people other than immediate family members may not be able to interpret meaning at all. The baby also begins to use different tones and vocal intensity, which makes the vocalization vaguely resemble adult speech. The interactions between babies and their parents can do much to enhance their developing language at this time. Parents often provide a great deal of reinforcement for word approximations such as praise in excited tones of voice or hugs. They also provide stimulus sounds and words for the baby to mimic, which gives the youngster considerable directed practice.

The timing of a baby's actual production of his or her first words is obviously open to interpretation, but it usually happens between nine and fourteen months. Often these words continue to involve echoing (repeating what has been heard) or mimic responses based on verbalizations by those around him or her. Initially the words may have little or no meaning, although they soon become attached to people or objects in the child's immediate environment such as Daddy, Mommy, or milk. It is not long before these words begin to have more perceptible intent, as the child uses them for requests and an apparent means of pleasing parents or siblings. Strings of two and three words that resemble sentences typically begin between eighteen and twenty-four months. At this stage, there is little question about meaning because the child can rather clearly indicate that he or she wants something. The child uses reasonably accurate syntax, usually with a word order involving subject–verb–object.

By three to four years of age, most children whose language is developing normally are using all basic syntactical structures. By the time they are five years old they have progressed to using six-word sentences, on the average. A child that is developing language normally articulates nearly all speech sounds correctly and in context somewhere between four and eight years of age.

As we have outlined the process of normal language development there have been variable age-ranges for each milestone. Some have been rather broad approximations. Several factors contribute to this variation. For one thing, children exhibit considerable variability in their rates of development, even those that are considered normal. Some of these differences are due to general health and vitality, some are inherited, and others relate to environmental influences, such as the amount of interaction with parents and siblings. Note also that age-ranges become more variable as one considers more advanced development (e.g., three to six months for babbling; eighteen to twenty-four months for two- and three-word strings). This is partially because there is more variation regarding when advanced developmental events occur than for earlier stages. It is also true, however, that these advanced developments are more complex, some involving subtleties that are not as singularly obvious as, say, the first "da-da." Therefore observation of when they first occur is perhaps less accurate.

The variability noted in normal language development will also be seen as we discuss abnormal language and speaking ability. In some cases, the same factors influence performance that is considered to be a disorder. In others, we will find that definitions differ in the literature, and characteristics vary between people, which we have encountered with other disorders.

SPEECH DISORDERS

Definitions of **speech disorders** vary greatly, some being quite detailed in terms of characteristics and others more general. A synthesis of definitions has been developed by Gelfand, Jenson, and Drew (1988):

> Defective speech or a speech disorder (which are terms often used interchangeably) refers to speech behavior which is sufficiently deviant from normal or accepted speaking patterns that it attracts attention, interferes with communication, and adversely affects communication for either the speaker or the listener (p. 203).

This definition is broad in that it refers to a wide range of specific speech disorders. Each of these disorders is designated by separate definitions that describe the condition. We highlight these descriptions and definitions in the following pages.

Speech is extremely important in contemporary society. Speaking ability can influence a person's success or failure in both the personal-social and professional arenas. Most people are about average in terms of their speaking ability. They may envy those who are unusually articulate, but also pity those who have a difficult time with speech. What is it like to have a serious deficit in speaking ability? Certainly it is different for each individual, depending on the circumstances in which he or she operates and the severity of the deficit. We caught a glimpse of what it may be like in the case of Doug, presented earlier.

Although we only saw a glimpse of Doug's day, it is obvious that his abnormal speech seriously affects his life. Doug carries some strong emotional reactions to his stuttering. Stuttering also significantly alters his behavior, as when he tries to wait until his father has left before coming to breakfast. It is easy to imagine the impact it must have on him in such settings as the classroom or social encounters with his peers. Speech is so central to functioning in society that such disorders often have a significant impact on affected individuals. As children, they may be ridiculed by peers, begin to feel inadequate in general, and suffer serious emotional distress.

There are many different speech disorders and considerable diversity in terms of theoretical perspectives regarding causes and treatment. Volumes much longer than this book have focused solely on the topic. We discuss here several speech disorders that represent major problems in this area.

Fluency Disorders

Normal speech is characterized by a reasonably smooth flow of words and sentences. It has a rhythm and timing that is, for the most part, steady, regular, and rapid. There is always a certain degree of variation, both between people and situations. Most of us also have times when we pause, to think about what we are saying, because we have made a mistake, or want to mentally edit what we are about to say. However, these interruptions are relatively infrequent and usually do not constitute an ongoing disturbance of the speech flow. In general, our speech can be considered fluent with respect to speed and continuity.

For some people, fluency of speech is a significant problem: they have a **fluency disorder.** The speech of a person with a fluency disorder is characterized by repeated interruptions, hesitations, or repetitions that seriously interrupt the flow of communication. Some people with a fluency disorder speak with what is known as cluttered speech, or **cluttering.** This type of fluency disorder is characterized by speech that is overly rapid (to the extreme), disorganized, and occasionally filled with unnecessary words—unrelated insertions that seem random. People with cluttered speech seem to be either unaware or indifferent to the problem. Another type of fluency disorder, where those affected are painfully aware of the problem, is **stuttering,** which we discuss at some length.

Stuttering. The most well-known fluency disorder is stuttering. Wood (1971) defined stuttering as "a disturbance of rhythm and fluency of speech by an intermittent blocking, a convulsive repetition, or prolongation of sounds, syllables, words, phrases, or posture of the speech organs" (p. 21). Stuttering may be the most studied of all speech disorders, and it has fascinated researchers for decades.

Stuttering is probably the most widely recognized type of speech problem. This recognition and interest is somewhat paradoxical, since stuttering occurs rather infrequently and has one of the lower prevalence rates compared to other speech disorders (Van Riper & Emerick, 1984). For example, articulation disorders (omitting, adding, or distorting certain sounds) occur in the United States many times more often than do stuttering problems.

The common view of stuttering partly comes from the nature of behavior involved in the problem. Stuttering is typically defined as a disturbance in the rhythm and fluency of speech. These may involve certain sounds, syllables, words, or phrases, and they may differ between stutterers. (Doug's diary described some of his specific problems as he thought about asking for breakfast.) Such interruptions in the flow of speech are very evident to both the speaker and listener. They are perhaps more disruptive to the communication act than other type of speech

FOCUS 2
What are three factors thought to be involved in the causation of stuttering?

disorders. Furthermore, listeners often become quite uncomfortable and may try to assist the stuttering speaker with missing or incomplete words. This discomfort may be magnified by physical movements, gestures, or facial distortions that often accompany stuttering. All this may make the experience a very vivid and easily remembered one for the listener, which accounts for part of the prominence of stuttering in the larger picture of speech disorders.

Parents often become unnecessarily concerned about stuttering as their children are learning to talk. Most children exhibit some fluency problems as they develop speech. These fluency problems involve disruptions in the rhythm and flow of speech and include some or all of the behaviors mentioned above (blocking, repetition, and prolonging of sounds, syllables, words, or phrases). Generally, such speech patterns represent normal fluency problems during early speech development, which diminish and cease as maturation progresses. However, these normal fluency problems have also historically played an important role in some theories regarding the causes of stuttering.

Causation of Stuttering. The search for a cause of stuttering has led behavioral scientists in many directions. One difficulty with these efforts has been that researchers have often sought a single cause for the disorder. Current thinking suggests that stuttering may have a variety of causes (Prosek et al., 1987; Rastatter & Dell, 1987), and the search for a single cause has been largely discarded. Theories regarding causes of stuttering seem to take three basic perspectives: (1) theories related to emotional problems; that is, stuttering as a symptom of some emotional disturbance; (2) theories that view stuttering as the result of a person's biological makeup or some neurological problem; and (3) theories that view stuttering as a learned behavior.

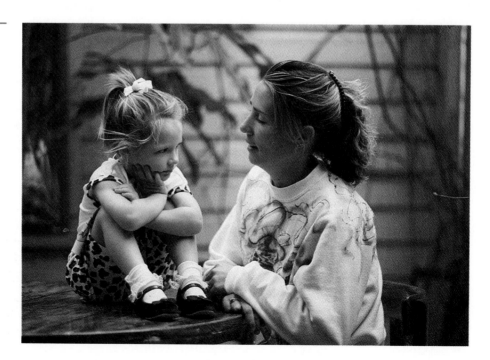

Parents often become unnecessarily concerned about their children's early speech patterns. (Frank Siteman/The Picture Cube)

Many professionals have become less interested in both the emotional and biological causation theories of stuttering. The emotional-problem theory tends to be held predominantly by psychiatrists and certain counseling psychologists. Van Riper and Emerick (1984) suggest that this may be "because their clinical practice brings them, not the garden variety of stutterers, but those with deep-seated emotional problems" (p. 268). Research in this area is scarce, and the topic is difficult to study due to measurement error in assessing deep emotional problems and trying to establish a causal relationship through such measurement.

A few studies have continued to appear on the biological-cause theory over the past fifteen years. Some research has indicated that the brains of stutterers may be organized differently from those of their fluent counterparts (Healey & Howe, 1987), but the nature of such differences remains unclear and a matter for speculation. Certain results suggest that stutterers and those with fluent speech use different sections of the brain to process material (Pindzola, 1987; Webster, 1988). Some evidence seems to indicate that stutterers may have brain hemisphere–dominance problems to a greater degree than nonstutterers; that is, they may have competition between the hemispheres in information processing (Rastatter & Dell, 1987; Rastatter & Loren, 1988). Conversely, other research suggests that brain hemisphere–dominance difficulties do not significantly influence stuttering (Gruber & Powell, 1974; Slorach & Noeher, 1973). Thus, as we view evidence on biological causes, some interest continues but the results are mixed.

One persistent theory over the years regarding the causation of stuttering relates to learning. This line of reasoning views stuttering essentially as a learned behavior that comes from the normal nonfluency evident in early speech development. Most young children exhibit nonfluent speech during the time they are developing their communication skills. From the learning causation point of view, a child may become a stutterer if considerable attention is focused on normal disfluencies at that stage of development, which may have occurred in Doug's case as his father focused on his speech and even labeled him a stutterer. The dysfluency of early stuttering may be further magnified by negative feelings about the self (Klinger, 1987) and anxiety (Kraaimaat, Janssen, & Brutten, 1988). Considerable current thinking and treatment follow this logic although the theory has been prominent for many years.

There has been some interest in the influence of heredity on stuttering. This has been approached from several perspectives, one of which is that it may be gender related. The logic of this theory has a certain appeal on the surface, since male stutterers outnumber females by about four to one. Thus, it is possible that under certain circumstances the genetic material that determines one's gender may also carry material that contributes to stuttering. However, this hypothesis is difficult to test and remains only speculation. Heredity has also been of interest because of the high incidence of stuttering within certain family lines as well as in twins (Sheehan & Costly, 1977). Once again, however, we are faced with the difficulty of separating hereditary and environmental influences, a problem that has long been evident in child development and behavioral disorders research (Ausubel, Sullivan & Ives, 1980; Gelfand, Jenson, & Drew, 1988).

In sum, the cause of stuttering has been an elusive and perplexing matter for professionals working in speech pathology. Researchers and clinicians continue their search for a cause, with the hope of identifying more effective treatment

Reflect on This 8–1

An Open Letter to the Mother of a Stuttering Child

Many years ago Wendell Johnson, one of the pioneers in speech disorder research, described the learning view of stuttering causation in a classic piece entitled *An Open Letter to the Mother of a Stuttering Child.* This letter provides cause for considerable thought because of the graphic manner in which it was written. It is presented in abridged form for your reflection as a beginning professional and/or parent. What do you think?

My Dear Mrs. Smith:

I thoroughly appreciate your concern over the speech difficulty of Fred, your four-year-old boy. You say that he is in good health, and that he is mentally alert, and is generally normal by any standards you know about. I note that you have been careful not to change his handedness, and that he is now generally right-handed. But in spite of all this he stutters.

It will interest you to know that the majority of four-year-old stutterers just about fit that description. I want to say to you very nearly the same things I should say to the mothers of thousands of other "Freds." There are some stuttering children who are not like your boy, and their mothers need somewhat different advice. But the "Freds" make up the majority. . . .

First of all, I want to put you at ease, if I can, by stressing that the most recent studies have tended strongly to discredit the popular view, which perhaps you share, that stutterers are generally abnormal or inferior in some very fundamental sense. Concerning this point, I should like to make as clear a statement as possible—and I make it on the basis of over one hundred scientific studies of stuttering in older children and adults, and five recent investigations involving over two hundred young children, stutterers and nonstutterers. . . .

We found, for example, that two-, three-, and four-year-olds—all the children of these ages in a large nursery school, somewhat better than average children by most standards—spoke, on the average, in such a way that one out of every four words figured in some kind of repetition! The whole word was repeated, or the first sound or syllable of it was repeated, or it was part of a repeated phrase. One out of four words was the average; about half of the children repeated more frequently than that. Another way to summarize the findings is to say that the average child makes 45 repetitions per thousand words. This was the average—the norm. . . .

Investigation seemed to show that a rose by any other name doesn't smell the same at all. If you call a child a stutterer you get one kind of speech—and personality—development, and if you call him a normal or superior speaker you get another kind of development—within limits, but

and prevention measures. The work of Perkins, Rudas, Johnson, and Bell (1976) is an example of such effort. These investigators studied subjects ranging in age from fourteen to sixty-seven. Their findings suggest that stuttering may be a function of voice coordination with articulation and respiration. One might view this as a physical dysfunction, but it could also be seen as a result of learning or a combination of the two.

Intervention.   Many different treatment approaches have been used with stutterers over the years, with mixed results. Techniques such as play therapy, creative dramatics, parental counseling, and group counseling with parents have they seem to be rather wide limits.

I can illustrate what I mean by telling you briefly about two cases. The first case is that of Jimmy, who as a pupil in the grades was regarded as a superior speaker. He won a number of speaking contests and often served as chairman of small groups. Upon entering the ninth grade, he changed to another school. A "speech examiner" saw Jimmy twice during the one year he spent at that school. The first time she made a phonograph record of his speech. The second time she played the record for him, and after listening to it, told him he was a stutterer.

Now, if you have ever tried to speak into a phonograph recording machine you probably suspect what is true. Practically all children who have done this—in studies with which I am familiar—have shown a considerable number of hesitations, repetitions, broken sen-

tences, etc. It is easy to see how the apparently untrained teacher misjudged Jimmy who was, after all, a superior speaker as ninth-graders go.

He took the diagnosis to heart, however. The teacher told him to speak slowly, to watch himself, and to try to control his speech. Jimmy's parents were quite upset. They looked upon Jimmy's speech as one of his chief talents, and they set about with a will to help him, reminding him of any little slip or hesitation. Jimmy became as self-conscious as the legendary centipede who has been told "how" to walk. He soon developed a quite serious case of stuttering—tense, jerky, hesitant, apprehensive speech.

The second case was Gene, a three-year-old boy. His father became concerned over the fact that now and then Gene repeated a sound or a word. Gene didn't seem to know he was doing it, and he wasn't the least bit tense about it. But the

father consulted the family doctor and told him that Gene was stuttering. The doctor took his word for it. (Practically all stutterers are originally diagnosed by laymen—parents and teachers—and "experts" almost never challenge the diagnoses!) He told the father to have Gene take a deep breath before trying to speak. Within forty-eight hours Gene was practically speechless. The deep breath became a frantic gasping from which Gene looked out with wide-eyed, helpless bewilderment. . . .

Source: "An Open Letter to the Mother of a 'Stuttering' Child," by Wendell Johnson, Appendix VII, pp. 558–67, abridged from *Speech Handicapped School Children*, Revised edition, by Wendell Johnson, Spencer J. Brown, James F. Curtis, Clarence W. Edney, and Jacqueline Keaster. Copyright 1948, 1956, by Harper & Row, Publishers, Inc. by permission of the publisher.

been useful in working with children who stutter. Even psychotherapy has been used to treat some cases of stuttering, but its success has been limited (Gelfand, Jenson, & Drew, 1988). Speech rhythm has also been the focus of some therapy for stuttering. In some cases, this approach has included the use of a metronome to establish a rhythm for the speaking act (Wohl, 1968). Relaxation therapy and biofeedback have also been used, since tenseness has typically been observed in stutterers (Hasbrouck et al., 1987). In all the techniques noted, outcomes are mixed, with some cases resulting in success and others being disappointing. It has been common for stutterers to repeat treatments using several approaches. The inability of any one treatment or cluster of treatments to consistently help stutterers to learn to speak fluently demonstrates the ongoing need for research in this area.

Thus a complete understanding of stuttering remains elusive. However, treatment approaches have increasingly focused on direct behavioral therapy that attempts to teach the stutterer to use fluent speech patterns. In some cases, children are taught to monitor and manage their stuttering (such as by speaking more slowly or rhythmically), and to reward themselves for increasing periods of fluency. Some behaviorally oriented therapies include providing knowledge regarding physical factors (e.g., regulating breathing) and direct instruction about correct speaking behaviors. Such research combines several dimensions to the overall therapy, such as an interview regarding the inconvenience of stuttering, behavior-modification training, and follow-up. Because stuttering is a complex problem, effective interventions are likely to be equally complex, perhaps combining different elements from several therapies.

Fluency disorders interfere significantly with spoken communication because they interrupt the flow of ideas. For people who stutter, the stream of communication is broken by severe rhythm irregularities. For people with cluttered speech, the flow of ideas is interrupted by extraneous words and disorganization. However, other people with speech disorders are not dysfluent; rather, they are delayed in their speaking ability.

Delayed Speech

FOCUS 3
What are two ways learning theory and home environment relate to delayed speech?

Definition. **Delayed speech** refers to a deficit in communication ability in which a person speaks like someone much younger. From a developmental point of view, this type of difficulty involves a delayed beginning of speech and language. Very young children are generally able to communicate, at least to some degree, before verbal behaviors are learned. They use gestures, facial expressions, other physical movements, and vocalizations that would not be considered speech, such as grunts or squeals (Tiegerman, 1985). This early behavior development illustrates the interrelationships between communication, language, and speech. Although it is difficult to distinguish among the three functions at this stage, we are concerned here only with speech delay. Delayed speech is considered a failure of speech to develop at the expected age and is often associated with other maturation delays, such as crawling or sitting up alone later than most children (Bishop & Edmundson, 1987). Delayed speech may also be related to hearing impairment, mental retardation, emotional disturbance, or brain injury. Delayed speech may occur for many reasons and take various forms, and treatment differs accordingly.

Children with delayed speech often have few or no verbalizations that can be interpreted as conventional speech. Some communicate solely through physical gestures. Others may use a combination of gestures and vocal sounds that are not even close approximations of words. Still others may speak, but in a very limited manner, perhaps using single words (typically nouns without auxiliary words, like *ball* instead of *my ball*) or primitive sentences that are short or incomplete (such as *get ball* rather than *would you get the ball*). Such communication behavior is normal for infants and very young children, but here

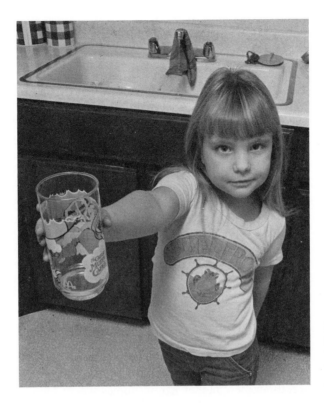

Some children with delayed speech communicate solely through physical gestures. (John Telford)

we are referring to children who are well beyond the age at which they should be speaking in at least a partially fluent fashion.

The differences between stuttering and delayed speech are obvious. However, the distinctions between delayed speech and **articulation disorders** are not as clear. In fact, children with delayed speech usually have many articulation errors in their speaking patterns. However, their major problems lie in grammatical and vocabulary deficits, which are more matters of developmental delay (Van Riper & Emerick, 1984). Powers (1971) discussed delayed speech in the following manner:

> There are two general types of disorder which both fall within the broad category of speech immaturity. These are *delayed speech*, which is a more complex and profound disorder, and **infantile perseveration.** Delayed speech is the more inclusive of the two. Indeed, infantile perseveration can be thought of as the articulatory aspect of delayed speech, but there is no sharp distinction between the two. If a child's speech immaturity is confined largely to sound omissions and substitutions, if he has learned to rely mainly on speech as his means of communication, if there is considerable output of speech, if the onset of speech has been fairly typical, if he attempts sentences as well as words and phrases, his speech deviation can best be referred to as *infantile perseveration*. If, however, there has been little or no attempt at speech until past two years of age, if gestures and nonspeech vocalizations are used extensively, if speech is limited mainly to nouns, with little use of qualifying, connective, or auxiliary words, if vocabulary

is meager, if single words are used for sentences or phrases, most speech clinicians would tend to call the disorder *delayed speech*. The distinction between *infantile perseveration* and *delayed speech* is thus both qualitative and quantitative, but there is considerable overlap between them in symptomatology (p. 843).

The current prevalence of delayed speech is very unclear, and new government estimates do not even provide data regarding provision of services for delayed speech during 1987–1988 (U.S. Department of Education, 1989). There has been confusion in the past regarding distinctions between incidence and prevalence. The two terms have been used interchangeably when, in fact, **incidence** refers to the number of *new* cases identified during a particular period of time (often one school year), whereas **prevalence** includes all of the cases existing at a given point in time—the newly diagnosed plus those previously identified. Such problems, plus definition differences between studies, have led many to place little faith in existing prevalence figures (Van Riper & Emerick, 1984).

Causation.   As discussed above, cases of delayed speech may take a variety of forms, so it is not surprising that the causes of these problems also vary greatly. Several types of environmental deprivation contribute to delayed speech. For example, partial or complete hearing loss may cause an individual to experience serious delay (or absence) of speech development. Since the auditory stimulus and modeling is deficient, learning to speak is extremely difficult.

For those with normal hearing, the environment may be a factor in delayed speech. Some children live in homes where there is little opportunity to learn speech, such as in families where there is minimal conversation or chance for the child to speak. Other problems may contribute to delayed speech, such as cerebral palsy and emotional disturbances. Even less severe emotional problems may result in delayed speech, such as negativism, which can be viewed as an emotional problem stemming from interpersonal difficulties between parents and child.

Negativism involves a conflict between parents' expectations and a child's ability to perform, which often occurs in some form as children develop speech. There is a great deal of pressure on children during the period when they are normally developing their speaking skills: to go to bed when told, to control urination and defecation properly, and to learn appropriate eating skills—among other things. The demands are great, and they may exceed a child's performance ability. There are many ways to react when more is demanded than one is able to produce, and refusal is one way children may respond to excessive performance demands. They may simply not talk, seeming to withdraw from family interactions, remaining silent. In normal development, children occasionally refuse to follow the directions of adults. One very effective area of refusal is speaking; the parents' reprisal options are few and may be ineffective. As a parent, it is relatively simple to punish refusal misbehaviors when they involve such acts as refusing to go to bed or not cleaning one's room. However, it is a different matter when parents encounter the refusal to talk. It is not easy to force a child to talk through conventional punishment techniques. Delayed speech may occur in extreme cases where negativism related to talking is prolonged.

Viewing the problem from another angle, there are other situations where children may be punished *for* talking. Parents may see a child's attempt to communicate as an irritant. A child may speak too loudly or at inappropriate times, such as when adults are reading, watching television, resting, or talking with other adults (even more rules to learn at such a tender age).

From these descriptions, we can see that some children might have delayed speech as a result of environmentally controlled learning due to refusal or rebellion. Not speaking may be rewarded in some instances, and in others it may be a way of expressing refusal that is unlikely to result in punishment. Thus in some cases children may *not learn to speak* and in others they may *learn not to speak*. Imagine the effect on a baby who is yelled at for practicing his or her babbling (perhaps loudly) while mother is on the telephone. Frightened, the child begins to cry, which further angers mother, who screams, "Shut up!" Of course the baby does not understand, and this episode escalates and becomes even more frightening to the child. Such situations may be alternated with more calm periods, when the mother hugs the baby and talks in soothing tones. A baby in this type of environment is likely to become very confused about the reaction to vocal output; sometimes it is punished, and other times it is rewarded. If such circumstances exist at the time a child normally develops speech and persist for a substantial length of time, seriously delayed speech may result.

As mentioned earlier, delayed speech may emerge from experience deprivation, in which the environment either limits or hinders the opportunity to learn speech. Basic principles of learning suggest that when one is first learning a skill, the stimulus and reward circumstances are important. A skill that is just beginning to develop is fragile. Stimuli and reinforcement must be reasonably consistent, appropriate, and properly timed. If such conditions do not exist, the skill development may be retarded or even negated. A child who is left alone for many hours each day, perhaps with only a single light bulb and four walls as stimuli, is not being rewarded for cooing, babbling, or approximating the first word. Over a long period of time, this baby falls behind his or her peers who are being hugged for each sound and hearing adults talk as models. This does not mean that the home environment must be an orchestrated language-development program. Most households involve adequate circumstances to permit and promote speech learning.

Learning to speak is no different from learning other skills. There are homes where conversation is abnormally infrequent, and parents may speak rarely to either each other or to the child. In such cases, a child may have infrequent speech modeling and little reinforcement for speaking, so delayed speech may result. It is also possible that verbal interchanges between parents reflect a strained relationship or emotional problems. The environment in such situations may be unpleasant, tense and troubled, involving threats, arguments, and shouting. A child learning to speak in this type of setting may learn that speech is associated with unpleasant feelings or even punishment. Seriously delayed speech may result from these environmental circumstances. When such contingencies are combined with infrequent interchanges, the learning (not to speak or not learning to speak) may be particularly potent.

The environment just described represents an unpleasant set of circumstances, one in which learning speech may be impaired. One might be concerned about the amount of love and caring in such a situation. But delayed speech may also occur in families where there is great love and caring, at least with respect to observable behavior. In some environments there may be little need for a child to learn speech. Most parents are concerned about satisfying their child's needs or desires. Carrying this desire to the extreme, a "superparent" may anticipate the child's wants (such as toys, water, or food) and provide them even before the child makes a verbalized request. Such children may only gesture and their parents immediately respond, thereby rewarding gestures and not promoting the development of speech skills. Learning to speak is much more complex and demanding than making simple movements or facial grimaces. If gesturing is rewarded, speaking is less likely to be learned properly.

If delayed speech is a complex phenomenon, causation is equally complicated—as complicated as the speech development process itself. If you are a new parent, or anticipating parenthood, you should know that the vast majority of children learn to speak normally. Certainly parents should not become so self-conscious that they see a problem before one exists.

Intervention.   Treatment approaches for delayed speech are as varied as the causes. Whatever the cause, an effective treatment is one that teaches the child appropriate speaking proficiency for his or her age-group. In some cases, matters other than just defective learning, such as hearing impairments, must be considered in the treatment procedures. Such cases may involve surgery and prosthetic appliances like hearing aides, as well as specially designed instructional techniques aimed at teaching speech.

If delayed speech is caused primarily by defective learning, treatment may

Effective treatment for delayed speech succeeds in teaching the child appropriate speaking proficiency for his or her age-group. (John Telford)

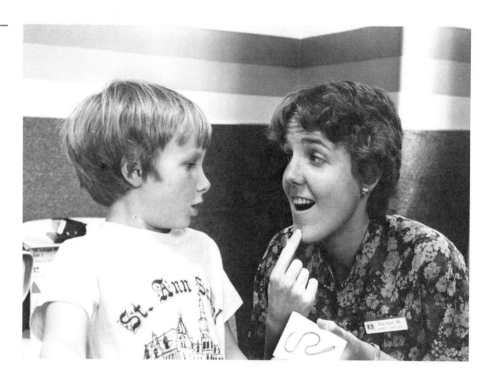

focus on the basic principles of learned behavior. In a general sense, the stimulus and reinforcement patterns that contributed to delayed speech must be changed. These circumstances must be rearranged so that appropriate speaking behaviors can be learned. This process sounds simple, but the identification and control of such contingencies may be complex. There has been some success over the years with specific teaching interventions using direct instruction, as well as other procedures aimed at increasing spontaneous speech (Cole & Dale, 1986; Raver, 1987). Such instruction places a heavy emphasis on the reinforcement of speaking, attempting to modify the child's behavior toward more normal speech. Other interventions involve collaborative efforts between speech clinicians, teachers, and parents (Hornby & Jensen-Proctor, 1984), focusing on modifying not only the child's speech but also the family environment that contributed to the problem. Because each case has different elements that cause the delay, therapies must be individually tailored to fit the situation. Further research on treatment is needed to evaluate the relative effectiveness of different procedures.

Articulation Disorders

Definition.   Articulation disorders represent the largest category of all speech problems. For most of those affected, the label **functional articulation disorders** is used. This term refers to articulation problems that are not due to structural physiological defects such as **cleft palate** or neurological problems, but are likely a result of environmental or psychological influences. An articulation disorder is an abnormality in the speech-sound production process resulting in inaccurate or otherwise inappropriate execution of the speaking act. This group includes omissions, substitutions, additions, or distortions of certain sounds. Omissions most often involve the dropping of consonants from the ends of words (such as *los* for *lost*), although they may occur in any position in the word. Substitutions frequently include saying a *w* for *r* (as in *wight* for *right*), *w* for *l* (such as *fowo* for *follow*), and *th* for *s* (*thtop* for *stop*). These represent only illustrations; misarticulations come in many forms and combinations.

Articulation disorders are a prevalent type of speech disorder. Emerick and Haynes (1986) indicate that the majority of speech problems seen by public school clinicians involve articulation disorders. Van Riper and Emerick (1984) estimate that articulation problems represent about 80 percent of the speech disorders encountered by such professionals. Although most of these difficulties are functional articulation disorders, not disorders caused by a conspicuous physiological defect, a certain number of articulation disorders do not fit into the functional type and may be attributed to physiological abnormality.

There is some controversy about the treatment of articulation disorders, due in part to the large number that are functional in nature. A predictable developmental progression occurs in a substantial number of functional articulation disorders. In such cases, articulation problems diminish and may even cease to exist as the child matures. For instance, the *r, s,* or *th* problems disappear for many children after the age of five. This phenomenon made many school administrators reluctant to treat functional articulation disorders in younger students, basically because of limited school resources. In other words, if a significant proportion of articulation disorders are likely to correct themselves as the child

FOCUS 4
Give two reasons why some professionals are reluctant to treat functional articulation disorders in young schoolchildren.

continues to develop, why expend precious resources to treat them now? The logic is obvious and has a certain amount of appeal, but it can be applied only with caution. In general, improvement of articulation performance continues until a child is about nine or ten years of age. If articulation problems persist beyond these ages, they are unlikely to improve unless intense intervention occurs. Furthermore, the longer such difficulties are allowed to continue, the more difficult treatment becomes, and the probability of success is reduced in this case (Cruz & Ayala, 1987). Thus the decision whether or not to treat articulation problems in young children is not an easy one. One solution is to combine articulation training with the other instruction for all very young children. This may serve as an interim measure for those who have continuing problems, facilitate the growth of articulation for others, and not overly tax school resources. It does, however, require some training for teachers of young children.

Causation. What causes articulation disorders? As with many other speech problems, there are many causes. Some are caused by physical malformations, such as mouth, jaw, or teeth structures that are abnormal. In other cases, articulation disorders are the result of nerve injury or brain damage. Functional articulation disorders are often seen as caused by defective learning of the speaking act in one form or another (Mecham & Willbrand, 1985). However, such categories of causation are not as distinct in practice as may be suggested by textbook discussion. There is definitely a blurring between even such broad types as functional and structural. Function and structure, although often related, are not perfectly correlated, as illustrated by the fact that some people with physical malformations that should result in articulation problems do not, and vice versa.

Despite this qualifying note, we examine causation of articulation performance deficits in two general categories: those due to physical oral malformations and those that are clearly functional because there is no physical deformity. These distinctions remain useful for instructional purposes, since it is the unusual individual who overcomes a physical abnormality and articulates satisfactorily. Even with general types of causes there may be a variety of specific circumstances that result in articulation difficulties.

We examine physical abnormalities of the oral cavity, noting, however, that other types of physical defects can affect articulation performances, such as an

WINDOW 8–1 *I Think I Talk Okay*	My name is Timothy. I am almost seven and a half years old. Mondays after school I go to the university where I meet with a lady who helps me talk betto. It was my teacha's idea because she said I couldn't say "l" and "r" good. I kinda like it [coming here] but I think I talk okay. I can say "l" good now all the time and "r" when I reeeally think about it. I have a lot of friends, fow, no—five. I don't talk to them about coming hea, guess I'm just not in the mood. Hey, you witing this down, is that "mood"? You know the caw got hit by a semi this mowning and the doow handle came off. I'm a little dizzy 'cause we wecked. *Timothy, Age 7½*

abnormal or absent **larynx.** Speech formulation involves many different physical structures that must be interfaced with learned muscle/tissue movements, auditory feedback, and a multitude of other factors. Although these coordinated functions are almost never perfect, they occur for most of us in an unbelievably successful manner. Malformed oral structures alter the manner in which coordinated movements must take place. With certain deformities, normal or accurate production of sounds is extremely difficult, if not impossible.

One oral malformation that most people recognize is the **cleft palate,** often referred to by speech pathologists as *clefts of the lip* or *palate* or both. The cleft palate is a gap in the soft palate and roof of the mouth, sometimes extending through the upper lip. The roof of the mouth serves an important function in accurate sound production. There is a reduced division of the nasal and mouth cavities with a cleft palate, which influences the movement of air so important to articulation performance. Clefts occur **congenitally** in about one out of every 750 births (Morris & Greulich, 1968) and may take any of several forms. Figure 8–2 shows a normal palate in configuration (A) and unilateral and bilateral cleft palates in (B) and (C). In cases of the cleft palates, it is easy to see how articulation performance would be impaired. These problems are caused by developmental difficulties **in utero** and are often later corrected by surgery.

Dentral structure also plays a significant role in articulation performance. Because the tongue and lips work together with the teeth in an intricate manner to form many sounds, dental abnormalities may result in serious articulation disorders. Some dental malformations are side effects of cleft palates, as portrayed in (B) and (C) of Figure 8–2. But other dental deformities, not associated with clefts, also cause articulation difficulties.

The natural meshing of the teeth in the upper and lower jaws is important

Figure 8–2
Normal and Cleft Palate Configurations

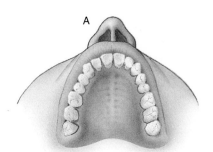

Normal palate configuration

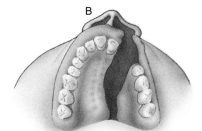

Unilateral cleft palate

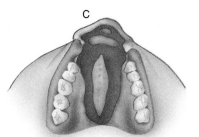

Bilateral cleft palate

to speech production. The general term used for referring to the closure and fitting-together of dental structures is **occlusion** or *dental occlusion.* When the fit is abnormal, the condition is known as a **malocclusion.** Occlusion involves several factors, including the biting height of the teeth when the jaws are closed, the alignment of teeth in the upper and lower jaws, the nature of curves in upper and lower jaws, and the positioning of individual teeth.

A normal adult occlusion is portrayed in (A) of Figure 8–3. The teeth of the upper jaw normally extend slightly beyond those of the lower jaw, and the bite overlap of those on the bottom is about one-third for the front teeth (incisors) when closed.

Although abnormalities take many forms, we discuss only two here. When the overbite of the top teeth is unusually large, the normal difference between the lower and upper dental structure is exaggerated. Such conditions may be due to the positioning of the upper and lower jaws. (B) of Figure 8–3 illustrates a malocclusion of the type where there is a misalignment of the jaw structures. In other cases, nearly the opposite situation occurs. This is illustrated in (C) of Figure 8–3 and is once again a jaw misalignment. Both exaggerated overbites and underbites may also be the result of abnormal teeth positioning or angles as well as jaw misalignment. All of these may result in articulation difficulties.

Functional articulation disorders are generally thought to be caused by faulty learning. In many cases, the sources of defective speech learning are difficult to identify (Mecham & Willbrand, 1985; Van Riper & Emerick, 1984). Like other articulation problems, those of a functional nature have many specific causes (Cruz & Ayala, 1987). In some cases, the existing stimulus and reinforcement contingencies may not be appropriate for developing accurate articulation. It is not uncommon for unthinking adults to view the normal inaccuracies of speech

Figure 8–3
Normal and Abnormal
Dental Occlusions

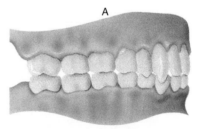

Normal dental occlusion

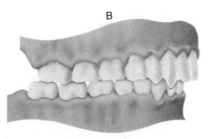

Overbite malocclusion

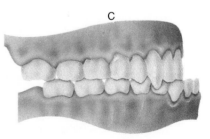

Underbite malocclusion

in young children as cute or amusing. Consequently such "baby talk" may be reinforced in a powerful manner, as when asking the young child to say a particular word in the presence of grandparents or other guests. This can be very rewarding for the young child, who is then on center stage and may be reinforced by laughter and physical affection like hugs and kisses. Such potent rewards can result in misarticulations that linger long beyond the time when normal maturation would diminish or eliminate them. Related defective learning may come from modeling. Parent (or other adult) modeling can result in articulation disorders when they imitate the baby talk of young children. If parents, grandparents, or friends realized the potential results of such behavior, they would probably alter the nature of verbal interchanges with young children. Modeling is generally a potent tool in shaping learned behavior (Harlan & Tschiderer, 1987), although the influence of baby talk between parents and children has been questioned (Cromer, 1981).

In certain cases, parental reinforcement for accurate articulation may simply be unsystematic. Parents are busy in their daily routines, and encouraging their children to speak properly may not be high among their conscious ordering of priorities. However, such encouragement is important, particularly if misarticulation begins to emerge as a problem.

Intervention.   Treatment of articulation disorders takes many forms. Clearly the treatment for disorders due to physical abnormalities is different from the treatment for disorders that are functional. However, in many cases treatment may include a combination of procedures.

In recent years considerable progress has been made in the surgical repair of cleft palates. Such techniques may involve several different procedures because of the dramatic nature of the structural defect. Some procedures include Teflon implants in the hard portion of the palate, as well as stretching and stitching together the fleshy tissue. As suggested by Figure 8–2, surgery is often necessary for the upper lip and nose structures too, and corrective dental work may be undertaken as well. It may also be necessary to train or retrain articulation in the individual, depending on the patient's age at the time of surgery. A child's continued development may result in later problems; for example, the physical growth of the jaw or mouth may create difficulties for someone who underwent surgery at a very young age. Although early correction has resulted in successful healing and speech for a very high percentage of treated cases, the permanence of such results is questionable in light of later growth spurts.

Treatment for cleft-palate cases has also involved the use of **prosthetic** appliances; for example, a device that basically serves as the upper palate or at least covers the fissures. Such an appliance may be attached to the teeth to hold it in position and can be visualized in terms of the palate portion of artificial dentures.

Dental malformations other than those associated with clefts are also often treated by means of procedures aimed at correcting the physical defect. Surgery may be undertaken to alter jaw structure and alignment. In some cases, orthodontic treatment may involve the repositioning of teeth through extractions and pressure applied using braces. Prosthetic appliances such as full or partial artificial dentures may also be used. As in other types of problems, the articulation patient who has orthodontic treatment often requires speech therapy to learn proper speech performance.

Treatment of people who have functional articulation disorders typically focuses on relearning the speaking act. Specific causation of the defective learning is difficult to identify precisely, but the basic assumption in such cases is that there was an inappropriate configuration of stimulus and reinforcement contingencies in the environment during speech development (e.g., inappropriate modeling by parents). Treatment attempts to rearrange those contingencies so that accurate articulation can be learned. Several behavior modification procedures have been employed successfully in treating functional articulation disorders (Mowrer & Conley, 1987). In all cases, treatment techniques are complex to implement because interventions must teach proper articulation plus the generalization of that learning to a variety of settings—beyond the treatment setting to the home and other places.

Voice Disorders

Definition. **Voice disorders** involve unusual or abnormal acoustical qualities in the sounds made when a person speaks. All voices differ significantly in pitch, loudness, and other qualities from others of the same sex, cultural group, and age. All people have varying acoustical qualities in their voices. However, voice disorders involve characteristics that are habitually and sufficiently different that they are noticeable and may divert a listener's attention from the content of a message.

Voice disorders have received relatively little attention compared to other speech problems. This lack of attention is due to several factors. First, voice normalcy represents a great deal of subjective judgment. And what is normal varies considerably according to the circumstances (e.g., football games, barroom conversation, or seminar discussion) and geographical location (such as western, rural, New England, or Deep South), as well as family environments, personality, and physical structure of the speech mechanism. Another factor contributing to the lack of attention to voice disorders is related to the acceptable ranges of normal voice. Most individuals have voices within our acceptable tolerance ranges. Finally, voice disorders have received relatively little attention from professionals in speech pathology. Knepflar (1976) noted, "I believe that voice problems constitute the most overlooked area in the diagnosis of communication disorders and that most training programs for speech pathologists are weaker in the area of voice than any other aspect of the field" (p. 14).

Children with voice disorders often speak with an unusual nasality, hoarseness, or breathiness. Nasality either involves too little resonance from the nasal passages (**hyponasality** or **denasality**), which sounds like the child has a continual cold or stuffy nose, or too many sounds coming through the nose (**hypernasality**), which causes a twang in the speech. People with voice disorders of hoarseness have a constant husky sound to their speech, as though they had strained their voices by yelling. Breathiness in a voice disorder tends to have a very low volume, somewhat like a whisper, and sounds like the person is not sending enough air through the vocal cords. Other voice disorders include overly loud or soft speaking and pitch abnormalities such as monotone speech.

The nature of voice disorders varies greatly. The description above provides considerable latitude, but it also outlined the general parameters of voice disorders often discussed in the literature: pitch, loudness, and quality. An individual with a voice disorder may exhibit deviation in one or a combination of these factors, significantly interfering with communication. Interference occurs when the abnormal voice results in listener attention being focused on the sound rather than on the message being conveyed.

Causation.   Hutchinson, Hanson, and Mecham described voice pitch: "An efficient, appropriate pitch is suited to the situation, the speaker's **laryngeal** structure and to the speech content. It allows for upward and downward inflections without undue strain or voice breaks. It varies within the sentence and within longer units of speech, according to meaning and emotions the speaker wishes to convey. It does not call undue attention to itself" (1979, p. 207). The acoustic characteristics of voice quality include such factors as degree of nasality, "breathy" speech, and hoarse-sounding speech. As with the other parameters of voice, loudness is a subjective determination. The normal voice is not habitually characterized by excessive loudness or unusual softness. Loudness depends a great deal on circumstances surrounding the communication.

Pitch disorders may take several forms. The voice may have an abnormally high or low pitch, it may be characterized by pitch breaks or a restricted pitch range, or it may be monotonal or monopitched. Many of us experienced pitch breaks as we progressed through adolescence. Although these are more commonly associated with young males, they also occur in females. Such pitch breaks are a normal part of development, but if they persist much beyond adolescence they may signal laryngeal difficulties. Abnormally high- or low-pitched voices may be due to a variety of problems. They may be learned through imitation, as when a young boy attempts to sound like his older brother or father. They may also be learned from certain circumstances that the individual is in, such as when those placed in positions of authority believe a lower voice pitch is necessary to suggest the image of power. Organic conditions, such as a hormone imbalance, may also result in abnormally high- or low-pitched voices.

Voice disorders involving loudness may likewise have varied causes. Excessively loud or soft voices may be learned either through imitation or through perceptions of the environment, much like those mentioned for pitch disorders. An example of this is mimicking the soft speaking of a female movie star. Other cases of abnormal vocal intensity occur because an individual has not learned to monitor loudness. Beyond learning difficulties, however, some intensity voice disorders occur because of organic problems. For example, abnormally low vocal intensity may result from such problems as paralysis of vocal cords, laryngeal trauma (including larynx surgery for cancer and damage to the larynx through accident or disease), and pulmonary diseases (like **asthma** or **emphysema**). Excessively loud speech may occur as a result of such organic problems as hearing impairments and brain damage.

Voice disorders having to do with quality-of-speech problems include such production deviances as those of abnormal nasality as well as the hoarse and breathy speech noted earlier. Abnormal nasality may take the form of a voice that sounds overly nasal (hypernasality) or a voice with reduced acoustic sound (denasality or hyponasality) that dulls the resonance of consonants. Hypernasality occurs "primarily because the back door of the nose fails to close sufficiently" (Van Riper & Emerick, 1984, p. 242). Such conditions can be due to improper tissue movement in the speech mechanism, or they may result from such organic defects as an imperfectly repaired cleft palate. Excessive hypernasality may also be acquired through learning, as in the case of country music or speech that represents an extreme form of the hillbilly dialect. Denasality is a type of voice quality that we all experience when we have a severe head cold or hay fever. The sounds produced are congested and/or dulled, with reduced acoustic resonance. In some cases, however, denasality in voice production is the result of learning or abnormal physical structures rather than these more common problems.

Intervention. Approaches to voice disorder treatment depend on causation. In some cases, when abnormal tissue and/or dental structures result in unusual voice production, surgical intervention may be necessary. In other situations, treatment may involve direct instruction to help the affected individual's learning or relearning of acceptable voice production. Such interventions often include counseling regarding the effects of unusual voice sounds on others and behavior modification procedures aimed at retraining the person's speaking. These efforts are more difficult if the behavior has been long-standing and is well ingrained as a learned habit. We have discussed interventions such as these previously, under other speech disorders. Interested readers may wish to consult other volumes focusing solely on speech problems (Emerick & Haynes, 1986; Mecham & Willbrand, 1985; Van Riper & Emerick, 1984).

Prevalence

We have already encountered the difficulties involved in estimating the prevalence of other disorders, due to differences in definitions and data-collection procedures. The field of speech disorders is very vulnerable to these problems and thus prevalence estimates vary considerably. The most typical prevalence figures cited for speech disorders indicate that between 7 and 10 percent of the population is affected (Emerick & Haynes, 1986). These figures do not deviate greatly from other estimates over the years, although some data suggest substantial differences between geographic locales (e.g., significantly higher percentages in some areas of California than in parts of the Midwest). These figures present difficulties when one considers the overall 12 percent ceiling for services to *all* disabled specified in P.L. 94–142. Obviously some speech disorders of a milder nature cannot be eligible for federally funded services. In the Eleventh Annual Report to Congress on the implementation of P.L. 94–142, 23.2 percent of those receiving special services during 1987–1988 were classified as speech impaired (U.S. Department of Education, 1989).

The frequency with which speech problems occur diminishes in the population as age increases. Speech disorders are identified in about 12 to 15 percent of the children in kindergarten through grade four. For children in grades five through eight, the figure declines to about 4 to 5 percent. The 5-percent rate remains somewhat constant after grade eight unless treatment intervenes. Thus age and development serve to diminish speech disorders considerably, more so with certain types of problems (such as articulation difficulties) than with others.

LANGUAGE DISORDERS

Language has assumed many forms throughout history. Early Native Americans communicated through systems of clucking sounds made with the tongue and teeth. Such sounds were also used in combination with hand signs and spoken language that often differed greatly between tribes. (These language systems have been described in historical documents. An excellent portrayal of such language differences is found in *Sacajawea* by A. L. Waldo, 1984.) Current definitions of language reflect the breadth necessary to encompass diverse communication systems. For example, Lucas (1980) noted that language reflects "a system of symbols agreed upon by two or more people and governed by the linguistic properties inherent in phonology, syntax, morphology, and semantics" (p. 242). Bernstein (1985) defined language as "the system of rules governing sounds, words, meaning, and use. . . . These rules underlie both linguistic comprehension (the understanding of language) and linguistic production (the formulation of language)" (p. 6).

The variety of speech disorders discussed earlier all involved problems related to verbal production; that is, vocal expression. Language disorders pertain to serious difficulties in the ability to understand or express *ideas* in the communication system being used. The distinction between speech and language disorders is like the difference in the *sound of a word* and the *meaning of a word*. As we examine language disorders we discuss difficulties in meaning, both expressing it and receiving it.

Definition

Language disorders occur when there is a serious disruption of the language process. Such malfunctions may occur in one or more of the components of language. Because language is one of the most complex sets of behaviors exhibited by humans, language disorders are complex and present some perplexing assessment problems (Allen & Bliss, 1987; Groshong, 1987; Wnuk, 1987). Language involves memory, learning, message reception and processing, and expressive skills. An individual with a language disorder may have deficits in any of these areas, and it may be difficult to identify precisely the nature of the problem. In addition, language problems may arise in the form of language delays or language disorders. The term **language delay** is used when the normal *rate* of developmental progress is interrupted but the systematic *sequence* of development remains essentially intact; that is, when the development follows a normal pattern or course of growth but is substantially slower than in most children of the same age. The term *language disorder* is different in that it refers to circumstances when language acquisition is not systematic and/or sequential. "A language disordered child is not progressing systematically and sequentially in any aspect of rule-governed and purposive linguistic behavior" (Lucas, 1980, pp. 52, 54). We use here the

FOCUS 5
What are two ways language delay and language disorder are different?

term *language disorder* in a general sense and discuss several types. Where evidence suggests that a delay may be a major contributor, we discuss it as such.

Classification

There is a wide range of terminology used to describe the processes involved in language as well as disorders in those processes. In many cases, language disorders have been classified according to their causes, which may be known or only suspected. In other cases, specific labels tend to be employed, such as *aphasia*. One common approach is to view language disorders in terms of *receptive* and *expressive* problems (Ewing-Cobbs, 1987). We examine both these categories, as well as **aphasia**, a problem that may occur in both children and adults.

Receptive Language Disorders.   **Receptive language disorders** result from difficulties in comprehending what others say. "Children with receptive language problems are often noticed when they fail to follow directions given by an adult. Often these children appear to be inattentive or may seem as though they do not hear or listen to directions" (Cole & Cole, 1981, p. 20). Individuals with receptive language disorders have great difficulty understanding the messages of others and may process only part (or none) of what is being said to them. They have a substantial problem in language processing, which is basically half of language (the other part being language production). Language processing is essentially listening and interpreting spoken language (Wiig & Semel, 1984).

Expressive Language Disorders.   **Expressive language disorders** are exhibited when individuals have difficulty in language production or formulating and using spoken language (Wiig & Semel, 1984). Those with expressive language disorders may have a limited vocabulary and rely on "the same core of words no matter what the situation" (Cole & Cole, 1981, p. 21). Expressive language disorders may appear as immature speech and often result in personal interaction difficulties. People with expressive language disorders also rely on hand signals and facial expressions to communicate.

Aphasia.   Definitions of aphasia have varied over time, but still have employed strikingly consistent themes. For example, Wood (1971) noted that aphasia was the "partial or complete loss of the ability to speak or to comprehend the spoken word due to injury, disease, or maldevelopment of the brain" (p. 11). Wiig and Semel (1984) viewed aphasia as involving those who have acquired a language disorder because of brain damage resulting in impairment of language comprehension, formulation, and use. Thus definitions of aphasia commonly link the disorder to brain injury, either through mechanical accidents, as we saw in the case of Millie, or other damage such as that caused by a stroke. Over the years, many different types of aphasia and/or conditions associated with aphasia have been identified and labeled, such as agnosia, paraphrasia, and dysprosody. Aphasic language disturbances have also been classified in terms of receptive and expressive problems.

Aphasia may be present both in childhood and during the adult years. The term **developmental aphasia** has been widely used with affected children despite the long-standing connection of such problems with neurological damage. Aphasic children often begin to use words at age two or later and phrases at age four. The link between aphasia and neurological abnormalities in youngsters has been of continuing interest to researchers, with some evidence suggesting a connection. For example, Geschwind (1968) found significant differences in the sizes of the **auditory cortex** in aphasics' right and left hemispheres. Such findings have prompted continued investigation exploring the neurological makeup of aphasic children (Cooper & Flowers, 1987). Despite the theories and assumptions, direct and objective evidence connecting specific neurological dysfunction to aphasia has been difficult to acquire.

Adult aphasia has had as many different definitions as childhood aphasia. Eisenson (1971a) suggested that there is likely to be more agreement between professionals with regard to identifying an aphasic individual than "agreement as to definitions of aphasia or to the *essence* of aphasic involvement" (p. 1220). According to Eisenson (1971a), the following observations are important in identifying persons with aphasia:

1. At some stage in their involvement, persons designated as aphasic indicate impairment for intake of sequential verbal events as well as for verbal sequential output. Intake disturbances are often labeled as memory or attention span defects. Output sequential disturbances are manifest in syntactical defects for formulations that are appropriate and relatively specific to the situation.

2. On a probability basis, aphasic involvements are in general expressed in a reduced likelihood that a given linguistic formulation will be understood (appropriately evaluated), or produced (appropriately formulated) in kind and manner consistent with the situation (events associated with the linguistic formulation). In general, the more intellectual and abstract the expected linguistic reaction, the less likely it is that the reaction will occur (p. 1220).

My name is Laura. As a Communication Specialist in a large district I am often faced with pupils in the second or third grades who speak much like children in kindergarten. By this time, their communication level has begun to seriously interfere with academic performance as well as peer social interaction. Often I am not certain exactly what to do. These children could be exhibiting delayed speech, or they could be suffering from an expressive language disorder. The assessment techniques I have at my disposal do not always help a great deal in distinguishing precisely. Yet my supervisor maintains that we have to provide an accurate diagnosis in order to serve such youngsters and receive funding. Frankly, there are times when I either flip a coin or check the list to see which category has room and make a decision that way. In this state one category brings more money into the budget than the other, and our administration likes to have as many students as possible labeled that way. This doesn't seem right, but then I'm not sure it matters anyway.

Laura, *Communication Specialist*

WINDOW 8–2

Which Is It and What to Do?

Causation

FOCUS 6
What are three factors thought to be involved in the causation of language disorders?

Identifying the precise cause of different language disorders can be difficult. The answers are not clear regarding what contributes to normal language acquisition, exactly how those contributions occur, or how malfunctions influence language disorders. We do know that certain sensory and other physiological systems must be intact and developing normally for language processes to progress normally. For example, if hearing is seriously impaired, a language deficit may result. Likewise, serious brain damage might deter normal language functioning. Learning must also progress in a systematic and sequential fashion for language to develop appropriately. For example, children must first attend to the communication around them before they can mimic it or attach meaning to it. Language-learning is like other learning; it must be stimulated and reinforced in order for the behavior to be acquired and mastered.

In our discussion of other communication disorders we encountered many of the physiological problems that may also cause language difficulties. Neurological damage that may affect language functioning can occur prenatally, during birth, or anytime throughout one's life. For example, oxygen deprivation before or during birth or an accident later in life can also cause language problems. Serious emotional disorders may be accompanied by language disturbances if an individual's perception of the world is substantially distorted.

Learning opportunities may be seriously deficient or otherwise disrupted and result in language disorders. As with speech, youngsters may not learn language because the environment is not conducive to such learning. Modeling in the home may be so infrequent that a child cannot learn language in a normal fashion. This might be the case in a family where no speaking occurs because the parents are deaf, even when the children have normal hearing. Such circumstances are rare, but when they occur a language delay is likely. The parents cannot model language for their children, nor can they respond to and reinforce such behavior. It should be emphasized, however, that learning outcomes are variable. In situations that seem normal, we may find a child with serious language difficulty. In circumstances that seem dismal, we may find youngsters whose language facility is normal. Gelfand et al. (1988) cite an example involving four brothers with normal hearing, who were born to and raised by parents who were both deaf and had no spoken language facility. These boys seemed to develop language quite normally, although they could not explain that development. They have distinguished themselves in various manners, ranging from earning Ph.D.s and M.D.s (one holds both degrees) to becoming a millionaire through patented inventions.

This example represents a rare set of circumstances, but it is a good illustration of how variable and poorly understood language-learning is. The assumption has long been that language-deprived environments place children at risk for exhibiting language delays or disorders. For example, it has been thought that language acquisition may be delayed when parents use baby talk in communicating with their young children. Such a view is based on the fundamental principles of learning theory that youngsters learn what is modeled and taught. There is little question that this perspective is sound with most skill acquisition. Many clinical reports of language problems uphold such a notion, and research also supports certain relationships between parental verbalizations and child language development (Fitzgerald & Karnes, 1987; Richard, 1986; MacDonald & Gillette, 1986). From another view, however, Cromer (1981) reviewed research on language acquisition and concluded that "most studies of baby talk fail to explain the acquisition of [language] structure" (p. 70). The effects of parent modeling on child language development may not be clear and simple.

An assumption of brain damage is usually associated with aphasia during adulthood. The causes of such brain damage are diverse. Various physical traumas may result in aphasia, such as automobile and industrial accidents or shooting incidents. This type of circumstance was illustrated in the vignette about Millie at the beginning of this chapter. Other factors, such as strokes, tumors, and diseases that affect brain tissue may have the same result. In most cases, aphasic trauma seems to be associated with damage to the left hemisphere of the brain.

The distinctions between speech and language problems are blurred because they overlap as much as do functions. Receptive and expressive language disorders are as intertwined as speech and language. When an individual does not express language well, is it because there is a receptive problem or an expressive problem? These cannot be separated cleanly, and thus causation also cannot be clearly divided into categories.

WINDOW 8–3

We Didn't Know They Were Different

My name is Cy and I am one of the four brothers mentioned. Both of my parents were deaf from a very early age: they never learned to speak. When you ask me how we learned speech I can't really answer, knowing what I now know about how those very early years are so important in this area. When we were really young we didn't even know they were deaf or different (except for Dad's active sense of humor). Naturally we didn't talk, we just signed. We lived way out in the country and were pretty isolated—all four of us just played together and didn't have other playmates. Grandma and Grandpa lived close by, and I spent a lot of time with them. That is when I began to know something was different. We probably began learning to talk there.

When we were about ready to start school we moved into town. My first memory related to school is sitting in a sandbox, I guess on the playground. We had some troubles in school but they were fairly minor as I recall. I couldn't talk or pronounce words very well. I was tested on an IQ test in the third grade and had an IQ of 67. Both Mom and Dad worked, and so we were all sort of out on our own with friends, which probably helped language, but now I wonder why those kids didn't stay away from us because we were a bit different. Probably the saving grace is that all four of us seem to have pretty well-developed social intelligence or skills. We did get in some fights with kids, and people sometimes called us the "dumby's kids." I would guess that all four of us pretty much caught up with our peers by the eighth grade. One thing is for certain, I would not trade those parents for any others in the world; whatever they did, they certainly did right.

Cy, *Ph.D.*

Intervention

FOCUS 7
Describe two ways that treatment approaches for language disorders generally differ for children and adults.

Language disorder treatment must take into account the nature of the problem and the manner in which an individual is affected. Intervention is an individualized undertaking, just as with other types of disorders. Some causes are more easily identified than others and may or may not be remedied by mechanical or medical intervention. Other types of treatment basically involve instruction or language training. Cole and Cole (1981) outlined several sequential steps in effective language training: (1) Identifying the child, (2) Assessing the child, (3) Establishing the instructional objectives, (4) Developing the language intervention program, (5) Implementing the language intervention program, (6) Reassessing the child, (7) Reteaching if necessary (p. 81). These steps are very similar to the general stages involved in special education interventions for other disorders. Thus the customary approach to language disorder intervention follows the basic steps for treatment as outlined in P.L. 94–142. Specific programs of intervention obviously include details not evident at this level.

Language training programs are tailored to an individual's strengths and limitations. In fact, current terminology labels these **individualized language plans (ILPs)**, similar in concept to the individualized educational plans (IEPs) mandated by P.L. 94–142. These intervention plans include long-range goals (annual), a set of more short-range and specific behavioral objectives, a statement of the resources to be used in achieving the objectives, a description of evaluation methods, program beginning and ending dates, and an evaluation of the individual's generalization of skills. For young children, such interventions often focus on beginning language stimulation. Such treatment is intended to mirror the conditions under which youngsters normally learn language, but the conditions may be intensified and taught more systematically (Chapman & Terrell, 1988). In many cases, parents are trained and involved in the intervention.

Many approaches have been used to remediate aphasia, but consistent and verifiable results have been slow to emerge. As with other disorders, remediation typically involves the development of an individual's profile of strengths, limitations, age, and developmental level (Ylvisaker, 1986). From this profile an individualized treatment plan can be designed. Several questions or points immediately surface, including what to teach or remediate first and whether teaching should focus on an individual's strengths or weak areas. These questions have been raised from time to time with respect to many disorders. Nearly all clinicians have their own opinions or carry with them some personal formula for balancing the extremes. Cooper and Griffiths (1978) made an interesting point concerning the latter question with respect to aphasic children: Teaching exclusively to one's deficit areas may result in more failure experiences than are either necessary or helpful to a child's overall progress. This may occur because, being taught solely in the weakest areas, the child receives so little success and reinforcement that he or she becomes discouraged about the whole process. Good clinical judgment needs to be exercised in balancing remediation attention to the aphasic child's strengths and weaknesses.

Remediation for adults with aphasia begins from a perspective different from that for children, in that the task involves *relearning or reacquiring* language function. Views regarding treatment have varied over the years. Early approaches included the expectation that adult aphasics would exhibit spontaneous recovery if left alone. This approach has largely been replaced by the view that patients are more likely to progress when direct therapeutic instruction is available.

Therapy for adults with aphasia has some predictable similarities to treatment for children. Areas of strength and limitation must receive attention when an individualized remediation program is being planned. However, development of a profile of strengths and deficits may involve some areas different from those of children because of age differences. For example, social, linguistic, and vocational readjustments represent three broad areas needing attention for most adult aphasics. Although children need attention beyond just language therapy, some aspects of adult treatment are not relevant, such as vocational readjustment; and the notion of readjustment differs substantially from initial skill acquisition. An individualized treatment program for adult aphasics also involves evaluation, profile development, and teaching in specific behavioral areas within each of the broad domains. Such training should begin as soon as possible, depending on the patient's condition. Some spontaneous recovery often occurs during the first six months after an incident resulting in aphasia. However, waiting beyond two months to begin treatment may not only be unnecessary but also seriously delay recovery to whatever degree may be possible.

REVIEW

FOCUS 1: What are four ways speech, language, and communication are interrelated?

☐ Both speech and language are part, but not all, of communication.

☐ There are components of communication that involve language but not speech.

☐ There may be speech that does not involve language.

☐ In humans, the development of communication, language, and speech overlap to some degree.

FOCUS 2: What are three factors thought to be involved in the causation of stuttering?

☐ Emotional problems, neurological problems, and learned behavior can contribute to stuttering.

☐ Some research has suggested that stutterers have a different brain organization.

☐ Stutterers may learn their speech patterns as an outgrowth of the normal nonfluency evident when speech development is first occurring.

FOCUS 3: What are two ways learning theory and home environment relate to delayed speech?

☐ The home environment may provide little opportunity to learn speech.

☐ The home environment may interfere with speech development when speaking is punished.

FOCUS 4: Give two reasons why some professionals are reluctant to treat functional articulation disorders in young schoolchildren.

☐ Many articulation problems evident in young children are developmental in nature, and speech may improve with age.

☐ Articulation problems are quite frequent among young children, and resources are limited.

FOCUS 5: What are two ways language delay and language disorder are different?

☐ In language delay, the sequence of development is intact but the rate of development is interrupted.

☐ In language disorder, the sequence of development is interrupted.

FOCUS 6: What are three factors thought to be involved in the causation of language disorders?

☐ Defective or deficient sensory systems.

☐ Neurological damage occurring through physical trauma or accident.

☐ Deficient or disrupted learning opportunities during language development.

FOCUS 7: Describe two ways that treatment approaches for language disorders generally differ for children and for adults.

☐ Treatment for children generally addresses initial acquisition or learning of language.

☐ Treatment for adults involves relearning or reacquiring language function.

Debate Forum

Role of the Speech and Language Specialist

There are millions of people in the United States affected by speech and language disorders, many of them school-age youngsters. This places a severe strain on the schools' ability to provide complete services. Likewise, it raises certain questions regarding the role of speech and language specialists—how they can most efficiently and effectively be employed. It also has ramifications for the nature of their professional training. Choose a position and defend it.

Point Speech and language specialists should be trained and employed to operate independently. They should be involved in direct treatment of speech- and language-disordered youngsters. This takes the best advantage of their knowledge and expertise and ensures that clients receive the most appropriate intervention for their problems. It also relieves other personnel, such as teachers and counselors, from any need to consider and deal with speech or language disorders. Further, it relieves the speech/language specialist from having to consider the outside environment where a youngster has to survive.

Counterpoint Speech and language specialists should be trained and employed to operate in an integrated, crossdisciplinary fashion with other educational professionals. They should be training others to assist with or provide service in school settings, limiting their direct-treatment activities to those more severe cases requiring lengthy intervention. It would make more efficient use of school district funds and also ensure interdisciplinary interaction between the professional components of the educational system. It would naturalize the intervention setting for many youngsters.

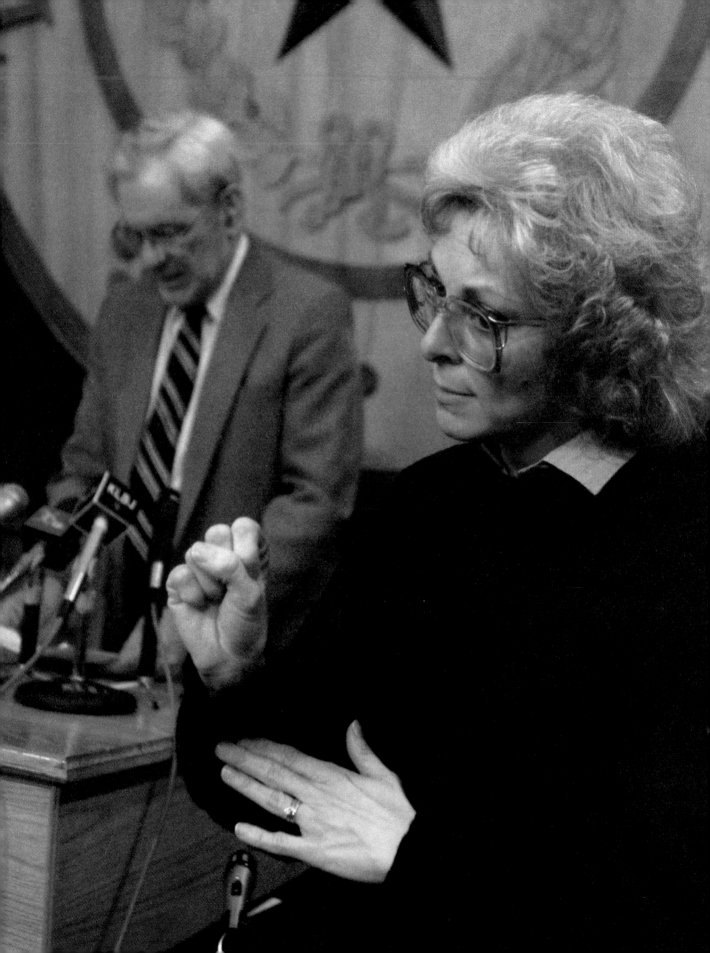

9 Hearing Disorders

To Begin With...

■ Hearing impairment is among the top five chronic health disorders in the United States. Seven out of every 100 people in this country are deaf or hearing impaired (Sullivan & Bourke, 1980).

■ In 1985, the Salem Shopping Mall in Dayton, Ohio, announced the availability of a Santa who could use sign language. More than 250 hearing impaired children visited Mr. Claus. One problem occurred: Santa's bushy beard got in the way for children who also used lip reading to communicate! (*Good Housekeeping*, 1985).

■ Closed-caption television programs including "The Cosby Show," "Sesame Street," news programs, and sports activities are now being used to teach reading to both hearing and hearing-impaired students (National Captioning Institute, n.d.).

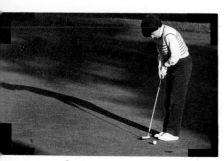

Rosa

Rosa is the oldest of three children. She was born with normal hearing, but at the age of eight she developed **spinal meningitis**. The disease resulted in a severe hearing loss in both ears. Rosa's parents worked diligently with her to retain the precious speech that had been acquired prior to the loss of hearing. Their work was reinforced through her educational experiences. Rosa spent the remainder of her elementary-school years in a special class for children with hearing disorders, and as an adolescent she went on to her neighborhood high school, where she graduated with honors. She continued her education at the university level, receiving an undergraduate degree in philosophy and completing law school. Rosa is now a successful real-estate lawyer and is very active in civic and charitable endeavors. Her leisure time is spent oil painting, reading history books, and relaxing at the local golf course.

INTRODUCTION

Although Rosa is unable to hear a single word, her life is one of independence and fulfillment. In Rosa's case, as well as those of many people with a hearing disorder, the obstacles presented by the loss of hearing are not insurmountable.

In a world that is often controlled by sound, the ability to hear and speak is a critical link in the development of human communication. Children who can hear learn to talk by listening to those around them. Our everyday communication systems would make little sense without sound. Telephones, loudspeakers, car horns, musical instruments, alarm clocks, fire alarms, radios, stereos, and intercoms would be useless in a world without sound. Our sense of hearing is an important factor in the way we learn to perceive our world and in the way the world perceives us.

How difficult is it, then, for the person who cannot hear to adjust to a hearing world? Most people with a hearing disorder, such as Rosa, can and do adjust successfully to life within their local communities. In some cases, people with a hearing disorder may become outsiders in a world "created and controlled by those who hear" (Higgins, 1980, p. 22). The term *outsider* implies that these people may be shunned by society, and if that is so, they must find some way to compensate. Higgins suggests that individuals with a hearing disorder may deal with the stigma in a number of ways. Some may try to adjust as much as possible to the demands of the hearing world. Others live a life of isolation, with few contacts with the hearing world. Still others become a part of organized groups whose members share the common bond of hearing loss.

Our discussion of hearing disorders begins with a look at the process of hearing. What is the structure of the mechanism through which we hear, and how is sound collected, processed, and transmitted to the brain?

The Hearing Process

FOCUS 1
Describe the process of transmitting sound.

Audition is defined as the act or sense of hearing. The auditory process involves the transmission of sound through the vibration of an object to a receiver. The process originates with a vibrator, such as a string, reed, membrane, or column of air, that causes a displacement of air particles. In order for a vibration to become sound, there must be a medium to carry it. Air is the most common carrier, but vibrations can also be carried by metal, water, and other substances. The displacement of air particles by the vibrator produces a pattern of circular waves that move away from the source. This movement is referred to as a *sound wave* and can be illustrated by imagining the ripples resulting from a pebble dropped in a pool of water. Sound waves are patterns of pressure that alternately push together and pull apart in a spherical expansion. Sound waves are carried through a medium (e.g., air) to a receiver. The human ear is one of the most sensitive receivers there is; it is capable of being activated by incredibly small amounts of pressure. Perkins and Kent (1986) suggest: "Considering its puny size, the ear is a prodigious instrument. With equipment that could almost be packaged in a sugar cube, we can distinguish all the sounds of speech, along with nearly a half a million other sounds" (p. 245).

The ear is the mechanism through which sound is collected, processed, and transmitted to a specific area in the brain that decodes the sensations into a meaningful language. The anatomy of the hearing mechanism is discussed in terms of the external, middle, and inner ears. These structures are illustrated in Figure 9–1.

The External Ear. The external ear consists of a cartilage structure on the side of the head called an *auricle,* or *pinna,* and an external ear canal referred to as the *meatus.* The auricle is the only outwardly visible part of the ear and is attached to the skull by three ligaments. The purpose of the auricle is to collect sound waves and funnel them into the meatus. The meatus secretes a wax called *cerumen,* which protects the inner structures of the ear by trapping foreign materials and lubricating the canal and eardrum. The eardrum, or tympanic membrane, is located at the inner end of the canal between the external and

FOCUS 2
What are the basic functions of the external, middle, and inner ear?

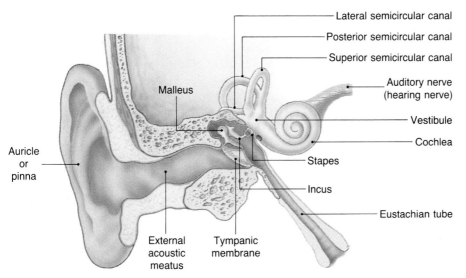

Figure 9–1
The Structure of the Human Ear

Lateral semicircular canal
Posterior semicircular canal
Superior semicircular canal
Auditory nerve (hearing nerve)
Vestibule
Cochlea
Stapes
Incus
Eustachian tube
Malleus
Auricle or pinna
External acoustic meatus
Tympanic membrane

middle ear. The concave membrane is positioned in such manner that when struck by sound waves it can vibrate freely.

The Middle Ear. The inner surface of the eardrum is located in the air-filled cavity of the middle ear. This surface consists of three small bones that form the **ossicular chain.** These bones are the malleus, incus, and stapes, often referred to as the *hammer, anvil,* and *stirrup* because each shape is similar to those common objects. These three bones transmit the vibrations from the external ear through the cavity of the middle ear to the inner ear.

The **eustachian tube** is a structure that extends between the throat and the middle-ear cavity. Its purpose is to equalize the air pressure on the eardrum with that of the outside. This is accomplished by controlling the flow of air into the middle-ear cavity. Although air conduction is the primary avenue through which sound reaches the inner ear, it is possible for conduction to occur through the bones of the skull. Bone conduction appears comparable to air conduction in that the patterns of displacement produced in the inner ear are similar.

The Inner Ear. The inner ear consists of a multitude of intricate passageways. The **cochlea** lies horizontally in front of the vestibule (a central cavity where sound enters directly from the middle ear), where it can be activated by movement in the ossicular chain. The cochlea is filled with fluid similar in composition to cerebral spinal fluid. Within the cochlea is **Corti's organ,** a structure of highly specialized cells that translate vibration into nerve impulses that are sent directly to the brain.

The other major structure within the inner ear is the **vestibular mechanism,** containing the semicircular canals that control balance. The semicircular canals have enlarged portions at one end and are filled with fluid that responds to head movement. The vestibular mechanism integrates sensory input passing to the brain and assists the body in maintaining its equilibrium. Motion and gravity are detected through this mechanism, allowing the individual to differentiate between sensory input associated with body movement and that from the external environment. Whenever the basic functions of the vestibular mechanism or any of the structures in the external, middle, and inner ear are interrupted, a hearing loss may occur.

DEFINITIONS AND CLASSIFICATION

Definitions

FOCUS 3
How are sound intensity and sound frequency measured?

A hearing disorder may be defined according to the degree of hearing loss. This is accomplished by assessing a person's sensitivity to loudness (sound intensity) and pitch (sound frequency). The unit used to measure sound intensity is the *decibel* (db), and the range of human hearing is approximately 0 to 130 dbs. Sounds louder than 130 dbs are extremely painful to the ear. Table 9–1 illustrates various common environmental sounds and their measurable decibel level.

The frequency of sound is determined by measuring the number of cycles that vibrating molecules complete per second. The unit used to measure cycles

TABLE 9–1 Common Environmental Sounds with Estimated Decibel (db) Level

Decibel Level (Sound Intensity)	
140 db	Jet aircraft (80 feet from tail at takeoff)
130 db	Jackhammer
120 db	Loud thunder
110 db	Live music
100 db	Chain saw
90 db	Street traffic
80 db	Telephone ring
70 db	Door slam
60 db	Washing machine
50 db	Conversational speech (40–60 db)
40 db	Electric typewriter
30 db	Pencil writing
20 db	Watch ticking
10 db	Whisper
0 db	Lowest threshold of hearing for the human ear

per second is the **hertz** (Hz). The higher the frequency, the higher the hertz. The human ear can hear sounds ranging from 20 to approximately 15,000 Hz. The pitch of speech sounds is 300 to 4000 Hz, whereas a piano keyboard ranges from 27.5 to 4186 Hz. Although it is possible for the human ear to hear sounds at the 15,000 Hz level, the vast majority of sounds in our environment range from 300 to 4000 Hz.

Deafness and Hard-of-Hearing. Two terms, **deaf** and **hard-of-hearing** (or partially hearing), are commonly used in definitions of hearing disorders. *Deaf* is often overused and misunderstood. Although this term is commonly applied to a wide variety of hearing disorders, it should be used in a more precise fashion. Deafness, as defined by the rules and regulations of Public Law 94–142, means "a hearing impairment which is so severe that the child is impaired in processing linguistic information through hearing, with or without amplification, which adversely affects educational performance" (Federal Register, 1977, p. 42478). A deaf person is unable to recognize sound or the meaning of sound-pressure waves. However, the degree of loss as measured on an audiometer should not be the sole criterion for defining deafness. Ross and Calvert (1984) suggest that the definition of deafness must be "a functional description, based on a person's ability to comprehend spoken language auditorily" (p. 129). Berg (1976) states:

> The deaf child typically has profound or total loss of auditory sensitivity and very little or no auditory perception. Under the most ideal listening and hearing

FOCUS 4
Distinguish between deaf and hard-of-hearing.

aid conditions, he either does not hear the speech signal or perceives so little of it that audition may not serve as the primary sensory modality for the acquisition of spoken language or for the monitoring of speech (p. 5).

From an educational perspective, the definition above strongly implies that the sense of hearing cannot be used as a functional source for acquiring new information.

For persons defined as hard-of-hearing, the sense of hearing is defective but remains somewhat functional. "A hard-of-hearing person is one who, generally with the use of a hearing aid, has residual hearing sufficient to enable successful processing of linguistic information through audition" (Brill, MacNeil, & Newman, 1986, p. 67).

A person who is described as hard-of-hearing generally has residual hearing that, with the use of a hearing aid, allows the processing of linguistic information through the auditory channel.

Berg (1976) suggests that what the person who is hard-of-hearing perceives at any given moment depends on several factors, including "hearing sensitivity, faintness of sound, distance between speaker and listener, noise background, language proficiency, past experience, environmental awareness, and corresponding lack of compensatory judgments" (p. 3).

The distinction between deaf and hard-of-hearing, based on the functional use of residual hearing, is not as clear as many traditional definitions would imply. New breakthroughs in the development of hearing aids, as well as improved diagnostic procedures, have made it possible for many children labeled as deaf to use their hearing functionally under limited circumstances.

In addition to measuring a person's sensitivity to loudness and pitch, there are two other factors in defining a hearing disorder: the age of onset and the anatomical site of the loss.

FOCUS 5
Why is it important to consider age of onset when defining a hearing disorder?

Age of Onset. A hearing disorder may be present at birth (congenital) or acquired at any time during one's life. The distinction between congenital and acquired disorders is an important one. The age of onset is a critical variable in determining the type and extent of intervention necessary to minimize the effect of the individual's disorder (McAnally, Rose, & Quigley, 1987). This is particularly true in relation to speech and language development. As was the case for Rosa in our opening vignette, her parents and teachers worked diligently to maintain the speech and language skills she had acquired prior to her hearing loss. The maintenance of these skills had a crucial effect on Rosa's subsequent pattern of intellectual development, communication, academic achievement, and social adaptation. In contrast, a person who is born with a hearing disorder has significantly more problems, particularly in the area of communication and social adaptation.

Rosa's experiences clearly reflect the need to distinguish between pre- and postlingual disorders. McAnally et al. (1987) identified **prelingual disorders** as occurring prior to the age of two, or about the time of speech development. **Postlingual** disorders occur at any age following speech development. Sanders (1980) stresses that "the critical factor appears to be whether or not the hearing deficit occurs before the acquisition of verbal language, or at least before language learning processes have been activated" (p. 227).

The Anatomical Site of the Loss. The two primary types of hearing loss based on anatomical location are peripheral and central auditory problems. There are three types of peripheral hearing loss: **conductive, sensorineural,** and **mixed.** Conductive hearing losses result from poor conduction of sound along the passages leading to the sense organ (inner ear). The loss may result from a blockage in the external canal, as well as from an obstruction interfering with the movement of the eardrum or ossicle. The overall effect is a reduction or loss of loudness. A conductive loss can be offset by amplification (hearing aids) and medical intervention. Surgery has proven to be effective in reducing or even restoring a conductive loss.

Sensorineural hearing losses are a result of an abnormal sense organ and a damaged auditory nerve. A sensorineural loss may distort sound, affecting the clarity of human speech. At present, sensorineural losses cannot be treated adequately through medical intervention. A sensorineural loss is generally more severe than a conductive loss, and it is permanent. Losses of greater than 70 dB are usually sensorineural and involve severe damage to the inner ear. One common way to determine whether a loss is conductive or sensorineural is to administer an air and bone conduction test. An individual with a conductive loss would be unable to hear a vibrating tuning fork held close to the ear, because air passages to the inner ear are blocked. However, if the same fork were applied to the skull, the person with a conductive loss may be able to hear it as well as someone with normal hearing. An individual with a sensorineural loss would not be able to hear the vibrating fork regardless of its placement. However, this test is not always accurate and must therefore be used with caution in distinguishing between conductive and sensorineural losses. Davis (1978) suggests that "there are practical pitfalls. Some skulls and the skin and soft tissues over them do not conduct sound as well as others" (pp. 93–94).

Mixed hearing loss, a combination of conductive and sensorineural problems, may also be assessed through the use of an air and bone conduction test. In the case of a mixed loss, abnormalities are evident in both tests.

Although most hearing losses are peripheral, such as conductive and sensorineural problems, some disorders occur where there is no measurable peripheral loss. This type of loss is referred to as a central auditory disorder and occurs when there is a dysfunction in the cerebral cortex. The cerebral cortex is the outer layer of gray matter of the brain. It governs thought, reasoning, memory, sensation, and voluntary movement. Consequently, a central auditory problem is not a loss in the ability to hear sound but a disorder of symbolic processes, including auditory perception, discrimination, comprehension of sound, and language development (expressive and receptive).

Classification

Hearing disorders, like other disorders, may be classified according to the severity of the condition. Table 9–2 illustrates a symptom-severity classification system and presents information relative to a child's ability to understand speech patterns at the various severity levels. In addition, it highlights implications for educational placement.

Classification systems based solely on a person's degree of hearing loss

FOCUS 6
Distinguish between conductive, sensorineural, and mixed hearing losses.

FOCUS 7
Classify hearing disorders according to the severity of the condition.

TABLE 9–2 Classification of Hearing Disorders

Average Hearing Loss in Better Ear as Measured in Decibels (db) (ISO[a]) at 500–2,000 Hertz (Hz)	Severity Level	Effect on Ability to Understand Speech	Typical Classroom Setting and General Language Characteristics of Students with a Hearing Loss
0–25 db	Insignificant	No significant difficulty with faint or normal speech	Individual is likely to be fully integrated into regular education setting. Support services, if any, would be minimal.
25–40 db	Mild (hard-of-hearing)	Frequent difficulty with faint sounds; some difficulty with normal speech (conversations, groups)	Individual is likely to be integrated into regular education setting with support services available to develop/maintain speech and language. Hearing aid is recommended.
40–60 db	Moderate (hard-of-hearing)	Frequent difficulty with normal speech (conversations, groups); some difficulty with loud speech	Individual is likely to be placed in special class for deaf students during significant part of the day, but can be integrated for at least some portion of the day. Individual exhibits language delays, articulation problems, and omission of consonants.

should be used with a great deal of caution when determining appropriate intervention strategies. These systems do not reflect the capabilities, background, or experiences of the individuals; they merely suggest parameters for measuring a physical defect in auditory function. Bitter (1981) suggests that professionals involved in the assessment process should be "very cautious in delimiting definitions of hearing impairment to avoid the mistake of inflexible classifications and stereotypes which include quantitative measurements in decibels or percentages" (p. 5). As a child, Rosa was diagnosed as having a severe hearing loss in both ears. Yet, throughout her life, she successfully adjusted to both school and community experiences. She went on to college and now has a successful career as a lawyer. Consequently, there are many factors beyond severity that must be assessed in the process of determining the potential of individuals with a hearing loss. In addition to severity of loss, such factors as general intelligence, emotional stability, scope and quality of early education and training, and the family environment must also be considered.

PREVALENCE

FOCUS 8
Why is it difficult to determine accurately the prevalence of hearing disorders?

It has been difficult to determine accurately the prevalence of hearing disorders in this country. The major problems with the prevalence estimates appear to be (1) inconsistent definitional criteria and (2) methodological problems in the

Average Hearing Loss in Better Ear as Measured in Decibels (db) (ISO[a]) at 500–2,000 Hertz (Hz)	Severity Level	Effect on Ability to Understand Speech	Typical Classroom Setting and General Language Characteristics of Students with a Hearing Loss
60–80 db	Severe (range includes hard-of-hearing and deaf)	Frequent difficulty with even loud speech; may have difficulty understanding even shouted or amplified speech	Individual is likely to be placed in special class with little or no integration into regular education setting. Even with amplification, person is unable to process ordinary conversational sound. Individual will likely have severe speech and language disorder.
80 db or more	Profound (deaf)	Usually cannot understand even amplified speech	Individual is likely to be placed in special class or school for the deaf. Individual will have severe speech and language disorder or may have no oral speech.

[a] International Standards Organization

surveys. Hoemann and Briga (1981) stated, "Unfortunately, the various surveys that have been undertaken have used different criteria for defining terms, both for the severity of the loss and for the age of onset. Moreover, some of the samples have been biased in that they have underrepresented populations of lower socioeconomic status, multiply handicapped groups, and racial and ethnic minorities" (p. 224). Other factors must also be taken into consideration when analyzing investigations of prevalence. Did the study differentiate between unilateral (one ear) and bilateral (two ear) loss? From what population was the sample drawn? School-age? Prevocational? Adult? Total?

The most accurate data source may well be the U.S. Department of Education in its Eleventh Annual Report to Congress (1989). This report indicates there are 56,937 hard-of-hearing and deaf students between the ages of six and twenty-one who are receiving specialized services in our Nation's schools. These students account for approximately 1.4 percent of the over 4 million students labeled as handicapped. It is important to note that these figures only represent students who are receiving special services. There are a number of students with hearing losses who would benefit from additional services but are not being served. About 20 percent of the students are being served in regular classrooms full-time, 24 percent in regular classes with resource-room support, 35 percent in separate special education classes, about 10 percent in separate public or private day schools for students with hearing disorders, and 11 percent in public or private residential living facilities.

In the News 9–1

Gallaudet Students Are Heard in Washington

Gallaudet University, the nation's only liberal arts college for the deaf, was the scene of an emotionally charged student protest in March of 1988. Evoking images of the civil rights rallies of the 1960s, one student proclaimed, "This is the Selma of the deaf." But unlike those in earlier marches, these protestors marched in silence, communicating their anger with scribbled posters, banners, and sign language.

The protest was launched when the school's trustees ignored the students' call for a deaf president and instead chose Elisabeth Ann Zinser, an educator from the University of North Carolina at Greensboro. Zinser was not only sound of hearing, she was unable

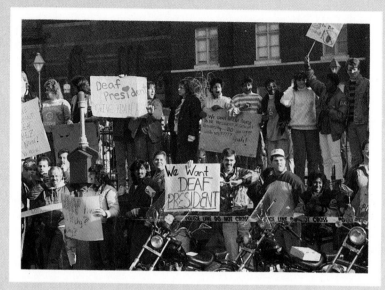

(Wide World Photos)

CHARACTERISTICS

In this section we examine some of the general characteristics of people with hearing disorders, including intelligence, speech and language skills, educational achievement, and social development. We emphasize that the effect of a hearing disorder on the learning or social adjustment of the individual is extremely varied. The influence may be far-reaching, as in the case of prelingual sensorineural deafness, or quite minimal, as in the case of a mild postlingual conductive disorder. Fortunately there has recently been increased emphasis on prevention, early detection, and intervention, which has resulted in a much-improved prognosis for individuals with hearing disorders.

Intelligence

FOCUS 9
Why is the research on the intelligence of people with a hearing disorder considered inconclusive?

The intelligence of people with hearing disorders has been a subject of controversy for the better part of this century. Although intellectual functioning has been studied extensively, the validity of these investigations has been questioned by several authors (Davis, 1977; McConnell, 1973; Meadow, 1980). Early investo communicate in sign language and had no experience in educating the deaf. In response to the decision, most of Gallaudet's 2,200 students angrily marched on the streets of Washington, D.C., rallying at the U.S. Capitol. They forced the cancellation of classes for the week and demanded the resignation of the new president and the board of trustees.

For the students at Gallaudet, the trustees' decision reflected a clear message: a deaf person was not capable of running the school. Since Gallaudet's founding in 1864, no hearing impaired person had ever held the position of president. In fact, at the time of the

protest, just four deaf members sat on the twenty-one-seat board of trustees. The students reacted angrily to what they viewed as the school's "paternalistic" attitude. Said one student, "Prejudice is believing that hearing people have to take care of deaf people."

Disabled groups across the United States cheered the efforts of the Gallaudet students. Politicians in Washington voiced their support of the protest and exerted pressure on the trustees to reconsider their decision. They reminded the trustees that Congress might be reluctant to increase the school's $76 million annual budget in view of the conflict.

Faced with such opposition, Zinser resigned her new position after four days of protests. Irving King Jordan, who is deaf, was chosen to be Gallaudet's new president. In March of 1988, the deaf were heard—loud and clear—in Washington, D.C.

Sources: Townsend Davis, "Hearing Aid," *The New Republic*, September 12, 1988, pp. 20–22.

David Brand, "This Is the Selma of the Deaf," *Time Magazine*, March 21, 1988, p. 64.

"A Cry From the Deaf Is Heard in Washington," *U.S. News & World Report*, March 21, 1988, pp. 9–10.

tigations (Pinter, Eisenson, & Stanton, 1941) reported that hearing-disordered individuals scored in the low 90s when tested on standard IQ scales. However, later reviews of the research (Meadow, 1980; Vernon, 1969; Vernon & Brown, 1964) suggest that hearing-disordered children have approximately the same distribution of IQ scores as hearing children, although the mean score is slightly lower. Meadow also indicates that the equal distribution of scores for hearing-disordered and normal children occurs only when the intelligence test involves the use of nonverbal instructions and does not require oral responses from the student. Davis suggests that test developers and administrators have not fully accounted for the relationship between atypical linguistic development and performance on the IQ test. Meadow further states: "Baseline data on language ability, spoken and signed, should be accumulated for deaf subjects and used in designing and administering test instruments, and in interpreting the test performance results" (p. 71).

A study conducted by Schlesinger and Meadow (1976) revealed that hearing children were superior to deaf children on three major tests of intellectual development. One striking find, however, was that the pattern of performance was consistent across the two populations. Deaf children, despite attaining concepts

Reflect on This 9–1

Aristotle Was Wrong

Society consistently has confused lack of hearing with lack of intelligence, and deaf people have been socially and spiritually isolated because of it. Aristotle hypothesized that without hearing, people could not learn. And so, from ancient times through the Middle Ages, deaf people were never educated. The ancient Greeks left deaf babies in the wild to die, as they did with any baby deemed "defective." In the Middle Ages, priests believed that people born deaf could not have faith and barred them from churches. In much of Europe, the deaf weren't allowed to marry or own property. It wasn't really until the 16th cen-

tury that a few clerics became interested in teaching the deaf and until nearly 300 years later that schools were set up. During the 19th century, deaf people founded and became superintendents and principals of 22 schools in at least 18 states. But by this century, according to Jack Gannon, a deaf Gallaudet administrator who wrote *Deaf Heritage*, things weren't going so well for them: In many schools, hearing people took over, and deaf teachers were banned from classrooms. There were no longer any deaf superintendents; today there are at most two in the U.S.

Even so, when permitted, the

deaf have made an impact on society. Samuel F. B. Morse developed his code by tapping out messages with his deaf wife. Alexander Graham Bell's mother and wife were deaf, and he invented the telephone because he was trying to come up with something that would help deaf people hear. (Ironically, his invention became an overwhelming barrier to deaf people, because most jobs require the ability to use a phone.)

Source: L. A. Walker (1989, April 23), I Know How to Ask for What I Want, *Parade,* 4–6.

at a later stage than normal, appear to learn them in approximately the same sequence as hearing children.

The findings of the past two decades suggest that intellectual development for people with hearing disorders is more a function of language development than of cognitive ability. These individuals learn concepts in the same way as their hearing peers. Their difficulties in performance appear to be more closely associated with reading and writing the English language.

Speech and Language Skills

FOCUS 10
How does the effect of a hearing disorder on speech and language differ for people with a mild loss as opposed to those with a more severe loss?

Speech and language skills are the areas of development most severely affected in those with a hearing disorder. Markides (1983) indicates that over 150 original papers have been published within the last fifty years on just the speech skills of deaf children. These publications clearly suggest that the effects of a hearing disorder on language development varies considerably. For people with mild and moderate losses, the effect on speech and language may be minimal. Even for individuals born with a moderate loss, effective communication skills are possible because the voiced sounds of conversational speech remain audible. Although individuals with a moderate loss cannot hear unvoiced sounds and distant speech, language delays can be prevented if the hearing loss is diagnosed

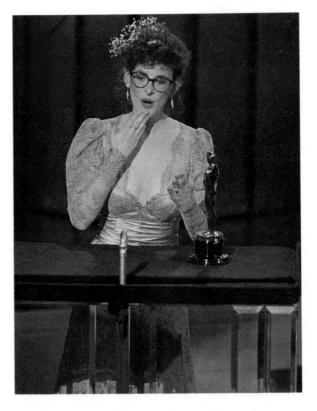

Hearing disorders present severe—but not insurmountable—obstacles in dealing with the hearing world. Here, Marlee Matlin uses sign language to accept an Oscar for her role in *Children of a Lesser God.* (Wide World Photos)

and treated early (Ling & Ling, 1978). The majority of people with a hearing disorder are able to use speech as the primary mode for language acquisition.

For the person who is congenitally deaf, most loud speech is inaudible, even with the use of the most sophisticated hearing aids. These people are unable to receive information through the speech process unless they have learned to lip (speech) read. Sound production by the deaf person is extremely low in intelligibility (McAnally et al., 1987). Oyers and Frankmann (1975) reported significant articulation, voice quality, and tone-discrimination problems in deaf children.

I was born with a bilateral, profound hearing loss that was not identified until I was nearly three years old. However, I have always been actively involved in the life of my family, church, community, and school in very meaningful ways. I think of myself as a person, not as a deaf person. I learned speech and speech-reading, and I learned to use spoken language. After all, the important people in my life—family, friends, neighbors, schoolmates—communicated that way. I consider my hearing impairment an inconvenience, not a tragedy. Success in the world of work and in society as a functional, independent citizen is so satisfying and exhilarating.

Coleen, *a person with a hearing disorder*

WINDOW 9–1

I'm Making It in a Hearing World

Jensema, Karchmer, and Trybus (1978) surveyed teachers of hearing-disordered children from across the Nation, and more than 42 percent of the students were rated as having barely intelligible or unintelligible speech. In addition, the survey indicated that approximately 13 percent of these hearing-disordered students would not even speak.

Persons who are congenitally deaf have a great deal of difficulty communicating adequately with the hearing world. In order to have any chance of overcoming this severe handicap, they must have access to early and extensive training in language production and comprehension. Ling and Ling (1978) indicate that "hearing impairment is a serious barrier to verbal learning, and with those whose hearing impairment is more than minimal, it can only be gained through deliberate programming" (p. 31).

Educational Achievement

FOCUS 11
Describe the effects of a hearing disorder on academic skills.

The educational achievement of students with a hearing disorder may be significantly delayed in comparison to their hearing peers. It should come as no surprise that this population has considerable difficulty succeeding in a system that depends primarily on the spoken word and written language to transmit knowledge. Low achievement is characteristic of deaf students, who average three to four years below their age-appropriate grade level (Mandell & Fiscus, 1981). However, even students with mild to moderate losses achieve below expectations based on their performance on tests of cognitive ability.

Reading and Arithmetic Skills. Reading is the academic area most negatively affected for students with a hearing disorder. Brooks (1978) indicates that "despite dedicated and tireless efforts by educators of the deaf, early severe hearing loss persists as a promissory for reading failure" (p. 87). Poor reading achievement for hearing-disordered students has been well documented in the literature (Cole, 1987; Kodman, 1963; Ling, 1972; Trybus & Karchmer, 1977). "Even when subgroups of deaf children are examined and differences found among those with varying characteristics, the students performing at a higher level still do not score at levels equivalent to their hearing peers" (Meadow, 1980, p. 55).

To counteract the difficulty with conventional reading materials, specialized instructional programs have been developed especially for deaf students. One such program is the Reading Milestone series (Quigley and King, 1984). The program uses content that focuses on the interests and experiences of deaf children, while incorporating linguistic controls. Controls include the careful pacing of new vocabulary, the clear identification of syntactic structures, and the move from simple to complex in the introduction of new concepts such as idioms, inferences, and the like. In less than a decade, Reading Milestones has become the most widely used reading program for deaf students (LaSasso, 1985).

The development of arithmetic-computation skills has also been investigated and found to be deficient for deaf students in comparison to the norm. Meadow (1980), in a review of studies focusing on academic achievement, reported that "the highest average achievement by any deaf age group on arithmetic computation was at grade level 6.7" (p. 72).

Written Language. A few studies (Boothroyd, 1971; Heider & Heider, 1940) have investigated the written language utilized by deaf students. These investigations basically agree that, compared to the norm, the vocabulary of the deaf student is simple and limited. Written sentences are generally shorter and more rudimentary, resembling sentences of less mature hearing students.

Allen (1986) examined the overall academic achievement of students who are deaf to see if there was any improvement in scores over a nine-year period. He evaluated student scores from achievement tests taken in 1974, and then did the same evaluation on a different set of students in 1983. He reported that achievement scores for students with hearing disorders were behind those of their hearing peers in both years. However, a comparison of both the 1974 and 1983 data indicate that the scores of students with hearing disorders had improved over the nine-year period, and the gap was closing. This is an encouraging trend that may reflect advances in instructional techniques for these students.

Social Development

A hearing disorder results in modification of the individual's capacity to receive and process auditory stimuli. People with a hearing disorder receive a reduced amount of auditory information, which is also distorted compared to the input received by those with normal hearing. Consequently, perceptions of auditory information are different from the norm. Sanders (1980) states:

> The problem is not simply one involving a reduction of sensitivity to sound; it concerns the whole process of structuring an awareness and understanding of things, events, people, and even self. The hearing-impaired child must develop his perceptions using an auditory system which distorts or even eliminates information that the normal developing child uses to build his understanding of the world (p. 219).

Meadows (1980) reviewed the literature on social and psychological development in deaf children and reported that such children appear to be less socially mature than hearing children. Delayed language acquisition may lead to more limited opportunities for social interaction (Cole, 1987). Deaf children may have more adjustment problems than their hearing counterparts. In spite of these findings, Meadow also suggests: "It would be a mistake to conclude that there is a single 'deaf personality type.' *There is much diversity among deaf people, and it is related to education, communication, and experience*" (pp. 96–97; emphasis added).

The generalization that individuals with a hearing disorder may be less mature socially than their hearing peers has received some support (Altshuler, 1964; Cole, 1987; Meadow, 1976; Myklebust, 1960; Schlesinger, 1978), but there is little consensus regarding the reasons for the immaturity. Schlesinger poses these questions: "Does the absence of early auditory stimulation, feedback, and communication in itself create a propensity toward these behavioral and achievement patterns, or does early profound deafness elicit particular responses from parents, teachers, siblings, and friends that contribute to a particular set of cognitive and behavioral deficiencies?" (p. 158).

FOCUS 12
Describe the effects of a hearing disorder on social adjustment.

Social maladjustment patterns are also positively correlated with the severity of the loss and the type of impairment. The more severe the loss, the greater the potential for social isolation and resulting social maladjustment. However, it is important to note that most individuals with severe hearing losses, such as Rosa from our opening vignette, are socially well adjusted.

CAUSATION

A number of conditions may result in a hearing disorder. These conditions are generally classified as congenital (existing at birth) or acquired factors. In 1982, the American-Speech-Language-Hearing Association listed several conditions that place an individual in the high-risk category for a hearing loss:

1. Family history of childhood hearing impairment
2. Congenital or perinatal infection
3. Anatomic malformations involving the head and neck
4. Birth weight of less than 1,500 grams
5. **Bacterial meningitis**
6. Severe **asphyxia** at birth.

Our discussion focuses on some of these factors while highlighting causal factors related to anatomical site of loss (external, middle, or inner ear).

Congenital Factors

FOCUS 13
Identify factors existing at birth that can result in hearing disorders.

Heredity.   Although there are more than sixty types of identified hereditary hearing disorders, the cause of 25 percent of all hearing loss remains unknown (Morgan, 1987). Morgan reports that about one-third to one-half of all profound sensorineural losses result from genetic inheritance. Trybus (1985) sampled 55,000 school-age students with a hearing loss, and found that approximately 11 percent of all cases were associated with hereditary factors.

Prenatal Disease.   One of the more common diseases that affects the sense of hearing is **otosclerosis.** The cause of this disease is unknown but it is generally believed to be hereditary. Otosclerosis is characterized by the destruction of the capsular bone in the middle ear and the growth of weblike bone that attaches to the stapes. The stapes is restricted and unable to function properly. Hearing disorders occur in about 15 percent of all cases of otosclerosis, and the incidence is twice as high for females as for males. Victims of otosclerosis suffer from high-pitched throbbing or ringing sounds known as **tinnitus,** a condition associated with disease of the inner ear.

Several conditions, although not inherited, can result in a congenital sensorineural loss. The major cause of nongenetic congenital deafness is infection, of which **prenatal rubella, cytomegalic inclusion** disease, and **toxoplasmosis** are the most common.

The rubella epidemic of 1963–1965 dramatically increased the incidence of deafness in the United States. Abroms (1977) indicates that during the 1960s approximately 10 percent of all congenital deafness resulted from women's contracting rubella during pregnancy. Morgan (1987) reports that for about 40 percent of the individuals who are deaf, the cause is rubella. About 50 percent of all children with rubella have a severe hearing disorder. Most hearing disorders caused by rubella are sensorineural, although a small percentage may be mixed. In addition to hearing disorders in rubella children, it is not uncommon to find heart disease (50 percent), **cataracts** or **glaucoma** (40 percent), and **psychomotor retardation** (40 percent) (Abroms, 1977). Since the advent of rubella vaccine, the elimination of this disease has become a nationwide campaign, and the incidence of rubella has dramatically decreased. "The hope for prevention of congenital rubella lies in immunization of susceptible populations with the currently available vaccines" (Morgan, 1987, p. 29).

Cytomegalic inclusion disease is a condition in newborns due to infection by cytomegalovirus (CMV). It is characterized by jaundice, microcephaly, hemolytic anemia, mental retardation, hepatosplenomegaly (enlargement of liver and spleen), and hearing disorders. There are some significant barriers to prevention of this virus. Experimental vaccines are available, but due to limited research they have not been approved by the government for general use (Morgan, 1987).

Congenital toxoplasmosis infection is characterized by jaundice and anemia, but frequently the disease also results in central nervous system disorders such as seizures, hydrocephalus, and microcephaly. Approximately 15 percent of the infants born with this disease are deaf.

Other factors associated with congenital sensorineural hearing disorders include maternal **Rh-factor incompatibility** and the use of **otoxic drugs.** Maternal Rh-factor incompatibility does not generally affect a first-born child, but as antibodies are produced during subsequent pregnancies multiple problems can result, including deafness. Fortunately, deafness as a result of Rh-factor problems is no longer common. With the advent of an **anti-Rh gamma globulin (RhoGAM)** in 1968, the incidence of Rh-factor incompatibility has significantly decreased. If injected into the mother within the first seventy-two hours after the birth of the first child, she does not produce antibodies that harm future unborn infants.

Ototoxic drugs are so labeled because of their harmful effects on the sense of hearing. If these drugs are taken during pregnancy, the result may be a serious hearing disorder in the infant. Although rare, congenital sensorineural disorders can also be caused by congenital syphilis, maternal chicken pox, **anoxia,** and birth trauma.

A condition known as **atresia** is a major cause of congenital conductive disorders. **Congenital aural atresia** results when the external auditory canal is either malformed or completely absent at birth. A congenital malformation may lead to a blockage of the ear canal due to an accumulation of cerumen. This wax hardens and blocks incoming sound waves from being transmitted to the middle ear.

Acquired Factors

Postnatal Disease. The most common cause of hearing disorders in the postnatal period is infection, although it has shown the most significant decrease in this century (Meadow, 1980). Postnatal infections, such as measles, mumps,

FOCUS 14
Identify conditions acquired later in life that can result in hearing disorders.

influenza, typhoid fever, and scarlet fever, are all associated with hearing loss. Remember that Rosa acquired a condition known as spinal meningitis at the age of eight. Meningitis is an inflammation of the membranes that cover the brain and spinal cord and is a cause of severe hearing disorders in school-age children. Loss of hearing, sight, paralysis, and brain damage are all complications of this disease. However, there has been a recent decrease in the incidence of meningitis due to the development of antibiotics and chemotherapy.

Another common problem that may result from postnatal infection is known as **otitis media,** an inflammation of the middle ear. This condition is the result of severe colds and spreads from the eustachian tube to the middle ear. Otitis media has been found to be highly correlated with hearing problems. Olmstead, Alvarez, Moroney, and Eversden (1964) studied eighty-two children with acute otitis media and found that 77 percent had some degree of hearing loss within a six-month period following the illness. Of this population, 12 percent suffered a persistent loss.

Environmental Factors.   Environmental factors, including extreme changes in air pressure caused by explosions, physical abuse of the cranial area, foreign objects, and loud music are also factors that contribute to postnatal hearing disorders. Loud noise is rapidly becoming one of the major causes of hearing problems. All of us are being subjected to hazardous noise, such as jet engines and loud music, more often than ever before. With the increasing use of headphones, such as those on portable cassette players, many people (particularly adolescents) are being subjected to damaging noise levels. Occupational noise (such as jackhammers, tractors, and sirens) is now the leading cause of sensorineural hearing loss. Other factors associated with acquired hearing disorders include the degenerative process in the ear as a result of aging, cerebral hemorrhages, allergies, and intercranial tumors.

Understanding the cause of a hearing loss helps us to take preventive measures, as well as to put in place the necessary interventions to support the individual in adjusting to the disability. In the next section we examine three principal areas of assessment and intervention for people with a hearing disorder: medical, social, and educational. Although these areas are discussed independently, the effective collaboration of professionals in all these areas is absolutely necessary if the comprehensive needs of the individual are to be met.

ASSESSMENT AND INTERVENTION STRATEGIES

Medical Services

FOCUS 15
Why is the early detection of a hearing loss so important?

Medicine plays a major role in the prevention, early detection, and remediation of hearing disorders. Several specialists are integrally involved in the medical assessment and intervention process. These include the **genetics specialist,** the **otologist,** the pediatrician, the family practitioner, the neurosurgeon, and the **audiologist.**

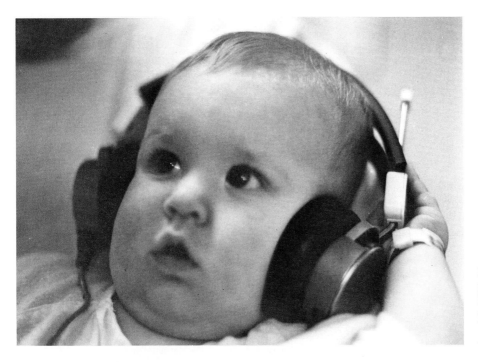

Early detection of a hearing problem can minimize its impact on an individual's overall development. (John Telford)

The Genetics Specialist.   Prevention of hearing disorders is a primary concern of the genetics specialist. A significant number of hearing disorders are inherited or occur during prenatal, perinatal, and postnatal development. Consequently, the genetics specialist is an important link in preventing disorders through family counseling and prenatal screening.

The Pediatrician and Family Practitioner.   Early detection of a hearing problem can prevent, or at least minimize, the impact of the disorder on the overall development of an individual. Generally, it is the responsibility of the pediatrician or family practitioner to be suspicious of a problem and to refer the family to an appropriate hearing specialist. Dipietro, Knight, and Sams (1981) suggest that the role of the physician is to "encourage early and accurate diagnostic testing whether the patient is an infant, a child, or an adult. Referral to specialists who can diagnose and treat hearing impairments and provide special services is almost always necessary" (p. 109). In order to meet their responsibilities, these physicians must be aware of family history. It is imperative that the physician also conduct a thorough physical examination of the child. The physician must be alert to any symptoms (such as delayed language development) that indicate potential sensory loss.

The Otologist.   An otologist is the medical specialist who is most concerned with the hearing organ and its diseases. Otology is a component of the larger specialty of diseases of the ear, nose, and throat. The otologist, like the pediatrician, screens for potential hearing problems, but the process is much more specialized and exhaustive. The otologist also conducts an extensive physical examination

Reflect on This 9–2

Developing the Artificial Ear

Over the past several years, researchers have been working on the development of a device that could at least partially restore hearing to individuals who suffer from sensorineural deafness. One such device, known as Ineraid,* has been under investigation at the

_____

* Ineraid is a trademark of Symbion, Inc., Salt Lake City, Utah. Symbion, Inc. designs, develops, and manufactures artificial organs and related devices, including the Jarvik-7 artificial heart.

University of Utah Institute for Biomedical Engineering and the Division of Artificial Organs.

The Ineraid artificial ear is a multichannel cochlear implant that protrudes through the skin. It consists of an implanted electrode assembly and an external microphone with a sound processor. Sound enters through the microphone and is relayed through a cable to the sound processor. The sound processor separates the sounds and directs them to the appropriate electrodes implanted in the cochlea. The electrodes imi-

tate the function of the (damaged) sensory hair cells in the ear. As a result, electrical information can be transmitted to the auditory nerve of the brain, where the signals are interpreted as meaningful information by the individual.

Presently, the Ineraid artificial ear is an experimental device that requires several more years of analysis before we fully understand its capabilities. However, it is possible that as much as 60 to 80 percent of a deaf individual's hearing could be restored through the artificial ear.

of the ear to identify syndromes that are associated with conductive or sensorineural loss. This information, in conjunction with family history, provides data regarding appropriate medical treatment. This treatment may involve medical therapy or surgical intervention. Common therapeutic procedures include monitoring aural hygiene (such as keeping the external ear free from wax); blowing out the ear (a process to remove mucus blocking the eustachian tube); and the use of antibiotics to treat infections. Surgical techniques may involve the cosmetic and functional restructuring of congenital malformations such as a deformed external ear or a closed external canal (atresia). **Fenestration** is the surgical creation of a new opening in the labyrinth of the ear to restore hearing. A **stapedectomy** is a surgical process conducted under a microscope whereby a fixed stapes is replaced with a prosthetic device capable of vibrating, thus permitting the transmission of sound waves. A **myringoplasty** is the surgical reconstruction of a perforated tympanic membrane (ear drum).

A **cochlear implant** is a surgical procedure that has proven to be highly successful. The purpose of the implant is to restore hearing through electronic stimulation of the auditory nerve. The implant consists of a receiver coil, electrodes (internal), a microphone, **transducer,** and transmitter (external). Cochlear implants are becoming more widely used with both adults and children. However, Simmons (1985) suggests that cochlear implants may be inappropriate for some children who are unable to benefit from conventional amplification. Additionally, caution

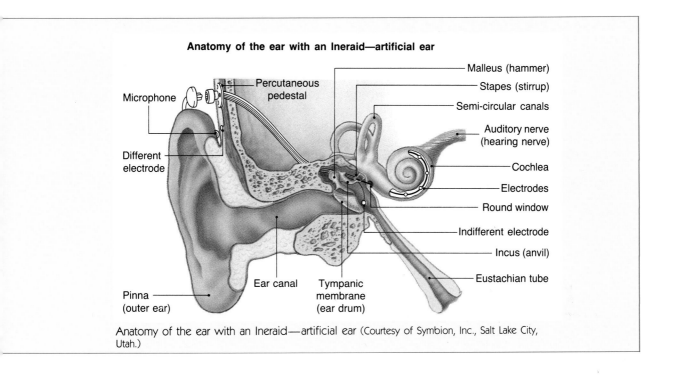

Anatomy of the ear with an Ineraid—artificial ear

Microphone

Percutaneous pedestal

Different electrode

Pinna (outer ear)

Ear canal

Tympanic membrane (ear drum)

Malleus (hammer)

Stapes (stirrup)

Semi-circular canals

Auditory nerve (hearing nerve)

Cochlea

Electrodes

Round window

Indifferent electrode

Incus (anvil)

Eustachian tube

Anatomy of the ear with an Ineraid—artificial ear (Courtesy of Symbion, Inc., Salt Lake City, Utah.)

should be exercised because of the risk of possible damage to an ear that has some residual hearing and the risk of infection from the implant.

The Audiologist. The degree of hearing loss, measured in decibel and hertz units, is ascertained by using a process known as audiometric evaluation. The audiometric evaluation is conducted by an audiologist, who presents the listener with tones that are relatively free of external noise (**pure-tone audiometry**) or spoken words, in which speech perception is measured (**speech audiometry**). An electronic device (**audiometer**) is used to detect a person's response to sound stimuli. A record (**audiogram**) is obtained from the audiometer that graphs the individual's threshold for hearing at various sound frequencies.

Whereas the otologist presents a biological perspective on hearing disorders, the audiologist emphasizes the sociological and educational impact of a hearing loss. Hodgson (1987) suggests:

> The first purpose of an audiologist in dealing with children is to identify an auditory disorder. If a hearing loss is found, its nature and magnitude must be determined. The audiologist must ask whether the disorder, as measured, is sufficient to explain observed behavior. The social, educational, and vocational implications of the disorder must be explored (p. 185).

Although audiologists are not specifically trained in the field of medicine, these professionals interact constantly with otologists to provide a comprehensive

FOCUS 16
What is an audiometric evaluation?

FOCUS 17
Distinguish between an otologist and an audiologist.

Reflect on This 9–3

Testing for a Hearing Loss

Figure A is an example of an audiogram before a hearing test. It shows several things: The numbers along the top show the frequency of the tone to be tested. The frequency may be indicated by Hertz (Hz), which is another way of describing how many vibrations happen each second. The numbers along the side are shown in decibels (dB). As the numbers go from zero to ten to twenty to thirty, the intensity (strength) increases.

When an audiologist tests hearing using the air-conduction test, he or she marks the audiogram with *X* for the left ear and *O* for the right ear.

Don

Figure B shows Don's audiogram. The line connecting the *X*s shows the hearing level in Don's left ear. The line connecting the *O*s shows the hearing level in his right ear. Don's hearing level is normal. This means he can hear very soft speech sounds with no difficulty. The dark part on Don's audiogram (0–25 dB) shows the area that is "within normal limits." Even if a person has a loss in this

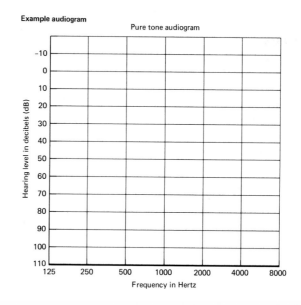

Example audiogram

Pure tone audiogram

area, he or she can still follow a normal conversation. People who are talking to each other usually speak at a volume of 55 dB. This helps you to see why a slight loss can be within normal limits.

Bill

Bill had his hearing tested also. The audiologist first used the air-

conduction test and marked Bill's audiogram. Then the audiologist used another test—a bone-conduction test—to find out where the problem might be. In this test, the sound goes past the middle ear. The test tells if the inner ear is working properly. For the bone conduction test, the audiologist uses a small device called a *vibra-*

assessment of hearing. The audiologist is trained in audiometry, the measurement of hearing. Patrick (1987) identified the goals of audiometry: "to identify those individuals who have sufficient hearing loss to compromise communication and/or learning in the typical classroom; 2) to find and send for medical management those students who have middle ear pathologies; and 3) to perform these tasks in the most cost-effective and efficient manner" (p. 402).

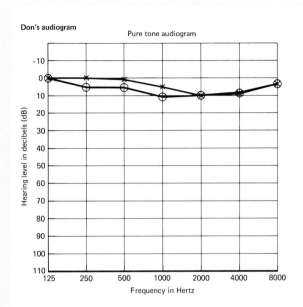

Don's audiogram

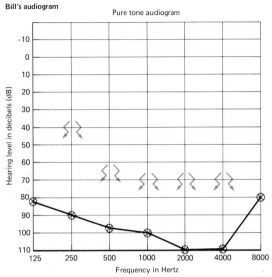

Bill's audiogram

tor, which makes the same kind of tones as the earphones. He places the vibrator behind the ear or on the forehead. The individual must respond when he hears a sound from the vibrator. The audiologist marks this response on the audiogram. He may use < for the left ear, and > for the right ear. An arrow (→) added to either symbol means that the person cannot hear the sound from the vibrator. The bone-conduction test tells if the inner ear is working properly.

Figure C is Bill's audiogram. It shows the results of both tests. We can see that Bill did not respond at all to the bone-conduction test. His hearing problem results from trouble in the inner ear or along the auditory nerve. This type of loss is a sensorineural loss.

Bill's audiogram shows that he is profoundly deaf. For Bill, this means that he cannot hear or understand speech. With a hearing aid, he can hear some speech sounds, but he may not be able to understand them. Bill became deaf when he was two years old, as a result of spinal meningitis.

Source: Adapted from *You and Your Deafness* by permission of Gallaudet College Press, 800 Florida Ave. N.E., Washington, D.C., 20002. Copyright 1982 by Gallaudet College.

Another important function of the audiologist and otologist is to provide assistance regarding the selection and use of hearing aids. At one time or another, most people with a hearing disorder wear a hearing aid. In a sample of hearing-impaired children in the United States, Karchmer and Kirwin (1977) found that over 80 percent of this population wore an amplification device. They reported that almost 90 percent of all children with moderate or severe losses (41–90 dB) consistently used a hearing aid. Nonwearers were found in greatest proportion among those children with a profound loss. Even so, approximately 77 percent of this population used a hearing aid.

Hearing aids are instruments used to make sounds louder, but they do not correct hearing. Butler (1981) indicates: "The hearing aid is like a public address system. It makes the sound louder, but the student does not hear all sounds even with the aid" (p. 167). Hearing aids have been used for centuries. Early **acoustic aids** included cupping one's hand behind the ear and the ear trumpet. Modern **electroacoustic aids** do not depend on the loudness of the human voice to amplify sound, but utilize batteries to increase volume. Electroacoustic aids come in two main types: body aids (strapped to the body) and behind-the-ear aids. These aids may be fitted monaurally (on one ear) or binaurally (on both ears). Although the quality of commercially available aids has improved dramatically in recent years, they do have distinct limitations. The criteria for effectiveness must be measured against wearability, the individual's communication skill, and educational achievement (Garwood, 1987). Another factor that must be considered is whether the aid is working correctly. According to studies by Bess (1971) and Chial (1977), about 30 percent of all hearing aids tested in the schools were not performing up to specification, and 50 percent were malfunctioning.

The stimulation of residual hearing through a hearing aid enables most people with a hearing disorder to function as hard-of-hearing. However, as Ross and Calvert (1984) pointed out, it must be done as early as possible, before the sensory deprivation takes its toll on the child. It is the audiologist's responsibility to weigh all the factors involved (including convenience, size, and weight) in

Most people with a hearing disorder wear some type of amplification device. (© Jeffrey Sylvester/FPG International)

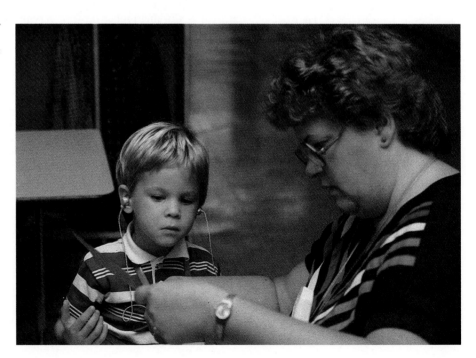

the selection and use of an aid for the individual. The individual should then be directed to a reputable hearing-aid dealer.

Social Services

The social consequences of a hearing disorder are highly correlated with the severity of the impairment. For the deaf individual, social integration may be extremely difficult because societal views of deafness have reinforced social isolation. The belief that a deaf person is incompetent has been a predominant theme from the time of the early Hebrews and Romans, who deprived deaf persons of their civil rights, to twentieth-century America, where in some areas it is still difficult for deaf adults to obtain a driver's license, buy adequate insurance coverage, and be gainfully employed. Moores (1987) indicates that people who are deaf remained significantly underemployed in the 1980s. The population that has had the greatest difficulty are those born with congenital deafness. The inability to hear and understand speech has often isolated these people from their hearing peers.

People who are deaf tend to marry other deaf persons (Woodward, 1982). Schein and Delk (1974) reported that eight out of ten deaf marriages are between two deaf partners. However, this phenomenon declines substantially for those who are postlingually deaf or hard-of-hearing. Even in marriages where both partners are deaf, only 12 percent of the offspring are deaf. Therefore, deaf parents are usually in a situation of presiding over a household of children whose hearing is normal.

A segment of the deaf population is actively involved in organizations and communities specifically intended to meet the needs of deaf people. The National Association for the Deaf (NAD) was organized in 1880. The philosophy of the NAD specifies that, "All deaf persons have the right to life, liberty, and the pursuit of happiness and . . . this right must be evidenced in ways that meet the satisfaction of the deaf persons themselves rather than that of their teachers and parents, who do not live with the condition" (Schreiber, 1979, p. 565). The NAD serves the deaf population in many capacities. Among its many contributions, the NAD publishes books on deafness, sponsors cultural activities, and lobbies around the country for legislation promoting the rights of deaf persons.

Another prominent organization is the Alexander Graham Bell Association for the Deaf. This association promotes the integration of persons with a hearing disorder into the social mainstream. The major thrust is the improvement of proficiency in speech communications. The Alexander Graham Bell Association is also a clearinghouse for information for deaf persons and their advocates. The association publishes widely in the area of parent counseling, teaching methodology, speech-reading, and auditory training. In addition, it sponsors national and regional conferences focusing on a variety of issues pertinent to the social adjustment of deaf persons.

Because of the unique communication problems of persons with a hearing disorder, many are unable to benefit from mental health services in their community. Tucker (1981) indicated that most mental health professionals are unaware of the communication barriers that prevent this population from obtaining service.

FOCUS 18
Identify factors that may impede the social integration of people who are deaf into a hearing world.

Mental health professionals must be trained to work with the unique problems of hearing-disordered persons. These professionals should be working with parents as early as possible to assist young children in adjusting to the sensory limitation. As children with hearing disorders become older, counselors must be available to help them explore their feelings regarding their disorders and cope with the reactions of parents, family, and peers. Finally, it is extremely important for mental health personnel to realize that "each individual's disability will be unique" (Boulton, Cull, & Hardy, 1974, p. 182).

Educational Services

FOCUS 19
Why are educational services for hearing-disordered students described as being in the process of change?

In the United States, educational programs for hearing-disordered children emerged in the early nineteenth century, and the residential school for the deaf was the primary model for educational service delivery. The residential school was a live-in facility where the student was segregated from the family environment. In the latter half of the nineteenth century, day schools were established, in which students lived with their families while receiving an education in a special school for the deaf. As the century drew to a close, some public schools established special classes for hearing-disordered children, located within the regular education facility.

The residential school continued to be a model for educational services well into the twentieth century. However, with the introduction of electrical amplification, advances in medical treatment, and improved educational technology, more options became available within the public school system. Today, educational programs for hearing-disordered students range from the residential school to regular class placement with support services.

The delivery of educational services to students with a hearing disorder is in the process of change. With the advent of the 1986 early childhood amendments, Public Law 99–457, there has been an expanding emphasis on early intervention. Newton (1987) emphasizes that "early identification is essential, for without it no further intervention will occur. Hearing-impaired children should be identified as close to birth as possible, but at least by one year of age" (p. 323). There is little disagreement among educators that the education of the child with a hearing disorder must begin at the time of the diagnosis.

Educational goals for students with a hearing disorder are comparable to those of their hearing peers. Butler (1981) indicates: "The hearing-impaired student faces the same problems and adjustments in the classroom that every other student faces. Hearing-impaired students bring the same strengths and weaknesses and the same creativity" (p. 171). The most formidable problem for the educator is the student's communication deficits.

FOCUS 20
Identify four approaches to teaching communication skills to persons with a hearing disorder.

Teaching Communication Skills. There are four common approaches to teaching communication skills to students with a hearing disorder: auditory, oral, manual, and total communication. There is a long history of controversy regarding which approach is the most appropriate for students with a hearing disorder. However, as Ling (1984a) indicates, no single method or collection of methods can meet the individual needs of all children with hearing disorders.

Reflect on This 9–4

Athletes and Poets: The World Heard Them

Most likely the football huddle was invented at Gallaudet in the 1890's so opposing teams could not see what plays were being worked out. And baseball owes some umpires' calls to the deaf: Raising the right arm to signify a strike was created for William Ellsworth "Dummy" Hoy, a deaf outfielder for Cincinnati and Washington. In one game in 1889, he threw out three runners at home plate, a record that still stands. At least fourteen other pro baseball players have been deaf, as well as pro boxers and wrestlers.

Erastus "Deaf" (pronounced deef) Smith was a Texas soldier, scout, and spy under Sam Houston. He led his men to victory in a famous battle, and a Texas county is named after him.

The French poets Pierre de Ronsard and Joachim duBellay became deaf as young men. And Beethoven, Goya, and Thomas Alva Edison all became profoundly deaf in later life. Helen Keller, of course, was an advocate for the rights of all disabled people.

These days there are deaf doctors, accountants, lawyers, and artists. Actress Marlee Matlin won the Oscar as Best Actress for 1986. In 1976, Kitty O'Neil, a deaf Hollywood stunt woman, set a land speed record for women in a rocket-powered racer. She also set a record in 1970 for the fastest woman on water skis. David Michalowski performed through the 1980s as a world-class figure skater—skating to music by memorizing beats.

Source: L. A. Walker (1989, April 23), I Know How to Ask for What I Want, *Parade*, 4–6.

It is not our purpose to enter into the controversies regarding these approaches, but to present a brief description of each approach.

The auditory approach emphasizes the use of amplified sound and residual hearing to develop oral communication skills. The auditory channel is considered the primary avenue for language development, regardless of the severity or type of hearing loss. Students are strongly encouraged to learn normal speech production, and the use of manual communication (other than natural gestures) is discouraged. In addition to the common body-type and behind-the-ear hearing aids, the approach utilizes a variety of electroacoustic devices to enhance residual hearing. Although the traditional portable desk trainer may still be found in schools, the general trend is more toward the "high-powered frequency modulated radio-frequency (FM-RF) body units" (Garwood, 1987, p. 440). These units use a one-way wireless system on radio-frequency bands. The receiver unit is worn by the student, and a microphone-transmitter-antennae unit is worn by the teacher. Although these body units have the advantage of "presence" (the child's ears are only inches away from the teacher's mouth), they are seldom preferred by students due to their conspicuousness (Garwood, 1987).

The oral approach to teaching communication skills also emphasizes the use of amplified sound and residual hearing to develop oral language. According to Ling (1984b), "The philosophy of oral education is that hearing-impaired children should be given the opportunity to speak and to understand speech, learn through spoken language in school, and later function as independent adults in a world in which people's primary mode of communication is speech" (p. 9). In addition to electroacoustical amplification, the teacher may employ speech-reading, reading and writing, and **motokinesthetic** speech training (feeling an individual's face and reproducing breath and voice patterns). Speech-reading (sometimes referred to as lip-reading) is the process of understanding another person's speech by watching lip movement and facial and body gestures. This skill is difficult to master, especially for the prelingually deaf person. It has been estimated that only about 4 percent of deaf adults are proficient speech readers (Pahz & Pahz, 1978). Problems with speech-reading are that many sounds are not distinguishable on the lips, and the reader must attend carefully to every word spoken, a difficult task for preschool and primary-age children. Additionally, the speech reader must be able to see the speaker's mouth at all times.

The oral approach is often combined with the auditory method and may be referred to as the **auditory-oral,** or **aural-oral,** method. Silverman, Lan, and Calvert (1978) suggest that all the above terms are "synonyms for the same fundamental method, or they designate variations within the same general framework" (p. 442). These authors coined the phrase **auditory global method** to describe any approach where the "primary, although not always exclusive, channel for speech and language development is auditory and . . . the input is fluent, connected speech" (p. 442).

The manual approach to teaching communication skills stresses the use of signs in teaching deaf children to communicate. The use of signs is based on the premise that many deaf children are unable to develop oral language and consequently must have some other means of communication. **Manual communication** systems are divided into two main categories: sign languages and sign systems.

Sign languages are a systematic and complex combination of hand movements that communicate whole words and complete thoughts, rather than sign the letters of the alphabet. One of the most common sign languages is the **American Sign Language (ASL).** American Sign Language has a vocabulary of about 6,000 signs. Examples of ASL signs are shown in Figure 9–2. ASL is currently the most widely used sign language among many deaf adults because it is easy to master, and historically it has been the preferred mode of communication. It is a language, but it is not English. In fact, it is more similar to Chinese in that its signs represent concepts rather than single words (Fant, 1972).

Sign systems are different from sign languages in that they attempt to "create manual-visual equivalents to oral languages" (Mayberry, 1978, p. 407). **Finger-spelling** is a signing system that incorporates all twenty-six letters of the alphabet. Each letter is signed independently, on one hand, to form words. Figure 9–3 illustrates the manual alphabet. In recent years, finger-spelling, probably the oldest form of signing, has become more of a supplement to ASL. It is not uncommon to see a deaf person use finger-spelling in a situation where there is no ASL sign for a word. The four sign systems used in the United States are Seeing Exact English, Signing Exact English, Linguistics of Visual English, and Signed Exact English. Today few educators rely solely on the manual system to teach communication skills. However, the system is in common use as a component of the fourth, combined approach to teaching communication skills, known as total communication.

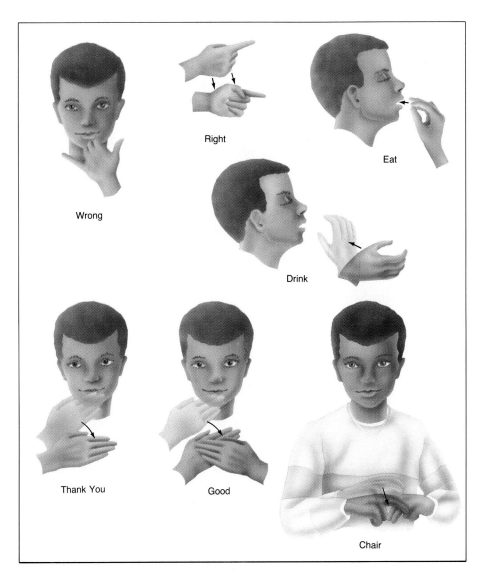

Figure 9-2
Examples of American Sign Language Signs

Total communication, often described as a new concept in the teaching of communication skills to the hearing disordered, actually has roots that can be traced to the late 1800s (Scouten, 1983). During this period, many professionals advocated an instructional system that employed every method possible to teach communication skills. This approach was known as the *combined system* or *simultaneous method.* The methodology of the early combined system was imprecise, and essentially any recognized approach to teaching communication was used as long as it included a manual component. The concept of total communication differs from the older combined system in several ways:

For the most part the combined system usually began with two strikes against it—that is, with an oral failure and after critical learning periods had passed. A

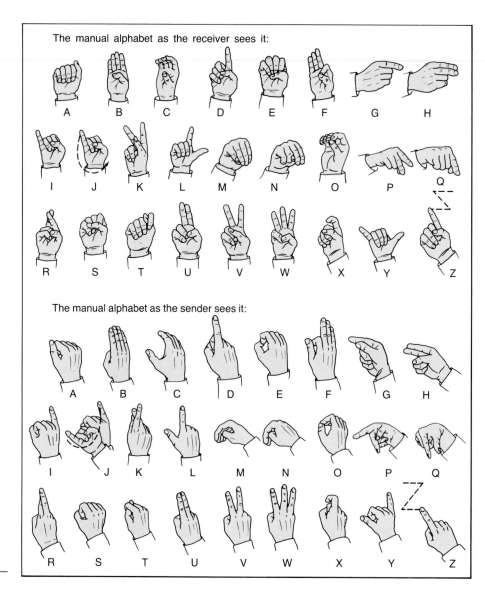

The manual alphabet as the receiver sees it:

The manual alphabet as the sender sees it:

Figure 9-3
The American Manual Alphabet

total communication approach starts at the beginning, even before the child is emerging from his infancy. *More important, total communication is not a system, but a philosophy* that incorporates the combined system and the oral system and whatever else is necessary to put the child at the center of our attention. In some instances, it might not be appropriate to utilize such procedures as sign language; in many cases it would be appropriate (Pahz & Pahz, 1978, p. 62; emphasis added).

The philosophy of total communication is that the simultaneous presentation of signs and speech enhances each child's opportunity to understand and use both more effectively (Ling, 1984a). Total communication programs use residual hearing, amplification, speech-reading, speech-training, reading, and writing in combination with manual systems. A method that may be used as an aid to total communication, but is not a necessary component of the approach, is **cued**

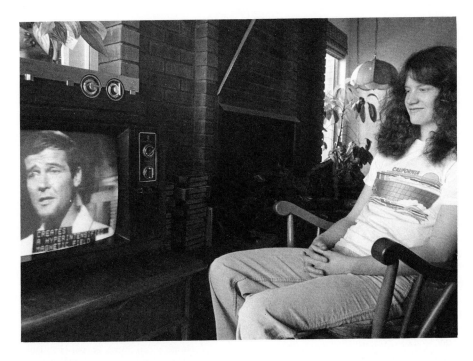

Closed-caption television programs for people with hearing impairments have increased steadily since 1980. Today, even live programs such as the evening news are available with closed captions. (John Telford)

speech. Cued speech is intended to facilitate the development of oral communication by combining hand signals with speechreading. Gestures provide additional information concerning sounds not identifiable by lipreading. The result is that an individual has access to all the sounds in the English language through either the lips or the hands.

Technological Advances. Educational and leisure-time opportunities for people with hearing disorders are being greatly expanded through technological advances such as **closed-caption** television and computer-assisted instruction. The closed-captioning process translates the dialogue from a television program into captions—subtitles. These captions are then converted to electronic codes that can be inserted into the television picture on sets that are specially adapted with decoding devices. The process is called the **line-21 system,** because the caption is inserted into blank line 21 of the picture.

Captioning is not a new idea and was in fact first used on motion picture film in 1958. Currently, there are over sixty libraries in the United States that distribute captioned films for the deaf. Closed-captioning on television has experienced steady growth in a short period of time. The service has been available only since 1980. Caldwell (1981) indicates that during its first year of operation, national programming was available at least thirty hours a week; more than seventy advertisers committed themselves to having specials and commercials captioned; and closed-captioned videotapes for classroom instruction and home entertainment were being introduced into retail markets.

> Evidence is mounting that closed captioning is far more than a technological breakthrough; it is a sociological and psychological triumph as well. Hearing-impaired people of all ages are already enabled to communicate more freely with

FOCUS 21
What are some of the widely used technological advances for people with hearing disorders?

Reflect on This 9–5

Is Captioned Media Really Important to People with a Hearing Disorder?

Absolutely! Much of the entertainment for the general public depends upon the sense of hearing. We see and *hear* movies, television, theatrical plays, lectures, concerts, etc. Some of these media forms are made more accessible through sign language interpreters. However, interpreter services won't help those who don't understand sign language. It is also expensive and in short supply. Thus, captioned materials assure people with a hearing disorder much greater access to entertainment and information.

Did you know that by 1983 over 70,000 homes in the United States were equipped to receive closed-captioning programs? The viewing audience is over 300,000 people. New viewers to closed-caption television are being added at over 4,000 subscribers per month. More than 40 hours of closed-caption programs are offered each week on the major networks, cable, and in television syndication. Over 100 closed-captioned movies are now available on home video cassettes.

What does it cost to close caption a TV program? For one hour of programming the cost is about $2,200, and takes about 30 hours of work to produce. The cost of a Telecaption color television runs about $400, and Telecaption decoders can be purchased through Sears Department Stores.

Sources: Did You Know? (Fall 1983) *Caption.* Falls Church, Va.: National Captioning Institute.
Home Video Scores Smash Hit. (Fall 1984). *Caption.* Falls Church, Va.: National Captioning Institute.

their hearing peers as they share information and entertainment gleaned from the television screen" (Caldwell, pp. 629–30).

Computer-assisted instruction offers an exciting dimension to learning for persons with a hearing disorder because it responds to touch and has no auditory requirements (Stepp, 1982). Through telephone lines, an individual can send and receive vast amounts of visual information that is stored in computer systems across the United States. But computer use in deaf education programs is expanding for many reasons besides the fact that there is no auditory requirement. The computer places the student in an interactive setting with the subject matter. It is a powerful motivator: Most students find computers fun and interesting to work with on a variety of tasks. Additionally, it allows for individualized instruction for the student who is hearing impaired. Students are able to gain independence by working at their own pace and level. In a survey of over 200 programs for deaf students by Rose and Waldron (1984), the investigators found that 50 percent used computer-assisted instruction.

The **videodisc** combines the computer-assisted system and the television video display. The videodisc, which is a recordlike platter, allows individuals to work with instructional material at their own pace and convenience. Another major advance is the development of **telecommunication devices for the deaf (TDD)**. TDD systems send, receive, and print messages through thousands of stations located across the United States. "The TDDs may also provide an excellent tool for the production and improvement of written language skills in

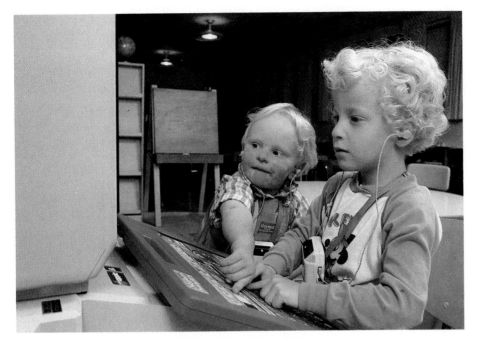

Computer-assisted instruction offers an exciting learning option for people with hearing disorders because the computer responds to touch and has no auditory requirements. (© Jeffrey Sylvester/FPG International)

deaf children. Coupling the graphic display with the written dialogue is extremely helpful in the development of language forms" (McAnally et al., 1987). The **teletypewriter and printer (TTY)** is also an effective use of technology for people who are deaf. The TTY allows people who are deaf to communicate by phone with a typewriter that converts typed letters into electric signals through a modem. These signals are sent through the phone lines and then translated into typed messages and printed on a typewriter connected to a phone on the other end.

From captioning to TDD systems, a new world of technology is opening up for people with hearing disorders. Through this technology, along with advances in medical, social, and educational services, a person with a hearing disorder is becoming less of an outsider in a hearing world. This is not to ignore the many problems (including underemployment and social isolation) still facing the person with a hearing disorder, but certainly much has been accomplished.

REVIEW

FOCUS 1: Describe the process of transmitting sound.

- A vibrator, such as a string, reed, or column of air, causes a displacement of air particles.
- Vibrations are carried by air, metal, water, or other substances.
- Sound waves are displaced air particles producing a pattern of circular waves that move away from a source to a receiver.

- The human ear collects, processes, and transmits sounds to the brain, where they are decoded into meaningful language.

FOCUS 2: What are the basic functions of the external, middle, and inner ear?

- The external ear consists of the auricle and an ear canal known as the *meatus*.

❑ The auricle collects sound waves and funnels them into the ear canal.

❑ The eardrum, located between the external and middle ear, vibrates freely when struck by sound waves.

❑ The inner surface of the eardrum is located in the cavity of the middle ear.

❑ The three small bones of the inner surface of the eardrum transmit the vibrations from the external ear through the cavity of the middle ear to the inner ear.

❑ The eustachian tube equalizes the air pressure on the eardrum with that of the outside air.

❑ The cochlea and the vestibular mechanism are the two major structures of the inner ear.

❑ Within the cochlea, specialized cells translate vibrations into nerve impulses that are sent directly to the brain.

❑ The vestibular mechanism contains canals that control balance.

FOCUS 3: How are sound intensity and sound frequency measured?

❑ Sound intensity (loudness) is measured in units known as decibels.

❑ Sound frequency (pitch) is measured using a unit known as the hertz.

FOCUS 4: Distinguish between deaf and hard-of-hearing.

❑ A person who is deaf typically has profound or total loss of auditory sensitivity and very little, if any, auditory perception.

❑ For the person who is deaf, the primary information input is through vision; speech is not received through the ear.

❑ A person who is hard-of-hearing (partially hearing) generally has residual hearing through the use of a hearing aid, which is sufficient to process language through the ear successfully.

FOCUS 5: Why is it important to consider age of onset when defining a hearing disorder?

❑ Age of onset is critical in determining the type and extent of intervention necessary to minimize the effect of the hearing disorder.

FOCUS 6: Distinguish between conductive, sensorineural, and mixed hearing losses.

❑ Conductive hearing losses result from poor conduction of sound along passages leading to the inner ear.

❑ The effect of a conductive hearing loss is the reduction or loss of loudness.

❑ Sensorineural hearing losses are the result of an abnormal sense or a damaged auditory nerve.

❑ Sound is distorted with a sensory hearing loss, thus affecting the clarity of human speech.

❑ Mixed hearing losses are a combination of conductive and sensorineural problems.

FOCUS 7: Classify hearing disorders according to the severity of the condition.

❑ The classification levels according to the severity of the condition include (1) insignificant, (2) mild (hard-of-hearing), (3) moderate (hard-of-hearing), (4) severe (hard-of-hearing and deaf), and (5) profound (deaf).

FOCUS 8: Why is it difficult to determine accurately the prevalence of hearing disorders?

❑ Prevalence estimates are difficult to determine because definitions are inconsistent, and there are problems with how surveys of people with hearing disorders are conducted.

FOCUS 9: Why is the research on the intelligence of people with a hearing disorder considered inconclusive?

❑ Although early investigations reported that hearing-disordered individuals scored lower on intelligence tests when compared to hearing individuals, more recent studies generally reported no significant difference between the two groups.

FOCUS 10: How does the effect of a hearing disorder on speech and language differ for people with a mild loss as opposed to those with a more severe loss?

❑ For people with mild and moderate losses, the effect on speech and language may be minimal.

❑ Although individuals with a moderate loss cannot hear unvoiced sounds and distant speech, language delays can be prevented if the hearing loss is diagnosed and treated early.

❑ The majority of people with a hearing disorder are able to use speech as the primary mode of language acquisition.

❑ People who are congenitally deaf are unable to receive information through the speech process unless they have learned to lip (speech) read.

❑ The sound production of the deaf person is extremely low in intelligibility.

FOCUS 11: Describe the effects of a hearing disorder on academic skills.

❑ The educational achievement of students with a hearing disorder may be significantly delayed in comparison to hearing peers.

❑ Reading is the academic area most adversely affected.

FOCUS 12: Describe the effects of a hearing disorder on social adjustment.

☐ There is some support, through research, for the idea that some individuals with a hearing disorder may be less mature socially than their hearing peers.

☐ There is little agreement as to why some people with a hearing disorder may be less socially mature, but there is a relationship between the severity and type of hearing loss and social problems.

FOCUS 13: Identify factors existing at birth that can result in hearing disorders.

☐ There are more than sixty types of hereditary hearing disorders.

☐ A common hereditary disorder is otosclerosis, bone destruction in the middle ear.

☐ Nonhereditary hearing problems existing at birth may be associated with infections (e.g., rubella), anemia, jaundice, central nervous system disorders, the use of drugs, venereal disease, maternal chicken pox, anoxia, and birth trauma.

FOCUS 14: Identify conditions acquired later in life that can result in hearing disorders.

☐ Acquired hearing disorders are associated with postnatal infections, such as measles, mumps, influenza, typhoid fever, and scarlet fever.

☐ Environmental factors associated with hearing disorders include extreme changes in air pressure caused by explosions, head trauma, foreign objects in the ear, and loud noise.

FOCUS 15: Why is the early detection of a hearing loss so important?

☐ Early detection of a hearing loss can prevent or minimize the impact of the disorder on the overall development of an individual.

FOCUS 16: What is an audiometric evaluation?

☐ An audiometric evaluation measures the degree of hearing loss in an individual.

☐ An electronic device known as an *audiometer* measures a person's response to sound stimuli.

☐ An audiometer records the responses of the individual that are graphed on an audiogram.

FOCUS 17: Distinguish between an otologist and an audiologist.

☐ An otologist is a medical specialist who is concerned with the hearing organ and its diseases.

☐ The audiologist is concerned with the sociological and educational impact of a hearing loss on an individual.

☐ Both the audiologist and otologist assist in the process of the selection and use of hearing aids.

FOCUS 18: Identify factors that may impede the social integration of people who are deaf into a hearing world.

☐ Social integration with hearing peers has been difficult for persons who are deaf.

☐ The inability to hear and understand speech has isolated some people who are deaf from their hearing peers.

FOCUS 19: Why are educational services for hearing-disordered students described as being in the process of change?

☐ There is an ongoing increase in the availability of educational services for students with hearing disorders from preschool through adolescence.

☐ Educational programming is becoming more individualized in order to meet the needs of each student.

FOCUS 20: Identify four approaches to teaching communication skills to persons with a hearing disorder.

☐ The auditory approach to communication emphasizes the use of amplified sound and residual hearing to develop oral communication skills.

☐ The oral approach to communication emphasizes the use of amplified sound and residual hearing, but also may employ speech-reading, reading and writing, and motokinesthetic speech training (feeling an individual's face and reproducing breath and voice patterns).

☐ The manual approach stresses the use of signs in teaching deaf children to communicate.

☐ Total communication employs the use of residual hearing, amplification, speech-reading, speech training, reading, and writing, in combination with manual systems, to teach communication skills to the child with a hearing disorder.

FOCUS 21: What are some of the widely used technological advances for people with hearing disorders?

☐ Closed-caption television translates the dialogue from a television program into captions (subtitles) that are broadcast on the television screen.

☐ Closed-caption television provides the person with a hearing disorder greater access to information and entertainment than was previously thought possible.

☐ Computer-assisted instruction allows access, through telephone lines, to vast amounts of information stored in computer systems throughout the country.

☐ TDD systems provide efficient ways for people who are deaf to communicate over long distances.

☐ TTY devices allow people who are deaf to use a typewriter, modem, and printer to communicate over the phone.

Debate Forum

Living in a Deaf Community

The inability to hear and understand speech may lead an individual to seek community ties and social relationships primarily with other deaf individuals. Deaf individuals may choose to isolate themselves from hearing peers and live, learn, work, and play in a social subculture known as "a deaf community." An example of this strong sense of community occurred in 1988, when the appointment of a hearing person as president of Gallaudet University, a university for the deaf, resulted in widespread student protest and the eventual appointment of the university's first deaf president. The following are two points of view on life in the deaf community.

Point The deaf community is a necessary and important component of life for many individuals who are deaf. The individual who is deaf has a great deal of difficulty adjusting to life in a hearing world. Through the deaf community, this person can find other individuals with similar problems, common interests, a common language (e.g., sign language), and a common culture. Membership in the deaf community is an achieved status that must be earned by the deaf individual. The individual must demonstrate a strong identification with the deaf world, understand and share experiences that come with being a deaf person, and be willing to actively participate in the deaf community's activities. The deaf community gives the individual an identity that can't be found among their hearing peers.

Counterpoint Participation in the deaf community only further isolates deaf individuals from their hearing peers. A separate subculture of deaf individuals unnecessarily accents the differences between hearing and deaf people. The life of the deaf individual need be no different from that of anyone else. Hearing and deaf individuals can live side by side in local communities, sharing common bonds and interests. There is no reason why they can't participate together in the arts, enjoy sports, and share leisure-time and recreational interests. Membership in the deaf community may only further reinforce the idea that disabled people should grow up and live in a culture away from non-handicapped people. The fact is, the majority of deaf people do not seek membership in the deaf community. These individuals are concerned that the existence of such a community makes it all the more difficult for them to assimilate into society at large.

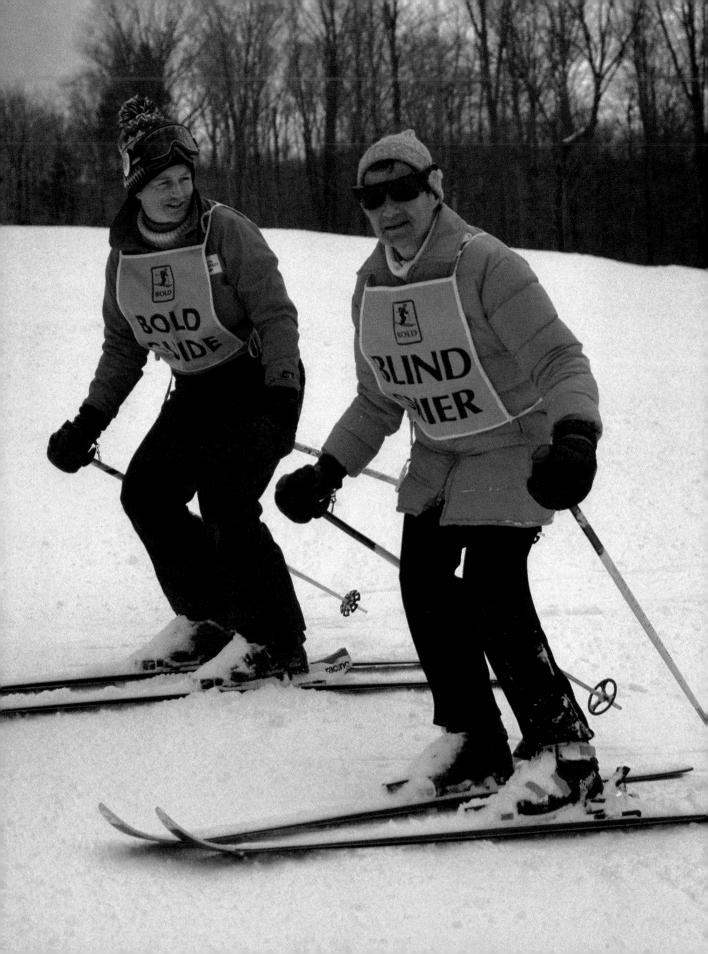

10 Visual Disorders

To Begin With...

- A daily frustration of blindness: Not being able to scope out the shortest check-out line at the grocery store (Susan, personal communication).

- In 1970, the Library of Congress began producing Braille editions of magazines, including *Playboy*. In 1985, Congress cut funds that largely supported the production of Braille *Playboy*. Blind subscribers went to court and won. The judge reasoned that blind persons have a fundamental constitutional right to read *Playboy*. Printing of the Braille edition resumed (Kilpatrick, 1986).

- Kent Cullers, a young physicist at NASA, is congenitally blind. He designs equipment whose purpose is to isolate intelligent signals from the random radio noise of the galaxies. Cullers uses a computer that automatically speaks each word he types. He is also assisted by a scanner which transfers printed documents to the computer screen and reads them aloud (Rogers, 1989).

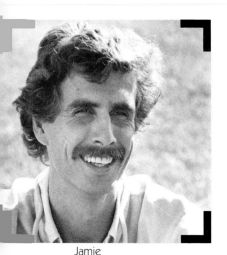

Jamie

By the time Jamie was three months old it was evident that he was not responding to objects within his visual field. His parents became concerned and sought the help of a medical specialist. The ophthalmologist confirmed their suspicions: "Your child has a visual disorder caused by a congenital cataract." As a young child, Jamie learned what it meant to move through his world with limited vision. He stumbled and fell frequently as he attempted to orient himself to people and objects around him. On entering school, it was clear that Jamie would need assistance from a vision specialist, but he could still remain with his age-mates in a regular classroom setting. The vision specialist worked with Jamie and his teacher on basic adaptive techniques in the classroom, such as the elimination of unnecessary glare on table and books, the removal of objects that might impede mobility and learning, and the introduction of special lighting to enhance his residual vision. Today, at the age of twenty-eight, Jamie's visual disorder has not prevented him from pursuing career and leisure-time interests. He is currently a successful sales representative for a local department-store chain. His leisure time is spent hiking, enjoying a good novel, and attending college sporting events.

INTRODUCTION

FOCUS 1
What are two misconceptions that sighted people have about people without sight?

Through the visual process we observe the world around us and develop an appreciation for and a greater understanding of the physical environment. Vision is one of our most important sources for the acquisition and assimilation of knowledge, but we often take it for granted. From the moment we wake up in the morning, our dependence on sight is obvious. We rely on our eyes to guide us around our surroundings, inform us through the written word, and give us pleasure and relaxation.

What if this precious sight were lost or impaired? How would our perceptions of the world change? The fear of losing one's sight is often nurtured by the misconception that persons with a visual disorder are helpless and unable to lead satisfying or productive lives (Bishop, 1987). It is not uncommon for people with sight to have little understanding of those who are visually impaired. Sighted people may believe that most adults who are blind are likely to live a deprived socioeconomic and cultural existence. Sighted children may believe that their peers who are blind are incapable of learning many basic skills, such as telling time or using a computer, or enjoying leisure-time and recreational activities, such as swimming or television. Another attitudinal barrier is the religious belief that blindness is a punishment for sins (Bishop, 1987). However, as our vignette about Jamie strongly suggests, these negative perceptions of people with a visual disorder are often inaccurate. Jamie is an independent adult, with a successful career, who did not allow his visual disorder to keep him from the work and leisure activities that we all value.

In order to more clearly understand the nature of visual disorders within the context of normal sight, we begin our discussion with an overview of the

Reflect on This 10–1

Contributions of Notable Blind or Partially Sighted Persons

Since the days of ancient Greece and the achievements of the blind poet and scholar, Homer, there have been innumerable people with visual disorders who have made outstanding advances in the fields of science, music, literature, medicine, law, and the humanities. For example, Ludovigo Scapinelli, born in 1585, was an eminent Italian philologist and poet. The great English poet of the seven-teenth century, John Milton, pro-duced his most notable works, *Paradise Lost, Paradise Regained*, and *Samson Agonistes*, after he lost his sight at age forty-five. Nicholas Saunderson was a re-nowned English mathematician and teacher at Cambridge Univer-sity. He invented the first arithme-tic board for individuals who were blind. From the United States, there was Helen Keller, an out-standing writer of prose who was both blind and deaf. William Hick-ling Prescott, American writer and scholar, wrote such works as *The History of the Conquest of Mexico* during the early nineteenth century. And, of course, two of the most famous American popu-lar musicians of the twentieth cen-tury, Ray Charles and Stevie Wonder, were both blinded early in life.

visual process. Since vision is basically defined as the act of seeing with the eye, we first review the physical components of the visual system.

The Visual Process

The physical components of the visual system include the eye, the visual center in the brain, and the **optic nerve,** which connects the eye to the visual center. The basic anatomy of the human eye is illustrated in Figure 10–1. The **cornea** is the external covering of the eye, and in the presence of light it reflects visual stimuli. These reflected light rays pass through the **pupil,** which is an opening in the **iris.** The pupil expands or contracts to control the amount of light entering the eye. The iris is the colored portion of the eye and consists of membranous tissue and muscles whose function is to adjust the size of the pupil. The lens focuses the light rays by changing their direction so they strike the **retina** directly. As in a camera lens, the lens of the eye reverses the images. The retina consists of light-sensitive cells that transmit the image to the brain by means of the optic nerve. Images from the retina remain upside down until they are flipped over in the visual center of the brain.

FOCUS 2
Briefly describe the anatomy of the eye.

The visual process is a much more complex phenomenon than is shown by a description of the physical components of vision. Schrock (1978) proposes that vision be viewed in a much broader context. He describes vision as "the result of the integration of a number of subskills that allow the individual to process and appropriately respond to the information contained in the light energy that reaches his eyes" (p. 31). Getman (1965) emphasized that vision is dependent on a number of subsystems, including (1) an antigravity process that allows the person to stand and move erect through the environment; (2) a centering subsystem that assists the person in locating objects in space relative

FOCUS 3
Why is it important to under-stand the visual process as well as know the physical components of the eye?

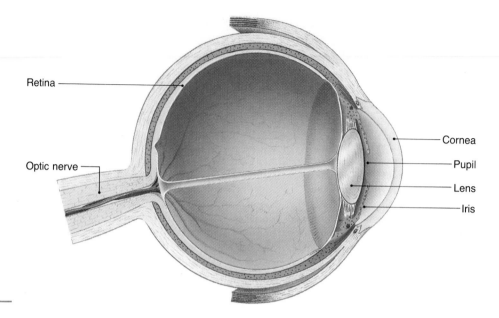

Retina

Optic nerve

Cornea

Pupil

Lens

Iris

Figure 10–1
Basic Anatomy of the Human Eye

to his or her own position; (3) an identification subsystem that integrates information from several sources and matches current visual experiences with past experiences; and (4) a speech-auditory system that matches vision with the language system of the individual, facilitating the development of a code that can be stored and more efficiently retrieved.

Vision is an important link to the physical world, helping us to gain information beyond the range of other senses, while also helping us to integrate the information acquired primarily through hearing, touch, smell, and taste. For example, our sense of touch can tell us that what we are feeling is furry, soft, and warm, but only our eyes can tell that it is a brown rabbit with a white tail and pink eyes. Our nose may perceive something with yeast and spices cooking, but our eyes can confirm that it is a large pepperoni pizza with bubbling mozzarella and green peppers. Our hearing can tell us that a friend sounds angry and upset, but only our vision can perceive the black scowl, clenched jaw, and stiff posture. The way we perceive visual stimuli shapes our interactions with, and reactions to, the environment while providing a foundation for the development of a more complex learning structure.

DEFINITIONS AND CLASSIFICATION

Definitions

FOCUS 4
Distinguish between medical-legal and educational definitions of blindness.

The term *visual disorder* or *visual handicap* includes people who are **blind** as well as **partially sighted.** Barraga (1983) defined a visually handicapped child as "one whose visual impairment interferes with his optimal learning and achievement, unless adaptations are made in the methods of presenting learning experiences, the nature of the materials used, and/or in the learning environment" (p. 25).

The word *blind* has many diverse meanings. In fact, there are over 150 citations for *blind* in Webster's Unabridged Dictionary. Definitions of blindness may be categorized using a medical-legal orientation or an educational orientation.

The Medical-Legal Definition. The medical-legal definition of blindness, adopted by the American Medical Association, states:

> A person shall be considered blind whose central **visual acuity** does not exceed 20/200 in the better eye with correcting lenses or whose visual acuity, if better than 20/200, has a limit in the central field of vision to such a degree that its widest diameter subtends an angle of no greater than twenty degrees (Connor, Hoover, Horton, Sands, Sternfeld, & Wolinsky, 1975, p. 240).

Most people considered legally blind have some light perception; only about 20 percent are totally without sight.

The above definition of blindness employs two basic criteria: visual acuity and the **field of vision.** A person's visual acuity is indicated by the use of an index that refers to the distance at which an object can be recognized. The person with normal eyesight is defined as having 20/20 vision. However, if an individual reads at 20 feet what a person with normal vision reads at 200 feet then his or her visual acuity would be described as 20/200. A person is also considered blind if his or her field of vision is limited at its widest angle to 20 degrees or less (see Figure 10–2). A restricted field is also referred to as tunnel vision, pinhole vision, or tubular vision. A restricted field of vision severely limits a person's ability to participate in athletics, read, or drive a car.

Educational Definitions. Educational definitions of blindness focus primarily on the student's ability to use vision as an avenue for learning. Children who are unable to use their sight and rely on other senses, such as hearing and touch, are described as educationally blind. Craig and Howard (1981) indicate that **educational blindness,** in its simplest form, can be defined by whether the student muse use braille when reading. Regardless of the definition used, the purpose of labeling a child as educationally blind is to ensure an appropriate instructional program. This program must assist the blind student in utilizing other senses as a means to succeed in a classroom setting and in the future as an independent, productive adult.

Blind versus Partially Sighted. A variety of terms are used to describe levels of visual dysfunction, and this has created some confusion among professionals in various fields of study. The rationale for the development of various definitions is directly related to their intended use. For example, in order to be eligible for income-tax exemptions or special assistance from the American Printing House of the Blind, individuals with a visual disorder must fall into one of two general subcategories: blind or partially sighted. Partially sighted is defined as "persons with a visual acuity greater than 20/200 but not greater than 20/70 in the better eye after correction" (National Society for the Prevention of Blindness, 1966, p. 10).

The field of education also distinguishes between blind and partially sighted, in order to determine the level and extent of additional support services required

FOCUS 5
Define *partially sighted.*

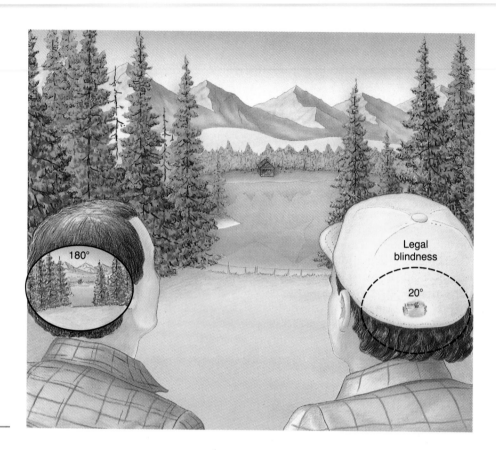

Figure 10–2
The Field of Vision

by a student. Partially sighted describes students who are able to use their vision as a primary source of learning. Jamie, the individual in our opening vignette, is a partially sighted individual. While in school, the vision specialist worked with Jamie to make the best possible use of his remaining vision. This assistance included the elimination of unnecessary glare in the work area, removal of obstacles that could impede mobility, the use of large-print books, and special lighting to enhance visual opportunities.

Suran and Rizzo (1979) suggest that "educational goals for the partially sighted child include maximal use of the child's functional residual vision by means of magnification, illumination, specialized teaching aids (such as large-print books and posters), as well as exercises designed to increase visual efficiency" (p. 149). The position of these authors is contrary to the traditional philosophy of **sight conservation** or sight saving, which advocates the restricted use of the eye. It was once believed that students with a visual disorder could keep what vision they had much longer if it was used very sparingly. However, several studies conducted during the 1960s demonstrated that extended reliance on residual vision, in conjunction with visual stimulation training, actually *improved* a person's ability to use sight as an avenue for learning (Barraga, 1964; Ashcroft, 1966).

The distinction between blind and partially sighted has not significantly minimized the confusion related to the terminology associated with visual problems.

In an attempt to refine the terminology and to group various levels of visual problems functionally, Barraga (1986) proposes the following descriptors:

1. Profound visual disability: The performance of the most gross visual task may be very difficult, and vision is not used at all for detailed tasks.

2. Severe visual disability: More time and energy are needed to perform visual tasks. Additionally, performance level may be less accurate than that of sighted individuals even though visual aids and modifications may be in use.

3. Moderate visual disability: Visual tasks may be performed with the use of special aids and lighting. Performance level may be comparable to that of students with normal vision.

Classification

Visual disorders may be classified according to the anatomical site of the problem. Anatomical disorders include impairment of the refractive structures of the eye, muscle anomalies in the visual system, and problems of the receptive structures of the eye.

Refractive Eye Problems. Refractive problems are the most common type of visual disorders and occur when the refractive structures of the eye (cornea, **aqueous humor, lens,** and **vitreous fluid**) fail to focus light rays properly on the retina. The four types of refractive problems are (1) **hyperopia,** or farsightedness; (2) **myopia,** or nearsightedness; (3) **astigmatism,** or blurred vision; and (4) **cataracts.**

FOCUS 6
Identify the four types of refractive eye problems.

Hyperopia occurs when the eyeball is excessively short (has a flat corneal structure), forcing the light rays to focus behind the retina. The person with hyperopia is able to visualize objects at a distance clearly but unable to see them at close range. This individual may require reading glasses.

Myopia occurs when the eyeball is excessively long (has increased curvature of the corneal surface), forcing the light rays to focus in front of the retina. The person with myopia is able to view objects at close range clearly but unable to see them from any distance (such as 100 feet). These individuals require eyeglasses to assist them in focusing on distant objects. Figure 10–3 shows the myopic and hyperopic eyeballs and compares them to the normal human eye.

Astigmatism occurs when the surface of the cornea is uneven, or the lens is structurally defective, preventing the light rays from converging at one point. The rays of light are refracted in different directions, and the visual images are unclear and distorted. Astigmatism may occur independently of or in conjunction with myopia or hyperopia.

Cataracts occur when the lens becomes opaque, resulting in severely distorted vision or total blindness. Surgical treatment for cataracts has advanced rapidly in recent years, preventing many serious visual problems. Remember that Jamie was born with congenital cataracts; as a result of surgery, he has been able to retain some vision throughout his life.

Muscle Disorders. Muscular defects of the visual system occur when the major muscles within the eye are inadequately developed or atrophy, resulting

FOCUS 7
What are the three types of muscle disorders of the visual system?

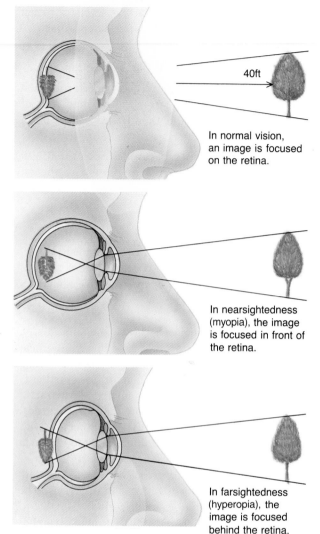

40ft

In normal vision, an image is focused on the retina.

In nearsightedness (myopia), the image is focused in front of the retina.

In farsightedness (hyperopia), the image is focused behind the retina.

Figure 10-3
The Normal, Myopic, and Hyperopic Eyeballs. The image is focused on the retina upside down, but the brain immediately reverses it.

in a loss of control and an inability to maintain tension. People with muscle disorders are unable to maintain their focus on a given object for even short periods of time. The three types of muscle disorders include **nystagmus** (uncontrolled rapid eye movement), **strabismus** (crossed eyes), and **amblyopia** (loss of vision due to muscle imbalance).

Nystagmus is a continuous, involuntary rapid movement of the eyeballs. The nystagmus pattern may be either circular or in a side-to-side sequence.

Strabismus occurs when the muscles of the eye are unable to pull equally, and the eyes therefore cannot focus together on the same object. Internal strabismus occurs when the eyes are pulled inward toward the nose. External strabismus occurs when the eyes are pulled out toward the ears. The eyes may also shift on a vertical plane (up or down), but this is rare. Strabismus can be corrected through surgical intervention. Persons with strabismus often experience a phenomenon known as double vision. In order to correct the double vision and reduce visual confusion, the brain attempts to suppress the image in one eye. As a result, the unused eye atrophies and loses its ability to see. This condition is known as *amblyopia*. Amblyopia can also be corrected by surgery, or by forcing the affected eye into focus by covering the unaffected eye with a patch.

Receptive Eye Problems.   Disorders associated with the receptive structures of the eye occur when there is a degeneration of, or damage to, the retina and the optic nerve. These disorders include **optic atrophy, retinitis pigmentosa, retinal detachment, retrolental fibroplasia,** and **glaucoma.** Optic atrophy is a degenerative disease that results from the deterioration of nerve fibers connecting the retina to the brain. Retinitis pigmentosa is a hereditary condition resulting from a break in the choroid, a vascular membrane containing pigment cells that lies between the retina and the sclera. The condition appears initially as night blindness but eventually results in total blindness.

Retinal detachment is a condition that occurs when the retina is separated from the choroid and the sclera. This detachment may result from such disorders as glaucoma, retinal degeneration, or extreme myopia. It can also be caused by trauma to the eye, such as a boxer's receiving a hard right hook to the face.

Until recently, retrolental fibroplasia (RLF) was one of the most devastating eye disorders in young children. This disorder occurs when too much oxygen is administered to premature infants. Scar tissue forms behind the lens of the eye and prevents light rays from reaching the retina. Retrolental fibroplasia gained widespread attention in the early 1940s, with the advent of improved incubators for premature infants. These incubators substantially improved the concentration of oxygen available to an infant but resulted in a drastic increase in the number of visually disabled children. The disorder has also been associated with neurological, speech, and behavior problems in children and adolescents. Now that a relationship has been clearly established between increased oxygen levels and blindness, premature infants are protected by carefully controlling the amount of oxygen received in the early months of life.

FOCUS 8
Identify the disorders associated with the receptive structures of the eye.

PREVALENCE

The prevalence of various visual disorders is often difficult to determine. For example, Reynolds and Birch (1982) indicate that at least 20 percent of the population have some visual problems, but most of these defects can be corrected to a level where they do not pose a handicap to the learning process. The figure of 0.1 percent is the most frequently cited prevalence for school-age children who meet the legal definitions of blindness and partially sighted. Based on the U.S. Department of Education's Eleventh Annual Report to Congress (1989), there are approximately 23,000 school-age children and youth with visual disorders receiving specialized services in the public schools.

Thousands of blind children born during the **maternal rubella** epidemic in 1963 and 1964 constituted a significant percentage of the enrollment in special education and residential schools for the blind in the 1970s and 1980s. Maternal rubella is now essentially under control, due to the introduction of a rubella

FOCUS 9
What is the prevalence of visual disorders?

vaccine. Retrolental fibroplasia, another major etiological factor in the 1960s, has also declined. However, a large percentage of the cases of blindness still have unknown causes. Lowenfeld (1980) suggests that this is proof that "our knowledge of causes of blindness is still far from satisfactory" (p. 259).

Thus far we have focused on prevalence figures as they relate to school-age children. Blindness also occurs as a function of increasing age. Approximately 75 percent of all blind people are over forty-five years old.

We now turn our attention from prevalence to characteristics. In the next section we examine some of the general characteristics associated with intelligence, speech and language skills, educational achievement, social development, orientation and mobility, and perceptual-motor development.

CHARACTERISTICS

FOCUS 10
Why is age of onset of a visual disorder significant to an individual's development?

As we begin our discussion of characteristics, it is again important to emphasize that a disorder present at birth has a more significant effect on the development of the individual than one that occurs later in life. Several investigators confirm that useful visual imagery disappears if sight is lost prior to the age of five (Lowenfeld, 1980; Schlaegel, 1953; Toth, 1983). If sight is lost after the age of five, it is possible for the person to retain some visual frame of reference. This frame of reference may be maintained over a period of years, depending on the severity of the visual problem. Lowenfeld delineates six gradations of visual disorders, according to their impact on the person's memory and sensory functions:

1. Total blindness, congenital or acquired, before the age of five years
2. Total blindness, acquired after five years of age
3. Partial blindness, congenital
4. Partial blindness, acquired
5. Partial sight, congenital
6. Partial sight, acquired (1980, p. 260).

These categories are in order of the degree of influence on the individual. Total blindness that occurs prior to age five has the greatest negative influence on overall functioning. However, these categories are merely generalities, and many people who are blind from birth or early childhood are able to function at a level consistent with sighted persons of equal ability.

Intelligence

FOCUS 11
In what ways can a visual disorder affect intellectual growth and development?

For a child with a visual disorder, perceptions of the world may be based on input from senses other than vision. This is particularly true of the blind child, whose learning experiences are significantly restricted by the lack of vision. Consequently, everyday learning experiences that we take for granted are substantially diminished. Warren (1984) reviewed the literature on intellectual development and reported that blind children differ from their sighted peers in some areas of intelligence. These areas range from understanding spatial concepts to a general knowledge of the world. Several investigators have confirmed that intellectual development and performance can be negatively affected by a visual disorder (Barraga, 1974; Lowenfeld, 1974; Parsons & Sabornie, 1987; Scholl, 1974). However, the comparisons of sighted to sightless individuals on such tests may not be appropriate if sighted students have an advantage. The only fair way to compare the intellectual capabilities of sighted and blind children is on tasks in which the visual disorder does not interfere with performance. Kirtley (1975) suggests that intellectual differences existing between visually disordered and sighted people may be attributed to a number of external factors, including unfavorable home environments and neurological or physical handicaps. In addition, he states, "There is no correlation of intelligence with the age at which sight has been lost" (p. 141).

Speech and Language Skills

For children with sight, speech and language development occurs primarily through the integration of visual experiences and the symbols of the spoken word. Depending on the degree of loss, children with visual disorders are again at a distinct disadvantage in developing speech and language skills because they are unable to visually associate the word with the object. This child cannot learn speech by visual imitation and must rely on hearing or touch for input. Consequently, speech may develop at a slower rate for those who are congenitally blind. Once these children have learned speech, however, it is typically fluent.

There is some conflicting evidence regarding the differences between children with a visual disorder and their sighted peers in overall language development. Warren (1984) reports, "For blind children without additional handicaps, there is little evidence of developmental differences from sighted children in some areas of language development. . . . The new work of the past several years strongly suggests that, while blind children may use words with the same frequency count as sighted children, the meanings of the words for the blind are not as rich or as elaborated" (p. 277). However, Parsons and Sabornie (1987) report that preschool-age children with low vision performed significantly lower than their sighted peers on a language scale in the areas of auditory comprehension, verbal ability, and overall language. The preschool-age visually disordered child may develop a phenomenon known as **verbalisms.** Verbalisms are the excessive use of speech (wordiness), in which individuals use words that have little meaning to them. Finally, Anderson, Dunlea, and Kekalis (1984) report that the language development of six blind children studied over three years appeared to be comparable to that of their sighted peers. The investigators were, however, concerned that in terms of quality, children who were blind seemed to have more difficulty understanding words as "symbolic vehicles" and formed hypotheses about word meaning significantly slower than sighted peers.

Educational Achievement

The educational achievement of students with a visual disorder may be significantly delayed when compared to that of sighted peers (Lowenfeld, 1980). Some of the variables influencing educational achievement may include excessive school

FOCUS 12
Why do many children with a visual disorder develop speech and language skills at a slower rate than their sighted peers?

FOCUS 13
Identify five factors that may influence the educational achievement of children with a visual disorder.

In the News 10-1

8 Budding Ballerinas Learn to Dance Without Sight and Without Fear

Guided by squeezes and whispers from her ballet teacher and an inexact sense of the people and objects around her, Ivonne Mosquera curtsied, turned and let her hand fall gracefully on the hand of a waiting prince.

"I felt like I was in clouds, nice soft clouds," said Ivonne, an 11-year-old who lost her sight to an eye tumor when she was 2. "I felt like I was floating."

The prince in this rehearsal was Jacques d'Amboise, a 54-year-old former star of the New York City Ballet and known in the arts community as the city's Pied Piper of Dance, a title that describes his ef-

forts over 13 years to bring dance to schoolchildren.

Those efforts have now reached the blind and visually impaired. . . .

In their class on Thursday at the Lighthouse, a center for the blind on East 59th Street near Park Avenue in Manhattan, the girls stretched and warmed up and practiced prancing across the floor in a session opened to spectators by Mr. d'Amboise and the students' regular teachers, Lori Kalinger and Katherine Oppenheimer.

One 11-year-old girl, Jasmine Bayron, said she quickly sensed three things when she walked into the room: the people in the back

of the room, the cameras clicking around her and heat "because I was nervous," she said.

The girls, ages 8 to 14, said their chief fears in dancing are making mistakes and looking silly.

"In ballet, if you make mistakes, they'll point you out," Melissa Malament, 13, said. Blindness adds to the problem, the girls said, because a knee can sometimes feel straight when it is bent or a foot can feel correctly placed when it is not.

They know where everything is in their practice room and are rarely worried about bumping into things. Although a partial or full

absences due to the need for eye surgery or treatment, as well as years of failure in programs that do not meet the student's specialized needs.

On the average, blind children are two years older than sighted children in their same grade. Thus any direct comparisons of visually disordered students to sighted students would indicate significantly delayed academic growth. However, this age phenomenon may result from entering school at a later age, absence from school due to medical problems associated with the eye, lack of appropriate school facilities, and use of **Braille.** Kirtley (1975) suggests that touch-reading is at least three times slower than visual reading. "Sole reliance on braille reading means a relatively slow acquisition of knowledge" (p. 142).

Social Development

FOCUS 14
What are three factors that may lead to greater social difficulties for individuals with a visual disorder?

The ability to adapt to the social environment depends on a number of factors, both hereditary and experiential. It is true that each of us experiences the world in his or her own way, but there are common bonds that give us a foundation on which to build perceptions of the world around us. One such bond is vision. Without vision, perceptions about ourselves and those around us would be drastically different. For the person with a visual disorder, these differences in loss of sight poses difficulties in learning ballet, "we want to do it because we want to know that we can do everything everybody else can do," Jasmine said.

A major problem is that students often learn dance by imitating others, and "you can't ask them to watch what I do and copy," Ms. Kalinger said.

As the girls moved their arms, Ms. Oppenheimer suggested that they imagine gently pushing away something soft. When she asked them what they were pushing, Ivonne said she was pushing snow. Another girl said she was pushing rain. Then a third said ice cream.

"Well O.K., but make sure you're pushing it away, not toward you," the teacher said.

The students are also working on "muscle memory," in which certain body movements become instinctive. In an eating motion, for example, the hand moves to the mouth without any conscious guidance, Ms. Kalinger said.

. . . This year's dance will depict what Washington and Lafayette might have done had they ever spent a night on the town in Paris. During their evening, they see a play titled "The Three Musketeers."

The play within the dance moves to the court of King Louis XIII, who reigned at the time of the Musketeers. That is where the girls come in, dancing to the music of an 18th Century French composer and to the voice and lyrics of the folk singer Judy Col-

lins, whose father was blinded by glaucoma when he was 4.

For Mr. d'Amboise, seeing the eight girls among his thousand young dancers will be a special treat.

"They're going to be able to come across the stage and not be afraid," he said at Thursday's class, moving across the floor with effortless grace.

Then he asked the girls to envision the stage, "where it will be bright and beautiful and the people will have come to see you."

perception may result in some social and emotional difficulties. For example, visually disordered people are unable to imitate the physical mannerisms of others and therefore do not develop one very important component of a social communication system: body language. The subtleties of nonverbal communication may significantly alter the intended meaning of spoken words. A person's inability to develop a nonverbal communication system through the acquisition of visual cues (such as facial expressions or hand gestures) has profound consequences for interpersonal interactions, not only for the visually disordered person's reception or interpretation of verbal language, but also for what he or she expresses to others. The sighted person may misinterpret the intended meaning because visual cues are not consistent with the spoken word.

Social problems may also result from the exclusion of persons with a visual disorder from social activities that are integrally related to the use of vision (such as sports or the movies). Individuals are often excluded from such activities, without a second thought, because they cannot see. This only serves to reinforce the mistaken idea that they do not want to participate and would not enjoy these activities (Tuttle, 1984). However, as we learned from Jamie, many people who have visual disorders seek out activities in which vision may be viewed as necessary, such as hiking, golfing, and spectator sports. Exclusion of the visually impaired individual from social experiences is more often a product of the negative attitude of the public toward visual disorders than the person's lack of social adjustment skills.

Lowenfeld (1980) reviewed the literature on public attitudes toward blindness and concluded that although many studies support the contention that people who are blind are perceived to be helpless and dependent, attitudes are changing. He further suggests that much of the information generated by the research is inconclusive and that more in-depth studies are needed. Lowenfeld's optimism concerning the growth of a social consciousness in regard to the blind is certainly a welcome perception, but it is not entirely supported in the literature. Attitudes of the general public are not necessarily those of acceptance and integration. Willis, Groves, and Fuhrman (1979) suggest "a visual disability may well be the most difficult exceptionality for sighted persons to accept" (p. 354).

Orientation and Mobility

FOCUS 15
What effect does a visual disorder have on orientation and mobility?

A visual disorder may impair orientation and mobility in several ways. The individual may be unable to orient to other people or objects in the environment simply because he or she cannot see them. Lack of sight may prevent persons with a visual disorder from understanding their own relative position in space, and consequently prevent them from moving in the right direction. They may develop a fear of injuring themselves and attempt to restrict their movements to protect themselves. In addition, parents and professionals may contribute to such fears by protecting them from everyday risk. Any unnecessary restrictions hinder the individual's acquisition of independent mobility skills and create an atmosphere for life-long dependence.

A visual disorder may also have an effect on fine motor coordination and interfere with the ability to manipulate objects. Poor eye–hand coordination interferes with learning how to use the tools, such as eating utensils, a toothbrush, or a screwdriver, necessary for everyday functioning and occupational efficiency. In order to prevent or remediate fine-motor problems, many people with visual

---

WINDOW 10–1

I Never Had the Chance to Know Any Blind Kids

Blind people have always evoked negative and frightening feelings in me. I guess part of my reaction stems from my fear of becoming blind. I really believe that such feelings come from my lack of experience with the blind. When I was in school, I never had the chance to get to know a blind person. There was a class of blind children in my school, but they never seemed to be around. I remember that they came to school at a different time, had different lunch periods, and never participated in school activities. I don't know whether this bothered them, but I know it never gave me the chance to know even one of my blind schoolmates.

Jeff, *an adult with sight*

WINDOW 10–2

*Sure I Know
Some Blind Kids*

Sure, I know some kids who can't see. They go to my school, and some are in my class. Jenny is in my reading group. Her face almost touches the book when she reads. My teacher tries to give her books where the words are bigger on the page. Sometimes she works with another teacher who helps her because she can't see. When school started, I used to walk with her to the library or the bathroom, so she wouldn't get lost. She doesn't need help anymore. She knows where everything is in our class and goes all over the school with no help.

Malcolm, *a child with sight*

disorders require extensive training, which must begin early and focus directly on experiences that enhance opportunities for independent living.

Perceptual-Motor Development

Perceptual-motor development is essential to the development of locomotion skills, but it is also important in the development of cognition, language, socialization, and personality. In a comprehensive review of the literature, Warren (1984) reports that the blind child's perceptual discrimination abilities in such areas as texture, weight, and sound are comparable to those of sighted peers. However, the blind do not perform as well on more complex tasks of perception, including form identification, spatial relations, and perceptual-motor integration. Early visual experience prior to the onset of blindness or partial loss of sight may provide a child with some advantage in the acquisition of manipulatory and locomotor skills.

A popular misconception regarding the perceptual abilities of persons with a visual disorder is that because of their diminished sight they develop greater capacity in other sensory areas; for example, that they are able to hear or smell things that people with normal vision cannot perceive. This empirically invalid notion is known as sensory compensation. Telford and Sawrey (1981) reviewed the literature on sensory compensation and reported:

> Studies have consistently shown that persons with vision are either equal or superior to the blind in their ability to identify the direction or distance of the source of a sound, to discriminate the relative intensities of tones, to recognize tactile forms, and to discriminate relative pressures, temperatures or weights, as well as in their acuteness of smell, taste, and the vibratory sense. . . . Any superiority of the blind in the perceptual areas is the result of increased attention to small cues and is a source of information and guidance. It is apparently not the result of a lowering of sensory thresholds (p. 353).

FOCUS 16
What effect does a visual disorder have on perceptual development?

CAUSATION

Visual disorders may result from a multitude of circumstances. For our purposes, we classify the causes of visual disorders in young children into two general areas: (1) genetically determined disorders, and (2) acquired disorders.

Genetically Determined Disorders

FOCUS 17
Identify at least seven congenital factors that may result in a visual disorder.

A number of genetic conditions may result in a visual disorder. These include **choroido-retinal degeneration** (a deterioration of the choroid and retina), **retinablastoma** (a malignant tumor in the retina), **pseudoglioma** (a nonmalignant intraocular disturbance resulting from the detachment of the retina), optic atrophy (loss of function of optic-nerve fibers), cataracts, myopia associated with retinal detachment, lesions of the cornea, abnormalities of the iris (e.g., coloboma or aniridia), **microphthalmus** (abnormally small eyeball), **anophthalmos** (absence of the eyeball), and **buphthalmos** (abnormal distention and enlargement of the eyeball). In addition, a visual disorder may be a result of other malformations. For example, **hydrocephalus** (excess cerebrospinal fluid in the brain) may lead to optic atrophy.

Acquired Disorders

FOCUS 18
Identify at least six acquired factors that may result in a visual disorder.

Acquired disorders can occur prior to, during, or after birth. Several factors present prior to birth, such as radiation or the introduction of drugs into the fetal system, may result in a visual disorder. A major cause of blindness in the fetus is infection, which may be due to such diseases as rubella and syphilis. Ward (1986) estimates that about 14 percent of all cases of legal blindness are caused by infectious diseases. Other diseases which may result in blindness include influenza, mumps, and measles.

The leading cause of blindness in children during the 1940s and 1950s was retrolental fibroplasia, now known as **retinopathy of prematurity.** As previously noted, RLF results from the administration of oxygen over prolonged periods of time to low-birth-weight infants. Lowenfeld (1980) indicates: "In the peak years of this disease, some states reported that almost 80 percent of their preschool blind children has lost their sight as a result of RLF. It has been established that RLF caused blindness in more than 10,000 babies who have not reached adulthood" (p. 259). Visual disorders occurring after birth may be due to several factors. Accidents, infections, inflammations, and tumors are all associated with loss of sight. Although the majority of visual disorders occur prior to adolescence or the adult years and approximately 60 percent occur before the age of one, some visual problems are associated with factors occurring during adulthood, including injuries, disease, and degeneration.

We now move from causes associated with visual disorders to the areas of assessment and intervention strategies. Individuals with a visual disorder require specialized services if they are to achieve independence in their school and community environment. These support systems range from medical prevention in early life, to adult rehabilitation and education. The level of intervention depends on the severity of the disorder and the availability of qualified professionals.

ASSESSMENT AND INTERVENTION STRATEGIES

Medical Services

FOCUS 19
How is visual acuity measured?

Initial screenings for visual disorders are usually based on the individual's visual acuity. Visual acuity may be measured through the use of the **Snellen Test,** developed in 1862 by the Dutch ophthalmologist Herman Snellen. This visual

Reflect on This 10–2

New Evidence on the Effect of Exposure to Light on Premature Infants

Over the years, retrolental fibroplasia (RLF) has been primarily associated with exposure to elevated levels of oxygen in the newborn nursery. However, a recent study (Glass et al., 1985) at the Georgetown University Hospital and the Children's Hospital National Medical Center indicates that RLF may also be associated with prolonged exposure to hospital lights in the nursery.

The intensity of light in hospital intensive-care nurseries has increased by about five to ten times over what it was about twenty years ago. Premature infants are now exposed to additional sources of light such as heat lamps, raising the concern about what effect these lights have on the underdeveloped infant. Glass et al. found that there was indeed a higher incidence of RLF among premature infants exposed to hospital lights, in comparison to infants of normal birth weight. The authors recommend that safety standards with regard to current lighting practices in newborn intensive care units be reassessed.

---

screening test is used primarily to measure central distance vision. A person stands twenty feet from a letter or E chart and reads each symbol, beginning with the top row. The different sizes of each row or symbol represent what a person with normal vision would see at the various distances indicated on the chart. As indicated earlier in this chapter, a person's visual acuity is then indicated by the use of an index that refers to the distance at which an object can be recognized. The person with normal eyesight is defined as having 20/20 vision.

Since the Snellen chart only measures visual acuity, it must be used primarily as an initial screening device that is supplemented by more in-depth assessments, such as a thorough ophthalmological examination. Parents, physicians, school nurses, and educators must also carefully observe the child's behavior, and a complete history of any presenting symptoms of a visual disorder should be documented. These observable symptoms fall into three categories: appearance, behavior, and complaints. Table 10–1 describes some warning signs within these three categories. The existence of symptoms does not necessarily mean a person has a visual disorder, but it does indicate that an appropriate specialist should be consulted for further examination.

Prevention.   Prevention of visual disorders is one of the major goals within the field of medicine and falls into three categories: genetic screening and counseling, appropriate prenatal care, and early developmental assessment.

Since many causes of blindness are hereditary, it is important for the family to be aware of genetic services. One purpose of genetic screening is to identify those who are planning for a family and who may possess certain detrimental genotypes that can be passed on to their descendants. Screening may also be

FOCUS 20
What are three steps that can be taken to prevent visual disorders?

TABLE 10–1   Observable Symptoms of Visual Disorders

Appearance	Behavior	Complaints
Crossed eyes, or eyes not functioning together	Walks with extreme caution	Dizziness
Swollen eyelids	Blinks constantly	Frequent headaches
Red-rimmed, crusted eyelids	Trips or stumbles frequently	Pain in the eyes
Frequent sties	Rubs eyes frequently	Blurry letters or objects
Bloodshot eyes	Is overly sensitive to light	Double vision
Pupils of different sizes	Tilts head; shuts or covers one eye when reading	Burning or itching eyelids
Eyes in constant motion	Frowns when trying to see distant objects	
	Is unable to distinguish colors	
	Fails to see objects in peripheral (side) vision	
	Holds reading material at an abnormal distance—either very close or at a great distance	
	Distorts face when using concentrated vision	

Source: From R. H. Craig and C. Howard, "Teaching Students with Visual Impairments," in M. L. Hardman, M. W. Egan, and E. D. Landau, eds., *What Will We Do in the Morning? The Exceptional Student in the Regular Classroom,* p. 188. © 1981 Wm. C. Brown Company Publishers, Dubuque, Iowa. Reprinted by permission.

Visual examinations should be conducted regularly during childhood. (John Telford)

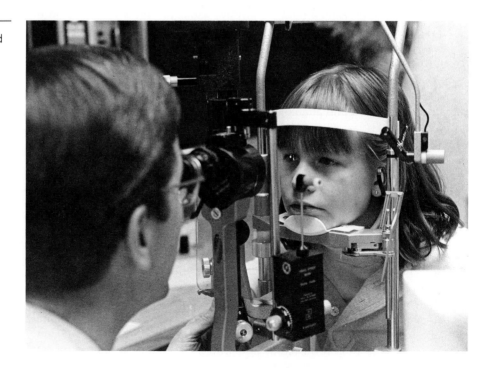

conducted after conception in order to determine whether the unborn fetus possesses any genetic abnormalities. Following the screening, a genetic counselor informs the parents of the results of the tests so that the family is able to make an informed decision about conceiving a child or carrying a fetus to term.

Adequate prenatal care is another means of preventing problems. Parents must be made aware of the potential hazards associated with poor nutritional habits, the use of drugs, and exposure to radiation (such as x-rays) during pregnancy. One example of preventive care during this period is the use of antibiotics to treat various infections, such as influenza, measles, or syphilis, thus reducing the risk of infection to the unborn fetus.

Developmental screening is also a widely recognized means of prevention. It was through early developmental screening that a medical specialist confirmed that Jamie had a serious visual disorder and would require the assistance of a trained vision specialist. Early screening of developmental problems enables the family physician to analyze several treatment alternatives and, when necessary, to refer the child to an appropriate specialist. The specialist conducts a more thorough evaluation of the child's developmental delays. Early visual screening, which also includes hearing, speech, motor, and psychological development, should be a component of this general development assessment. Raikes (1979) describes four periods during the early childhood years when visual screening should routinely take place. She suggests that a complete medical examination be conducted at birth and include the general physiological condition of the newborn, a family history, and information concerning any problems during gestation or delivery. When observing the general condition of the baby immediately after birth "[the] eyes should be examined for damage, infection and congenital abnormalities" (Raikes, 1979, p. 2). At six weeks of age, visual screening should be a component of another general developmental assessment. This examination should include input from the parents concerning how their child is responding (e.g., smiling and looking at objects or faces). The physician should check eye movement, as well as search for any infection, crusting on the eyes, or **epiphora** (an overflow of tears from obstruction of the lacrimal ducts). The next examination should occur at about six months of age. A defensive blink should be present at this age, and eye movement should be full and coordinated. If there is any imbalance in eye movements, a more thorough examination should be conducted. Family history is extremely important, since in many cases there is a familial pattern. Between the ages of one and five, visual evaluation should be conducted at regular intervals. A particularly important period is the time just prior to the child's entering school. Visual problems must not go undetected as these youngsters attempt to cope with the new and complex demands of the educational environment.

Treatment. In addition to medicine's emphasis on prevention of visual disorders, this profession has made significant strides in the treatment of these problems. The nature of medical intervention depends on the type and severity of the disorder. For partially sighted individuals, use of an optical aid can vastly improve access to the visual world. Most of these aids are in the form of corrective glasses or contact lenses, which are designed to magnify the image on the retina. Some aids are able to improve muscle control within the eye, while others clarify the retinal image. Appropriate use of optical aids, in conjunction

FOCUS 21
Identify three significant strides medicine has made in the treatment of visual disorders.

with regular medical examinations, not only helps correct existing visual problems but may also prevent further deterioration of existing vision.

Surgery and drug therapy have also played important roles in treating visual disorders. Treatment in these areas may range from the extremely complex surgical procedures associated with corneal transplants, to the process known as **atropinization**. Atropinization is the treatment for cataracts that involves washing out the eye with the alkaloid drug atropine, which permanently dilates the pupil.

Social Services

FOCUS 22
Why is the availability of appropriate mental health services important for people with a visual disorder?

Some individuals with a visual disorder may have social adjustment problems, which include poor self-concept and general feelings of inferiority. So it is important for mental health services to be available as early as possible in the person's life. These services may begin with infant stimulation programs and counseling for the family. As these children grow older, group counseling may assist them in coping with their feelings concerning blindness. In addition, the individual may need some guidance in the area of human sexuality. Limited vision may distort the perception of the physical body. Counseling eventually extends into matters focusing on marriage, family, and adult relationships. For the visually disordered adult, special guidance may also be necessary in preparation for employment and independent living.

Other services that facilitate the participation of people with a visual disorder in the community include specialized library and newspaper services, with books that have large print, are available on cassette, and are printed in braille. The *New York Times* publishes a special edition, with type three times the size of its regular type, once each week.

The mobility of the person with a visual disorder may be greatly enhanced in large cities by the use of auditory pedestrian signals at crosswalks. The "walk" and "don't walk" signals are indicated by an auditory cue such as different bird chirps for each signal. Restaurants can assist the person with a visual disorder through the availability of Braille menus.

Educational Services

FOCUS 23
What is the purpose of an educational assessment for students with a visual disorder?

Educational Assessment. In the area of education, the assessment process is no different for visually disordered students than it is for their sighted peers. The educational team is interested in assessing the cognitive ability, academic achievement, language skills, motor performance, and social/emotional functioning of the student. Assessment must also focus specifically on how the visually disordered student utilizes any remaining vision (visual efficiency) in conjunction with other senses.

The nature and severity of the visual problem determine the assessment instruments to be used. Some assessment instruments have been developed specifically for visually disordered students. Others are intended for sighted students, but have been adapted to visually disordered students. There are also instruments that have been developed for sighted students which are used in their original form with visually disordered students. Regardless of the instruments employed, educational assessment, in conjunction with medical and psychological data, must provide the diagnostic information that ensure an appropriate educational experience for the student.

Educational Placement. Historically, education of blind individuals was implemented primarily through specialized residential facilities. These segregated centers for the blind have traditionally been referred to as asylums, institutions, or schools. One of the first such facilities in the United States was the New England Asylum for the Blind, later named the Perkins School. This facility opened its doors in 1832 and was one of several Eastern schools that used treatment models borrowed from well-established institutions for the blind in Europe. For the most part, early institutions in this country operated as "closed" schools, where a blind person would live and learn in an environment essentially segregated from the outside world. The segregation policies went as far as separating blind males and females, allowing only a minimal level of closely supervised interaction. Lowenfeld (1975) suggests that the philosophy of the closed school was to retain blind people in "an environment that prepares them for future life but does not expose them to it" (p. 101).

More recently, some residential schools have advocated an "open" system of intervention, based on the philosophy that blind children should have every opportunity to gain the same kind of experiences that would be available if they were growing up in their own communities. Both open and closed residential facilities remain today as alternative intervention modes, but they are no longer the primary social or educational system for a blind person. As was true for Jamie in our opening vignette, the vast majority of blind and partially sighted individuals now live at home, attend local public schools, and interact within the community. However, in some instances a residential facility may still be an alternative, if the family is unable to cope with a visually disordered child and if a separate (usually temporary) living arrangement is determined to be in the best interests of the child and the family.

Educational programs for students with visual disorders are based on a principle of flexible placement. A wide variety of services are available for these students in the public schools, ranging from regular class placement with little or no assistance from specialists, to segregated residential schools. Between these extremes of delivery systems, the public schools generally offer several alternative classroom structures, including the use of a consulting teacher, resource rooms, part-time special classes, or full-time special classes. Placement of a visually disordered student into one of these delivery modes depends on the impact of the individual's disorder on his or her overall educational achievement. Many visually disordered students are able to function successfully within regular education if the learning environment is adapted to meet their needs. Craig and Howard (1981) suggest:

> Visually impaired children can listen, speak, think, and participate in many physical activities. Most of them can even see, though not as clearly as the other pupils. . . . Since the child's basic needs parallel those of sighted peers, the classroom teacher is capable of meeting them. Because one important avenue of sensory input is weak or absent, the mode of presentation of lessons must be altered occasionally, but not the content or the goal. The academic curriculum of the visually impaired child should match that of the sighted child (p. 189).

FOCUS 24
What is the range of educational services available to students with a visual disorder?

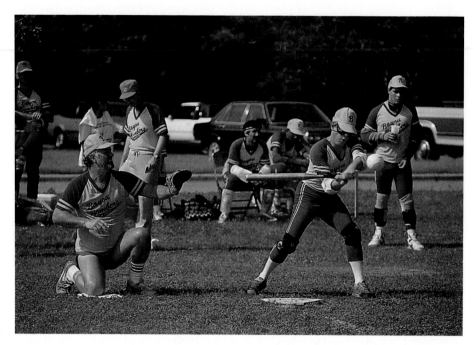

Visually impaired individuals can participate in many physical activities, including baseball. When playing beep baseball, a player can identify the ball and the bases by the sounds they emit. (© Bob Daemmrich/ Stock Boston)

Whether the student is integrated into the regular classroom or taught in a special class, a vision specialist must be available, either to support the regular classroom teacher or to provide direct instruction to the student. A vision specialist receives specialized training in the education of visually disordered students and holds professional certification in this area. This specialist, and the rest of the educational support team, must be knowledgeable concerning appropriate educational assessment techniques, specialized curriculum materials and teaching approaches, and the use of various communication media. Specialized instruction for students who are visually impaired may include a major modification in curricula, including teaching concepts that sighted children learn incidentally—walking down the street, getting from one room to the next in the school building, getting meals in the cafeteria, and using public transportation (Hatlen & Curry, 1987).

FOCUS 25
Identify two essential content areas that should be included in an educational program for a student with a visual disorder.

Mobility Training and Daily Living Skills. The educational needs of students with a visual disorder are comparable to those of their sighted counterparts. In addition, many of the instructional methods currently used with sighted students are applicable with the visually disordered. However, it is important for the educator to be aware of certain content areas that are essential to the visually disordered student's success in the educational environment but are usually not a focal point for sighted students. These areas include mobility and orientation training, as well as acquisition of daily living skills.

The ability to move safely and efficiently through the environment enhances one's opportunities to learn more about the world and thus to be less dependent on others for survival. A lack of mobility restricts individuals with a visual disorder in nearly every aspect of their educational life. Such a student may be unable to orient to physical structures in the classroom (such as desks, chairs, and aisles), hallways, restrooms, library, or cafeteria. Whereas a sighted person is able to establish a relative position in space automatically, the visually disordered person must be taught some means of compensating for the lack of visual input. This may be accomplished in a number of ways. Halliday and Kurzhals (1976) stress that "orientation and mobility should be emphasized in every situation of the school program" (p. 15). It is important for blind or partially sighted students not only to learn the physical structure of their own schools but also to develop specific techniques that can be employed to orient them in unfamiliar surroundings. These techniques involve using the other senses. For example, their sense of touch and hearing can help to identify cues that locate the bathroom in the school. Although it is not true that the blind are able to hear better than sighted persons, they may be able to learn to use their hearing more effectively, by focusing on subtle auditory cues that go unnoticed by sighted people. Efficient use of hearing, in conjunction with the other senses (including any remaining vision), is the key to independent travel for the visually disordered. Independent travel with a sighted companion but without the use of a cane, guide dog, or electronic device is the most common form of travel for young school-age children. As these children grow older, they may be instructed in the use of a long cane or **Mowat Sensor.** The Mowat Sensor, approximately the size of a flashlight, is a hand-held ultrasound travel aid that vibrates at different rates to warn of obstacles in front of the individual.

Guide dogs or electronic mobility devices may be appropriate for the adolescent or adult, since the need to travel independently significantly increases with age. A variety of electronic mobility devices are currently being used. These devices do everything from enhancing hearing efficiency to detecting obstacles. The recently developed **Laser cane** converts infrared light into sound as light beams strike objects in the path of the person who is blind. The **Sonicguide,** which is worn on the head, emits ultrasound and is able to convert reflections from objects into audible noise. The individual is then able to learn about the structure of an object through the characteristics of the sound that is echoed back to the Sonicguide. For example, loudness indicates size: the louder the noise, the larger the object.

The acquisition of daily living skills is another curriculum area that is important to success in the classroom and independence in society. Most sighted people take for granted many routine events of the day, such as eating, dressing, bathing, and toileting. An individual with sight learns very early in life the tasks associated with perceptual-motor development, including grasping, lifting, balancing, pouring, and manipulating objects. These daily living tasks become more complex during the school years as a child learns personal hygiene, grooming, and social etiquette. Eventually, sighted individuals acquire many complex daily living skills that later contribute to their independence as adults. Money management, grocery shopping, laundry, cooking, cleaning, repairing, sewing, mowing, and trimming are all a part of the daily tasks associated with adult life, which are learned from experiences that are not usually a part of an individual's formalized educational program. For someone with a visual disorder, however, routine daily living skills are not learned in the give-and-take of everyday experiences. In fact, visually disordered children may be discouraged from developing self-help skills and protected from the challenges and risks of everyday life by their parents, siblings, or other family members and friends. Chapman (1978) believes, "Systematic teaching is essential here although the child will need plenty of opportunities to find out for himself how to do things and do them the way that suits him best, as well as having guided help in mastering techniques" (p. 110).

Traditional Curriculum Content Areas. Mobility training and the acquisition of daily living skills are components of an educational program that must also concentrate on the traditional curriculum areas. Particular emphasis must be placed on developing receptive and expressive language skills. Students with a visual disorder must learn to listen in order to understand the auditory world more clearly. Finely tuned receptive skills contribute to the development of expressive language, which allows these children to orally describe their perceptions of the world. Oral expression can then be expanded to include handwriting as a means of communication. The acquisition of social and instructional language skills opens the door to many areas, including mathematics and reading.

Abstract mathematical concepts may be difficult for blind students, who usually require additional practice in learning to master symbols, number facts, and higher level calculations. As these concepts become more complex, additional aids may be necessary to facilitate learning. Specially designed talking microcomputers, calculators, rulers, compasses, and the Cranmer abacus have been developed to assist blind students in this area.

Reading is another activity that can greatly expand the knowledge base for visually disordered individuals. For the partially sighted, various optical aids are available. These include video systems that magnify print, hand-held magnifiers, magnifiers attached to eyeglasses, and other telescopic aids. Another means to facilitate reading for partially sighted students is the use of large-print books. These books are generally available through the American Printing House for the Blind and come in several print sizes (see Figure 10–4). Other factors that must be considered in teaching reading to partially sighted students include adequate illumination and the reduction of glare.

FOCUS 26
In what ways can communication media facilitate learning for people with a visual disorder?

Communication Media. For partially sighted students, limited vision remains a source of information. The use of optical aids, in conjunction with auditory and tactile stimuli, allows the individual an integrated sensory approach to learning. However, this approach is not possible for the blind student. A blind person does not have access to visual stimuli and must compensate for this loss through the use of tactile and auditory media. Through these media, blind children develop an understanding of themselves and the world around them. One facet of this development process is the acquisition of language, and one facet of language development is learning how to read.

The tactile sense represents a blind student's entry into the symbolic world of reading. Currently, the most widely used tactile medium for teaching blind people to read is the raised-line Braille system. This system, which originated with the work of Louis Braille in 1829, is a code that utilizes a six-dot cell. There are sixty-three different alphabetical, numerical, and grammatical characters.

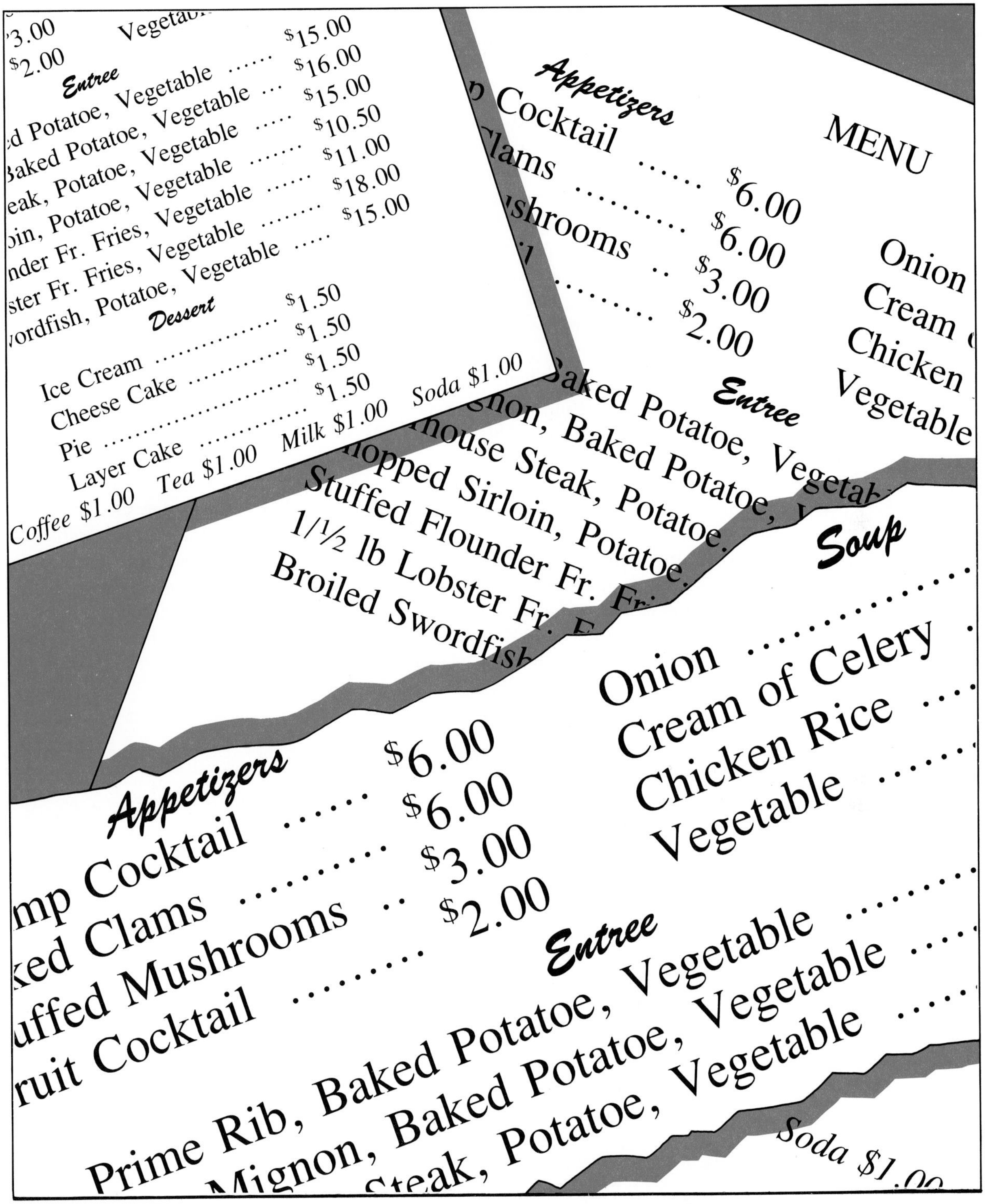

3.00   Vegetab... $15.00
$2.00   *Entree*
...d Potatoe, Vegetable $16.00
...Baked Potatoe, Vegetable ... $15.00
...eak, Potatoe, Vegetable $10.50
...oin, Potatoe, Vegetable $11.00
...nder Fr. Fries, Vegetable ... $18.00
...ster Fr. Fries, Vegetable $15.00
...ordfish, Potatoe, Vegetable ....
Dessert
Ice Cream $1.50
Cheese Cake $1.50
Pie $1.50
Layer Cake $1.50
Coffee $1.00   Tea $1.00   Milk $1.00   Soda $1.00

Appetizers
...Cocktail $6.00
...lams $6.00
...shrooms .. $3.00
... $2.00

MENU

Onion
Cream ...
Chicken
Vegetable

Entree
...gnon, Baked Potatoe, Vegetab...
...ouse Steak, Potatoe,...
...opped Sirloin, Potatoe....
Stuffed Flounder Fr. Fr...
1½ lb Lobster Fr. F...
Broiled Swordfis...

Soup

Onion ....
Cream of Celery ....
Chicken Rice ......
Vegetable ....

Appetizers
...mp Cocktail $6.00
...ked Clams $6.00
...uffed Mushrooms .. $3.00
...ruit Cocktail $2.00

Entree
Prime Rib, Baked Potatoe, Vegetable ......
...Mignon, Baked Potatoe, Vegetable ...
...Steak, Potatoe, Vegetable .....
Soda $1.00

Figure 10–4 Illustrations of Large-Print Type

In order to become a proficient Braille reader, one must learn 263 different configurations, including alphabet letters, punctuation marks, short-form words, and contractions. As illustrated in Figure 10–5, Braille is not a tactile reproduction of the standard English alphabet but a separate code for reading and writing. Braille is still considered by a significant number of people who are blind to be an efficient means for teaching reading and writing. Critics of the system note that Braille readers are estimated to be two or three times slower than print readers (Harley, Henderson, & Truan, 1979; Kirtley, 1975), and that Braille materials are somewhat bulky and tedious. It can be argued, however, that without Braille the person who is blind would be much less independent. The individual who is unable to read Braille is more dependent on sight readers or recordings. Simple tasks, such as labeling cans, boxes, cartons in a bathroom or kitchen, become nearly impossible to complete.

Braille writing is accomplished through the use of a slate and stylus. Using this procedure, a student writes a mirror image of the reading code, moving from right to left. The writing process may be facilitated by using a Braille writer. This hand-operated machine has six keys that correspond to each dot in the Braille cell.

A recent innovation for Braille readers, which may reduce some of the problems associated with the medium, is the **paperless brailler.** One such machine, the Rose Braille Display Reader, comes in a compact desk-top unit where Braille is recorded and retrieved on standard magnetic tape cassettes, thus significantly reducing the space necessary for storage. This machine is representative of the continuing research in the development of communication media for people who are blind. The Rose Braille Display Reader has been described by the National Federation for the Blind as "revolutionary as the development of the Braille system by Louis Braille more than a century and a half ago" (*Braille: An Overview*, 1982, p. 181). However, many newer systems do not incorporate

Figure 10–5
The Braille Alphabet

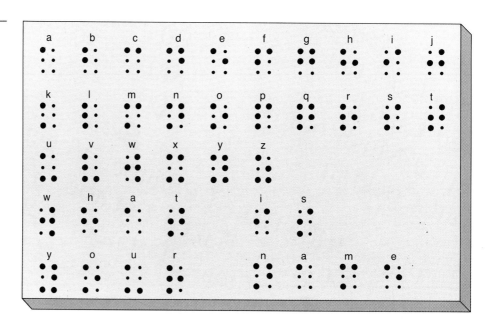

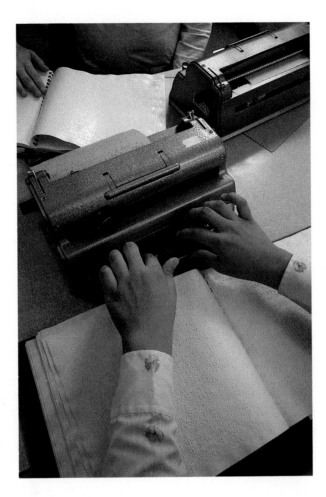

This teenager is using a Braille writer during class. (© Bob Daemmrich/Stock Boston)

Braille as the medium for communication. Although it is the most widely known tactile medium, Braille may not be functional for blind individuals who do not have tactile sensitivity (e.g., elderly blind people).

One of the most popular tactile devices that does not use the Braille system is the **Optacon** scanner. Printed material is exposed to a camera and then reproduced on a finger pad using a series of vibrating pins. These pins are tactile reproductions of the printed material. The Optacon was developed by J. C. Bliss and became available commercially in 1971. There are currently thousands of Optacons in use worldwide. Although the Optacon greatly expands a visually disordered person's access to the printed word, it has its drawbacks as well. First, it still requires tactile sensitivity. Second, reading remains a slow, laborious process. Jernigan (1982) describes the Optacon as not only slow, but requiring considerable training for the individual to become a skilled user. Tobin and James (1974) report that the reading rate on the Optacon after a short training session averages only about ten words per minute, although some subjects were able to maintain forty words per minute for short time-spans. Although the

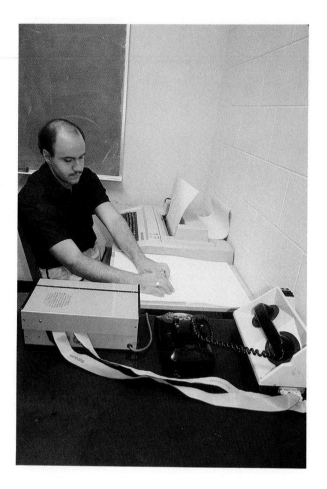

Computers offer unique opportunities for visually impaired people. This blind programmer uses a computer that prints out in Braille. (© Don Kryminec/ Photo Researchers, Inc.)

Optacon is nearly twenty years old, much research remains to be done, and many improvements are currently being evaluated (such as a self-contained hand-held model).

For some blind individuals, the tactile medium may not be the most functional or the most efficient means of acquiring information. Some blind people must rely solely on the auditory sense, while others are able to integrate tactile and auditory input. Specialized auditory media for blind people are becoming increasingly available. One example is the development of the **Kurzweil Reading Machine.** This machine, developed by the Kurzweil Computer Products Company, was first introduced in 1975. It converts printed matter into synthetic speech at a rate of approximately 250 words per minute. Models are presently being used nationwide. The original model was too expensive for an individual to afford, and it was not easily portable. However, a much smaller, portable model, introduced in 1988, is one sixth the original price. Another advance in the reading machine is the recent development of a hand-held device from International Business Machines. Other auditory aids that assist blind people include talking calculators, talking-book machines, compact disk players, and audio tape recorders.

Reflect on This 10–3

Why Not Braille?

The author of the following article, Ann Hollowell, lives in Portsmouth, Virginia, and is the parent of a blind child.

Having a visually handicapped child who is in the category of not totally sightless but legally blind can, as some may know, be very difficult. My son at age five was diagnosed as having macular degeneration, a disease that can leave only peripheral vision. In the past three years we have spoken with many doctors and professionals in the "vision field." Doctors, of course, offer very little if any hope for the future, while many of the professionals cannot agree on teaching skills or learning aids.

Our first professional, an employee of the Virginia Department for the Visually Handicapped, only stressed and assisted with large-print books, talking books, and magnifying aids. She was very adamant that a person should always use any remaining eyesight. To do otherwise would, in her words, "make him handicapped."

When I suggested Braille as a tool for learning and as a means of relieving severe eye strain, she became very upset and firmly stated that Braille skills would never help him.

Seeing my son struggle for two years in private school, always at the bottom of the class, was enough to make me realize that special education was needed. After contacting our public school and visiting the vision class, I knew more could be done. Again, the professionals felt that no special placement was needed. I recommended a regular classroom setting with visiting teachers. After much discussion I requested that my son be placed with the vision program in a school outside our immediate school zone.

During his first year in the new setting (a public school) Braille was introduced at my request and with the agreement of his teachers to see if he would want to learn it. His response was extremely positive, and his teachers agreed that Braille should become a part

of his regular education program.

This year has been wonderful. His self-esteem has improved. With Braille he feels he has a special talent, not a handicap. As a parent I see only positive points with his knowing Braille—a future job, ease and speed in reading, medically less strain, and therefore less medication for inflamed eyes.

I feel that no "professional" should be allowed to make all of the decisions about a child's future learning program. I know my child, and I want to be part of his education planning program. I have become involved and have learned much in a short time. By giving my child this added gift and skill, I feel that his future looks bright for the first time in many months. He will have a choice in the planning of his future with this added skill. I say, why not Braille?

Source: Reprinted from A. Hollowell (Spring, 1987). Why not Braille? *Newsletter* of the National Association to Promote the Use of Braille (NAPUB).

REVIEW

FOCUS 1: What are two misconceptions that sighted people have about people without sight?

☐ Most blind people live a deprived socioeconomic and cultural existence.

☐ Blind people are incapable of learning many basic skills or enjoying leisure-time and recreational activities.

FOCUS 2: Briefly describe the anatomy of the eye.

☐ The cornea is the external covering of the eye and reflects visual stimuli in the presence of light.

☐ The pupil controls the amount of light entering the eye.

☐ The iris consists of tissues and muscles whose function is to adjust the size of the pupil.

☐ The lens focuses light rays to strike the retina.

☐ The retina consists of light-sensitive cells that transmit images to the brain by means of the optic nerve.

FOCUS 3: Why is it important to understand the visual process as well as know the physical components of the eye?

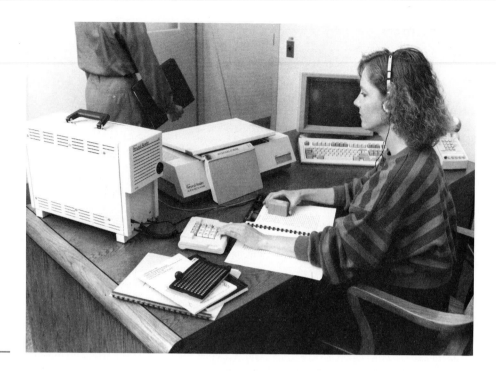

The Kurzweil Reading Machine converts printed matter into synthetic speech. (Courtesy of Kurzweil Computer Products)

□ Vision is the integration of many subskills that allow a person to process and respond to information that reaches the eyes.

FOCUS 4: Distinguish between medical-legal and educational definitions of blindness.

□ Medical-legal definitions are primarily concerned with the loss of visual acuity and central field of vision.

□ Educational definitions of blindness focus primarily on the individual's ability to use vision as an avenue for learning.

FOCUS 5: Define *partially sighted*.

□ A person who is partially sighted can still use vision as a primary means of learning.

□ A person who is partially sighted has a visual acuity greater than 20/200 but not greater than 20/70 in the better eye, after correction.

FOCUS 6: Identify the four types of refractive eye problems.

□ Hyperopia occurs when the eyeball is excessively short, forcing the light rays to focus behind the retina.

□ Myopia occurs when the eyeball is excessively long, forcing the light rays to focus on the plane in front of the retina.

□ Astigmatism occurs when the surface of the cornea is uneven or the lens is structurally defective, preventing light rays from converging at one point.

□ Cataracts occur when the lens becomes opaque, resulting in severely distorted vision or total blindness.

FOCUS 7: What are the three types of muscle disorders of the visual system?

□ Nystagmus is a continuous, involuntary rapid movement of the eyeballs.

□ Strabismus occurs when the muscles of the eye are unable to pull equally, and the eyes cannot focus together on the same object.

□ Amblyopia is the loss of vision due to the imbalance of the eye muscles.

FOCUS 8: Identify the disorders associated with the receptive structures of the eye.

□ Optic atrophy is a degenerative disease that results from deteriorating nerve fibers connecting the retina to the brain.

□ Retinitis pigmentosa is a hereditary condition resulting from a break in the choroid.

□ Retinal detachment occurs when the retina is separated from the choroid and the sclera.

□ Retrolental fibroplasia (RLF) occurs when premature infants are administered too much oxygen, resulting in the formation of scar tissue behind the lens.

FOCUS 9: What is the prevalence of visual disorders?

- At least 20 percent of the general population have some visual problems.
- About 0.1 percent of all school-age children meet the legal definition of blind or partially sighted.
- Approximately 75 percent of all blind people are over forty-five years of age.

FOCUS 10: Why is age of onset of a visual disorder significant to an individual's development?

- If an individual's sight is lost after the age of five, it is possible to retain some visual frame of reference.

FOCUS 11: In what ways can a visual disorder affect intellectual growth and development?

- A blind child's learning experiences may be significantly restricted by the lack of vision.
- A number of external factors may influence the intellectual differences between sighted and blind individuals, including unfavorable home environments and neurological and physical handicaps.

FOCUS 12: Why do many children with a visual disorder develop speech and language skills at a slower rate than their sighted peers?

- Children with a visual disorder are at a distinct disadvantage in developing speech and language skills because they are unable to visually associate a word with an object.
- Children with a visual disorder cannot learn speech by visual imitation, but must rely on hearing or touch for input.

FOCUS 13: Identify five factors that may influence the educational achievement of children with a visual disorder.

- Factors that may influence the educational achievement of a visually disordered student include: (1) late entry to school, (2) failure in inappropriate school programs, (3) loss of time in school due to illness, treatment, or surgery, (4) lack of opportunity, and (5) a slower rate of acquiring information.

FOCUS 14: What are three factors that may lead to greater social difficulties for individuals with a visual disorder?

- People with a visual disorder are unable to imitate the physical mannerisms of others and do not develop body language, an important form of social communication.
- A sighted person may misinterpret what is said by a person with a visual disorder because visual cues may not be consistent with the spoken word.
- People with a visual disorder are often excluded from social activities that are integrally related to the use of vision, thus reinforcing the mistaken idea that they do not want to participate.

FOCUS 15: What effect does a visual disorder have on orientation and mobility?

- The lack of sight may prevent people with a visual disorder from understanding their own relative position in space.
- A visual disorder may affect fine motor coordination and interfere with the ability to manipulate objects.

FOCUS 16: What effect does a visual disorder have on perceptual development?

- The blind child's perceptual discrimination abilities in the areas of texture, weight, and sound are comparable to those of sighted peers.
- People who are blind do not perform as well as sighted people on complex tasks of perception, including form identification, spatial relations, and perceptual-motor integration.

FOCUS 17: Identify at least seven congenital factors that may result in a visual disorder.

- Genetically determined factors that may result in a visual disorder include a deterioration of the choroid and retina, malignant tumors on the retina, detachment of the retina, loss of function of optic-nerve fibers, cataracts, myopia, lesions of the cornea, abnormalities of the iris, absence of the eyeball, and an enlargement of the eyeball.

FOCUS 18: Identify at least six acquired factors that may result in a visual disorder.

- Acquired factors associated with visual disorders include drug abuse, radiation, prenatal infections, prolonged use of oxygen with premature infants, accidents, tumors, inflammations, and vascular diseases.

FOCUS 19: How is visual acuity measured?

- Visual acuity is measured through the use of the Snellen Test.

FOCUS 20: What are three steps that can be taken to prevent visual disorders?

- Visual disorders may be prevented through genetic screening and counseling, appropriate prenatal care, and early developmental assessment.

FOCUS 21: Identify three significant strides medicine has made in the treatment of visual disorders.

- The development of optical aids, including corrective glasses and contact lenses, has greatly improved the individual's access to the visual world.

□ Medical treatment may range from extremely complex surgical procedures such as corneal transplants, to drug therapy such as atropinization (washing out the eye with the alkaloid drug atropine).

FOCUS 22: Why is the availability of appropriate mental health services important for people with a visual disorder?

□ The availability of mental health services is important because an individual's poor self-concept and general feeling of inferiority should be addressed.

□ Mental health services include infant stimulation programs, family counseling, and individual counseling relative to preparation for employment and independent living.

FOCUS 23: What is the purpose of an educational assessment for students with a visual disorder?

□ A multidisciplinary team assesses the student's cognitive ability, academic achievement, language skills, motor performance, and social/emotional functioning.

□ Assessment also focuses on how the visually disordered student uses any remaining vision in conjunction with other senses.

FOCUS 24: What is the range of educational services available to students with a visual disorder?

□ Residential facilities try to provide opportunities for blind children and youth to gain the same kind of experiences that would be available if these individuals were growing up in their own communities.

□ The vast majority of blind and partially sighted individuals live at home, attend local public schools, and interact within their local communities.

□ Within the public-school system, services range from regular class placement with little or no assistance, to special day schools.

FOCUS 25: Identify two essential content areas that should be included in an educational program for a student with a visual disorder.

□ Beyond a basic core curriculum, certain content areas are essential to the student's success, including mobility and orientation training and the acquisition of daily living skills.

FOCUS 26: In what ways can communication media facilitate learning for people with a visual disorder?

□ Through communication media, such as optical aids in conjunction with auditory and tactile stimuli, visually disordered individuals can better develop an understanding of themselves and the world around them.

□ Tactile media include the raised-line Braille system and the Optacon scanner.

□ Specialized auditory media include the Kurzweil Reading Machine, talking calculators, talking-book machines, record players, and audio tape recorders.

Debate Forum

Public Schools or Special Schools—Where Should Blind Children Be Educated?

In 1900, the first class for blind students in the public schools opened in the city of Chicago. Prior to this time, blind children in the United States were educated in state residential schools, where they lived away from their families. Up until 1950, the ratio of students attending schools for the blind to those in regular public schools was about 10 to 1. However, in 1950 children with retrolental fibroplasia increased the number of blind children attending public schools. By 1960, more blind children were being educated with their nonhandicapped peers in regular public schools than in schools for the blind.

The issue of what is the most appropriate educational environment for blind children continues to be debated in this country. The following are some representative points of view:

Point Blind children should be educated in the public schools alongside their seeing peers. This allows the child to remain at home with the family, which is just as important for these children as it is for their nonhandicapped friends. Schools for blind children have endeavored over the years to offer the best education possible and one that is intended to be equivalent to that for seeing children. However, these schools cannot duplicate the experiences of living at home and being a part of the local community. Although it can be argued that the special school is geared entirely to the needs of the blind child, there is much more to education than a segregated educational environment can provide. During the blind child's growing years, he or she must be directly involved in the "seeing world" in order to have the opportunity to adjust and become a part of society.

Counterpoint   The special school for blind children provides a complete education that is oriented entirely to individual needs. The teachers in these schools have years of experience in working exclusively with blind children and are well aware of appropriate educational experiences to help them reach their fullest potential. Additionally, these special schools are equipped with a multitude of educational resources developed for blind children. The public schools are not able to offer blind children the intensive and individualized programs in such areas as music, physical education, arts, crafts, and the like that are available through schools for blind children. The strength of a school for blind children is that it is entirely geared to the specialized needs of the blind and thus can more effectively teach the skills necessary to adapt to life experiences.

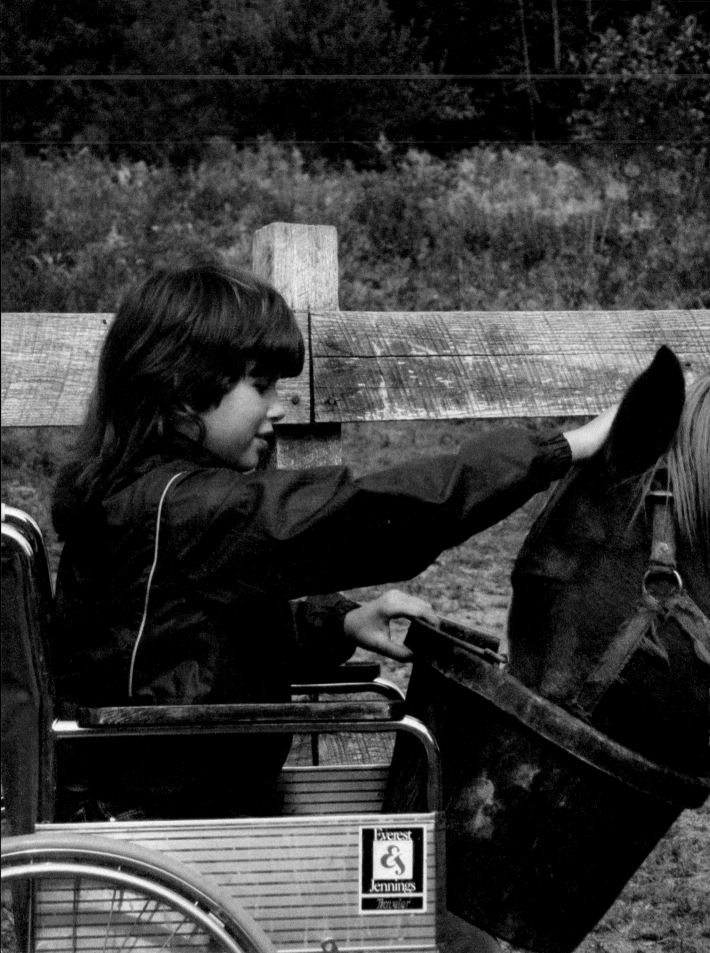

11 Physical Disorders

To Begin With...

- Five Reasons I Play Wheelchair Basketball
  by Jill Sager
  Because I enjoy the competition. Because I enjoy the speed. Because I like how my body feels. Because I like calling myself a jock. Because it makes me feel good about myself (Brown et al., 1985).

- Disabled persons who cannot speak or move their limbs can communicate through a computer called the Eyetyper. A camera scans the user's eyes and interprets the key the user has selected. The computer then prints that character. A voice synthesizer can speak the typed message aloud (*Education Daily*, 1984).

- Remember that using a wheelchair is not, in itself, a tragedy. The chair makes it possible for the user to be independently mobile and therefore offers opportunities to exercise personal freedom (Stroud & Sutton, 1988).

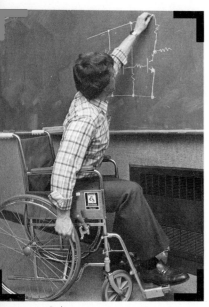

Rob

It was late August and very hot. This was the type of day that made the swimming hole the only place to be. Rob was a high school freshman, rather thin, and this year he had passed the magic six-foot-four-inch mark that was so essential to his first love—basketball. At this moment, however, he was intent on the pool of water below him as his friends cheered and shouted challenges for him to dive. He had jumped before, but swimming was not his strong suit, and a dive from this height was something new.

Rob does not remember leaving the rock overhang or hitting the water. His next conscious act involved an attempt to respond to his friend's frantic cry for him to move his legs.

Later on doctors pounded him with small mallets, pricked him with pins. He could see them doing these things, but could feel nothing. His spinal cord had been severed when he struck the large tree trunk below the surface of the water. Days later, after he had been transferred to the university hospital, he still could not believe that the damage was permanent. He kept telling himself that he would soon be up and moving around and that he would return to school within a few weeks.

More than two years elapsed before Rob returned to school. During that time, he remained in the hospital, although he had some brief visits home. He underwent many tests, and physical therapists worked with him daily. After two years Rob still could not move his legs, although he had some minimal control of his arms. The physicians told him that the upper part of his spinal cord had less severe damage, but the lower part of the spinal cord had been completely severed. He had no bladder or bowel control and soiled his clothes without even knowing it.

Rob's buddies were no longer in the same classes, and some of them had graduated. Consequently, he had virtually no social life, which in some ways was all right with him, because he was embarrassed by the many problems associated with his accident. The physical problems were bad enough, but they were compounded by his emotional difficulties. His depression was chronic and severely hampered his life in nearly every way. He had difficulty studying and generally felt like a loser, something that he had never experienced before. Rob's saving grace was his family. They supported him strongly, obtaining counseling and participating in the therapy sessions when necessary.

With the passage of time Rob made the necessary adjustments. He still loves basketball and attends every game at the university, where he now teaches. He finished his schooling and was awarded a Ph.D. in psychology at the age of twenty-eight. Last year he was promoted to the rank of associate professor and received tenure based on his active research and teaching effectiveness. Certainly his life is different, but it is one that he is proud of. His goals have changed, but he has no remorse, because Rob realizes that most people's goals change from time to time.

Defining Physical Disorders

The term **physical disorders** generally refers to impairments that interfere with an individual's mobility, coordination, communication, learning, or personal adjustment. These impairments are usually diagnosed by physicians early in a child's life. Primary care physicians (pediatricians or general practitioners) ordinarily refer children suspected of having serious physical impairments to other specialists. These specialists refine the diagnosis and recommend treatment. They are also responsible for determining the extent of an impairment and the consequences of the disability. A variety of medical and rehabilitation personnel may be involved in treatment, depending on the nature of the problem(s). As a youngster with physical disorders grows older, many different disciplines may be included in the total treatment program, including psychology, education, vocational rehabilitation, and social services.

FOCUS 1
What are physical disorders?

Factors That Influence the Impact of Physical Disorders

The overall impact of a physical disorder depends on several factors: (1) age of onset, (2) degree of disability, (3) visibility of the condition, (4) family and social support, (5) attitudes toward the individual, and (6) social status with peers (Lewandowski & Cruickshank, 1980). Each of these factors interacts with the others.

FOCUS 2
What are six factors that influence the overall impact of physical disorders on children and adolescents?

Age of Onset. A child born with paralyzed legs is likely to be severely limited in the number and types of exploratory activities he or she can pursue. The growth and development derived from crawling around household furniture and other items is missing to a certain extent. Likewise, the usual learning gained from being able to explore freely by walking, climbing, and running is absent in varying degrees. Skill acquisition in the social domain may also be impeded, because the child may not have the same level of opportunity to interact with peers and learn from them as do normal children.

Youth like Rob, who become paralyzed in lower body extremities, are faced with different problems. Such individuals must deal with a condition for which they have little or no preparation. By contrast, young children with congenital physical conditions have never really known what it is like to use their legs freely for running, jumping, and walking. These children adjust to the paralysis more gradually, while those injured later in life must deal with the stark realities of their preaccident and postaccident functioning. Also, those injured later may have already gleaned from their environment many of the basic academic and social skills necessary for successful participation in society. As noted above, the child with a congenital problem or one who is injured at a very young age must master these skills in a more restrictive environment.

Degree of Disability. Some physical disorders are very disabling, in that they have a pronounced effect on the individual's capacity to speak, move about independently, dress oneself, and engage in various motor activities. In Rob's case, the degree of his disability limited his mobility and some opportunities for socialization, but it had little, if any, impact on his ability to obtain an education.

Visibility of the Condition.   Some physical disorders are very visible. The presence of the disorder may be signaled by a wheelchair or other prosthetic device which the child, youth, or adult uses. For example, a young boy shopping with his mother may be very curious about a young adult with spastic cerebral palsy. The involuntary movement associated with this form of cerebral palsy may be a behavior that the boy has never before observed. In other cases, it may be very difficult to detect a disorder unless you have spent a lot of time with the individual. Such is often the case with seizure disorders or epilepsy. In our case study, Rob had a very visible condition resulting from his accident. The presence of him in his wheelchair provoked a lot of attention when he returned to school. This attention, however, gradually subsided. Over the next several years, he learned to adjust to the peculiar looks of young children and others as he went shopping, traveled to school, and attended various sporting events.

Family and Social Support.   Family and social support are essential to the long-term adjustment of children and youths affected by physical disorders. For example, the support Rob received from his family played a major role in his becoming an active participant in society. His attitude about himself was significantly influenced by his family and other friendships that he developed over time. His positive beliefs about himself played an important role in his becoming a highly skilled researcher and teacher. His disability, although psychologically painful at times, did not prevent him from succeeding and utilizing his abilities. Many colleges now offer specialized support to students with physical disorders and other handicapping conditions. These services are invaluable to all the students who are pursuing independence as well as professional training (Morfee & Morfee, 1987).

Attitudes toward the Individual.   Individuals with physical disabilities are very much impacted by the attitudes and expectations of others. Parent and sibling attitudes exert a strong influence on the strides a disabled child or youth makes in adjusting to a physical disorder. For example, Rob's eventual accomplishments as a teacher and researcher were very much an outgrowth of his parents' attitudes and expectations during the challenging years immediately following his injury. The attitudes of teachers and employers also play an important role in the success of persons with physical disorders throughout their life spans.

Social Status with Peers.   Physical disabilities often interfere with an individual's socialization and growth. Reduced physical mobility often prevents the person from participating in many of the social and physical activities available to those without disabilities. For example, think about the games you played as a child and what you learned about yourself and others while playing these games. Fortunately, some headway has been made in adapting games and toys to children with physical disabilities (Illinois State Board of Education, 1986; Shaeffer, 1988; Williams & Matesi, 1988).

The socialization and career-related goals of those with physical disabilities are similar to those of their nondisabled peers. Disabled adolescents often anticipate and think about completing school, preparing for a career, engaging in courtship activities, getting married, and becoming parents. Many, if not all, of these activities and goals are achievable for persons with physical impairments. However, their achievement is influenced by a number of variables.

Physically disabled girls experience unique problems in preparing for the world of work (Olsen, 1986). Major problems include a lack of strong female role models, insufficient transition planning, and inadequate interaction with nonhandicapped peers. Additionally, adolescent females with cerebral palsy have significantly lower levels of self-esteem, in comparison with like handicapped boys and nondisabled peers (Magill & Hurlbut, 1986).

It is worth noting in this regard that research on the interactions of able-bodied people with the physically disabled reveals several interesting findings. Able-bodied people in face-to-face interaction with disabled individuals tend to maintain more physical distance, terminate their conversations more quickly, feel less comfortable about the communication, display less variability in expressions, smile less, engage in less eye contact, and exhibit greater motor inhibition (Albrecht, 1976). All these factors have an immense impact on the communication process, the roles that people with physical disabilities assume, and the feedback they receive regarding their competency and adequacy.

In an interesting study conducted by Armstrong, Rosenbaum, and King (1987), gender-matched, able-bodied schoolmates were paired with forty-six physically impaired schoolmates for weekly social activities over a three-month period. Attitudes of 43 percent of the able-bodied children changed significantly, in a positive direction, over the time period. A secondary outcome of this project was significant positive changes in the attitudes of the mothers and fathers whose children were "buddies" to the physically impaired students.

Contemporary Western society tends to place great value on physical beauty, prowess, independence, and mobility. It is readily evident that these attributes and conditions are difficult for the individual with physical disabilities to achieve. However, with appropriate and comprehensive treatment, individuals with physical disorders can redefine their roles and pursuits and thereby achieve the independence and other goals needed for successful living. This notion was illustrated in our vignette of Rob.

Architectural and Transportation Barriers.   Architectural barriers in buildings, and transportation barriers, may cause difficulties in terms of both leisure activities and employment. Several advocacy organizations in the United States now have a so-called "adopt a curb" program. Advocacy leaders persuade businesses and other organizations to pay for the reconstruction of curbs. Newly remodeled curbs have ramps rather than steps, making crossing the street and moving independently much easier for those who travel by wheelchair.

Many physically disabled people would like to work but have no means of transporting themselves. Now many transit systems provide several options for individuals who need assistance in getting to work. However, although progress has been made, many older buildings remain inaccessible for those with physical disabilities.

There are a great number of physical disorders and diseases that affect

WINDOW 11—1

I'm Not Opposed to Miracles

My means of motion is one of two wheelchairs. One of these chairs is a typical wheelchair, not unlike many that you frequently see in hospitals for transporting patients. The other chair is a new, electronically driven model. It's powered by several batteries and is a real boon to me since I can direct the motion and speed of the chair by myself. Also, I can use this chair without an assistant. When I use my old wheelchair, I must be propelled by an aide, my wife, or one of my children.

I like my new chair and the freedom it allows me, but there are still a lot of barriers that interfere with my getting around. Take my church, for example. I have no trouble getting into the church. It has a very suitable ramp, and I have access to many areas in the church. But I can't easily attend my Sunday school class without considerable effort on the part of others, and I get tired of having people help me. I like to do things on my own. I like to be as independent as I can. This is one of the reasons I enjoy my new electronic chair so much. With it, I can get around without major assistance from others. However, the electronic chair isn't yet equipped with "stair climbers."

Let me put it this way. My Sunday school class is a mere six steps up from a major hallway in the church. In order to get to my Sunday school class, I need someone to lift me and my chair up six steps to the second level of the building. You might say to yourself, "What's the problem?" "Aren't the members of your church compassionate?"

The problem is basically this. If I choose to be independent by using my new electronic wheelchair, I can enter the church almost unaided. I can also move from one room to another on the main floor of the church without being propelled by someone else. But the electronic chair weighs about 120 pounds. If you add my weight to that of the chair's, you have the hefty sum of 250 plus pounds. Raising me the six steps vertically to attend my Sunday school class is nothing short of a modern-day miracle. I'm not opposed to miracles. I just like to be independent.

Mark, *securities firm owner*

children, adolescents, and adults. We limit our coverage to a representative sample of major physical conditions. They have been subdivided into two areas: central nervous system disorders, and skeletal and muscular disorders. Typical of the central nervous system disorders are **cerebral palsy, seizure disorders (epilepsy), spina bifida,** and **spinal-cord injuries.** Conditions in the skeletal and muscular disorders category include **arthritis, amputations,** and **muscular dystrophy.**

CENTRAL NERVOUS SYSTEM DISORDERS

Cerebral Palsy

The whole time I was growing up I had friends who were older than I because kids my own age just never accepted me. I had braces on my legs until I was in the fourth grade. The kids were always making fun of me and being cruel. They would never let me join in games with them. I guess older kids tolerated me because they saw me as just a young kid hanging around with them. I was fat when I was younger, and because my cerebral palsy made it hard for me to go to the bathroom, I was always wetting my pants. That made things worse, because not only did I look terrible, I also smelled terrible.

My mother would get very upset when I wet my pants. She thought I did it because I was too lazy to go to the bathroom. I would get to the point where I was wetting my pants every day, and my mother would let it go for about a week and then she would explode. She was very hurt and angered by my problem, and she also was ashamed that I couldn't control myself better.

I had the same problem in school. My first-grade teacher . . . wouldn't let me use the bathroom by myself. She used to claim that I couldn't walk down the stairs alone, which was completely untrue. This meant I didn't get a chance to use the bathroom all day, and by the time I got home I had already wet my pants.

When I was in school, I would start crying if any of the other children started talking about my braces or the way I walked. I spent most of my elementary school years in the back of the classroom crying. The kids didn't even have to say anything malicious; they only needed to mention that I was different to start me crying. I just couldn't cope with hearing about how different I was.

In the seventh grade, when I was 11, I had an operation on my bladder. I finally had some control over myself and stopped wetting my pants. That improved my self-image a lot. I also started going to a new school—it was like I was making a new start in life. I took theatre and music lessons, and learned how to handle a camera.

Theatre was the best thing that happened at that time. For the first time in my life, I started seeing myself as a person and not just a fat, crippled girl. When you are involved in theatre you have to be very honest with yourself. I had to start coping with and accepting the fact that I was different. Once I could admit this, I was on my way to becoming able to deal with other people's reactions to me.

I know that I will never be able to do things that take a lot of physical strength or endurance. I've tried dance, skiing, roller skating, baseball, football—almost everything you could think of; I can't do any of these things well, but it's very important to me that I've been willing to try them.

I'll always have my funny gait. It's really very slight, and other people don't always notice it, but I do. And sometimes when I go to buy a dress, the hem will hang more on one side than the other because my body is slightly lopsided. I can start feeling very sorry for myself at times, but when I think how very far I've come since all that crying I used to do in the back of the room, I really feel very lucky (Education Development Center, 1975, pp. 58–9).

Definitions and Concepts.   Cruickshank (1976) defines cerebral palsy as a neurological syndrome evidenced by motor problems, general physical weakness, lack of coordination, and physical dysfunction. The syndrome is not contagious, progressive, or remittent. Its seriousness and overall impact can range from very mild to very severe. A variety of classification schemes have been used to describe the different types of cerebral palsy, but the two major schemes for classification focus on the motor and topographical characteristics of the syndrome. The motor scheme emphasizes the type and nature of physiological involvement or impairment. The topographical scheme focuses on the various body parts or limbs that are affected.

Several categories of motor involvement have been identified, each varying from the others according to the nature and extent of brain damage involved. They are:

1. *Spasticity.* An individual with spastic cerebral palsy experiences great difficulty in using muscles for movement. Involuntary contractions of the muscles occur when the individual attempts to stretch or use various muscle groups. Spasticity prevents the person from performing controlled, voluntary motion.

2. *Athetosis.* An individual with athetosis is characterized by constant contorted twisting motions, particularly in the wrists and fingers. Facial contortions are also common. The continual movement and contraction of successive muscle groups prevents any well-controlled use of muscular motion.

3. *Ataxia.* An individual with ataxia experiences extreme difficulties in controlling both gross and fine motor movements. Problems related to balance, position in space, and directionality make coordinated movement extremely difficult if not impossible.

4. *Rigidity.* An individual with rigidity has one of the most severe and rare types of cerebral palsy. This condition is characterized by continuous and diffuse tension as the limbs are extended. Walking or movement of any type is extremely difficult.

5. *Tremor.* An individual with tremors manifests motions that are constant, involuntary, and uncontrollable. The motions are of a rhythmic, alternating, or pendular pattern. They occur as a result of muscle contractions that are continuously taking place.

6. *Atonia.* An individual with atonia has little if any muscle tone. The muscles fail to respond to any stimulation. This condition is extremely rare in its true form.

7. *Mixed.* An individual with mixed cerebral palsy may manifest parts and combinations of all the conditions described above.

The topographical classification approach refers not only to designations given to individuals with cerebral palsy but also to those who have paralytic conditions that resulted from accidents or such neurological diseases as polio. The topographical classification system includes seven categories:

1. Monoplegia, which involves one limb
2. Paraplegia, which involves the legs only
3. Hemiplegia, which involves one side of the body in a lateral fashion
4. Triplegia, which involves three appendages or limbs, usually both legs and one arm

5. Quadriplegia, which involves all four limbs or extremities

6. Diplegia, which refers to a condition in which the legs are more involved than the arms

7. Double hemiplegia, which involves both halves of the body, with one side more involved than the other.

Cerebral palsy is a complex and perplexing condition. The affected individual is likely to have mild to severe problems in nonmotor areas of functioning as well. These difficulties may include hearing deficits, speech and language impairments, intellectual deficits, visual impairments, and general perceptual problems. Because of the multifaceted nature of this condition, many people with cerebral palsy are considered to be multihandicapped. Thus cerebral palsy cannot be characterized by a set of homogeneous symptoms. It is a condition in which a variety of problems may be present in varying degrees of severity (Lewandowski & Cruickshank, 1980). For instance, 45 percent of those with cerebral palsy are considered to be mentally retarded. On the other hand, 35 percent are average to above average in intellectual ability, with the remaining percentage falling slightly below average (Heilman, 1952).

FOCUS 3
Why are many individuals with cerebral palsy considered to be multihandicapped or multi-impaired?

Causation and Prevalence. The causes of cerebral palsy are varied. Any condition that can adversely affect the brain may cause cerebral palsy. Chronic diseases, maternal infection, birth trauma, fetal infection, and hemorrhaging may all be sources of this neurological/motor disorder.

The prevalence of cerebral palsy ranges from 1.5 to 5 per 1,000 live births (Anderson, 1986; Whaley & Wong, 1985). The figures fluctuate as a function of several variables. Many children born with cerebral palsy come from families who are unable to obtain medical care. Consequently, many of these children do not become known to physicians or the agencies that collect prevalence information. As noted above, cerebral palsy is often accompanied by other conditions, such as learning disabilities and mental retardation. This overlap of conditions complicates the categorization process and affects prevalence figures reported.

Intervention. A number of professionals are needed to diagnose and provide treatment for the multifaceted nature of cerebral palsy. The initial diagnosis of the condition generally occurs very early in life. Subsequent diagnosis of accompanying problems and deficits occurs in an ongoing fashion. The assessment process can often be quite difficult if a child's condition includes impairments that make it difficult or impossible for him or her to respond to test items. This is particularly true if the child's language and motor skills are greatly impaired. Some attempts have been made to adapt test items to evaluate the cerebral palsied more adequately (e.g., Haeussermann, 1952; Peters, 1964), but these efforts have met with mixed results.

Treatment of cerebral palsy and its attendant conditions is best undertaken in a multidisciplinary fashion. Medical and motor aspects are handled by orthopedic personnel. Surgery may be necessary for treatment of muscle and tendon problems. Physical therapists provide training in muscle use, including how to utilize prosthetic and bracing devices effectively. Medical and physical therapy are aimed at achieving

FOCUS 4
Why is the treatment of cerebral palsy often multidimensional?

more controlled mobility and psychomotor behavior. For example, Maxi-Move, a new family-based program for children one to eight years of age, is now being used by many children with cerebral palsy (Lotz, 1986). This program fosters motor development and exercise through entertaining and natural activities that are common to children's home environments and communities.

Speech and language clinicians provide therapies directed at developing the individual's communication skills. The speech synthesizer is beginning to play a major role in helping young people with cerebral palsy to communicate with their peers, teachers, and other individuals (Tranowski & Drabman, 1986). Communication inaccuracy, error rates, and response times have been cut practically in half through the use of voice synthesizers.

Educational Considerations. Professionals who provide educational services for young children with cerebral palsy must be aware of several factors. These children and their parents have spent considerable time and energy dealing with referral agencies, referral procedures, evaluations, and payment for interventions. The preparations for their children's entrance into school programs may have been quite exhausting as well as frustrating. In fact, having their children attend school is a tremendous accomplishment. Educators who understand these factors may be in a better position to understand and assist these children and their parents.

Students with cerebral palsy often require daily physical therapy sessions. A physical therapist is responsible for developing students' physical skills. Therapy includes techniques designed to strengthen muscles, teach muscle relaxation, and optimize students' physical functioning for ambulation, independent travel, and movement.

In some cases, students with cerebral palsy may require surgery when bracing and physical therapy have not been effective in preventing or correcting an existing or potential deformity. After surgery, students generally return to school with a cast. When arrangements are made for comfortable seating and means for toileting, they can again receive the benefits of attending school and participating in learning activities.

The location and type of educational treatment depends on an individual's unique learning needs. If the condition is accompanied by significant intellectual or other deficits, an individual may be served in one of several special education environments. If the child can be suitably served in a regular school environment, this should occur as early as he or she can profit from this placement.

As a rule, education and related services for cerebral palsied students must be provided by a diverse team of medical and education professionals. These services generally span the entire time the student is in school.

Seizure Disorders (Epilepsy)

Mike was seventeen and had recurring moments of blankness and staring that bothered him. He had been seen by the doctors at the Family Practice Clinic, who referred him to a specialist. The specialist told Mike that he had something like small seizures—she actually mentioned petit mal or absence seizures—but she couldn't tell him what caused them, so

Reflect on This 11–1

Biofeedback and Keeping One's Mouth Closed and/or Open Voluntarily

Biofeedback is a relatively new procedure for helping individuals develop control of a variety of biological functions. Biofeedback is simply making an individual aware of some aspect of his or her biological functioning through some visual representation. Gradually, by exposure to the visual feedback, the person learns to produce a desired pattern of biological functioning. For example, a person may learn to produce a brain-wave pattern that is synonymous with relaxed behavior using information provided from sensors that monitor brain-wave functioning. Using the visual information provided by the sensors, the individual learns how it feels biologically to be relaxed. Gradually, the person learns through the biofeedback how to produce this state of mind without the aid of the sensors and monitors.

A youth with cerebral palsy may find it difficult to control the muscles that are responsible for opening and/or closing the jaw or mouth. A physical therapist skilled in biofeedback therapy may place surface electrodes over the group of jaw muscles responsible for opening and closing the mouth. The youth is then able to see the various electrical patterns that are produced when the jaw is closed and open. Gradually, with visual feedback provided by the surface electrodes and a monitoring device, the youth is able to gain voluntary control of either contracting or relaxing the jaw muscles. He can then open his mouth when it is closed or close it when it is open.

This same approach has been used experimentally with seizure disorders. Certain brain-wave patterns are associated with various types of seizures, and some seizures, as you know, are preceded by auras. The biofeedback therapist helps the person with seizures to learn how to voluntarily produce brain-wave patterns that are normal and uncharacteristic of seizure patterns. Again, some visual feedback is provided so that the person can learn how to produce at will the desired pattern of brain-wave functioning. Then, when the affected individual experiences an aura (a distinct physical sensation such as hearing a sound) or warning of the onset of a seizure, he or she may be able to avoid the seizure by intentionally producing an alternative brain-wave pattern.

Because the clinical use of biofeedback is in its infancy, the usefulness of this treatment approach is extremely limited. Future experimentation and refinement of the instrumentation used to monitor biological functions and provide feedback to individuals with health conditions will ultimately validate or invalidate this treatment procedure.

Mike decided she didn't know what she was talking about. He became quite uncooperative with the medical personnel and was intent on concealing his condition. His school performance became erratic, and he often pretended to have completed an assignment when he had not. Further, Mike blamed others for his performance problems.

Mike's parents were quite protective. They would not allow him to stay home alone or travel by himself, even to school. They did not explain to Mike what his problem was, talking to medical personnel behind his back. Mike was aware of this behavior and was further frightened by all the mystery. He became increasingly secretive about his "spells," tried to hide the problems, and grew increasingly dependent on his parents.

Mike was also bothered by related conflicts generated by his condition. Although he was frightened and dependent on his parents, he wanted to be more independent, to be like his peers, to hold a job. He had participated in counseling sessions at school for some time, but he could not admit openly that he had a problem, despite the fact that other students were able to talk about their disabilities. As he listened to them, Mike began to wonder whether he could also admit that he had difficulties, and if that would help him enter the world of his peers. Finally he mustered all his courage and nearly shouted to the group, "I have seizures too! Small ones." At that point everyone turned to him, but with supportive looks rather than the ridicule he had expected. He began to cry, and then talked about his fears for the entire session.

That was a turning point for Mike. He began to cooperate with the medical personnel and soon was receiving treatment, with excellent results. His seizures were dramatically reduced, and his feelings about himself were greatly enhanced. Although Mike's parents remained apprehensive, he insisted on continuing treatment and getting a part-time job.

Mike is now successful in insurance sales, and his supervisor anticipates a promising career. Mike has come a long way from when we first met him at age seventeen.

FOCUS 5
What are seizures?

Definitions and Concepts. The terms *seizure disorders* or *epilepsy* are used to describe a variety of disorders of brain function characterized by recurrent seizures. Seizures are clusters of behavior that occur in response to abnormal neurochemical activity in the brain. They typically have the effect of altering the individual's level of consciousness while simultaneously resulting in certain characteristic motor patterns (Dreifuss, 1988). Several classification schemes have been employed to describe the various types of seizure disorders. We briefly discuss two types of seizures, tonic/clonic and absence seizures (Dreifuss, 1988).

Tonic/clonic seizures, formerly identified as grand mal seizures, are often preceded by a warning signal known as an aura. The individual experiencing an aura senses a unique sound, odor, or physical sensation just prior to the onset of a seizure. In some instances the seizure is also signaled by a cry or other similar sound. With a loss of consciousness, the affected individual falls to the ground; this is the tonic phase of the seizure. Initially, the trunk and head of the body become rigid. This rigidity is followed by involuntary muscle contractions (violent shaking) of the extremities, which is the clonic phase of the seizure. Irregular breathing, blueness in the lips and face, increased salivation, loss of bladder and bowel control, and perspiration may occur to one degree or another. The nature, scope, frequency, and duration of such seizures vary greatly from person to person. Such seizures may last as long as twenty minutes or less than one minute. One of the more dangerous aspects of tonic/clonic seizures is potential injury from falling and striking objects in the environment. In responding to this type of seizure, it is best for observers to ease the person to the floor, if possible, remove any dangerous objects from the immediate vicinity, place a soft pad under the person's head (e.g., a coat or blanket), and allow the person to rest after the seizure has terminated. A period of sleepiness and confusion usually follows the seizure.

A person who has experienced a tonic/clonic seizure may exhibit drowsiness, nausea, headache, or a combination of these symptoms. Such symptoms should be treated with appropriate rest, medication, or other therapeutic remedies. Each individual's seizure characteristics and attendant aftereffects vary along a number of dimensions and should be treated with this variability in mind.

Absence seizures, formerly identified as petit mal seizures, often appear as a form of daydreaming. They are characterized by brief periods (moments or seconds) of inattention that may be accompanied by rapid eye blinking or head twitching. During these seizures "the brain's normal activity shuts down" (Dreifuss, 1988, p. 3). The individual's consciousness is altered in an almost imperceptible manner. Youngsters with this type of seizure disorder may experience these mini-seizures as often as one hundred times a day. Such inattentive behavior may be viewed as daydreaming by a teacher or work supervisor, but the suspected daydreaming is really a momentary burst of abnormal brain activity that the child or adult does not consciously control. The lapses in attention caused by this form of epilepsy can greatly hamper the individual's ability to respond properly to or profit from a teacher's presentation or a supervisor's instruction. Treatment and control of absence seizures is generally achieved through prescribed medication.

Diagnosis of the various types of seizure disorders occurs in a number of ways. As a rule, the actual medical diagnosis takes place after one or several seizure incidents have been observed in the person. The peak ages at which seizures are most likely to begin are in the newborn period, late infancy, pre-adolescence, and early adolescence.

Information provided by someone who has observed the seizure or seizures is absolutely essential in establishing an accurate diagnosis of seizure disorders. Such an observer may provide valuable information regarding the nature, duration, and circumstances surrounding the seizures. The informant may also provide additional information about the child's or youth's development and medical history. If necessary, recordings of seizure activity with an **EEG** (**electroenceph-alogram**) may provide additional information for the neurologist in developing appropriate treatment plans for the affected individual (Dreifuss, 1988).

Causation and Prevalence.   Exact causation of the various types of epilepsy remains unclear, but any condition that may adversely affect the brain and its functioning (head trauma, neural chemical irregularities, inflammation, and tumors) is a potential cause. Similarly, precise reasons for the actual triggering of a seizure are also unknown. In some instances, a seizure may be instigated by repetitive visual stimuli to which the seizure-prone individual is exposed. Seizures may also occur in normal individuals as a function of a fever, brain tumor, or disease.

Prevalence figures for seizure disorders vary. This is a function of the social stigma associated with them. Studies indicate that 0.6 to 0.9 percent of the population is directly affected by seizure disorders (Dreifuss, 1988). Seventy-five percent of all individuals who are affected by seizures experience their first one prior to their eighteenth birthday (Dreifuss, 1988).

Prevalence estimates also fluctuate according to the types of groups investigated and the time period selected for review. Children with cerebral palsy or moderate to severe mental retardation are much more likely to have seizure disorders than are their normal counterparts. Also, adults who have reached the stage of senescence (sixty to eighty years of age and older) are much more likely to have problems with convulsions. With regard to various time periods, the prevalence of seizure disorders caused by head injuries resulting from automobile accidents declined in the United States when the speed limit was reduced from 65 or 70 to 55 miles per hour. With the increased use of motorcycles for transportation, however, many youngsters and adults have developed seizures as a result of head injuries from motorcycle accidents.

The stigma associated with seizure disorders also plays a role in the accuracy of prevalence estimates. Many parents are reluctant to reveal that someone in their family has epilepsy. Consequently, they often do not share this information with school and other officials responsible for collecting data concerning prevalence levels. This is also true of those who develop the condition. They may be reluctant to report it for fear that they will lose their jobs, be unable to retain their driver's license, or suffer social rejection.

FOCUS 6
What three interventions are used with persons with seizure disorders?

Intervention. Treatment of the several epileptic conditions takes a variety of forms. Once a referral has been made by a general practitioner, pediatrician, or internist, the patient is interviewed and examined by a neurologist. During the interview, the neurologist attempts to (1) identify potential causes for the condition, (2) determine the exact nature and extent of seizure difficulties, and (3) determine the circumstances and events surrounding each seizure incident. The interview is accompanied by a thorough neurological exam. The electroencephalograph is fundamental to the diagnostic process and assists the neurologist in assessing brain-wave activity. This instrument is also helpful in identifying potential structural abnormalities within the brain. It should be noted that many seizure disorders are not detectable through electroencephalographic measures. A **CAT scan x-ray** of the brain is usually obtained to rule out the presence of a structural abnormality (brain tumor, hemorrhaging, etc.) that may account for the seizure. Using information from the interview and results derived from neurological measures, the neurologist may be able to prescribe an effective treatment program for the epileptic individual. Many types of seizures can be successfully treated with careful medical and drug management.

Anti-epileptic drugs must be chosen very carefully. Parents and affected individuals must balance the risk–benefit proportions of each medication. Once an anti-epileptic drug has been prescribed, parents and affected children should be educated in its use. They should be aware of the side effects of the drug and the necessity for regular administration. As you might guess, maintaining a regular medication regimen can be very challenging for children, teenagers, and their parents. In some instances, medication may be discontinued after several years of seizure-free behavior (Dreifuss, 1988). This is particularly true for those young children who do not have some form of underlying brain pathology.

As with other neurological conditions, some individuals with seizure disorders also have serious accompanying problems, such as mental retardation, cerebral palsy, and emotional or psychological difficulties. Each individual with a seizure disorder must be treated with an array of medical, educational, social, and psychological strategies. Special education is not generally required for children with seizure disorders unless the seizures are symptomatic of other, more serious impairments that adversely affect their academic and social functioning. Seizure-disordered individuals need responses from others that are calm and supportive. The treatment efforts of various professionals and family members must be carefully orchestrated to provide affected individuals with an optimal chance to profit from their abilities and talents (Reisner, 1988).

Educational Considerations. Perhaps the most important consideration in dealing with seizures disorders in classrooms and other settings are teachers' attitudes. To a great extent, these attitudes are mirrored in the ways in which they prepare children and youth for the occurrence of a seizure. Moreover, the modeling they provide for students in dealing with a seizure is incredibly important. A seizure incident can actually be turned into a rich learning experience for all concerned. Young children need to be given a simple explanation of what seizures are and how they are generally treated through various types of medication. Additionally, they need to know that seizures are not contagious. Last, teachers need to encourage understanding but not pity. Teachers' behaviors, more than anything else, serve as the guide to their students'.

Spina Bifida

I just turned twenty-one. I never thought I would actually reach the official age of adulthood, but it has come and gone; and I am, at least according to law, a little more responsible for my behavior. Actually, I've been responsible for a lot of my behavior since I was a young child. For reasons that I don't completely understand, I've always had a personal resilience that helped me deal with the challenges that have been an integral part of my life. My mother, who is an exquisitely beautiful woman, was very excited about my birth. I was her first child. The expectations she had for me were wonderful. But, within moments of my delivery, it was discovered that I had a serious birth defect known as spina bifida. This discovery altered many of my mom's expectations for me. Although my parents didn't know a great deal about spina bifida at the time, they shortly became specialists.

Their major concern at the time of my birth was not my physical appearance, even though the sack on my spine was quite gross, but the prevention of infection, my intellectual capacity, and the degree of paralysis.

The sack and related nerve tissue were surgically cared for very early in my life through several operations. Fortunately, the infection that was an ever-present threat during the first days and months of my existence was successfully prevented. Because of the location of the sack with neural tissue, I'm paralyzed from the waist down. I walk with the aid of crutches now.

As for my intellectual capacity, I've just completed my Bachelor's degree. I wasn't an academic superstar, but I did hold my own in my major, which is fashion merchandising.

To be frank with you, my greatest challenge hasn't been my paralysis per se, but my lack of bowel control. I'd love to have the facility that most normal people have, but I don't. I'm working on my attitude about this particular problem. I'm not nearly as sensitive about it as I once was.

This month I will be getting married. My husband is aware of the challenges that I will pose as his spouse, but I have a feeling that he will provide a few challenges that are totally unique to him as well.

FOCUS 7
What is spina bifida?

Definition and Concepts. Spina bifida is a birth defect of the nervous system. Until about the twelfth week of pregnancy, the backbone of a developing fetus remains open. If for some reason certain bones of the spinal column fail to close properly, an opening is formed. The abnormal opening may allow the contents of the spinal canal to flow between the bones that did not fully close. Spina bifida may or may not influence intellectual functioning, but it frequently involves some paralysis of various portions of the body, depending on the location of the opening. There are two types of spina bifida: **spina bifida occulta** and **spina bifida cystica.**

Spina bifida occulta is a very mild condition in which a small slit is present in one or several of the vertebral structures. Most people with spina bifida occulta are unaware of its presence unless they have had a spinal x-ray for some other condition. Spina bifida occulta has little if any impact on the developing infant. There are usually no other abnormalities of any kind.

There are two subdivisions of spina bifida cystica (see Figure 11–1). They are spina bifida meningocele and spina bifida myelomeningocele. The meningocele type presents itself in the form of a tumorlike sack on the back of the infant. This sack contains spinal fluid but no nerve tissue. In contrast, the myelomeningocele does contain nerve tissue. It is also the most serious variety of spina bifida in that it generally includes, as part of its debilitating effects, paralysis or partial paralysis of certain body areas, lack of bowel and bladder control, and mental retardation. There are two types of myelomeningocele: one in which the tumorlike sack is open, revealing the neural tissue, and one in which the sack is closed or covered with a combination of skin and membrane.

Children with spina bifida occulta exhibit the normal range of intelligence. Children with myelomeningocele generally have IQs in the low-average to mildly retarded ranges. For affected children whose learning capacity is normal or above average, no special educational programming is required.

Causation and Prevalence. The exact cause of spina bifida is unknown. There is a slight tendency for the condition to run in families. In fact, myelo-meningocele appears to be transmitted genetically through an **autosomal recessive trait** (Swaiman & Jacobsen, 1984). It probably occurs as a function of certain prenatal factors interacting with genetic predispositions. It is also possible that certain agents taken by the mother prior to or during the first few days of pregnancy may be responsible for the defect. The neural tube closes about the fourth week of embryonic development; thus **teratogens** present in the body before or during the fourth week of an infant's development may adversely affect the neural tube. Teratogens that may induce malformations in the spine include

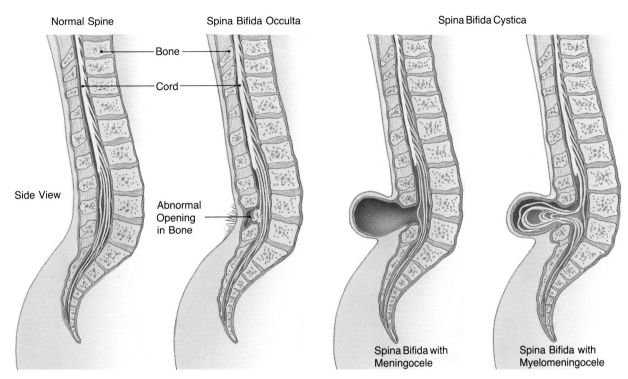

Normal Spine   Spina Bifida Occulta   Spina Bifida Cystica

Bone

Cord

Side View

Abnormal
Opening
in Bone

Spina Bifida with
Meningocele

Spina Bifida with
Myelomeningocele

Figure 11–1
Side Views of a Normal Spine, Spina Bifida Occulta, and Spina Bifida Cystica

radiation, maternal hyperthermia (high fever), vitamin A deficiency, excess glucose, and folic acid deficiency (Dobling, 1983; Swaiman & Jacobsen, 1984).

The prevalence figures for spina bifida (myelomeningocele and meningocele) vary markedly. The highest prevalence rate occurs in Ireland, with a figure exceeding 4 in 1,000 individuals. The lowest rate is found in tropical countries, where the condition occurs in 0.5 in 1,000 individuals or less. In the United States, estimates range from 0.3 to 0.9 in 1,000 live births (Shurtleff, Lemire, & Warkany, 1986). More females seem to develop the condition than males, with a ratio of about 3 to 1. Future research may reveal the reasons for these marked differences.

Intervention.   It is now possible to identify babies with myelomeningocele before they are born by means of certain sophisticated instruments and techniques: ultrasonic scanning of the fetus late in pregnancy to identify major defects; **fetoscopy,** a moderately risky procedure to identify small defects; and **amniocentesis,** a procedure in which the level of alphafetoprotein (AFP), a chemical marker of neurological defects, in the amniotic fluid is assessed. AFP is not a marker specific to spina bifida; it is a marker for neurological defects in general.

Immediate action is often called for when the child with myelomeningocele is born. Depending on the nature of the lesion, its position on the spine, and

FOCUS 8
What treatments are used to assist children with spina bifida?

the presence of other related conditions such as hydrocephalus, the parents and the consulting physician must determine whether immediate medical action should be taken. Such decisions are extremely difficult, for they often entail problems and issues that are not easily or quickly resolved. For example, 80 percent of the children with spina bifida myelomeningocele have an area of the spinal cord that is exposed. This places them at great risk for developing meningitis, which has a mortality rate of over 50 percent (Freeman, 1973; Lorber, 1974). The decision to undertake surgery is often made quickly if the tissue sack is located very low on the infant's back and there is no presence of hydrocephalus. In cases where the myelomeningocele is relatively high on the spine and other conditions are present, such as meningitis, surgery may not be performed.

Children with spina bifida myelomeningocele have little if any bowel or bladder control. The lack of control is directly attributable to the paralysis caused by the malformation of the spinal cord. In addition, children with this condition will be paraplegic and have no sensation of temperature or pain in their legs. As these children mature, they can be trained to regulate their bowel movements through the use of suppositories. Once this training has been achieved, the individual no longer needs to worry about the problems associated with accidental soiling (Williamson & Szczepanski, 1987).

Physical therapists play a critical role in helping these children, particularly younger children, as they learn to cope with the paralysis caused by myelomeningocele. This paralysis limits the child's exploratory activities, which are critical to later learning and sensory-motor performance. With this in mind, many such children are fitted with a modified skateboard, which allows them to explore their surroundings. Utilizing the strength in their arms and hands, they may become quite adept at exploring their home environments. Gradually they graduate to leg braces, crutches, a wheelchair, or a combination of the three.

Most children with spina bifida who have no signs of hydrocephalus have normal intelligence. Like other children, they may be average, below average, or above average in their intellectual performance. Consequently, they receive their education in a normal school environment. Exceptions relate to the physical environment of the school and the coordinated support needed by these youngsters. The facilities within the school should be suited to the children's physical needs. Coat hooks, lockers, and water sources may need to be lowered to accommodate those who are confined to wheelchairs. Specialized seating, tables, and desks may also be necessary.

Educational Considerations. Young students with the severe forms of spina bifida are often absent from school for significant periods of time for surgery, therapy, and other related medical appointments. If hospital or home stays are lengthy, homebound or hospital teachers may be beneficial in helping students stay current in their studies.

If a student uses a wheelchair or other walking aid, the physical environment of the classroom should be such that the student may move freely from one area to another. Also, provision should be made for emergency situations in which the student may need some assistance in exiting the classroom or building.

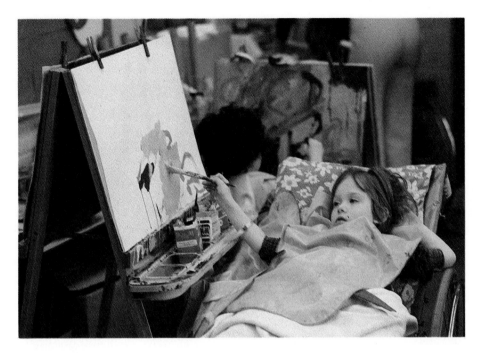

Most children with spina bifida who have no signs of hydrocephalus are of normal intelligence. (William Lupardo)

Spinal-Cord Injuries

Definitions and Concepts.   The spinal cord is the conduit through which the brain transmits messages to various parts of the body. It is basically a cable of nerve cells. The spinal cord controls both the motor and sensory functions of various parts of the body, in conjunction with peripheral nervous systems. Without adequate pathways, the messages and sensations generated from the nerve endings are not communicated to the brain. The spinal cord is enclosed by the spinal column, which is made up of thirty-three vertebrae. These vertebrae, together with the muscles attached to them, provide the protection for this invaluable communication network.

Spinal-cord injury occurs when the spinal cord is traumatized or transected (severed). The cord can be injured through extreme extension or flexion resulting from a fall, an automobile accident, or a sports injury. Transection of the cord may occur as a result of the same types of accidents, although such occurrences are extremely rare. Usually in such cases the cord is bruised or otherwise injured. Within a short time after the injury the cord appears to swell, and within hours hemorrhaging (bleeding) often occurs. Gradually, a self-destructive process ensues in which the affected area slowly deteriorates and the damage becomes irreversible. The greatest number of spinal-cord injuries occur between the ages of sixteen and thirty.

The overall impact of injury on an individual depends on the site and nature of the insult. If the injury occurs in the neck or upper back, the resultant paralysis and effects are quite extensive. If the injury occurs in the lower back, paralysis is confined to the lower extremities.

The physical characteristics of spinal-cord injuries are similar to those of spina bifida myelomeningocele. The terminology (paraplegia, quadriplegia, and hemiplegia) used to describe the impact is identical. It is worth noting however, that the terms *paraplegia, quadriplegia,* and *hemiplegia* are global descriptions of functioning and not precise enough to accurately convey the actual level of an individual's functioning. For example, the degree of paralysis in two paraplegics may be substantially different, depending on the location and nature of the injury. In general, we can assume that the person with a spinal-cord injury experiences some level of paralysis from the point of the injury downward through the body. The amount of sensation lost and the degree of paralysis experienced by the individual depends on the amount of damage to the spinal cord and nerve roots at the point of insult.

As we saw with Rob, the losses of voluntary movement and sensation are often staggering to the injured individual. Some quadriplegics are not able to move or change their body position without the aid of an assistant or mechanical device. Even sitting is difficult for some quadriplegics. The paraplegic who has good use of one or both arms is able to compensate in part for paralysis of the lower extremities. Injury to the spinal cord also affects other bodily systems. Bowel and bladder control are often lost. The individual may be incapable of perspiring in the affected areas due to sensorial loss, which seriously hinders the body's natural cooling system. The respiratory system may also be affected if the injury occurs in the neck region. In such cases, the individual may need to rely on a respirator or rocking bed for assistance in breathing.

Causation and Prevalence.   While falls, accidents, and sports injuries can cause spinal-cord injury, various diseases can have the same result. Cancer, tumors, infections, abscesses of the spine, arthritis, multiple sclerosis, and poliomyelitis can all cause spinal-cord injury. Motor vehicle accidents are responsible for approximately half of all spinal-cord injuries. Twenty-five percent of the injuries are derived from falls. Ten percent are a function of sports-related injuries. Some 5,000 to 10,000 new cases appear each year, 75 percent of which involve males. Individuals in the age-range from fifteen to thirty-four are most likely to incur such an injury. The overall prevalence rate for spinal-cord injuries is 3 for every 100,000 individuals (Yashon, 1986).

FOCUS 9
What are seven treatments provided to individuals with spinal-cord injuries?

Intervention.   The immediate care rendered to a person with a spinal-cord injury is critical. If proper procedures are not employed early after the accident or onset of the condition, the impact of the injury can be magnified.

The first phase of treatment, provided by a receiving hospital or specialized center, is the management of shock. Quickly thereafter the individual is immobilized in order to prevent movement and further damage. As a rule, surgical procedures are not undertaken immediately. The major goal of medical treatment at this point is to stabilize the spine and prevent further complications. Catheterization may be employed to control urine flow, and steps may be taken to reduce swelling and bleeding at the injury site. Traction may be utilized to stabilize certain portions of the spinal column and cord. Medical treatment of spinal-cord injuries is long and often tedious. Once physicians have successfully stabilized

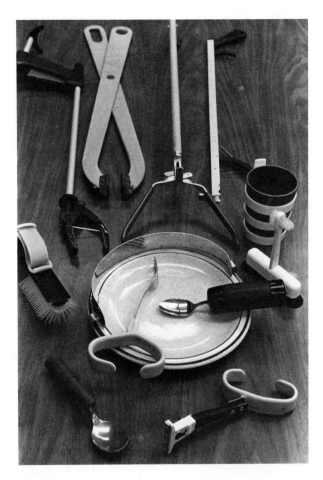

A variety of orthotic devices (reachers, plate guards, modified eating utensils, etc.) have been devised to assist persons with physical disorders. (John Telford)

the spine and treated any other medical conditions, the rehabilitation process proceeds at an accelerated pace. The individual is taught to use new muscles and to take advantage of any and all residual muscle strength. The injured person is also taught to use orthopedic devices and equipment such as hand splints, braces, reachers, head sticks for typing, and plate guards. Together with an orthopedic specialist, occupational and physical therapists become responsible for the re-education and training process. Psychiatric and other support personnel are also engaged in the rehabilitation activities. Psychological adjustment to a spinal-cord injury and the impact of the injury on an individual's functioning can take a great deal of time (see Figure 11–2). The goal of all treatment is the achievement of independence to the maximum degree possible. This may take many months or years, and the medical expenses can be staggering given the type of equipment and treatment that is required.

As the individual masters necessary **self-care skills**, other educational and career objectives are pursued, with the assistance of the rehabilitation team. The members of this team change constantly as the skills and needs of the individual

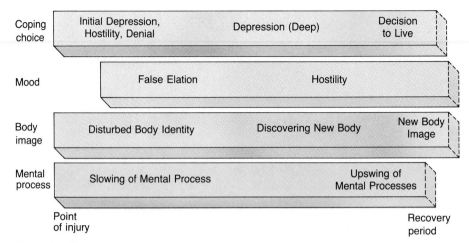

Figure 11–2
Psychological Changes after Spinal Cord Injury (*Source:* LeBaron, S., Currie, D., & Zeltzer, L. [1984]. "Coping with Spinal Cord Injury in Adolescents." In R. W. Blum [Ed.], *Chronic Illness and Disabilities in Childhood and Adolescence.* Orlando, Fla.: Grune & Stratton, Inc.)

change. Schooling for individuals with spinal-cord injuries is similar to that for any children or adults. Modifications are necessary in the school environment (providing grab-bars near chalkboards, doors, and stairs; lowering towel dispensers; changing stall-door widths and swinging directions for doors; ordering adapted utensils; etc.), and the methods by which these individuals express the learning they have acquired may have to be altered. Note takers may be necessary. The individual may use a tape recorder to verbally respond to test items or assignments. A word processor or other computerized device may be used to convey information if the individual has learned to use a head stick or other adaptive instrument.

Vocationally and professionally, an individual with a spinal-cord injury may need to be retrained or reeducated with assistance provided by vocational rehabilitation services. Some have limitations that make it necessary to have full-time attendant care. Such care providers assist with all the daily functions of bathing, grooming, dressing, shopping, and other activities. Recreational pursuits also need to be changed. Many people who are limited to wheelchairs enjoy bowling, swimming, square-dancing, basketball, and even golf. Since 1960, many wheelchair athletes have enjoyed participating in the Paraolympics. The adaptation process is often arduous and challenging, but with appropriate support the individual with a spinal-cord injury can lead a fulfilling and meaningful life.

Educational Considerations. Like other conditions we have discussed, teacher attitudes and behaviors are very important. For a youth who has been severely injured in a sporting or vehicle-related accident, the road to "full functioning" emotionally and socially can be very arduous and challenging. Teachers who understand the needs of such a student and respond appropriately contribute significantly to the healing process.

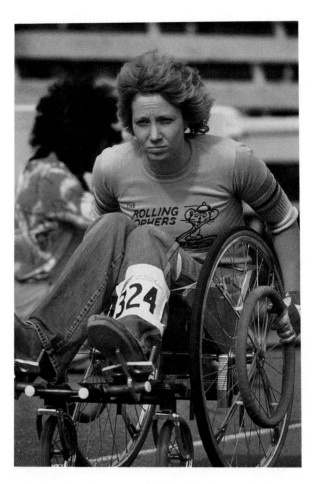

Recreational activities are important for people with spinal cord injuries. Many athletes in wheelchairs compete in distance races. (J. Myers/FPG)

SKELETAL AND MUSCULAR DISORDERS

Arthritis

Definition and Concepts. **Arthritis** is a disease typified by pain in and around the joints. Individuals of all ages can be affected by this condition. In children, the condition is known as **juvenile rheumatoid arthritis.** Usually it manifests itself between eighteen months and four years of age; however, it may present itself at any time during childhood (Schumacker, Klippel, & Robinson, 1988). Arthritis in children is often preceded by a respiratory infection and can affect the entire body. Juvenile rheumatoid arthritis is frequently masked by symptoms characteristic of other disorders. For example, instead of joint pain and swelling, the initial symptoms or signs may be fever, rash, eye pain, liver swelling, lung fibrosis, or blood-clotting abnormalities. Thus, in the early stages of the disease before there is clear joint involvement, the physician may have trouble arriving at the correct diagnosis. Children who develop this condition are influenced by its presence in several significant fashions. They may miss a considerable amount of school. They may not be able to participate fully in many of the activities pursued by others during recesses or physical education periods. Fortunately, half of all children who have arthritis experience a complete remission of symptoms without serious side effects, and another one-quarter experience a complete remission with only limited crippling side effects. Spondylitis of adolescence, a form of rheumatoid arthritis, affects the entire body rather than isolated joints or areas. It is characterized by pain in the legs and lower back which results from swelling vertebrae. It occurs during the teenage and young-adult years and can be physically debilitating.

Causation and Prevalence.   The exact causes of various arthritic conditions are not fully known. The initiating factors may be bacteria or viruses, and for reasons not completely understood, the body responds to these bacteria or viruses in a pathogenic (disease-producing) fashion. The actual pathogenic process is complicated and involves many interactions. Ultimately the critical components and fluids of the joints are altered, and the joints eventually become deformed. Spondylitis of adolescence appears to have some genetic basis, as it tends to be a familial condition passed from generation to generation.

About 1 percent of the adult population have rheumatoid arthritis (Rodnan & Schumacher, 1983). Five to 10 percent of this adult population are diagnosed as having arthritis during their childhood years. The Arthritis Foundation suggests that about 60,000 to 200,000 children are affected by this condition in the United States (Rodnan & Schumacher, 1983). Many more females than males (3:1) are affected during the first two decades of life.

FOCUS 10
What major intervention is used to aid children with arthritis?

Intervention.   Early diagnosis and treatment are important to minimize deformity and disability. The immediate goals of therapy are relief of symptoms as well as maintenance of joint position and strength and muscular function. Aspirin continues to be the most basic anti-inflammatory medication, although other medications are available. Anti-inflammatory medications can cause side effects, such as stomach upset, stomach bleeding, easy bruising, kidney damage, and anemia, which may substantially influence the individual's academic, social, and behavioral performance. Teachers, parents, and health personnel need to be aware of these potential influences and respond with sensitivity.

Other interventions for children and adolescents with arthritis include exercises to maintain or regain muscle and joint strength and range of motion and function; use of daytime and nighttime resting splits to reduce contractures at the wrists; daily adoption of the prone (lying-down) position for extended periods of time to reduce hip flexion contractures; and, when appropriate, active physical therapy (Schumacker, Klippel, & Robinson, 1988).

Rheumatoid arthritis is a condition that varies in intensity. During certain phases or time periods, affected individuals may have greater need for medication due to increased pain caused by the inflammation. In addition, those with arthritis should be encouraged to participate in activities requiring the use of all joints as much as possible. As with other impairments, care providers should avoid performing tasks for arthritic children that they can do for themselves. Overprotection on the part of others lessens the current and eventual ability of the arthritic individual to deal with the school and community and may lead to unnecessary dependency. As affected children move into adolescence, vocational and psychological counseling may be helpful.

Educational Considerations. Students with arthritis seem to be the least affected by their condition from midmorning to early afternoon. Soreness and stiffness in the distressed joints seem to increase in the later afternoon (Athreya & Ingall, 1984). Writing and other related physical activities may need to be adjusted accordingly. Additionally, extended sitting or writing may be difficult for these students. Consultation with parents may be very helpful in planning appropriate regimens. Also, teachers may play an important role in monitoring the effects of medication.

Amputations

Definitions and Concepts. There are two types of amputations: congenital and acquired. Congenital amputations are apparent at birth. They occur for a variety of reasons, which are not fully understood. As a normal fetus develops, tiny arm buds appear on the twenty-sixth day after conception. Shortly thereafter, these buds begin to develop into the arm and hand components. At the end of the first month the fetus develops leg buds, which progress in a similar fashion. When a child is born with an amputation, it means that some portion of the budding process was terminated prematurely. Children may be born with minor congenital malformations or the complete absence of limbs. Their adjustment to the condition is generally less traumatic than those who acquire an amputation later in life, as teenagers or young adults. Children with congenital amputations also accept and respond more favorably to the use of prosthetic devices than those who experience amputations later on.

Acquired amputations are generally the result of an injury or a therapeutic surgical procedure. Relatively few children have acquired amputations. Children who have cancer of the bone in an extremity may have to undergo surgery to remove the affected limb. Most acquired amputations occur as a function of accidents or injuries later in a child's life.

Causation and Prevalence. The causes of congenital amputations are not completely understood. Over the years, we have become aware of a variety of teratogens that adversely affect the development of fetuses. Thalidomide, quinine, aminoprotein, and Myleran have all been implicated in congenital amputations in children whose mothers used these substances during pregnancy. All drugs during pregnancy are considered potentially harmful, including abused drugs. Certain genetic or inherited predispositions for congenital abnormalities in the limbs have also been identified. The reasons for the actual triggering of these predispositions remain unknown, but the presence of certain agents, such as those mentioned, heightens the chances for birth defects. The same is true of the presence of the rubella virus.

Accurate prevalence figures are difficult to obtain. "Sampling techniques are notoriously inadequate" (Friedman, 1978b, p. 3). The current prevalence rate is 1.7 to 8.6 amputees per 1,000 people (Sanders, 1986). Prevalence figures

Jim Abbott's Field of Dreams

"Phenom" is used to describe only the best of baseball's new rookies, the rising stars. In the Spring of 1989, no one embodied the word more than California Angels rookie pitcher Jim Abbott.

Born twenty-one years ago to teenage parents, Abbott played quarterback for his Flint, Michigan, high school football team and was the star pitcher on the baseball team. In his senior year, Abbott finished with a 10–3 won-lost record, and a 0.76 earned run average. He went on to pitch for the University of Michigan with a 26–8 won-lost record in three years. He earned the 1987 Sullivan Award as America's best amateur athlete. He led the U.S. baseball team to a gold medal in the 1988 Olympics in Seoul and was the Angel's first-round draft choice later that year. He bypassed the minor leagues and went straight to the majors in 1989. In one of his first appearances he out-pitched Roger Clemens, two-time Cy Young Award winner, to shut out the Boston Red Sox, 5–0. His fastball has been clocked at 93 m.p.h. But there is one fact that you won't find in James Anthony Abbott's biographical profile: He was born with only one hand.

Jim Abbott's right arm ends with a stump and one rudimentary finger where his wrist and hand should be. It is ten inches shorter than his left arm. For most people, such a handicap would limit their aspirations. But according to Abbott, neither of his parents ever treated him as disabled when he was growing up. He was fitted with a hooklike prosthesis when he was four. He threw it out when he was five.

"I *hated* that hand," he says, "it limited the things I could do. It didn't *help* me do anything. It was ugly. It drew attention to me, and I threw it out."

His parents never told him he couldn't do the things his friends did, they just reminded him that he would have to work harder to succeed. He says, "Growing up, I always pictured myself as a baseball player, but I can't remember how many hands I had in my dreams. I never thought to myself, 'Wow, I only have one hand. Can I eat with a certain fork?' I just did things."

So Abbott learned to play baseball with his friends. Soon he became the best in the neighborhood. He learned to juggle the glove between his "good" and "bad" hands in the time it takes his fastball to reach the batter: Throw the ball. Switch the glove. Catch. Tuck the glove under the arm. Take the ball out. Throw again.

"The transfers aren't that difficult," he says. "There's no dramatic story that goes with it. Just a matter of learning to do things a little differently. I never told myself, 'I want to be the next Pete Gray' [a one-armed outfielder for the St. Louis Browns in 1945]. I said, 'I want to be the next Nolan Ryan.'"

And he may well be the next Nolan Ryan. The 1989 season has proven to cynics that the California Angels didn't bring Abbott into their lineup just to sell more tickets. There is even some talk about the Cy Young Award, along with offers from book publishers and movie producers for his life story. He has received thousands of fan letters, many from youngsters with physical disabilities who see Abbott as a hero. Thanks to Abbott, they now dream of being baseball players instead of spectators.

Some of the attention from fans and the press bothers Abbott. "As much as you appreciate

regarding children suggest that there are 15 in every 100,000 children who have amputations (Jones, 1988). Females per capita have far fewer amputations than do males (Mensch & Ellis, 1986). The ratio of congenital to acquired amputations in children is 3.7 to 1 (Jones, 1988). Some 75 percent of the amputations in children age five to sixteen result from injuries and accidents. The other 25 percent are due to malignant diseases (Friedman, 1978b).

it," he says, "you wonder whether it's just because they feel sorry for you. . . . When they realize that I'm here for the pitching, then maybe some of the tiresome questions will stop."

For now, Abbott is concentrating only on perfecting his fastball, practicing his fielding skills, and developing an off-speed pitch.

Says Doug Rader, California Angels manager: "Anyone who approaches Jim as an oddity, believe me, is on the wrong path. Jim is the most *un*handicapped person I know."

And Milwaukee Brewers star Paul Molitor, after being struck out by Abbott, says, "If he can look past his disability the way he has, then my advice to batters who face him is that they better do the same thing."

Jim Abbott may not be a hero, but according to people who have watched baseball players come and go through the years, he *is* a phenom.

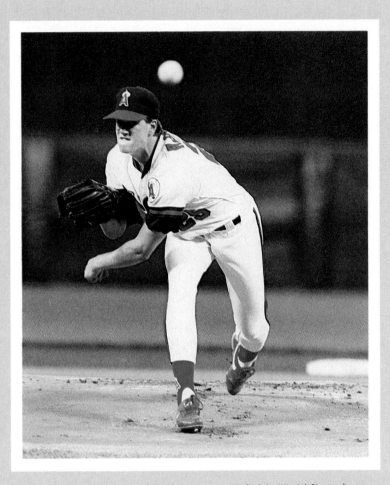

(Wide World Photos)

Sources: Charles Leerhsen with Tim Padgett, "The Complete Jim Abbott: One Hell of an Angel," *Newsweek*, June 12, 1989, p. 60.

Dave Anderson, "How Abbott Has Changed Baseball," *The New York Times*, May 25, 1989, p. D23.

Tom Callahan, "Dreaming the Big Dreams," *Time*, March 20, 1989, p. 78.

Dave Anderson, "Jim Abbott: Baseball's Real Phenom," *The New York Times*, March 9, 1989, p. B11.

Mike Lupica, "The Kid Who Wins One-Handed," *Parade Magazine*, March 2, 1986, pp. 4–5.

Intervention.   As already noted, children born with congenital amputations generally have an easier time adjusting to the treatments and therapies provided by the orthopedic physician and occupational and physical therapists than do children, youths, and adults who undergo amputations later in their lives. Children with congenital amputations also adjust more readily to prosthetic equipment and are less reluctant to utilize it in public settings. Utilization of various prostheses

FOCUS 11
What are six goals of treatment for individuals with congenital and acquired amputations?

occurs in a developmental fashion. Young children born with incomplete legs may be provided with customized skateboards to assist them with crawling activities. Later they may be fitted with artificial legs tailored to their physical dimensions. As such children grow and develop, the prosthetic devices must be redesigned and modified according to their emerging physical needs. Maintenance and replacement of the devices is very costly. Early encouragement of the use of prostheses is based on the notion that exposure and practice early in a child's life significantly influences the skill with which he or she eventually performs and his or her acceptance of the process.

Schooling for children with congenital amputations should proceed in a fashion commensurate with their intellectual capacity. Most children with congenital amputations profit from education provided in normal school settings. The teacher's role in responding to students with both types of amputations is multifaceted. A child with a missing body part or parts often produces an avoidance reaction in others, particularly children. Teachers who display and encourage appropriate physical and social contact with the young amputee provide an excellent model for their students to imitate.

Individuals who acquire an amputation later in life (e.g., during their teen or adult years) generally experience shock, consternation, and adjustment problems. The first step in treatment is typically medical. The orthopedic surgeon has the

---

WINDOW 11–2

I Was Always Chosen Last

I can still remember the half hour we had for recess twice a day in elementary school. On good-weather days, the main sport was softball. I was in the third grade when I really grew interested in recess softball. I didn't own a softball mitt, and wouldn't have known how to use it if I had one. I lost most of my right arm in a clothes washer motor when I was ten months old. The boys always brought their mitts to recess, and the best players were elected to be the captains who chose the teams. In the third grade I was always chosen last.

When I told my dad what was happening, he immediately took me to buy a first baseman's mitt. I began to practice every night, throwing a tennis ball against the garage door and finding a way to get my mitt back on before the ball returned. I tried everything with that mitt: putting it on the ground after I had caught the ball, throwing it in the air and trying to get the ball to drop out of it, and other awkward systems.

I eventually found that after catching the ball with my left hand, I could put my mitt under my right arm in one motion and pull the ball out in a second motion and throw it. I worked every night on this method with my dad and brothers and many hours just throwing the ball against the door myself.

Between the third and fourth grade, I moved up from being chosen last at recess to being a captain who chose the teams. I eventually played in the Little League as a pitcher and first baseman, was an all-star in our Babe Ruth League and captain of a Yankee baseball team in northern England. I still use the technique I developed in third grade for playing on our over-the-hill church softball team.

Richard Johns, Jr., M.D.

responsibility for preparing the rest of the arm or leg for its eventual use in conjunction with a prosthetic device. Following the completion of surgical procedures, the second step of the treatment process is begun. This step involves helping an individual cope with the feelings and self-perceptions that emerge as a result of the loss of a limb or limbs. The third step of the treatment process is rehabilitation. During this phase, the orthopedic specialist, prosthetist, occupational therapist, physical therapist, and rehabilitation personnel work together to help amputees adjust to their condition and their prosthetic devices.

In the future, biomedical engineers, in conjunction with other health professionals, will have a profound effect on the lives of individuals with amputations. Presently there are a variety of environmental control systems that allow the individuals with amputations and other physical impairments to operate home appliances and other devices (Dickey & Shealey, 1987). Typically these systems have several important components. They include a visual display, a central processing unit (CPU), and a transducer (control switch). The transducer allows individuals to activate various peripheral devices in their home environments, without using hands in some cases. The transducer may be activated by a dual control, sip-puff switch, an input controller from a powered wheelchair, a computer, an electronic communication aid, or a voice-recognition component. Using these switching devices, individuals with physical disorders may operate telephones, radios, stereos, televisions, video equipment, electronic beds, call signals for requesting assistance, intercoms, and even page turners. The visual display allows the individual to see if the outside doors are locked, if the lights were left on in the kitchen, and if the alarm clock has been set. If the kitchen lights have been left on, the individual may, with a voiced command, turn them off.

Another interesting device is the no-hands toothbrush developed by the Northern Electric Company (1988). The dental-care system never requires more than a 65-degree turn of the head of its user. The on and off switch, toothpaste, brushes, and water are easily controlled by the lips, tongue, and teeth. Thus those with little or no arm movement may brush without the aid of an assistant or care giver.

Educational Considerations.   Acquired amputations pose far more significant challenges to affected individuals than to those born with congenital amputations. Again, the attitudes and behaviors teachers and parents exhibit in response to these individuals is very important. Providing positive support for the use of prosthetics and expecting students to perform at a rate commensurate with their abilities contribute greatly to their adjusting to an amputation.

Muscular Dystrophy

Definition and Concepts.   **Muscular dystrophy** is a term used to describe a variety of conditions. "Muscular dystrophies are a group of chronic, inherited disorders characterized by progressive weakening and wasting of the voluntary skeletal muscles" (U.S. Department of Health and Human Services, 1980, p. 1). Each dystrophy condition varies from the others in intensity and manifestations. The seriousness of the various dystrophies is influenced by hereditary antecedents, the age of onset, the physical location and nature of onset, and the rate at which

FOCUS 12
What is muscular dystrophy?

Reflect on This 11–2

The Utah Artificial Arm

Intensive communication and collaboration among engineers, physicians, prosthetists, and amputees have produced the Utah Artificial Arm. The arm has been developed for persons with amputations above the elbow. As with any new and innovative venture, the creators and designers of the arm and its various modular components are continually refining its features and functions.

One of the amazing features of this arm is its capacity to sense and respond to electrical signals provided by antagonist muscles of the upper arm or shoulder of the amputee. The sensing takes place with skin electrodes that are located in upper portions of the artificial arm that attaches to the amputee's body (see Figure 11–3). Signals from these electrodes provide input controls for the movement of the arm. The control system in the arm is designed to give the user rapid motions as well as delicate, manipulative arm movements. Muscle signals provided by the amputee also control the locking or unlocking of the elbow of

the arm. This signaling capacity makes it possible for the amputee to lift heavy loads without seriously depleting the electrical output of the power pack.

The arm is capable of actions that are quite astounding. The arm itself is capable of lifting three pounds without seriously draining the electrical capacity of the batteries that power other functions of the arm. When the elbow of the arm is automatically locked, it is structurally capable of sustaining loads up to fifty pounds. The elbow module of the arm is able to produce a normal day's flexions on a single rechargeable battery. Furthermore, the elbow of the arm can be locked in twenty-one different positions depending on the use that is being made of the arm. All of the internal components of the arm are modular. Therefore, if a module is malfunctioning the arm can easily be serviced with a screwdriver and a new modular insert.

The exterior components of the arm are made of rugged yet light-

weight, fiber-reinforced plastic. The electrical control system of the arm allows the arm to swing naturally while it is not in direct use, which amputees appreciate. You might be wondering whether the arm makes any mechanical noises as its various drive mechanisms are activated. The answer is yes, but users describe it as being reasonably quiet and unobtrusive.

The designers of the arm are in the process of developing drive systems for the wrist rotation for the arm. There are still incredible challenges ahead for the development team in refining and improving the arm, but their tenacity has already benefited a number of amputees. The day may come when many will benefit from the efforts of this team and others who are interested in using the emerging technologies to aid and assist people with physical impairments.

Source: Reproduced courtesy of The Center for Engineering Design, University of Utah, and Motion Control, Inc.

the condition progresses. Actual causes of the different types of muscular dystrophy are unknown, and there are no known cures for any of the conditions. It affects the muscles of the hips, legs, shoulders, and arms. Afflicted individuals progressively lose their ability to walk and to use their arms and hands. The loss of ability is attributable to fatty tissue that gradually replaces muscle tissue. Heart muscle may also be affected, in which case symptoms of heart failure may occur.

There are several types of muscular dystrophy, four of which are outlined here (Turek, 1984). The first, pseudohypertrophy, is found most frequently in males. It is also known as Duchenne muscular dystrophy. It develops rapidly between the ages of two and six. The muscles usually increase in size; later, atrophy sets in. Children affected by this condition show a reluctance to walk

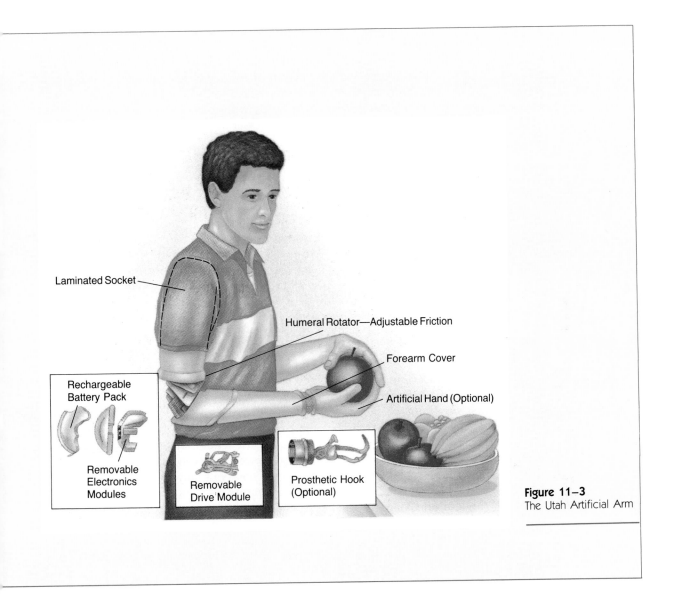

Laminated Socket

Humeral Rotator—Adjustable Friction

Forearm Cover

Rechargeable Battery Pack

Artificial Hand (Optional)

Removable Electronics Modules

Removable Drive Module

Prosthetic Hook (Optional)

Figure 11–3
The Utah Artificial Arm

or run. Eventually all strength in the hip, knee, ankle, shoulder, and elbow is lost. The atrophy gradually spreads outward to the hands and feet. Limb-girdle muscular dystrophy represents a second type. It typically manifests itself as muscle degeneration in the pelvic girdle, affecting the legs; or in the shoulder girdle, affecting the arms. The third type, facioscapulohumeral muscular dystrophy, affects muscles in the facial area, shoulders, and upper arms. Myotonic muscular dystrophy, the fourth type, is initially characterized by weakness in the hands, feet, neck, and face.

Causation and Prevalence. The exact cause of muscular dystrophy remains unknown, but it is viewed as a hereditary disease. However, about 50 percent of the cases develop without any clear hereditary antecedents (Whaley & Wong, 1985). The etiology of muscular dystrophy may be related to enzyme disturbances that subsequently affect muscle metabolism. Abnormalities in red blood cell membranes also suggest that the condition is a systemic disorder. About 2 hundred thousand people are affected by muscular dystrophies and other neuromuscular disorders. Some estimates indicate that about 0.14 in 1,000 people develop muscular dystrophy (Whaley & Wong, 1985). One-third are between the ages of three and thirteen, and eight out of ten are males.

FOCUS 13
What four interventions are employed in treating individuals with muscular dystrophy?

Intervention. There is no known cure for muscular dystrophies. The focus of treatment is directed at maintaining or improving the individual's functioning and preserving his or her ambulatory independence as long as possible (Shock, 1985). The first phases of the maintenance and prevention processes are handled by a physical therapist. The therapist is responsible for preventing or correcting (to the degree possible) contractures, which are a permanent shortening and thickening of muscle fiber. As the condition becomes more serious, treatment generally includes prescribing supportive devices such as walkers, braces, night splints, surgical corsets, and hospital beds. Eventually the individual with muscular dystrophy may be confined to a wheelchair, which should be tailored to the individual's needs (Kamenetz, 1986). For example, consideration must be given to the following: the age and size of the individual; the places in which the chair is to be used; the kind of support required; the method by which the chair will be propelled; the overall comfort of the chair; the chair's durability and attractiveness; the individual's present capacities; the degree to which the chair can contribute to the individual's independence; and the collapsibility, weight, and size of the chair.

The individual with muscular dystrophy is frequently given some type of medication in hopes of increasing muscle strength or counteracting the disease's effect on the heart. If the child or adolescent is receiving medication, parents and teachers play an important role in observing any peculiar reactions that occur. As the condition advances, respiratory muscles are often affected, and the individual may be unable to cough strongly enough to expel mucus and phlegm, which sometimes leads to recurrent pneumonia. People with muscular dystrophy should be encouraged to participate actively in all activities for which they have the skill. In fact, long periods of sitting should be avoided because inactivity leads to increased muscle wasting.

One of the major problems for the individual with muscular dystrophy is the appearance of contractures (permanent shortening of muscle fibers that decreases joint mobility), which seriously interfere with the individual's ability to walk or move in other manners. The best treatment for prevention of such contractures is physical therapy and the avoidance of classroom activities that involve prolonged periods without movement.

Education of individuals with muscular dystrophy may take place in a variety of settings, depending on the educational and physical needs of each student. Some are served in special classes for the physically disabled, others are served in the regular classroom. Because of the progressive nature of muscular dystrophy, the life span for many affected individuals is relatively short. Consequently, parents, teachers, and others should prepare themselves (and the patient) as best they can for the advent of death. Several excellent books have been designed for this purpose (Arnold & Gemma, 1983; Backer, Hannon, & Russell, 1982; Buckingham, 1983; Kalish, 1985; Krulik, Holaday, & Martinson, 1987; Poss, 1981; Wass & Corr, 1982).

Educational Considerations. Children and adolescents with muscular dystrophy are living much longer than they used to. Their presence in school, which used to be a rarity, is now quite common, particularly during the early phases of the disease. The key to success in dealing with children with this condition is collaboration. Parents, medical personnel, physical and occupational therapists, and teachers need to work together. Dealing with increased falling, providing adapted equipment, encouraging adjustments to new wheelchairs, coping with diminished energy, and helping these students maintain a sense of direction as their bodies gradually deteriorate are some of the tasks of the team of parents and professionals.

REVIEW

FOCUS 1: What are physical disorders?

- ☐ Physical disorders refer to impairments that interfere with an individual's mobility, communication, coordination, learning, and adjustment.

FOCUS 2: What are six factors that influence the overall impact of physical disorders on children and adolescents?

- ☐ Age of onset
- ☐ Degree or severity of the physical disability
- ☐ Visibility of the condition
- ☐ Family and social support
- ☐ Attitudes of others toward the affected individual
- ☐ Social status among peers

FOCUS 3: Why are many individuals with cerebral palsy considered to be multihandicapped or multi-impaired?

- ☐ Often, individuals with cerebral palsy have several impairments.
- ☐ They may have hearing deficits, speech and language problems, intellectual deficits, and visual and perceptual problems.

FOCUS 4: Why is the treatment of cerebral palsy often multidimensional?

- ☐ Because of the multifaceted nature of cerebral palsy, many professionals may be involved in treating the various aspects of the condition.

FOCUS 5: What are seizures?

- ☐ Seizures are clusters of behavior that occur in response to irregular neurochemical activity in the brain.

FOCUS 6: What three interventions are used with persons with seizure disorders?

- ☐ The primary medical treatment for seizures is anticonvulsant drug therapy.
- ☐ Treatment may also include individual and family therapy, career development counseling, and special education, if necessary.
- ☐ Another therapy technique currently being investigated is biofeedback.

FOCUS 7: What is spina bifida?

- ☐ Spina bifida is a defect in the spinal column.
- ☐ The defect is an opening in the spinal column that allows the contents of the spinal canal to flow between bones (vertebrae) that did not fully close or grow normally. Spina bifida myelomeningocele, the most serious form of this condition, causes paralysis.

FOCUS 8: What treatments are used to assist children with spina bifida?

- ☐ Surgical treatment is often performed to repair the opening in the spine.
- ☐ The repair often prevents the infection that otherwise might occur.
- ☐ If the site of the myelomeningocele is high on the back, surgery may not be indicated.
- ☐ Paralyzed children profit greatly from the services of physical therapists, who help them make full use of their physical capacities.

FOCUS 9: What are seven treatments provided to individuals with spinal-cord injuries?

- ☐ Immediate stabilization of the spine is critical to the overall outcome of the injury.
- ☐ Once the spine has been stabilized, the rehabilitation process begins.
- ☐ Physical therapy helps the affected individual make full use of any and all residual muscle strength.
- ☐ The individual is also taught to use such orthopedic devices as hand splints, braces, reachers, and head sticks.
- ☐ Psychological adjustment is aided by psychiatric and psychological personnel.
- ☐ Rehabilitation specialists aid the individual in becoming retrained or re-educated. They may also assist the individual in securing new employment.
- ☐ Some individuals need part-time or full-time attendant care for assistance with daily activities, such as bathing, dressing, and shopping.

FOCUS 10: What major intervention is used to aid children with arthritis?

- ☐ Anti-inflammatory drug therapy is the major intervention used in treating children and youth with arthritis.

FOCUS 11: What are six goals of treatment for individuals with congenital and acquired amputations?

- ☐ Children with congenital amputations are fitted with prosthetic devices as soon as they can profit from them. As these children grow, their prosthetic devices are modified and customized to their specific needs. Individuals with acquired amputations are treated surgically.
- ☐ The surgeon treats the affected limb area and prepares

it for eventual use in conjunction with a prosthetic device. Generally, people with acquired amputations experience greater difficulties in adjusting to the challenges inherent in their injuries than do children who have had the limb defects since birth.

- ☐ Occupational, physical, and other therapists play critical roles in helping people with congenital and acquired amputations realize their full potential in a variety of domains.

FOCUS 12: What is muscular dystrophy?

- ☐ Muscular dystrophy is a group of chronic, inherited disorders that are characterized by the progressive weakening and wasting of voluntary skeletal muscles. Each dystrophy varies from the others in its intensity and its manifestations.
- ☐ Affected individuals progressively lose their ability to walk and use their arms and hands effectively.

FOCUS 13: What four interventions are employed in treating individuals with muscular dystrophy?

- ☐ There is no known cure for muscular dystrophy.
- ☐ The first goal of treatment is to maintain or improve an individual's physical functioning and to prevent contractures.
- ☐ Physical therapists play an important role in maintaining physical function and preventing contractures.
- ☐ As the condition progresses, treatment includes prescribing supportive devices, such as walkers, braces, and night splints.
- ☐ Treatment also includes preparing parents and other loved ones for the shortened life span of individuals with severe forms of muscular dystrophy.

Debate Forum

Surgery: Should They Go Ahead with It?

The decisions faced by parents of a newborn who has been diagnosed as having a serious birth defect are often overwhelming. In addition, the time frame for making the decisions is usually very limited. Sometimes immediate surgical or other medical action must be taken. Before a medical team or physician can proceed with any substantive action, the parents must provide consent. In order to give informed consent, they must

know the risks, potential benefits, and possible side effects of the medical intervention. They must also be apprised of the long-term prognosis for the child's condition. Many would argue that parents who are under stress of this magnitude are not in a position to provide informed consent.

Another aspect of this dilemma involves the nature of the information that might be provided by the physician. Consciously or unconsciously, a physician may guide the decision outcome by underplaying or overemphasizing certain risks or benefits. Furthermore, the physician certainly has his or her own biases that may shape the counsel given. What values should govern the ultimate decision that is made? What do you think? The following is an abbreviated case study of a newborn by the name of Linda.

Linda is only several hours old, and already her life seems to be filled with frenzy. During her delivery it was discovered that she had spina bifida. The location of the opening in Linda's spine is in the upper back region, and the sack contains nerve tissue. Thus, she is likely to be paralyzed in her lower extremities. Moreover, she will most likely be unable to control her bowel and bladder functions. There is also potential risk of her developing hydrocephalus. However, Linda's intelligence may turn out to be completely normal.

The medical personnel have discussed the options available to the parents. Immediate surgery for repair of the spine and prevention of infection is one of the options. Linda's father and mother are in their late twenties. They were married shortly after their graduation from high school and have two other children, Joshua and Sarah. Although they have both made significant headway in their vocational pursuits since high school, they do not make a great deal of money. In fact, they struggle to pay their bills on a monthly basis. They recently moved into their first home, which created additional financial pressures. The complications that have arisen in conjunction with Linda's birth were not anticipated.

The medical personnel have been candid about the future costs and care that will be part of rearing Linda.

She will probably require neurosurgical, orthopedic, and other types of specialized medical care throughout her life. All of these services will be very expensive. What obligation do they have to their other children? What about their futures? Could they live with themselves if they chose not to proceed with the surgery? If Linda does not have the surgery, she will very likely develop meningitis and die. The decision to intervene must be made quickly. Who should make the decision? What decision should be reached? Should Linda be represented by someone other than her parents?

Point Linda's parents are morally and legally obligated to care for their children. They are also responsible for providing for their children's welfare during their formative years. They must bear the expenses involved in caring not only for Linda, but also for their other children. If they are well informed about the immediate and long-term potential outcomes of Linda's congenital condition, the issues surrounding her eventual quality of life, and the needs of their present family, they are in the best position to decide what interventions should or should not be employed in treating Linda, in spite of the time limitations.

Counterpoint Interventions for Linda should not be determined solely by her parents, particularly if the decision is to withhold treatment. If the withholding of treatment may result in Linda's death, other informed people should be involved. Linda's life should not be altered or terminated by individuals who may not have her ultimate interests at heart. Intervention facilities should have committees of three whose members are professionally prepared to represent the child and legally engage in binding arbitration with the parents.

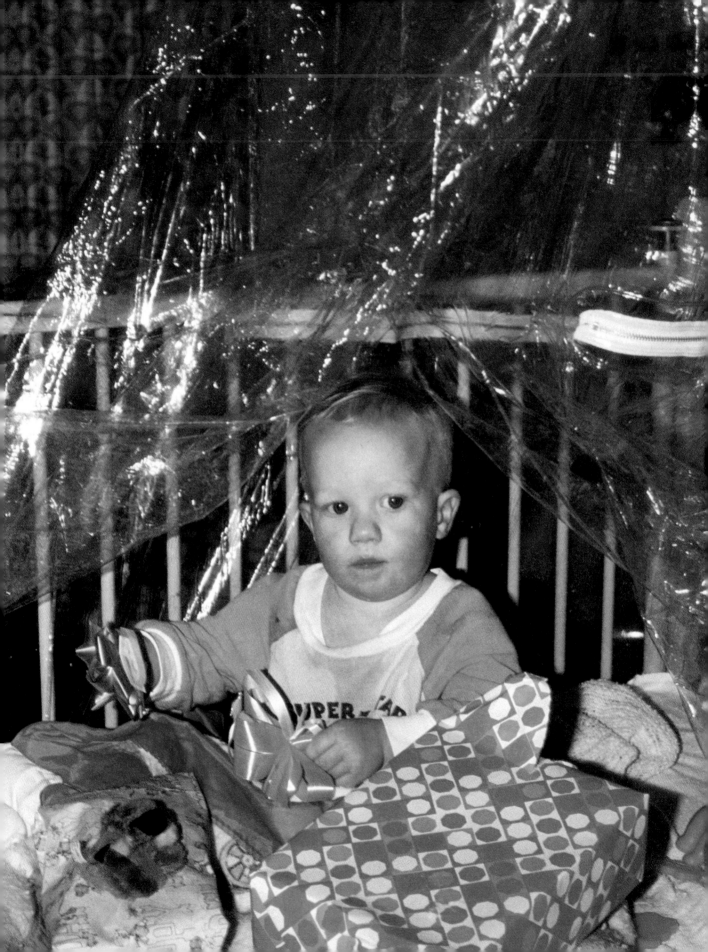

12 Health Disorders

To Begin With...

■ Approximately 10 to 15 percent of children under the age of 18 are chronically physically ill (Pless & Perrin, 1985).

■ Given an estimated 62 million children under the age of 18 in the United States, nearly one million have health disorders which are classified as severe (Hobbs, Perrin, & Ireys, 1985).

■ The most important thing to remember about chronic illness is that it is exactly that: chronic. It never goes away (Robert Massey, age 29, who has hemophilia; Patterson, 1988).

■ Adults and children suffer and die from AIDS. The epidemic also makes "orphans" of those children who are not infected but lose their parent(s) to the disease. Predictions are that during this generation, in the city of New York, between 50,000 and 100,000 will lose at least one parent to AIDS (*Herald Times*, 1987).

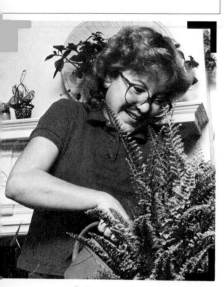

Patty

atty had always been the sick one in the family. As a diabetic, her childhood had been disrupted. Her physical development was delayed, and she was behind her peers in school because of frequent absences. Yet Patty achieved a great deal—for any youngster, let alone one with health problems. When her mother died, Patty was only fifteen, but she assumed responsibility for most of the household chores and cared for her younger brother and sister.

Despite all Patty did for the family, she received little in return. Her brother and sister ridiculed her because she was "sick," and her father believed she would never be able to get a job or a husband. Patty basically held the same opinion of herself. At the age of twenty, she finally graduated from high school but had no goals for further education. Her aunt tried to convince Patty that a local vocational rehabilitation program would be exciting and good for her. Patty finally agreed, and her father reluctantly acquiesced.

The results were astonishing to all. It took time, but Patty began to believe in herself, dressed more attractively, performed well, and soon gained full-time employment outside the home. Patty has been gainfully employed now for nearly two years and recently received her company's employee-of-the-year award.

INTRODUCTION

It is 2:00 A.M. You are suddenly awakened by a physical sensation in your body. Your chest feels like someone is sitting on it, and you know there will be no more sleep tonight. Asthma is only one of many health problems that have significant impacts on people's lives. When a person's health severely restricts daily activities, what he or she can eat, or his or her social contacts, the impact is significant. Most of us give little thought to our health on a daily basis, but for those with serious health disorders, health status may be the most significant factor in their lives.

Defining Health Disorders

The term **health disorders** refers to conditions or diseases that interfere with a person's functioning. A number of health disorders present serious problems for both youngsters and adults. These health disorders significantly alter not only the lives of the individuals who develop them but also the lives of the individuals' families and others around them. In this chapter, we discuss various health disorders and conditions under the categories of systemic disorders, stress-related disorders, life-endangering diseases, and other health conditions.

Unlike physical disorders, health disorders do not generally hinder the person's ability to move about in various settings. Architectural barriers do not seriously restrict the activities of persons with health disorders. Resulting limitations are usually related to such conditions as reduced alertness and participation, fatigue, pain, fear, and stress. For example, a child with a heart condition may have to limit the amount of time spent in highly active games or team sports. In advanced stages, however, certain conditions seriously affect an individual's mobility.

Factors That Influence the Impact of a Health Disorder

The impact of a health disorder on an individual depends on such factors as (1) the seriousness of the condition, (2) the age at which the condition appears, (3) the support of the family and friends, (4) the quality of medical treatment provided, and (5) the nature of the condition—whether it remains about the same or worsens over time. Referral and treatment processes for health disorders are similar to those for physical disorders. **Primary-care physicians** refer the affected individual to a specialist or several specialists for further diagnosis and/or treatment. Treatment for certain chronic health conditions can be lifelong.

The prevalence of social and psychological problems in children who have serious health disorders is somewhat higher than that in normal children. A serious health problem seems to heighten an individual's chances for experiencing personal adjustment difficulties. The higher prevalence of emotional problems occurs as a function of several factors. Children with serious health disorders spend a considerable amount of time away from home, receiving hospital care. Such hospitalization often hampers the development of satisfying social relationships with siblings, parents, and peers, thus complicating the process of building friendships. Physical restrictions may also be a factor. Activity limitations exist with a variety of health conditions, including asthma, diabetes, and sickle cell anemia. It is easy to see how discouraged a child might become about not being able to participate with peers in physically demanding activities.

FOCUS 1
What five factors influence the impact of a health disorder on individuals?

SYSTEMIC DISORDERS

Diabetes

> "Boy, your mom must be real mad at your sister. You got a Snickers and she only got an orange."
> "Mom's not mad. It's just my sister is sugarless."

This is a cute response for a six-year-old, unaware of how wise his statement is. Most nondiabetics fear the injection of insulin, but the quest to be "sugarless" is much more difficult and critical. *Sugarless* means a correct balance between food, exercise, sleep, and medication, not simply going without candy bars. For most people, continual calculation of these items is overwhelming at first. It is important for the person with diabetes to be aware of the danger that comes from not sticking to regimens, especially diet:

> At camp I was too afraid to say I needed fruit with my dinner and that the Lifesavers taken out of my suitcase were medicinal. As a result I went into severe insulin reaction. This episode not only frightened the counselor and campers, but shouted to the others, "I'm different from you!" which was hard for a thirteen-year-old.

Diabetes does not have to limit one's life. With discipline, patience, and honest communication, management of the disease can increase awareness of good nutrition and health.

FOCUS 2
In addition to disordered metabolism, what three other problems may a child, youth, or young adult with diabetes eventually experience?

Definition and Concepts. Diabetes influences the way in which the body uses food. **Glucose** (a sugar), one of the end products of digesting carbohydrates, is used by the body for energy. Some of this glucose is used right away and some is stored in the liver and muscles for later use. However, muscle and liver cells cannot absorb and store the energy produced by glucose without **insulin,** a **hormone.** It converts glucose into energy that can be used in cells of the body to perform their various functions. Without insulin, glucose accumulates in the blood. Insulin, a secretion of the pancreas, assists the body by allowing glucose to enter the body's cells.

Increased concentrations of glucose in the blood (**hyperglycemia**) and in the urine (**glycosuria**) prior to the discovery of insulin caused many individuals with this condition to experience diabetic **ketoacidosis** and the progressive development of a coma (severe unconsciousness). Typical symptoms associated with glucose buildup in the blood are extreme hunger and thirst and frequent urination. Although much headway has been made in addressing the insulin side of diabetes, the prevention and treatment of the accompanying complications (blindness, cardiovascular disease, and kidney disease) still pose tremendous challenges for the internist or diabetic specialist.

Juvenile diabetes is particularly challenging. Compared to adult diabetes, juvenile diabetes tends to be more severe and progresses more quickly. Generally, the symptoms are easily recognized. The child develops an unusual thirst for water and other liquids. The child's appetite also increases substantially, but listlessness and fatigue occur despite the increased food and liquid intake.

Adults with diabetes generally develop the disease between the ages of forty and fifty, with another increase in the incidence occurring in the late seventies. They also experience complications from the disease, but the full onset of structural abnormalities related to heart disease, kidney disease, or eye problems does not occur as rapidly as it does in children and adolescents with juvenile diabetes. Obesity is a very common characteristic of adults with diabetes. The vast majority of adult diabetics can control their condition by simply modifying their diets (Davidson, 1981; Podolsky, Krall, & Bradley, 1980).

Causation and Prevalence. Although considerable research has been devoted to determining the biochemical mechanisms responsible for diabetes, the causes remain obscure. As with other disorders, an individual's environment and heredity interact in determining the severity and the long-term nature of the condition. Juvenile diabetes appears to be more clearly linked to hereditary factors than the adult forms of the disease. The course of diabetes is greatly influenced by such factors as an individual's degree of obesity, level of personal stress, and the type of diet a prediabetic or diabetic maintains. The multiple causes of diabetes are gradually becoming clearer through ongoing research.

It is estimated that 5 percent of the U.S. population has diabetes. The prevalence rate for children for insulin-dependent diabetes is approximately 10 per 100,000 children. The peak incidence periods occur between 11 and 14 years of age (Greenberg, 1987). Recent studies indicate that by age 18, approximately 1 in 300–400 Caucasian children in the United States have insulin-dependent diabetes (Ross, Bernstein, & Rifkin, 1983). The prevalence rate of diabetes in non-Caucasian children is half that found in Caucasian children (Krolewski & Warram, 1985).

Intervention. Medical treatment centers around the regular intake of insulin, which is essential for youngsters with juvenile diabetes. Several exciting advances have been made in recent years to monitor blood-sugar levels and deliver insulin to individuals with diabetes. Also, recent success with pancreas transplants has virtually eliminated the disease for some individuals.

Newly developed, home blood-glucose-monitoring devices provide young people and adults with diabetes an accurate means of assessing their blood glucose levels. These devices require a so-called **finger stick** to draw the blood. Using the information generated by the devices, many diabetics can maintain near-normal or normal levels of glucose in the blood (Ross, Bernstein, & Rifkin, 1983).

The maintenance of normal levels of glucose is now achieved in many instances with a continuous subcutaneous (below the skin) **insulin infusion pump,** which is worn and operated by affected persons and powered by small batteries. The infusion pump continuously delivers insulin in the amount determined by the physician and patient. This form of treatment is only effective if used in combination with carefully followed diets and exercise programs (Raskin, 1983). Reactions of the individuals who have been involved in studies dealing with the pumps and their effectiveness have been generally positive. Unfortunately, the present pumps are quite expensive, from $1000 to several thousand dollars. Furthermore, a great deal of patient and physician time is required to prepare the patient to effectively use the infusion devices. For these reasons, children under ten years of age are not fitted with infusion pumps.

Individuals with diabetes are now becoming more capable than in the past of managing their illness and its effects upon their lives. Because they are able to more closely monitor themselves and receive continuous or timely infusions of insulin, they have greater freedom in choosing the times when they want to eat, exercise, or engage in other physically intensive recreational activities such as skiing, dancing, running, or swimming. A great deal of energy is consumed during these activities. Having the right kinds of food available and the ability to precisely adjust the amount of insulin the body receives are great aids to those individuals with diabetes who enjoy participating in athletics and other physically demanding activities.

Juvenile diabetes is a lifelong condition that can have a pronounced effect on an individual's behavior in a number of areas. The family is greatly affected by the presence of a youngster with diabetes. Not only must the family members cope with the medical expenses, but they must also assist the child in monitoring glucose levels and maintaining the prescribed diet and exercise regimen.

Hypoglycemia (an abnormal decrease of sugar in the blood), which is usually caused by too much insulin, too much exercise, or insufficient amounts of food, frequently produces such symptoms as irritability, poor attention span, temper tantrums, and other related behaviors. Such behavior may be misinterpreted by school personnel or parents unless they have been adequately informed. Another factor that has a pronounced effect on the child is the limitation placed on various types of vigorous physical activity or exercise. However, if the exercise is regular and of the proper amount, rapid sugar depletion in the blood is not a problem. An appropriate snack or candy before vigorous activity and thirty minutes afterward lessens the chances of insulin shock. The snack supplies the glucose needed for the activity, or replaces the glucose used during the activity. Both of these strategies significantly lessen the possibility of abnormal buildups of insulin in the blood.

Educational Considerations. Children with diabetes benefit significantly from exercise and other physical activities. Glucose is burned through exercise without the aid of insulin, thereby keeping blood-sugar levels from rising. However, before or after strenuous or demanding physical activities, these children benefit from having a sugar snack (fruit juice, 6 ounces of regular soda pop, or three or four Lifesavers).

WINDOW 12–1

My World Has Come to an End

I was a junior in high school when I found out that I had diabetes. On that particular day, I became very ill, so ill that I went home. Within the next four hours, I was hospitalized.

I distinctly remember my first thoughts on hearing that I had diabetes. "My world has come to an end," I said to myself. I was then a member of my high school pep club. I loved performing at the games. I'd always enjoyed physical activity. At the time, I thought this disease would permanently alter all the wonderful dreams and aspirations I had for myself.

Unfortunately, I could not at the time hide the fact that I had diabetes. All of my close friends knew I had become very ill in school. They were also aware of my hospitalization. Although I wanted to keep my condition a secret, doing so was virtually impossible. I believed that everyone of any importance knew about my condition. Again, I remember saying to myself, "No one will want to date me if he knows I have diabetes." I began to feel much better about myself when a boy I liked but had never dated asked me out. This occurred several weeks after my hospitalization.

However, the fact that I was different from most everyone else practically killed me! I wanted to be accepted. I wanted to be like everyone else. For example, the foods everyone else loved and consumed without thought were taboo for me. My energy intake was never a spontaneous event. Every calorie I consumed was done with great care. I had a regimen to maintain. Malts, candy bars, soft drinks, and other sugar-rich commodities were simply out of the question.

At first, my illness controlled my every action and thought. I was virtually consumed by the disease and its treatment. Now, the diet regimen and other parts of my treatment have become second nature to me. I'm now focused on my children and my life as a wife and mother of two preschoolers. Needless to say, things have worked out very well for me in spite of my diabetes. Being different isn't easy, but it is manageable.

Susan, *a mother*

Teachers and others should be aware of the symptoms of hypoglycemia—dizziness, hunger, pallor, sweating, drowsiness, inattentiveness, and inappropriate behavior. If these symptoms are observed, the affected child should be provided with some form of sugar or food. If the symptoms persist longer than ten minutes, the child's parents should be notified.

The symptoms of **ketoacidosis** (frequent urination, dehydration, vomiting, drowsiness, and labored breathing) should be treated by encouraging the affected child to consume large volumes of sugar-free liquids. Also, insulin should be administered as quickly as possible. Parents should be contacted immediately when this condition arises. Unlike hypoglycemia, this condition may take several hours to subside.

Cardiac Disorders

Maria was born with a congenital heart condition. Openings in the heart wall were present at birth, allowing oxygenated and unoxygenated blood to mix. As a result, Maria was cyanotic, blue in appearance. She was immediately placed on a respirator, and additional diagnostic assessments were undertaken to identify the cause of the cyanosis. After the physicians determined that her heart had some congenital defects, Maria's parents were alerted and permission was obtained for surgery. Within a few hours of birth, Maria underwent surgery to correct her heart problems. Maria would have died in a few days if the condition had not been surgically corrected.

Since that time, Maria has undergone a series of operations for other complications associated with her heart condition. Several electronic heart pacemakers have been implanted at various times. She has responded to hospitalization, surgery, and the frequent medical checkups with considerable courage. Although she has had recurring medical problems, her schooling has proceeded in a normal fashion. She has had to restrict her activity at recess and during physical education periods, but she has taken creative dancing and enjoys quiet activities such as reading and drawing.

Recently, at age eleven, Maria's heart condition worsened, and her life has become somewhat tenuous. She now regularly experiences seizures, and her circulation is often poor. The circulation problems cause her legs to "fall asleep," as she describes it. Maria's pediatric cardiologist, in conjunction with other medical specialists, is attempting to resolve the present problems. Fortunately, Maria has extremely supportive parents, who have constantly encouraged and supported her.

Definitions and Concepts. Heart disease is a leading cause of death in the United States. A basic understanding of the anatomy and functions of the heart is a necessary preface to the identification and treatment of heart disease. The heart in people of normal stature is about the size of an adult's closed fist (see Figure 12–1). It is located between the lungs, just above the diaphragm and stomach, and weighs about half a pound. The heart is actually a double synchronized pump, with chambers on each side of the septum (dividing wall). The

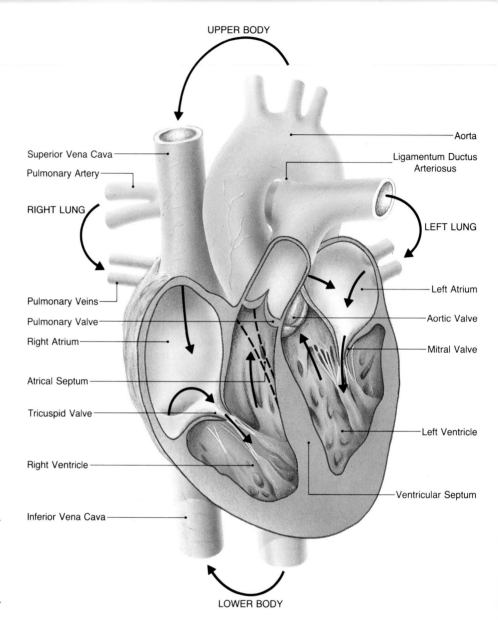

UPPER BODY

Aorta

Ligamentum Ductus Arteriosus

Superior Vena Cava

Pulmonary Artery

RIGHT LUNG

LEFT LUNG

Left Atrium

Pulmonary Veins

Pulmonary Valve

Aortic Valve

Right Atrium

Mitral Valve

Atrical Septum

Tricuspid Valve

Left Ventricle

Right Ventricle

Ventricular Septum

Inferior Vena Cava

LOWER BODY

Figure 12–1
Normal Heart. The arrows indicate the direction of blood flow through the four chambers and great vessels. (Adapted, by permission, from Clinical Education Aid No. 7, Ross Laboratories, Columbus, Ohio.)

"right heart" processes blood from the major veins and returns it to the lungs through the pulmonary artery. Blood returning from the lungs is processed by the "left heart" and is pumped to all parts of the body through the aorta. Each chamber of the heart is subdivided into the atrium (upper chamber) and ventricle (lower chamber). Between each chamber is the septum. The flow of blood from one area to another is controlled by a number of valves. A normal adult heart beats about 100,800 times in a twenty-four-hour period. The entire blood supply of an adult (about six quarts) passes through the complete cardiovascular system in less than sixty seconds.

There are four major types of **cardiac disorders:** (1) **congenital heart disease,**

(2) rheumatic heart disease, (3) heart attacks, and **(4) congestive heart failure.** We limit our discussion primarily to the factors related to congenital and rheumatic heart disease. Congenital heart disease is usually detected immediately after birth by medical personnel. Infants with anomalies in heart structure or functioning, like Maria, are often blue in appearance or have difficulty in breathing. The more common congenital heart defects involve openings in the wall of the atria (see Figure 12–2) or ventricles, inappropriate operation of the pulmonary valve, or excessive constriction of the major arterial channel. Recent advances in surgery, anesthesiology, and bioengineering have revolutionized the treatment of both congenital and acquired heart conditions. The heart can now be surgically repaired while a heart–lung machine carries on the individual's breathing and heart

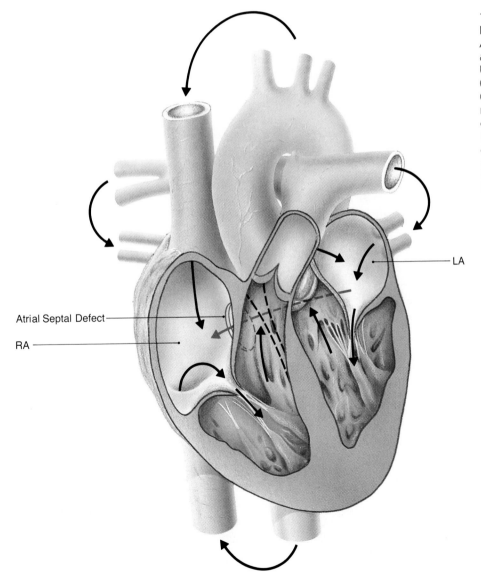

Atrial Septal Defect

RA

LA

Figure 12–2
Atrial Septal Defect. An arrow indicates flow of blood from the left atrium (LA) to the right atrium (RA), thus overloading the right heart, pulmonary circulation, and left heart. Left to right shunt: no cyanosis. (Adapted, by permission, from Clinical Education Aid No. 7, Ross Laboratories, Columbus, Ohio.)

functions. Or the heart can be removed and replaced by an artificial heart while the child or youth waits for an appropriate donor. Heart valves can be repaired or replaced, and even the electrical signal that triggers the pumping rhythm can be created with a pacemaker. The number of infants who die of congenital heart disease has been dramatically reduced as a result of these medical advances.

Rheumatic heart disease is a by-product of rheumatic fever. Although rheumatic fever affects the entire body, it has a pronounced impact on the heart and connective tissues of the body. The muscles, valves, and lining of the heart become inflamed and may be permanently damaged. About 33 percent of all individuals who have rheumatic fever suffer from residual side effects of heart damage. "Rheumatic fever licks the joints but bites the heart" was the way the French physician Laseque put it (Armington & Creighton, 1971, p. 43). If such damage is not corrected by surgery or other therapy, the person may experience congestive heart failure and early death.

Causation and Prevalence. Congenital heart conditions can be caused by a variety of factors, including drugs taken by the mother during critical periods of prenatal development, or the presence of rubella virus in the mother. In some

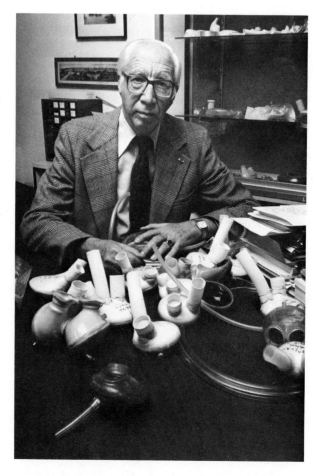

Willem Kolff, past head of the Division of Artificial Organs at the University of Utah, displays several of the artificial heart components that led to the development of the artificial heart that is now clinically used. (John Telford)

instances, the congenital condition may be hereditary, or it may be a function of a genetic predisposition that is triggered by certain environmental stimuli.

Congenital heart defects are present in approximately 1 out of 1,000 live births. A large number of those born with heart defects at birth die during the first year of life. Of all babies remaining alive at the end of the first year of life, only about 1 in 30,000 has an abnormal heart.

The prevalence of rheumatic heart disease in school-age children is between 0.7 and 2.0 per 1,000. Among college students and young military selectees, the prevalence is 5.7 to 8.8 per 1,000 (Silber, 1987).

Intervention.   Heart disease in children is treated with a variety of approaches. Cardiac failure or other problems may be prevented with nonsurgical measures. Surgery for congenital conditions is generally postponed, when possible, to reduce risk and to make the operation less technically difficult. Surgery for congenital heart conditions is generally corrective in nature. This is also true for rheumatic heart problems. Appropriate programs of rest and exercise prepare the child for further treatment. Fortunately, many children with congenital heart conditions naturally sense the time at which they should rest or reduce their physical activity. Sedatives may be provided to enhance the beneficial effects of rest. Other heart medicines, such as digitalis, may also play a critical role in the maintenance process. It is the physician's task to monitor the child who may be at risk for heart failure or other complications. Regular examinations are vital for the infant or young child with cardiac problems.

The child's age plays a significant role in the mortality rate. If a child is only a few days old, the mortality rate is very high, which is why most physicians wait for the child to grow and develop before initiating intensive surgery. Mortality risks involved in corrective surgery for older children (ages six to twelve) range from 1 to 5 percent for most conditions.

Corrective surgery for rheumatic heart disease may involve repair or replacement of vital valves. Repair of the heart generally involves closing abnormal openings in heart chamber walls or removal of extraneous tissue that prevents or interferes with blood flow. Valve replacement is a relatively common surgical procedure. Antibiotics, the heart–lung machine, and new surgical techniques, including the implantation of an artificial heart, have significantly reduced the number of deaths due to congenital heart malformations and rheumatic heart disease.

Educational Considerations.   Both younger and older individuals who have experienced chronic cardiac problems must carefully select the physical activities they pursue. Rest and appropriate exercise are vital, particularly during convalescence. Teachers, in cooperation with parents and the medical team, should set realistic goals for a child recovering from a heart condition. The goals should be such that the child is not overly restricted. Often children develop counterproductive psychological attitudes during the postoperative period, which may be detrimental to eventual performance in school. As these children progress through school, they should be provided with opportunities to match their skills and physical abilities with appropriate potential careers. Many students with cardiac conditions are eligible for vocational rehabilitation services provided by each state. The services provided by state agencies may be very beneficial in helping students to select suitable careers and receive medical assistance and support for technical or professional education.

STRESS-RELATED DISORDER

Asthma

Definitions and Concepts. Asthma is a "condition of altered dynamic state of respiratory passages due to the action of diverse stimuli, resulting in airways obstruction of varying degree and duration, and reversible partially or completely, spontaneously or under treatment" (Kuzemko, 1980, p. 1). This chronic respiratory disorder is characterized by not only difficulty in breathing but also excessive coughing, wheezing, and sputum. The severity and outcome of asthmatic episodes are greatly influenced by the interaction of a number of factors. And the clinical severity of asthma varies greatly from individual to individual.

FOCUS 3
What four factors appear to be related to the emergence of asthma in children?

Causation and Prevalence. The body produces **antibodies** in response to certain **antigens,** such as pollen. Individuals with asthma produce a surplus of these antibodies. When the antigens become responsible for allergic reactions they are identified as allergens. The intolerance of an asthmatic to these allergens is immense. Allergic antibodies do not insulate the body from an attack. As they react to offending allergens, harmful chemical substances, known as **histamines,** are produced or released. Histamines cause swelling in various affected areas, such as the bronchi, or airways (see Figure 12–3). Inflammation of these airways causes them to constrict, resulting in an insufficiency of air to the lungs.

The number of potential allergens is limitless. Certain foods, molds, drugs, insect stings, and bacteria can cause severe reactions.

There appears to be a strong relationship between psychological well-being and the presence of asthmatic conditions. Children with asthma tend to have more emotional difficulties than children who do not have asthma. Frequently, asthmatic episodes are preceded by psychologically stressful events. Family factors also seem to play a role in the emergence of asthma. Between 50 and 75 percent of individuals who develop asthma have a family history of allergic reactions to various allergens (Kuzemko, 1980). However, the exact nature of the genetic and inheritance factors responsible for asthma remains unknown.

Many children develop asthma after respiratory infections. Although the relationship between the infections and the development of asthma remains unclear, viral infections, in particular, seem to act as provocative agents for eventual onset of the condition. Exercise also often induces acute episodes, as do changes in temperature and season.

The actual prevalence of asthma remains somewhat elusive. It is estimated that 4.5 percent of the population in the United States have asthma. About one-third of all asthmatic patients are school-age children (Aaronson & Rosenberg, 1985).

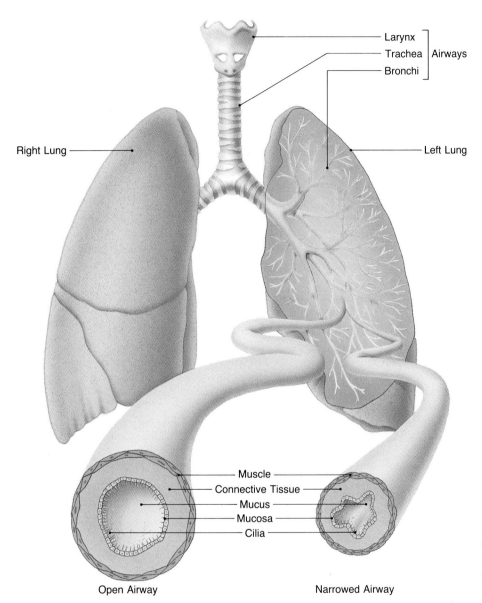

Larynx ⎤
Trachea ⎬ Airways
Bronchi ⎦

Right Lung

Left Lung

Muscle
Connective Tissue
Mucus
Mucosa
Cilia

Open Airway   Narrowed Airway

Figure 12–3
The Lungs, Trachea, and
Bronchi, with Examples of
Open and Closed Airways

Intervention.   The treatment of asthma requires a comprehensive diagnosis prior to intervention. Differentiating asthma from certain other conditions can be very challenging at times. Some children whose wheezing appears to be asthmatic may actually be suffering from other problems, including cystic fibrosis, congenital heart disease, and chronic adenoidal infection. A skilled physician who conducts a comprehensive diagnostic examination can successfully identify the asthmatic. Diagnosis typically includes skin-sensitivity tests, nasal and bronchial arousal tests, lung functioning, a review of family medical history related to

FOCUS 4
What six types of treatment can be provided to individuals with asthma?

allergies, and an investigation of the nature and precipitating causes of the asthmatic episodes.

Drugs play a significant role in relieving children from the effects of an attack. Medication may be administered as injections or suppositories. If an attack occurs at home, a parent may be responsible for rendering the first phases of treatment. A portable air compressor, which can provide a combination of inhalation and drug therapy (antihistamine medication administered through the breathing apparatus), may be used by parents. Hospital treatment of asthma also involves the extensive use of drugs and oxygen therapy. Long-term treatment of asthma may include a variety of therapies. The family and the affected child are encouraged to maintain accurate records of the peak expiratory flow rates so that the effects of various treatments can be evaluated. A treatment plan is initiated and then monitored two to four weeks following its implementation. Thereafter, monitoring varies according to the severity of the asthma and treatment success. Treatment is both medically and psychologically oriented. Drug treatments

---

WINDOW 12–2

We Never Know What to Expect

Since my child was eleven months old, we've known he is severely asthmatic. He is now seven years old. His father also has asthma and regularly takes medication to control his allergies. When Daniel was born he was the first grandson for both sets of grandparents. Given this distinctive position, he was lavished from day one with gifts and enormous amounts of attention. Because of this and other factors, he has a very strong attachment to his paternal grandfather. He and Daniel spend a lot of time together.

Recently, Daniel went with this grandfather to an indoor recreational facility. His grandmother also tagged along. Daniel enjoys these activities with his grandparents, and I enjoy having some time to myself. When the time came for the outing to end, Daniel refused to come home with me when I went to pick him up.

I finally got him in our family car. As we struggled, Daniel threatened me: "Mom, you'll be sorry, I'm going to start coughing and wheezing." By the time we got home, he was in the middle of a rather severe asthmatic episode—which he had produced to keep me from making an appointment downtown. I put him on our small air compressor and began to medicate the air he was processing through his respirator. This manipulative behavior on his part is a new challenge to us.

One last thing. I never thought I would pray for winter, but it's now a regular part of my routine in the fall. It takes three days of twenty-eight-degree weather to kill the weed pollen in our area. Last year we almost died waiting for three days of twenty-eight-degree weather. This year we had an early snow, and things were much better around our house.

We don't know exactly what causes Daniel's allergy problems, nor do we know how long each episode is going to be. Some nights we have made as many as three visits to the emergency room at the hospital. Even the slightest cough in the night produces an icy cold feeling in us. We never know exactly what to expect from Daniel.

Sharon, *Daniel's mother*

include **bronchodilators, steroid aerosols,** and **corticosteroids.** Psychotherapy, family therapy, and hypnosis are also used to aid individuals suffering from asthma. If personal or familial problems are aggravating the asthma, a psychiatrist or family therapist may be helpful in lessening personal or family tensions and problems. Some families are unable to respond adequately to all the demands (exceptionally clean home environments, diet modification, limitation of vigorous exercise) that must be met for the asthmatic child or adolescent. In some instances, the juvenile asthmatic must be removed from the family for a time and live in a specialized residential treatment center in order for treatment to succeed.

Educational Considerations.   As with juvenile diabetes and certain heart ailments, asthma is a condition that often dictates a limiting of various types of activity in youngsters. In fact, asthma is the primary reason cited for school absence by children. Youngsters may experience embarrassment and fear after an asthmatic attack. If the episodes are extremely serious or frequent, hospitalization may be required. Absence from peers, school involvement, and family due to hospitalization can have a marked impact on juvenile asthmatics. They may begin to regard themselves as being different, weak, sick, and of little value, either to themselves or to others. Extended school absences without appropriate homebound or hospitalized teaching assistance make it difficult for the asthmatic student to perform at grade level.

FOCUS 5
In addition to the physical effects of asthma, what three other elements of a child's life might be affected by this condition?

The majority of individuals with asthma who receive appropriate medical and psychological support successfully complete their schooling and lead normal lives. Teachers and others who must assist individuals with asthma should work cooperatively with parents and attending medical personnel. Such cooperation lessens many of the negative side effects of hospitalization, absence from school, and reduced physical activity.

LIFE-ENDANGERING DISEASES

Cystic Fibrosis

Sally appeared normal when she was born, although her stools were abnormal. Her feces had a greenish tint at first, and then became paler than normal. After the first few weeks of life, Sally's stools became soft, crumbly, and bulky, increased in frequency, and had a pungent, penetrating odor. Sally's mother said, "You could smell them a mile away."

Sally's mother and pediatrician became concerned when Sally failed to make minimal weight gains, even though she seemed "to eat like a champ." Sally also had recurring bronchitis. As all factors were considered, Sally's pediatrician believed that cystic fibrosis was a definite possibility. Subsequently, testing was undertaken at a regional children's hospital, and the diagnosis was confirmed.

Definition and Concepts.   Cystic fibrosis (CF) is an inherited, systemic, generalized disease that begins at conception. It is a disorder of the secretory (exocrine) glands. These glands produce abnormal amounts of mucus, sweat,

FOCUS 6
What is the impact of cystic fibrosis on the lungs and other affected organs of the body?

and saliva. Three major organ systems are influenced by the abnormal secretions: the lungs, pancreas, and sweat glands. The gluelike mucus in the lungs obstructs their functioning and heightens the chances for the development of infections. With repeated infections, the lungs are gradually destroyed. As lung deterioration occurs, the heart is also burdened, and heart failure may result.

The pancreas is affected in a similar fashion. Excessive amounts of mucus prevent critical digestive enzymes from reaching the small intestine. Without these enzymes, proteins and fats that are consumed by the individual with CF are lost in frequent, greasy, flatulent stools.

Individuals with CF produce sweat that is exceptionally high in salt content. The presence of these inordinate levels of salt are diagnostically very significant in identifying children or youth suspected of having CF. Activities that are physically demanding for the individual, when not accompanied by adequate salt intake, may cause heat prostration, exhaustion, or fatigue.

The prognosis for an individual with cystic fibrosis depends on a number of factors. The two most critical ones are early diagnosis of the condition and the quality of care provided from the time of the diagnosis. If diagnosis occurs late, preliminary damage, which is irreversible, may have already occurred. With early diagnosis and appropriate medical care, most individuals with CF can achieve weight and growth gains similar to those of their normal peers. Earlier diagnosis and improved treatment strategies have lengthened the average life span of children with cystic fibrosis. More than half of the children affected by this disease now live beyond their twentieth year (Cheney & Harwood, 1985).

Causation and Prevalence. The causes of cystic fibrosis are unclear, and there are many theories about its origin (Boat & Dearborn, 1984). It is known, however, that cystic fibrosis is an inherited disease (Cystic Fibrosis Foundation, 1988).

Cystic fibrosis is primarily a Caucasian phenomenon. Studies conducted in the United States have demonstrated a minimum prevalence range from 1 in 2000 Caucasian children to 1 in 17,000 Black children. Worldwide occurrence rates of cystic fibrosis range from 1 in 620 individuals with Dutch ancestry in southwest Africa, to 1 in 90,000 in an Asian population in Hawaii (Doershuk & Boat, 1987).

Intervention. The diagnosis of cystic fibrosis is based on a number of symptoms in the gastrointestinal and respiratory systems. Since the disease may emerge at nearly any age, there is great variability in the ways the condition presents itself. Thus a number of different diagnostic techniques are useful. Infants with cystic fibrosis may fail to thrive, have soft and greasy stools, and exhibit respiratory symptoms. School-age children may have recurrent abdominal pain, heat exhaustion following exercise on hot days, and chest infections. Diagnosis of adolescents and adults with cystic fibrosis occurs less frequently than during the younger years.

FOCUS 7
What six types of intervention are used in treating young people with cystic fibrosis?

Intervention for cystic fibrosis is varied and complex. Afflicted individuals must receive treatment throughout their lives. Consistent and appropriate application of medical, social, educational, and psychological aspects of the treatment process allows these individuals to live longer, with less discomfort and fewer complications. Treatment of cystic fibrosis is designed to accomplish a number of goals. The first is to diagnose the condition before any severe symptoms are exhibited. Other goals include control of chest infection, maintenance of adequate nutrition, education of the family regarding the condition, and provision of a suitable education for the child.

Management of respiratory disease caused by cystic fibrosis is critical. If respiratory insufficiency can be prevented or minimized, the youngster's life is greatly enhanced and prolonged. Vital components of treatment for respiratory disease include the regular administration of antibiotics and aerosols, intermittent inhalation therapy, **chest physiotherapy, postural drainage,** and the use of mechanical aids to assist with the postural drainage (Doershuk & Boat, 1987).

Diet management is also essential for the child with cystic fibrosis. Generally, individuals with this condition require more caloric intake than their normal peers. The diet should be high in protein and adjusted appropriately if the child fails to grow and/or make appropriate weight gains.

Management of cystic fibrosis by the family is challenging. Parents are often overwhelmed when informed of the diagnosis and consequences of the condition. With training and support, however, parents and other family members can learn to provide the care, structure, and support necessary for the affected youngster.

The major social and psychological problems of these children relate to chronic coughing, small stature, offensive stools, gas, delayed onset of puberty and secondary sex characteristics, and impaired social relationships because of the condition. Support provided by counseling or psychiatric personnel and a sensitive teacher may be helpful to the youngster who is burdened with these problems.

The prognosis for individuals with cystic fibrosis remains elusive. If we look only at the extension of life, without measuring the quality of life, we are missing some vital facts. Teenagers with CF often fail to maintain their treatment regimens. Gradually, the consequences of such behavior begin to appear. Depression is common, and the quality of life for such adolescents declines immensely. Nevertheless, future research related to promising diagnostic and treatment techniques may alleviate many of these problems. Some of the more interesting developments related to CF are heart–lung transplants (Cystic Fibrosis Foundation, 1987), **immunosuppressive drugs** (agents that discourage the body from rejecting implanted organs), and the identification of the gene that causes CF (Buchwald & Tusi, 1987; O'Connell, Leppert, Nakamura, Dean, Park, Woude, Farrall, Wainwright, Williamson, Lathrop, Lalouel, and White, 1987; Roberts, 1988; Williamson, Wainwright, Cooper, Scambler, Farrall, Estivill, & Pedersen, 1987).

Educational Considerations. Education for children with cystic fibrosis should occur, in most instances, in a regular school setting. Children with well-controlled cystic fibrosis have few if any problems participating in the activities of a regular school program. In fact, school for these children can be therapeutic (Stern, 1989).

A persistent cough is very common in CF children. The cough is not a function of some bacterial or viral infection; it is a symptom of the disease. Affected children and youth may profit from having easy access to restrooms and frequent opportunities for liquid intake.

Sickle Cell Anemia

Ray had a lot of problems. At age sixteen he was constantly complaining and blaming others for his misfortunes. He was an angry young man, angry about being Black, angry because the school system had unreasonable rules (especially when it came to assignment deadlines, attendance, and punctuality), and particularly angry at his family for their expectations.

Ray had been diagnosed as having sickle cell anemia when he was ten years old. He exhibited none of the more severe signs of the condition, but he experienced frequent stomach pains and periodic hospitalizations, when blood transfusions and medication were administered. Neither Ray nor his family viewed him as being seriously ill. His mother and father both thought Ray was lazy and moody. They argued with him a great deal and pressured him to behave.

At seventeen Ray was dead. His last complaints had fallen on the deaf ears of both his parents and his teachers. They had become accustomed to his complaints and largely discounted them as representing a difficult personality.

WINDOW 12–3

My Mornings Are a Real Bummer

I sometimes wonder what it must be like to have normal lungs. I often think about my friends. When they get up in the morning and get ready for school, they don't have to worry about taking forty or fifty pills. And they don't have to spend time having someone pound their chest in twelve different positions. My mornings are a real bummer. If I could just get up, eat my breakfast, and go to school, I'd be very happy. I just have to do what I'm supposed to or I can get very sick.

Luckily, CF can't be seen easily. It can be heard, which bugs me a lot. New kids in school ask me if I have a permanent cold. Or they ask what has happened to my teeth. "Did you start smoking at three?" The medicine I take to help my stomach digest food colors my teeth.

I also cough a lot. Because the coughing happens all the time, some of the kids wonder if I have a contagious disease. I just tell them I have funny lungs. I also tell them my coughing comes from a disease you're born with, not one you catch from someone else. Once they know they aren't going to get my cough, they're pretty understanding. By the way, some think I have asthma until we talk a little.

Right now I'm trying to increase my lung capacity by riding my bike regularly. I'm trying to work up to riding five miles per day.

One of the best helps to me is a group I belong to. Everyone in the group has CF. We meet regularly. We talk about things that are bothering us, and we try to help each other. I like helping the new group members who are younger. I know what they're feeling, and I try to make things better for them. CF is not something I'd want anyone to have, but I've learned to deal with it okay.

Lester, *an eighth grader*

Definitions and Concepts. Sickle cell anemia (SCA) is a chronic **hemolytic disorder;** that is, the disease has a profound impact on the function and structure of red blood cells. The hemoglobin molecule in the red blood cells of individuals with SCA is abnormal. More specifically, the hemoglobin molecule (of which there are millions in each red cell) is vulnerable to structural collapse when the blood-oxygen level is significantly diminished. As the blood-oxygen level declines, these blood cells become distorted into bizarre shapes. This distortion process is known as sickling. Cells that normally have a donutlike shape now appear as microscopic sickle blades.

People affected by sickle cell anemia experience unrelenting **anemia.** In some cases, this anemia is tolerated well; in others, the condition is quite debilitating (Huntsman, 1987). Another aspect of this condition involves periodic vascular blockage. These crises occur as a function of the sickled cells, which block microvascular channels. The blocking can often cause severe and chronic pain in the extremities, abdomen, or back. A fever may also accompany these crises, which may last for hours or even days. The pain and tenderness may appear to be that of appendicitis or another serious condition. In addition, the disease may affect any organ system of the body (Serjeant, 1985). Moreover, the disease has a significant negative effect on the physical growth and development of infants and children (Bunn & Forget, 1986).

Diagnosis of sickle cell anemia is usually made before a child reaches the age of two. The symptoms may include painful swelling of the hands and feet, and severe abdominal pain (Behrman & Vaughan, 1987). Clinical symptoms are infrequent during the first six months of life. The early-childhood period is a particularly dangerous time for affected children. In the past, many children died of this condition before the age of seven. Bacterial infection was the cause of most of the deaths.

Causation and Prevalence. Sickle cell anemia and **sickle cell trait (SCT)** are caused by various combinations of genes, which are inherited by the child. A child who receives a mutant S-hemoglobin gene from each parent exhibits SCA to one degree or another. The child receiving a mutant S-hemoglobin gene from only one parent and a normal hemoglobin gene from the other parent exhibits SCT. The child with SCT does not suffer the effects of the disease, but is a carrier of the condition. Only in rare instances would a child with SCT actually experience any of the ill effects from the disease.

The actual mechanisms responsible for onset of the primary and secondary clinical manifestations of sickle cell anemia are still unclear. The increased susceptibility to infection is likely due to the loss of functioning of the spleen, since the spleen is thought to be responsible for clearing microorganisms from the blood and providing antibody defense for incoming antigens.

The prevalence of sickle cell anemia varies, depending on geographic location. Studies conducted during the 1950s and 1960s identified specific populations with high prevalence rates of SCT. These populations were found across a broad belt of tropical Africa. High prevalence rates of SCT were also found in Sicily, southern Italy, Greece, Turkey, Arabia, and southern India (Conley, 1980). SCA occurs in about 0.1 to 1.3 percent of the American Black population (deGruchy,

FOCUS 8
What impact does the sickling of cells have on the tissues of the body?

FOCUS 9
What are two symptoms that commonly accompany crises directly related to vascular blockages?

1980). The actual prevalence of SCA in Black Americans is 141 per 100,000 (Wintrobe, Lee, Boggs, Bithell, Foerster, Athens, & Lukens, 1981).

Intervention. Diagnosis of sickle cell anemia is based on various hemoglobin tests that confirm the presence of sickled cells. The individual's health history is also reviewed. Of particular interest to the physician are the characteristics of the crises that may have preceded the diagnostic interview. The spleen may also be examined to determine if it is affected. The diagnosis is particularly critical for infants, since one in ten Black babies who have SCA die before they reach ten years of age. After the age of ten, less than 5 percent die during their succeeding decade (deGruchy, 1978).

A number of treatments are employed to deal with the problems and pain caused by sickle cell anemia. In fact, much of the morbidity and mortality experienced by people with this condition in the past has been reduced through improved health care and living conditions in many parts of the world. In the main, individuals learn to adapt to their anemia and lead relatively normal lives. When their lives are interrupted by crises, a variety of treatment approaches may be utilized. Medication may be helpful to those with severe anemia. Other medical procedures may be aimed at raising the hemoglobin level in the blood.

FOCUS 10
What five factors predispose individuals to SCA crises?

Several factors predispose an individual to SCA crisis. They include dehydration from fevers, reduced liquid intake, and hypoxia (air that is poor in oxygen content). Stress, fatigue, and exposure to cold temperatures should be avoided by those who have a history of SCA crises. Treatment of crises is generally directed at keeping the individual warm, increasing liquid intake, ensuring good blood oxygenation, and administering medication for infection. Support can also be provided for crisis periods by partial **exchange transfusions** with fresh, normal red cells. Transfusions may also be necessary for individuals with SCA who are preparing for surgery or are pregnant.

Educational Considerations. Children with sickle cell anemia require special attention and care on the part of school personnel. Teachers should be alert to signs of anemia and other conditions that may precipitate a crisis. These children have less energy because of their condition and consequently tire easily. Strenuous activities should generally be avoided by such youngsters. Sensitivity and careful management on the part of a teacher may prevent a crisis. If a crisis does occur, the teacher needs to take immediate action and secure prompt medical attention for the ailing child. Teachers and other school staff also play a critical role in helping the SCA child to adjust psychologically and physically to the challenges associated with this condition.

Cancer

Steve had recently recovered from a case of bronchitis. He was just beginning to feel better, although his parents noticed that he did not have the same energy he had before.

Shortly after his sixth birthday, Steve went to the dentist to have his teeth examined and cleaned. While at the dentist, Steve had a tooth removed, and he experienced persistent bleeding at the site of the tooth extraction. The dentist was also concerned about small ulcers in Steve's mouth and slight swelling in the gum tissue. He recommended that Steve's mother make an immediate appointment with the family pediatrician.

The next day, Steve and his mother met with Dr. Fletcher, their pediatrician. She gave Steve a routine physical and found that his sternum was very tender. Slight bruises were also evident on his legs and arms. His liver and spleen appeared to be enlarged. Dr. Fletcher gave Steve a blood test, which she sent off to the laboratory for analysis.

On receiving the results of the blood test, Dr. Fletcher promptly called Steve's parents. She asked them to take Steve to the university medical school for further tests. There, a bone-marrow biopsy was performed, as well as other blood tests. Gradually, the diagnosis was formulated: Steve had acute lymphocytic leukemia.

Definitions and Concepts.   The principal type of leukemia which affects children is **acute lymphocytic leukemia (ALL)**. ALL is a disorder of blood-cell production in which abnormal white blood cells accumulate in the blood and bone marrow. There are, however, two types of hematologic (of or relating to blood) cancer: the **leukemias** and the **lymphomas**. The leukemias are found throughout the body, and their impact is primarily on the blood-forming organs— bone marrow, liver, spleen, and lymph nodes. The lymphomas are localized. They are evidenced by swelling of the lymph nodes.

Individuals may develop leukemia at any age, although the peak period for emergence is between birth and the first six years of life. The actual onset of leukemia may be either abrupt or very slow, but in children the condition usually occurs abruptly. Symptoms of leukemia include anemia, pallor, bruises, pain, and infections. Frequently, a series of respiratory infections precede the apparent onset.

Because different types of leukemia affect the various blood-cell groups in the body, natural defenses are impaired, and the individual becomes susceptible to infection. Anemia occurs as a function of the reduced number of red blood cells that transport the life-giving oxygen to all cells of the body. Hemorrhaging occurs as a function of reduced platelet production. Platelets are necessary for normal blood-clot formation. The loss of these vital cell functions results in a child who is extremely ill (U.S. Department of Health and Human Services, 1988).

FOCUS 11
What are four serious outcomes of the various types of leukemia?

Causation and Prevalence.   Causation of the various leukemias remains obscure. Despite considerable research, no one knows why youngsters develop these cancers (U.S. Department of Health and Human Services, 1988). Several factors interact together or in sequence to produce leukemia, including a genetic predisposition for the condition, viral activity, and a variety of physical and chemical agents. Such factors have been collectively identified as triggering mechanisms. Other sources of leukemia have been identified as well. They include ionizing radiation, gamma rays, and atomic radiation. New research suggests that leukemias may be caused by certain retroviruses too. These viruses are known to cause leukemia in cats, cattle, and gibbon apes (Freeman & Brecher, 1985).

The incidence of leukemia is highest during the first six years of life; some 20 percent of all leukemias appear in children. Of these children, the highest mortality rate occurs between the ages of two and five (Grunz, 1980). About 12.5 in 1,000,000 Caucasian children and 9.8 in 100,000 Black children under the age of fifteen develop some form of leukemia (Freeman & Brecher, 1985). A slightly higher number of boys than girls are affected by this disease. Black children appear to be at less risk for developing acute lymphocytic leukemia than their Caucasian counterparts. Siblings of leukemia patients have a slightly greater risk of eventually developing leukemia than does the general pediatric population.

FOCUS 12
What are two major goals of treatment in combating the effects of various leukemias in children?

Intervention.   Once a leukemic condition is confirmed, treatment proceeds in a twofold fashion. The first step is to treat the conditions caused by the leukemia: anemia, bleeding, infections, and metabolic complications. **Transfusions** of packed red blood cells may be administered for anemia, or the child may gradually self-correct an anemic condition. Bleeding may be handled with **platelet transfusions.**

The second step in the intervention process is antileukemic therapy. The goals of therapy are to decrease the number of leukemic cells that are burdening the blood and to foster the repopulation of normal cells in the bone marrow. A variety of chemical agents are typically successful in achieving these goals. Adequate treatment of the predominant form of childhood leukemia (ALL) results in significant decreases in the number of leukemic cells in the body.

The major causes of death in leukemic children are infection and bleeding. Thus the control and management of infections are of critical importance in maintaining the lives of children with cancer. The underlying bacteria and fever are treated with a variety of broad-spectrum antibiotics.

Approximately 90 percent of the children with ALL experience substantial remissions, and approximately 50 percent of these children live five years or longer. In effect, some may be deemed cured of the disease. Children between the ages of three and seven are most likely to respond favorably to treatment (Klemperer, Rubins, & Lichtman, 1978). For those not so fortunate, death may occur in only a few weeks or months.

Educational Considerations.   After the young patient is released from the hospital, his or her parents should discuss with their physician the nature and types of activities in which the child can participate. The child should be allowed to pursue life as normally as possible. The same holds true with regard to the school environment. As a child with leukemia returns to school, he or she may still be easily fatigued and susceptible to infection. Teachers should take these and other factors into account (U.S. Department of Health and Human Services, 1987).

Teachers should also be aware of when treatments are to be administered and their potential side effects. With younger children, teachers may want to ascertain what these children know about the seriousness of their condition.

Moreover, teachers may need to determine what information, if any, should be shared with classmates.

If a child's death is expected soon, or even likely, appropriate action should be taken to prepare the other students for this eventuality (Spinetta & Deasy-Spinetta, 1981). Likewise, parents, siblings, and others who are potentially at risk emotionally may require help in coping with their feelings and behaviors (American Cancer Society, 1984; National Cancer Institute, 1987; U.S. Department of Health and Human Services, 1987). As with the other life-endangering diseases discussed in this book, there are a variety of written materials and other aids available: *Young People with Cancer: A Handbook for Parents*, U.S. Department of Health and Human Services; *Emotional Aspects of Childhood Leukemia*, Leukemia Society of America, Inc.; *Help Yourself: Tips for Teenagers with Cancer*, U.S. Department of Health and Human Services; *Youth Looks at Cancer: When Your Brother or Sister Has Cancer*, American Cancer Society. The Candlelighters may be particularly helpful in the case of leukemia. In addition, friends, psychiatric personnel, and clergy may play a critical role in the adjustment process.

Acquired Immune Deficiency Syndrome (AIDS)

Definition and Concepts.   AIDS is truly a modern-day medical syndrome. First reports regarding some of the features of this syndrome were received by the Centers for Disease Control in the spring of 1981. These reports dealt exclusively with young men who had a rare form of **pneumonia.** Simultaneously, reports were also received by the Centers regarding an increased incidence of a rare skin tumor, Kaposi's sarcoma. Individuals who had developed these conditions were homosexual men in their thirties and forties. Many died or were severely debilitated within twelve months of their diagnosis.

Prior to the spring of 1981, primary-care physicians in New York, San Francisco, and other large cities had seen many cases of swollen **lymph nodes** (persistent generalized lymphadenopathy or lymphadenopathy syndrome) in homosexual men. Many of these individuals exhibited this condition for months or even years after their initial diagnosis, without serious side effects. However, those who developed **opportunistic infections** (caused by germs that are not usually capable of causing infection in normal persons) often experienced severe side effects or even death. Eventually, these opportunistic infections were linked to a breakdown in the functioning of the **immune system.** Persons affected with these infections exhibit pronounced depletions of a particular subset of white blood cells, **T lymphocytes.** White blood cells fight infections; without sufficient numbers and kinds of them, the body is rendered defenseless. Such individuals become host to a wide range of opportunistic infections and tumors affecting the gastrointestinal system, central nervous system, and skin.

The term *AIDS*, or Acquired Immune Deficiency Syndrome, was coined in 1982 by the Centers for Disease Control. It has been described as a reliably diagnosed disease that is at least moderately predictive of a defect in cell-mediated immunity, occurring with no known cause of the diminished resistance to disease (Falloon, Eddy, Roper, & Pizzo, 1988).

FOCUS 13
What are the essential components of the definition of AIDS?

Reflect on This 12–1

What Can a Sibling Say or Do after Losing a Brother or Sister?

"Having to explain that my sister died isn't all that easy." "I think some kids act nice to me just because my brother died." "Ever since my sister, Sally, died, I haven't been myself. I think I might be depressed. I used to do so many things. Feeling this way is really a bummer, but I don't know what to do." "Since John died I haven't spent much time with my friends. Maybe they don't know what to say to me or how to react to John's death. I don't know what to do either."

Children and adolescents who have lost a brother or sister to cancer, cystic fibrosis, or other serious health disorders or accidents are often at a loss as to how to deal with their feelings, what to say to schoolmates and others about the death of a sibling, and what to do to feel better.

Sue N. Sauer has worked with groups of children who have lost a sibling due to a serious illness or accident. She has summarized the advice that they would give to others to become happier as follows:

1. Be around someone, but it matters who you want to be around.
2. Talk with other teens who have lost someone, because they are the only ones who know what you are feeling.
3. Know that you need someone, but not just anyone.
4. Go to a support group. If you try to do it by yourself, it doesn't work, and later it gets worse.
5. It helps to know you're not the only one thinking about death.
6. Think of comforting thoughts, such as "They had a good life, they're happy, or they are with God."
7. It's a comforting thought to know you helped another kid through it.
8. Keep occupied and try to forget. This helps in some ways, but if you aren't careful, it catches up with you.
9. It helps to be around someone you view positively, like my Sea Explorer Scout Leader. It helps me to try to see myself this way in the future. It gives me a direction and a feeling I'll be OK.
10. Don't think you should get better real soon. It takes a year.
11. Holidays need special preparation. It helped to think about why we can no longer watch the Muppets or the John Denver Family Christmas Show.
12. Be yourself, most of all.

Source: S. N. Sauer (1984), "Siblings of Children Who Have Died." In R. W. Blum (Ed.), *Chronic Illness and Disabilities in Childhood and Adolescence* (p. 187). Orlando, Fla.: Grune & Stratton.

FOCUS 14
What is believed to be the main cause of AIDS?

FOCUS 15
What are the most common ways in which infants and children receive the HIV virus?

Causation and Prevalence. With the naming of the syndrome, the scientific and medical communities focused their attention on identifying the cause(s) of AIDS. Late in 1983, scientists in France and the United States were able to isolate two retroviruses with affinities for T lymphocytes, that special subset of white blood cells. Several names were generated for these viruses, but eventually the designation that prevailed was **Human Immunodeficiency Virus (HIV).** This virus is passed from one person to another through blood, semen, unscreened blood products, cervical and vaginal secretions, and perhaps breast milk.

Children may receive the HIV virus through a number of pathways. Some children and teenagers have been exposed to the HIV virus through blood transfusions. Particularly those children and individuals with hemophilia were once at risk for receiving blood that contained the HIV virus. Today, tests are available to detect for its presence in donated blood.

Another way in which children acquire the virus is through their mothers. Mothers who are pregnant and have received the virus through intravenous drug use or other means transmit it to their yet-unborn children (Falloon, Eddy, Roper, & Pizzo, 1988). Many of these children develop AIDS and die before their second birthday.

In a very few cases, sexual abuse is the source of AIDS in children (Falloon, Eddy, Roper, & Pizzo, 1988). Unfortunately, children in some home and community environments are subjected to sexual activities with parents, siblings, or others that make them vulnerable to the HIV virus and the subsequent development of AIDS.

The virus has been found in tears and saliva; however, there is no evidence that contact or ingestion of these substances by another person produces AIDS. Some concern has been expressed about arthropods (mosquitoes and flies) as carriers of the disease. However, studies of African children and adults repeatedly bitten by arthropods in communities where the incidence of AIDS is exceptionally high show a remarkable absence of HIV infections (Goedert & Blattner, 1988).

Some controversy continues regarding the role of the HIV virus in the causation of AIDS. Some assert that the virus may be necessary but not entirely responsible for the development of AIDS. Others suggest that the HIV virus may itself be only an opportunist—a marker of infection by an unknown causal agent (Aggleton & Homan, 1988).

Currently, there are about 57,000 cases of AIDS in the United States (Fischinger, 1988). However, 1 to 1.5 million individuals are currently thought to be infected with the HIV virus (Lifson, 1988). It is estimated that by 1991 the United States will have 135,000 to 270,000 cases of AIDS (Goedert & Blattner, 1988). It is further predicted that between 1993 and 1996 a total of 10 million individuals worldwide will die of AIDS (Gotta, 1989). At least two factors will influence the incidence figures as well as deaths related to AIDS in the United States and elsewhere by 1991 and thereafter: the success or failure of various interventions and the emergence of new, related viruses (Goedert & Blattner, 1988).

The information regarding the prevalence of AIDS among children and infants is far less accurate and complete than for adults. In August of 1987, there were 558 confirmed cases of AIDS in children under thirteen years of age in the United States (Falloon, Eddy, Roper, & Pizzo, 1988). By 1991, it is anticipated that the number of AIDS cases in children will swell to at least 3000.

Sixty percent of the children who test positive for HIV and eventually develop AIDS die. "Which children or what proportion of children will progress to symptoms, opportunistic infections, malignancy or death cannot be predicted" (Falloon, Eddy, Roper, & Pizzo, 1988, p. 346). Children who develop AIDS earlier appear to have a shorter median survival rate than those who develop it when they are older.

Intervention. To date, there is no known cure for AIDS. Although much work is being done with new drugs (interferon, interleukin II, ribavain, zidovudine, & azidothymidine) and **antiretroviral agents,** no effective treatment has been

In the News 12–1

A Lesson in Quiet Caring

Wilmette, Ill.—Central Elementary School principal Paul Nilsen says he knows it's corny but he thinks maybe John Graziano was sent here to teach a lesson.

John Thomas Graziano died of AIDS on May 13, the day he would have celebrated his 10th birthday. After his funeral, his family and friends ate chocolate cake and sang "Happy Birthday." His sister Christine, 11, put Silly Putty and Juicy Fruit gum in the coffin and Tom and Mary Lou Graziano buried their adopted son on Martha's Vineyard, a favorite family vacation spot.

The story of John's last years is, his parents believe, proof that, sometimes, people do the right thing. In the beginning the Grazianos, out of fear, kept John's illness a secret. But by the time he died hundreds of people knew his identity. But until his obituary last month, no one—including at least several local reporters in the know—publicly revealed the name of the boy at the center of a story that attracted national attention.

School Sought Public Support

Unlike school authorities in some other communities, Wilmette officials not only allowed John to stay in school but worked aggressively to win public support for him. John's classmates, his neighbors and many others supported and cared for the little boy. Only one family pulled their child from school over a three-year period.

Wilmette, an affluent suburb north of Chicago, is, with its excellent schools, safe streets and beautiful parks, the model of a protected environment. Tom and Mary Lou Graziano came from New Jersey in 1985, three years after they were married and three years after Tom and his first wife, Joan, with four children of their own, had adopted John, the son of drug addicts. Mary Lou was John's caseworker. Tom married her after Joan died of cancer.

One day in April 1986, Mary Lou Graziano got a telephone call out of a mother's book of nightmares: John's natural mother had AIDS. Mary Lou Graziano knew in her heart that John had it too. AIDS would explain the little boy's constant colds and infections, his developmental lags in school, his increasing lethargy. "It was like: This is it. This is the key, as horrible as it is," she recalls.

Tom Graziano argued that the boy's illness should be kept secret from everyone. He thought of what had happened to Ryan White, an AIDS-stricken teenager barred from school the year before in Kokomo, Ind., and admitted only after a bitter court battle that led to his family being ostracized in the town.

But his wife began telling the parents of children with whom John played. She asked each neighbor to keep the secret and they honored her request.

FOCUS 16
What steps should be taken to assist infants and children with AIDS?

found (Polsky & Armstrong, 1988). However, progress is being made, and certain agents are now ready for testing or have been tested in human beings (Boyd, 1988; Fischinger, 1988).

Interventions for infants and children with AIDS are in their genesis. The medication most frequently used with infants and children with AIDS is immunoglobin. This medication is used to control, to the degree possible, the infectious diseases that attack infants and young children with AIDS. Eventually, more use will be made of the antiviral therapies that are being developed for adults (Falloon, Eddy, Roper, & Pizzo, 1988).

Prevention of AIDS in children and others is a multifaceted and very complicated process (Christi, Siegel, & Moynihan, 1988). Motivating people to actually change their behaviors, through public-information campaigns and ed-

"When I saw this, and when I saw that John was still being permitted to play with my neighbors' children, even though they knew he had AIDS, it became more and more difficult for me not to talk about it," Mary Lou Graziano says. "I hated keeping it a secret."

In November, seven months after John had been diagnosed, the Grazianos decided to move forward. First, they told John and the other children. Then, on Jan. 6, 1987, they took the irrevocable step. In a meeting with Central principal Nilsen and John's teacher, Marcia Yospin, they broke the news. They were prepared for the worst; they had retained a lawyer and would fight in court if school authorities rejected their son.

Principal 'Spoke Volumes'

Nilsen made it clear that wouldn't be necessary. "Paul said something that spoke volumes," recalls Tom. "As we were getting ready to leave, he said 'I'm glad you've come here. This is where your son belongs.'"

Nilsen, school superintendent William Gussner and school board president Don Stephen decided to disclose that a child with AIDS was attending Central but not identify him. In January, they mailed letters and packets of information about AIDS to 2,000 parents of children in the district, informing them that an unnamed child in the Central school had the disease. They set up a hotline to answer questions, dealt fully with reporters and answered parents' fears in two public forums, quickly winning overwhelming support for their actions.

Throughout John's three-year illness, his parents and school authorities worked to keep to a minimum the number of people who knew his identity. It was John himself who came close to revealing the secret, in the first early days of media attention. "He got kind of excited by all the commotion and he just started telling his friends 'It's me, guys. I'm the one. I have AIDS,'" says Yospin.

But John's classmates obeyed their teacher's instructions to not spread the secret outside of class. Their parents, told by the Grazianos in an emotional private meeting, also kept the secret and, except for a few, supported the decision to keep John in school. "It was hard," says Susie Roth, mother of John's best friend, Avi. "We had to reassure Avi that there was no danger, not the slightest danger when, at the beginning, really, we did not believe this ourselves."

Mary Lou says there is a lesson she would like others to draw from her son's illness: "I would like AIDS to be looked upon as simply tragic, like any other disease, without this repulsion and fear, so that many other mothers and fathers and husbands and sisters and brothers of AIDS victims don't have to hide."

Source: "A Lesson in Quiet Caring," by Michael Kelly, Boston Globe, June 27, 1989. Used by permission.

ucation programs, has met with some success (Homans & Aggleton, 1988). There appear to be reductions in new cases of AIDS, particularly in homosexual males. Less headway has been made in reducing the incidence figures for those who are also intravenous drug users. Unfortunately, many innocent children become victims of AIDS through drug abuse in mothers or their AIDS-infected partners.

Prevention at this juncture is the single most effective treatment for AIDS. At the heart of prevention is informed choice and the empowerment of individuals to make wise decisions regarding their own health and others'. Rather than mere information distribution about the causes and effects of AIDS, current health education programs emphasize health enhancement and an understanding

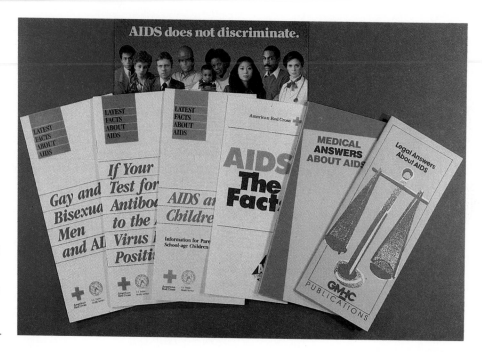

There is no known cure for AIDS. Intervention programs have focused on preventing AIDS through public information campaigns aimed at changing people's behavior. (© Martin M. Rotker/Taurus Photos)

of the personal, social, environmental, and economic factors that influence healthy behavior (Homans & Aggleton, 1988). In many parts of the country, counseling is now an integral part of any prevention program (Homans & Aggleton, 1988). Whether the choice is a more cautious selection of sexual partners, abstinence, use of prophylactics, or employment of safer sexual practices, individuals in greater numbers are making choices that favor good health for them and their intimates (McKusick, Horstman, & Coates, 1985; Silverman, 1986).

Educational Considerations.   Children, as well as others who have developed AIDS or have tested positive for the HIV virus, need to be treated with dignity and compassion. Children and youths should be allowed to attend school and associate with their peers and family members. Shaking hands, engaging in the customary family and school activities, and playing with children with AIDS do not place their siblings and/or peers at risk for developing the disease. Only those activities that result in the exchange of bodily fluids such as semen and blood place youngsters at risk for receiving the HIV virus. Saliva, airborne particles produced by sneezing or coughing, and sweat are not *documented* mediums through which the HIV virus is transmitted (Lerner, 1987; Lifson, 1988). "It is suggested that infected children attend school unless they lack control over body secretions, have uncoverable oozing lesions, have unacceptable behavior such as biting, or unless their risks of contracting infectious disease at school is felt to be unacceptable" (Falloon, Eddy, Roper, & Pizzo, 1988, p. 348).

OTHER HEALTH CONDITIONS

Child Abuse

Tyson was born on Christmas Eve. He left the hospital with his fifteen-year-old mother after two days of routine hospital care. Although Tyson's first home was sparsely furnished, it was adequate.

Tyson matured rapidly, was active, and loved to play with all the little colored statues on his mother's newly purchased coffee table. They were great fun, but Tyson was very confused. When his mother caught him playing with these little toys, she would scream at him and slap him very hard on the side of his head. One time it really hurt, and his ear started to sound funny.

When Tyson was four, he was helping his mother cook in the kitchen one day. He liked helping. He pushed a chair over to the stove. All of a sudden his mother screamed at him: "What do you think you are doing? That's hot!" Instinctively, Tyson put his hands over his ears to protect himself from the blow that always came. "Damn you, listen to me or else!" his mother shouted. "If you won't listen to me, then I'll show you what hot means!" She grabbed his right hand away from his head and jerked him up on the chair. She pushed his palm onto the burner of the stove. "There, you little bastard, now do you know what hot is?"

At the hospital, the physicians huddled in conference. The story regarding Tyson's "accident" was disturbing, mainly because of the physical evidence. Tyson's hand had second- and third-degree burns. It was unlikely that he would ever regain functional use of his right hand.

"It seems to me that a little kid would pull his hand back before it was burned that badly," said a young resident.

"I think we have a lot more here than an accident," noted another.

Definitions and Concepts. **Child abuse** and **neglect** can be regarded as a means of coping. All parents are confronted with many personal and family challenges. Some are able to cope with adaptive behaviors that are not detrimental to their children, while others, like Tyson's mother, respond with maladaptive behaviors that are harmful. Still others choose to deal with the pressures and strains of living by neglecting or abandoning their children. Child abusers come from all walks of life, all ethnic groups, and all socioeconomic strata. There is, however, a greater prevalence of child abuse among families of low socioeconomic status (Meier, 1985).

Helfer (1987) defines child abuse and neglect as "any interaction or lack of interaction between family members which results in non-accidental harm to the individual's physical and/or developmental states" (p. 61). Typically, state laws define abuse as inflicted, nonaccidental trauma or injury. Ample proof must be presented in order to substantiate that a parent has deliberately inflicted serious physical injury on a child.

Another form of child mistreatment is **sexual abuse**—incest, assault, or sexual exploitation. Sexual mistreatment occurs in all strata of society. Forty-four percent of sexual abusers are parents, members of the victim's immediate family, other relatives, neighbors, or close acquaintances of the family (Summit, 1985). Some refer to sexual abuse as a "psychological time bomb." The bomb may go off at any time, having profound psychological effects on children and youth as they become adults.

A variety of factors seem to influence the immediate impact and long-term effects of the bomb's impact (Brassard & McNeill, 1987). They include the youngster's age and developmental status, the relationship of the abuser to the victim, the intensity of the violence or force used by the abuser, the nature of the responses made by the parents and professionals relative to the abuse incident(s), and the degree of guilt felt by the victim.

Other forms of abuse are much more elusive to the investigator or health specialist than those already cited. The psychological and verbal abuse that some children experience is viewed by some to be just as serious as physical abuse. Verbal abuse in the form of put-downs and sarcasm can have a profound impact on a child's self-esteem and overall personality development. In contrast to the broken bones and bruises of a physically abused child, psychological and emotional injuries may never heal entirely.

Causation and Prevalence.   An immense number of variables may cause a parent to be abusive. In fact, some have suggested that the phenomenon is, in reality, the product of several constellations of interacting factors. Research indicates that about 30 to 35 percent of abusive parents were mistreated by their own mothers and fathers (Kaufman & Zigler, 1987). The intergenerational nature of child abuse is a causative factor that must be considered, but there are many other contributing factors as well. These may include crises caused by unemployment, unwanted pregnancy, and economic difficulties (Meier, 1985). An unwanted child often becomes a source of stress. "If I didn't have you, I wouldn't have all these problems" is a common rationalization of abusive parents.

Establishing accurate and precise prevalence estimates for child abuse is very difficult. Much of the difficulty is attributable to the criteria for child abuse and reporting procedures used in various states. Current prevalence estimates for physical abuse, neglect, or sexual exploitation of children eighteen years old and younger are 1.25 to 1.5 percent in the United States. Between 900,000 and 1 million children are abused yearly. Thirty percent of this number are repeat cases and 70 percent are new cases. Some 25 percent of the child abuse cases are classified as physical abuse. Ten percent of the cases are traced to sexual abuse, 55 percent are ascribed to nutritional deprivation, and 10 percent are unknown (Helfer, 1987). Cases of emotional or verbal abuse are not often reported because it is difficult to prove this type of abuse in court.

Approximately 2,000 children in the United States die as a result of physical abuse each year. The overall mortality rate traced to child abuse is approximately 3 percent (Meier, 1985). These figures represent a major cause of childhood death.

Intervention.   Diagnosis of the various forms of mistreatment can be difficult. At the heart of diagnosis are some profound philosophical and practical questions. When does discipline become abuse? What constitutes an accidental injury as opposed to an induced injury? Isn't child-rearing and the way parents treat their children a private affair? How can one determine if a child has been sexually abused? None of these questions is easily answered.

With regard to physical abuse, the presence of bruises which cannot be attributed to accidents may be grounds for taking immediate protective action. Other signs of physical abuse are burns, head injuries, fractures, abdominal injuries, and poisoning. Neglect, including nutritional neglect, failure to provide medical care, or failure to protect a child from physical or social danger is often difficult to detect because many families do not maintain regular contact with physicians or nurses. Gauntness, a lack of fatty padding on the cheeks and buttocks, and a voracious appetite are some of the characteristics of a child who fails to thrive.

Diagnosis of sexual abuse or sexual exploitation is extremely problematic and painful for the physician or counselor who must pursue the possibilities of this type of maltreatment. Complaints by children about their parents' fondling or exhibitionism must be taken seriously. Children who report being sexually assaulted or becoming involved in incest should be handled delicately.

Sexual abuse in young children often results in fears, sleeping difficulties such as nightmares or night terrors, clinging behavior, and developmental regression. The younger school-age child may exhibit other clinical symptoms, such as depression, insomnia, hysteria, anxiety, fear, sudden weight loss, sudden school failure, running away, or truancy. A variety of symptoms can surface in adolescents: serious rebellion against parents, serious delinquency, loss of self-esteem, chronic depression, social isolation, and running away.

Treatment of child abuse is a multifaceted process (Kempe, 1987). The children, parents, and siblings must be involved in treatment. The first goal is to treat abused children for any serious injuries and simultaneously prevent further harm or damage. Hospitalization may be necessary to deal with immediate physical injuries or other complications. During hospitalization, the child protection and treatment team, in conjunction with the family, develops a comprehensive treatment plan.

Once the child's immediate medical needs have been met, a variety of treatment options may be employed: individual play therapy, therapeutic play school, regular preschool, foster care, residential care, hospitalization, and group treatment. Individual play therapy is particularly well suited to hyperactive or aggressive children. The intent of play therapy is to provide these children with a stable, reliable, and understanding relationship with an adult.

Therapeutic play schools serve as temporary islands of reprieve for abused children and their families. Within these predictable school environments, children gradually learn to trust themselves and others, particularly adults. Their teachers or teacher-therapists serve as prototype parents. Special instruction may be provided in the areas of language and motor development.

Foster care used to be the predominant treatment for neglected or abused children, but this option is employed less frequently now. Foster-care placement is used as a temporary means of care while the family is experiencing a crisis or potentially volatile situation. It may also be employed to deal with cases of neglect where the child must be removed immediately to prevent further damage or injury.

A recent innovative but expensive option is the residential treatment center. Rather than placing the child in a foster home, the child, the child and mother, or the entire family enter a residential center for treatment. Hospitalization and institutional care are provided for children in need of extensive, long-term health or psychiatric care. Group treatment approaches have been particularly helpful to preadolescents and adolescents. Within the context of a group setting, they are able to share feelings and seek solutions to their problems.

Treatment for parents and families of abused children is similar to that provided for the children themselves. Treatment options include, but are not limited to, individual psychotherapy, marital and family therapy, group therapy, crisis hot lines, and crisis nurseries (Meier, 1985).

FOCUS 17
What significant obligations do educators and others have in responding to child abuse?

Educational Considerations. Educators and others who have regular or daily contact with children outside their homes have several important obligations. These include awareness of the state laws that deal with child abuse, the procedures to be followed in reporting abuse, and the symptoms of various kinds of abuse and neglect.

Additionally, teachers and other care providers play important roles in helping abused children make the necessary adjustments to lead happy lives. Teachers and others may contribute to the well-being of these children in several ways. One of the most important things that teachers can do is to provide a stable, positive environment. An integral part of this environment is the teacher–child relationship. Abused children have learned to distrust adults. Thus teachers play a critical role in helping them begin to trust again. This trust may be built through nurturing activities in which children learn that adults can be predictable and supportive. Teachers may also be instrumental in helping these children find adaptive ways of expressing anger, disappointment, and other strong feelings.

Adolescent Pregnancy

Kathy was an attractive fifteen-year-old. She began dating when she was eleven years old. Because she was outgoing and comfortable around boys, she dated with great frequency. Her mother, a somewhat cautious woman, did not know how to handle her daughter's popularity. Nor did she know what to tell her daughter about sex.

Kathy's home was not a very appealing place. Her mother had remarried when she was about twelve, and Kathy did not get along very well with her stepfather. In fact, she often argued with him about the clothing she wore, the makeup she used, and the hours she kept. Her mother was often a passive bystander during the arguments.

Slowly, Kathy's dating patterns changed. On weekends, she often did not come home until late the next day. Her mother's greatest fear was realized when Kathy announced one Sunday morning that she was pregnant.

Definition and Concepts.   Adolescent pregnancy is a serious social problem. For Kathy and others like her, the disruption of life activities is much more profound than can be illustrated in a brief vignette.

Adolescents undergo a number of developmental changes. These include the construction of an identity; the development of personal relationships and responsibilities; the gradual preparation for vocational or professional work through education; the emancipation from parents; and various adjustments to a complex society. Many, if not all, of these processes are affected by pregnancy in adolescence.

For adolescents who marry because of their pregnancy, the resulting levels of stress may also be great. Furstenberg (1976) studied adolescent marriages and found that 20 percent of the mothers were divorced within one year, 33 percent within two years, 50 percent within four years, and 60 percent within six years. The major impediments to success in adolescent marriages appear to be the financial and employment restrictions that beset the couples. These restrictions occur for a number of reasons, but the major factor is probably a lack of education. The ability to earn money and secure employment may be severely limited because of termination of schooling.

The risks of adolescent pregnancy are substantial if the mother is fifteen years old or younger. Children born to these mothers experience (1) higher rates of infant mortality, (2) higher rates of birth defects, (3) higher rates of mental retardation, (4) higher rates of central nervous system problems, and (5) increased potential for a reduction in intelligence (Delano, 1986).

Adolescent fathers often become fathers in absentia. Few adolescent fathers truly assume the role of a parent. It is the adolescent mother and her immediate family who shoulder most of the burden of caring for and supporting the child. Furstenberg (1976) found that only 25 percent of the adolescent mothers who expected to marry the fathers of their offspring actually did so. Some 25 percent of these mothers had completely lost contact with the fathers within one year of their deliveries. With these factors in mind, it becomes clear that the majority of adolescent mothers must plan for a family existence that does not include participation of the fathers of their children.

Causation and Prevalence.   There are a number of varied and complex reasons why adolescent girls become pregnant. Delano (1986) has suggested several different types of factors that contribute to it. These are general and societal factors. General factors include a lack of knowledge about conception and sexuality, lack of access to contraceptives, misuse of contraceptives, a desire to escape family control, an attempt to be more adult, a desire to have someone to love, a means of gaining attention and love, and an inability to make sound decisions.

Societal factors certainly play a role in the increased number of adolescents who become pregnant. Some of these factors include greater permissiveness and freedom, social pressure from peers, and continual exposure to sexuality through the media. Another factor is the earlier age at which girls in the United States reach sexual maturity: The average age of menarche has been falling by about four months per decade for the last 130 years.

FOCUS 18
What factors appear to contribute to the increased prevalence of adolescent pregnancy?

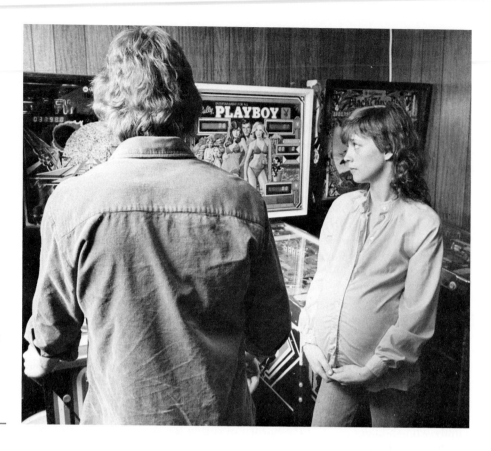

In the United States, 25% of all women will become pregnant before age 18. What are some of the reasons for this high prevalence rate? (John Telford)

The prevalence of adolescent pregnancy is staggering. In the United States, 25 percent of all women become pregnant before the age of eighteen, and about 45 percent by the age of twenty-one. For Black women, the statistics are even more overwhelming: 40 percent become pregnant by age eighteen, and nearly 66 percent by age twenty-one (Hayes, 1987). It is important to remember that not all pregnancies end in childbirth. In fact, about 40 percent of all teenagers choose abortion, and slightly more than 10 percent suffer miscarriages (Hayes, 1987).

Intervention.   The goals of treatment for the pregnant adolescent can be many and varied. The first goal for the prospective mother is to help her cope with the discovery that she is actually pregnant. What emerges from this discovery is a crisis—for her, for the father, and for the families of both individuals. Parents often react to the announcement with anger. Affected adolescents may respond with denial, disbelief, bitterness, disillusionment, or a variety of other feelings. Parents' anger is often followed by shame and guilt. "What did we do wrong?" is a question pondered by many.

Treatment during this period is focused on reducing the interpersonal and intrapersonal strain and tension. A wise case worker or counselor involves the family or families in crisis intervention. This is achieved through careful mediation and problem solving. For many adolescents, this period involves some very intense decision making: "Should I keep the baby?" "Should I have the baby and then put it up for adoption?" "Should I have an abortion?" If the adolescent chooses to have the baby, nutritional support for the developing infant, quality prenatal care, training for eventual child care, education, and employment skills become the focus of the intervention efforts (Delano, 1986).

Group processes have been used extensively in the rehabilitation and treatment for pregnant adolescents (Sadler, Corbett, & Meyer, 1987). They provide adolescents with an opportunity to develop some friendships based on mutual needs. Communication that takes place in such group settings is often uniquely suited to the needs and perspectives of the adolescents involved. Members of the group likewise provide a form of psychological support for each other. As relationships and friendships grow, other types of support also emerge.

Many group process techniques are integral parts of school-based programs. School systems across the United States now allow the majority of pregnant students to continue their enrollment in regular school settings with their peers. Some modifications must be made to accommodate these students, but they are usually limited to such adjustments as allowing for appropriate rest periods and reducing physical education activities.

Unfortunately, many services rendered to pregnant adolescents fade after the delivery of the child. This is most unfortunate, for the problem is one that requires ongoing attention and follow-up; problems do not cease with the delivery. The development of functional life skills for independent living is a long-term educational and rehabilitation process. If adolescents are not assisted in developing these survival skills, they are likely to return to the decision-making processes and behaviors of the past.

Educational Considerations.   Support and educational services are critical for pregnant adolescents. The great majority of pregnant adolescents benefit significantly from ongoing and continuous involvement in their normal school settings. Exceptions should be made on the basis of social or medical problems that might jeopardize the health of the developing child or prospective mother.

The greatest challenge for young mothers is the **postpartum period.** It is during this period that the fewest support services are available. Securing child care, responding to school assignments, transporting the child for various medical check-ups, and dealing with periodic illnesses force many young mothers to discontinue their schooling.

Teachers assist young mothers most effectively when they become part of an active support team. These teams work together to provide the integration and support that young mothers need throughout their pregnancies and thereafter. Sensitivity, understanding, and appropriate expectations on the part of teachers allow many young mothers to complete their high school educations rather than drop out.

Suicide in Youth

Tien was not his real name, but a nickname that he used when he came to the United States from Southeast Asia. His Cambodian name was far too difficult for his new acquaintances to pronounce.

Throughout his life, Tien had experienced a series of traumatic events. He was orphaned at the age of five, during the Khmer Rouge takeover of his small village in the center of Cambodia. During the next several years, he saw all kinds of human depravity. Starvation, killings, and brutal punishment were ever-present during his childhood.

Coming to America was a great blessing, but the transition had been extremely difficult for him. The language, the rapid pace of life, the climate, the lack of close family ties, few friends, the lack of a real identity, and no positive prospects for the future eventually had an impact on him.

Just after Christmas, Tien took his life by shooting himself. He was just about to complete his last year of high school. His teachers were shocked. They had no idea that he was struggling with so many issues. The American couple who had adopted him were severely traumatized by his death.

Definition and Concepts.   Suicide in youth is a means of satisfying needs, alleviating pain, and coping with the challenges and stress that are an inherent part of being a youth in today's society. Suicide is now the third most common form of death in youth fifteen to twenty-four years of age in the United States (Pfeffer, 1986). Well over 5,000 adolescents and young adults commit suicide each year in the United States.

FOCUS 19
What appear to be the major causes of suicide in youth?

Causation and Prevalence.   The causes of suicide are multidimensional (Pfeffer, 1986). As Novick (1984) suggests, "suicide is best viewed as the result of a complex interaction of many factors taking place over a long span of time" (p. 135). Suicide is rarely, if ever, an impulsive act. Generally, it is the culmination of serious, numerous, and long-standing problems (Curran, 1987). As a child moves into adolescence, these problems often become more serious. Another key antecedent is repeated failure. In spite of their best coping efforts in attempting to resolve problems, suicidal youth are not successful. Progressive failure over time leads to isolation from meaningful relationships. Often, just prior to the suicide, there is a dissolution of any remaining important relationships.

Obviously, the sequence of events varies for each youth; however, the antecedents are generally the same. Often, it is not the presence of certain critical events in the lives of these young people but their perception of the events that is so decisive. Some of these events include abandonment, divorce, death of a parent, remarriage of a parent, major moves, and school changes. Collectively, the events may be described as a series of losses and disruptions. Another important feature of these events is that they seem endless; they never seem to abate.

There are other causative factors that have been identified by researchers. Some believe suicide is a product of genetic inheritance triggered by overwhelming environmental stress (Ford, Rushforth, & Sudak, 1984; Kety, 1985). Suicide may also be an outgrowth of major depressive disorders. Studies indicate that many depressed youth who exhibit these disorders have accompanying abnormalities in several hormonal systems of the body (Ambrosini, Rabinovich, & Puig-Antich, 1984).

Reflect on This 12–2

What to Do if a Friend Is Thinking of Suicide

1. Do not be afraid to talk about suicide or to use the word. This will not put the idea in friends' heads or influence them to do it.

2. Try to get your friends to talk about what it is in their lives that makes them feel the way they do. The more talking on their part, the better.

3. Try to convince them that they need to speak to a trusted adult: their parents, a teacher, a coach, or a counselor. Tell them you want them to get more help than just you alone can give. Go with your friends to speak with an adult, if necessary.

4. Unless you are absolutely certain that a friend has spoken to an adult about suicide, you need to speak to an adult yourself about your concern. It is better if you tell your friend you intend to do this.

5. Confidentiality. If a friend asks you not to tell anyone, should you keep the secret? NO. There is no rule of confidentiality when it comes to potential suicide. It does no good to keep the secret and lose the person.

6. A friend may be angry and try to convince you that you will get him or her in trouble if you tell. If you still believe your friend is at risk, you must act now. All you can do is try to convey the idea that you are sincerely trying to help.

Source: D. K. Curran (1987), *Adolescent Suicidal Behavior* (pp. 187–88). Washington, D.C.: Hemisphere Publishing Corporation.

Substance abuse, of all forms, is also a contributor to suicide (Curran, 1987). It lessens a youth's effectiveness in dealing with the primary problems of adolescence and produces numerous secondary problems as well. Still another major contributor to the dramatic rise in suicide in youth may be the changes that have occurred over time in the structure and stability of the family (Fuchs, 1983).

The reported prevalence of suicide among youth is 8.7 per 100,000 (Curran, 1987). However, most professionals believe that this figure represents only a quarter to two-thirds of the actual number of suicides (Hawton, 1985). Far more young males than females commit suicide, the most conservative estimate suggesting that the ratio of male-to-female suicides is 3 to 1 (Curran, 1987).

Treatment and Prevention.   Treatment of suicidal youth is directed at protecting them from further harm, decreasing acute suicidal tendencies, decreasing suicide risk factors, and enhancing factors that protect against suicidal tendencies and decrease vulnerability to repeated suicidal behavior (Pfeffer, 1986). Hospitalization may be the first step. If the youth has physical injuries or complications that need to be dealt with, they are addressed first. Once these injuries or complications have been treated, a variety of professionals, together with parents, begin the planning process and then the implementation of a treatment plan. Therapies directed at decreasing the problems manifested by suicide attempters include individual, peer-group, and family therapy.

Prevention of suicide is a multifaceted process. Different levels and kinds of prevention may be implemented. For example, crisis intervention is directed at moving youth away from imminent suicide and making referrals for appropriate treatment. In contrast, prevention programs are designed to provide early intervention, assist students in developing coping skills, teach youth how to manage stress, and provide counseling and other therapeutic services for children and youth throughout their school years (Curran, 1987).

Prevention is a communitywide endeavor in many ways. The goal is to develop a network of social connections that give adolescents meaningful experiences with peers and other individuals. These connections may avert the problems that are often associated with loneliness and alienation.

Educational Considerations.   Teachers and others who spend a significant amount of time with youth play several critical roles. It may be a teacher, coach, or counselor who is first aware of an adolescent's deterioration. This may be exhibited in declining grades, social involvement, and attendance. A sensitive teacher may use these observations to make a referral to a school counselor or school psychologist. Furthermore, teachers are often among the first to know that an adolescent is thinking of suicide. The knowledge may be conveyed in a written assignment, a note, or by other informal means. In fact, teachers may be second only to friends in learning about an adolescent's intent or ideation about suicide.

Teachers can contribute to the prevention and education process by being knowledgeable about the services available in their school and community. They should also be aware of the procedures for securing these therapeutic services. Acting with dispatch in securing appropriate assistance and support may be one of the most important things a teacher can do for a student who is considering suicide.

REVIEW

FOCUS 1: What five factors influence the impact of a health disorder on individuals?

☐ Factors include the seriousness of the condition, the age of onset, the support of family and friends, the quality of medical care, and the nature of the condition.

FOCUS 2: In addition to disordered metabolism, what three other problems may a child, youth, or young adult with diabetes eventually experience?

☐ Structural abnormalities occur over time that may result in blindness, cardiovascular disease, and kidney disease.

FOCUS 3: What four factors appear to be related to the emergence of asthma in children?

☐ Sensitivity to various allergens is the basis of asthma.
☐ Asthmatic episodes are frequently preceded by stressful events.
☐ Fifty to 75 percent of individuals with asthma have family histories of allergic reactions to various allergens.

☐ Many children appear to develop asthma after respiratory infections.

FOCUS 4: What six types of treatment can be provided to individuals with asthma?

☐ Treatments include medications as injections or suppositories; inhalation therapy; intensive hospital treatment; psychotherapy and family therapy; and specialized residential treatment.

FOCUS 5: In addition to the physical effects of asthma, what three other elements of a child's life might be affected by this condition?

☐ Asthma may limit the types of strenuous activities in which an affected child may engage.
☐ The fear of having an asthma attack may inhibit the desire of some individuals to participate in certain activities that have caused attacks in the past.

□ Absence from school, home, and neighborhood activities may affect the child socially and academically.

FOCUS 6: What is the impact of cystic fibrosis on the lungs and other affected organs of the body?

□ Secretions from the exocrine glands obstruct the functions of the lungs and other vital organs.

□ Because of these secretions, the lungs become highly susceptible to infection.

□ If the lungs are not treated, they are gradually destroyed.

□ As lung deterioration occurs, the heart is also burdened and heart failure can result.

FOCUS 7: What six types of interventions are used in treating young people with cystic fibrosis?

□ Interventions include drug therapy for prevention and treatment of chest infections, diet management, family education regarding the condition, chest physiotherapy and postural drainage, inhalation therapy, and psychological and psychiatric counseling.

FOCUS 8: What impact does the sickling of cells have on the tissues of the body?

□ Sickled cells are more rigid, and as such, they frequently block microvascular channels.

□ The blockage of channels reduces or terminates circulation in these areas, and tissues in need of blood nutrients and oxygen die.

FOCUS 9: What are two symptoms that commonly accompany crises directly related to vascular blockages?

□ Symptoms include pain in the abdomen, extremities, and back.

□ A fever may accompany these conditions.

□ The symptoms may last for days or weeks.

FOCUS 10: What five factors predispose individuals to SCA crises?

□ Factors include dehydration from fevers and reduced liquid intake, hypoxia, stress, fatigue, and exposure to cold temperatures.

FOCUS 11: What are four serious outcomes of the various types of leukemia?

□ Outcomes include high susceptibility to infection, anemia, hemorrhaging, and illness resulting from untreated infections.

FOCUS 12: What are two major goals of treatment in combating the effects of various leukemias in children?

□ The first goal is to treat the conditions that the leukemia has caused: anemia, infection, and bleeding.

□ The second goal is antileukemic therapy: reduction of leukemic cells in the bloodstream and repopulation of normal cells in the bone marrow.

FOCUS 13: What are the essential components of the definition of AIDS?

□ AIDS is a reliably diagnosed disease.

□ AIDS is an acquired disease.

□ AIDS is presumably caused by a virus that affects the immune system of the body and, in particular, the T lymphocytes.

□ AIDS is a syndrome or disease with a pattern of problems with opportunistic infections.

FOCUS 14: What is believed to be the main cause of AIDS?

□ AIDS is presumably caused by the HIV (human immunodeficiency virus) or a variety of other DNA viruses.

FOCUS 15: What are the most common ways in which infants and children receive the HIV virus?

□ Common pathways include transfusions contaminated with the HIV virus, in utero via the mother who has AIDS from intravenous drug use or other causes, or other genital secretions from the mother.

FOCUS 16: What steps should be taken to assist infants and children with AIDS?

□ Infants and children should be provided with the most effective medical care (medications, vaccinations, etc.).

□ Children with AIDS should attend school unless they exhibit behaviors that are dangerous to others or they are at risk for developing infectious diseases that would exacerbate their condition.

FOCUS 17: What significant obligations do educators and others have in responding to child abuse?

□ Obligations include an awareness of the state laws that address child abuse, the procedures to be followed in reporting abuse, and the symptoms of various kinds of child abuse and neglect.

□ Additionally, teachers and others may contribute to treatment by providing a stable, positive classroom environment and by giving these children nurturing activities in which they learn that adults can be predictable and supportive.

FOCUS 18: What factors appear to contribute to the increased prevalence of adolescent pregnancy?

□ General factors include a lack of knowledge about conception and sexuality, a desire to escape family control, an attempt to be more adult, a desire to have someone to love, a means of gaining attention and love, and an inability to make sound decisions.

□ Societal factors include greater permissiveness and freedom, social pressure from peers, and continual exposure to sexuality through the media.

FOCUS 19: What appear to be the major causes of suicide in youth?

□ The causes of suicide are multidimensional. Suicide in adolescents is a culmination of serious, numerous, and long-standing problems. Other causative factors that have been implicated by researchers include a genetic predisposition triggered by overwhelming environmental stress and major depressive disorders accompanied by imbalances in several hormonal systems of the body.

Debate Forum

AIDS and the Public Schools

Guillermo is a first-grader. Unless you knew him well, you would assume that he was a very normal kid. He likes cold drinks and pizza, and watches cartoons every Saturday morning.

In school he performs reasonably well. He's not an academic superstar, but he is learning to read and write quite well. His teacher likes him and says that he is quite sociable for his age and size. Guillermo is a little on the small side, but he doesn't let that get in the way of his enjoying most things in life.

Since his foster parents have had him, he has been quite happy. The crying and whining that characterized his first weeks in their home has disappeared. He is now pretty much a part of the family.

His older foster brother, John, likes him a lot. John and Guillermo spend a good deal of time together. They are about sixteen months apart in age. John is a second-grader and a mighty good one at that. He has always excelled in school, and he loves to help Guillermo when he can.

Guillermo, from day one of his placement, has been ill regularly. He has one infection after another. Of course, his parents knew that this would be the case since Guillermo has AIDS. His biological mother could not care for him as she was a drug addict and has AIDS herself.

Keeping a secret is sometimes very hard, and such was the case for John. From the very beginning of Guillermo's placement in his home, John knew that there was something special about him. His parents have talked to him about Guillermo and his condition. It was a family decision to have Guillermo live in their home.

John is often scared, not for himself but for Guillermo. He wonders how long he will be able to play with his young friend and constant companion. Also, it is often hard to keep the family secret about Guillermo.

Guillermo attends his neighborhood school. Those who are aware of his condition are his classmates, their parents, his teacher, the principal, the school board members, and of course, John. Just about everyone kept the secret at first, and Guillermo was well received by the overwhelming majority of his classmates. He played with them, enjoyed stories with them, and had a good wrestle now and then with some of the boys in his class.

However, over time other parents and students learned about his condition. Then there was a big uproar about Guillermo being in school. The PTA was divided. The principal was in favor of Guillermo's continued attendance, but a few vocal parents began a petition to have Guillermo taught by a teacher for the homebound.

Point Given our current knowledge about the ways in which AIDS is spread in adults and children, there is no reason to remove Guillermo from his neighborhood school. His behavior and physical condition do not place other children at risk for receiving the AIDS virus or developing AIDS.

Counterpoint With the limited knowledge we have about AIDS and its transmission, we should not let children with AIDS or the HIV virus attend neighborhood schools. We should wait until we know a great deal more about the disease. The potential risks for other children are too great and far-reaching.

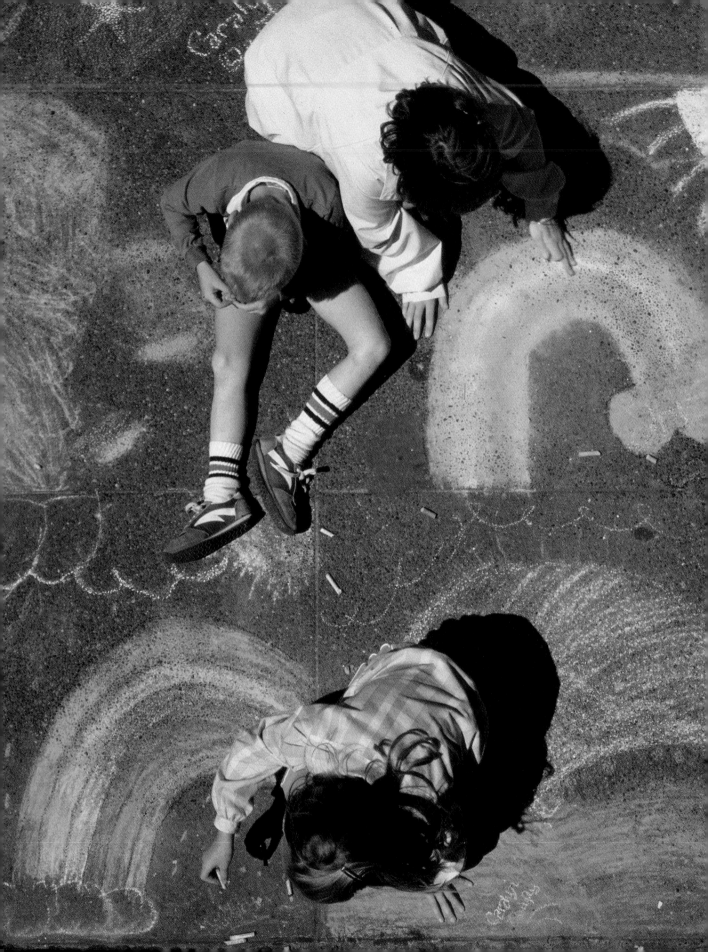

13 Children and Youth Who Are Gifted, Creative, and Talented

To Begin With...

- Interview questions composed by Samantha W., age 8, in a class for gifted and talented children:

  Dear Adam and Eve,

  Did you guys feel yourself being created?
  What did you eat beside the apple you weren't supposed to eat?
  Tell me, how did you keep fit and trim?
  Where is the garden now?

- One educator, commenting on the difficulty of identifying atypical gifted students using the conventional tests presently available: We're having a heck of a time finding kids (Landers, 1986).

- Physics professor and author of a *Brief History of Time*, Stephen W. Hawking is unable to speak but is able to move his eyes and three fingers of his right hand. Widely regarded as the most brilliant theoretical physicist since Einstein, his goal is the complete understanding of the universe (Adler et al., 1988).

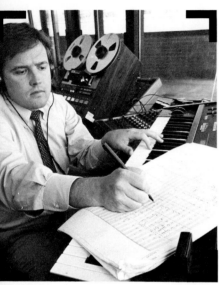

Dwight

Dwight spends most of his time in a variety of creative business endeavors. He is currently president of Broadcast International, a company that specializes in using satellite technologies to deliver information to businesses and consumers throughout the United States.

He is an exceptionally talented musician, composer, and arranger. He plays a number of instruments with great skill, including the bass viol, the fender bass, the guitar, the drums, and the piano. In addition, he has perfect pitch and sings well.

During his early twenties, he was the musical director for a popular rock group that performed on television and in concerts around the world. In this capacity, he wrote musical scores, arranged songs and instrumentals, and developed an extensive library of recordings for radio stations.

As a youngster, Dwight's siblings and classmates referred to him as "the little professor" or "Doc." Throughout his school years, Dwight easily mastered the content in his classes, from science to math, to creative writing. His interests were broad and school was sheer pleasure for him.

As a senior in high school, Dwight composed and arranged all types of musical scores. One example of his tremendous talent involved an audio tape that he created when he was seventeen. The tape included fifteen contemporary songs. Each song was systematically produced using the instruments he played himself. First he recorded the piano on one tape track, then drums on another track, and so on. The result was a musical presentation that would have impressed many professional producers.

Sarah is now twenty. She works as a motel clerk in a very small community in West Virginia. She is incredibly adept at her job, but it provides her with few if any challenges. She does most of the bookkeeping for the motel and manages its newly installed computer system.

She enjoyed her schooling in her rural community and often helped other students when they struggled with their studies. Everything seemed to come easily to her. Her teachers were always impressed with her prowess in reading, broad interests, and solid performance on achievement tests. However, she was not directly encouraged to further her schooling.

No one in her family has ever gone to a university or community college. Her dad and his family have always been involved in mining. Her mother is a homemaker. Two nights a week Sarah worked in a local cafe as a waitress. Earnings and tips from this job were used to take care of the family during the lean times when dad was out of work. When Sarah finished high school, she knew she could work full time at the motel.

Sarah had no idea she was gifted. Nor did she know that she had the "smarts" necessary for college or university training. Going to school after high school was not something that had been encouraged in her family. She had no role models or mentors.

Gifted, creative, and **talented** are terms associated with a special group of people who have extraordinary abilities in one or more areas of performance. In many cases, we admire such individuals and occasionally are a little envious of their talents. The ease with which they are able to master diverse and difficult concepts is impressive. Because of their unusual abilities and skills, we are often reluctant to provide them with the support they need to fully realize their potential.

For many years, behavioral scientists described children with extraordinarily high intelligence as being gifted. Only recently have researchers and practitioners included the adjectives *creative* and *talented* in their descriptions. These terms are typically employed to suggest domains of performance other than those measured by intelligence tests. Dwight is one of those individuals who is probably gifted, creative, and talented. Not only did he excel in intellectual (traditional academic) endeavors, but he also exhibited tremendous prowess with regard to producing and performing music. Certainly the behaviors and traits associated with these terms interact with one another to produce the various constellations of giftedness. Some individuals soar to exceptional heights in the talent domain, others achieve in intellectual areas, and still others excel in creative endeavors. Furthermore, a select few exhibit remarkable levels of behavior and aptitude across several domains or areas.

Unfortunately, some individuals who are gifted are unaware of their unique capacities. This lack of awareness may be attributable to a variety of factors. In Sarah's case, neither her parents nor her teachers were truly cognizant of her capabilities. Nor did she have anyone to encourage her or serve as a role model. No one in her family had ever completed more than a high-school education. Given these and other factors, her giftedness was not fully recognized or utilized.

Historical Background

Definitions describing the unusually able in terms of intelligence quotients and creativity measures are recent phenomena. Until the beginning of the twentieth century, there was no suitable method for quantifying or measuring the human attribute of intelligence. The breakthrough occurred in Europe when Alfred Binet, a French psychologist, constructed the first developmental assessment scale for children in the early 1900s. This scale was created by observing children at various ages to identify specific tasks that ordinary children were able to perform at each age level. These tasks were then sequenced according to age-appropriate levels. Children who could perform tasks well above that which was normal for their chronological age were identified as being developmentally advanced.

Gradually the notion of **mental age** emerged. The mental age of a child was derived by matching the tasks the child was able to perform to the age scale (i.e., typical performance of children at various ages) carefully developed by Binet and Simon (1905; 1908). Although this scale was initially developed and used to identify mentally retarded children in the Parisian schools, it eventually became an important means for identifying those who had higher-than-average mental ages as well.

FOCUS 1
Briefly describe several historical developments that are directly related to the measurement of various types of giftedness.

The Stanford-Binet Individual Intelligence Scale

Lewis M. Terman, an American educator and psychologist, expanded the concepts and procedures developed by Binet. He was convinced that Binet and his colleague, Simon, had developed an approach for measuring intellectual abilities in all children. This belief prompted him to revise the Binet instrument, adding greater breadth to the scale. In 1916, Terman published the Stanford-Binet Individual Intelligence Scale in conjunction with Stanford University. During this period, Terman developed the term **intelligence quotient,** or IQ. The IQ score was obtained by dividing a child's mental age by his or her chronological age and multiplying that figure by 100 (MA/CA × 100 = IQ). For example, a child with a mental age of 12 and a chronological age of 8 would have an IQ of 150 (12/8 × 100 = 150).

Terman and his followers aroused great interest in gifted individuals and their education. They also had a profound effect on how giftedness was initially defined. The intelligence quotient of an individual became the major gauge for determining one's eligibility for the designation of gifted.

Gradually, other researchers became interested in studying the nature and assessment of intelligence. They tended to view intelligence as an underlying ability or capacity that expressed itself in a variety of ways. The unitary IQ scores that were derived from the Stanford-Binet tests were representative of and contributed to this notion.

Over time, however, other researchers came to believe that the intellect of a person was represented by a variety of distinct capacities and abilities (Cattell, 1971; Guilford, 1959). This line of thinking suggested that each distinct, intellectual capacity could be identified and assessed. Several mental abilities then received attention through research, including memory capacity, divergent thinking, vo-

What is intelligence? Can it be accurately measured by an IQ test? (William Lupardo)

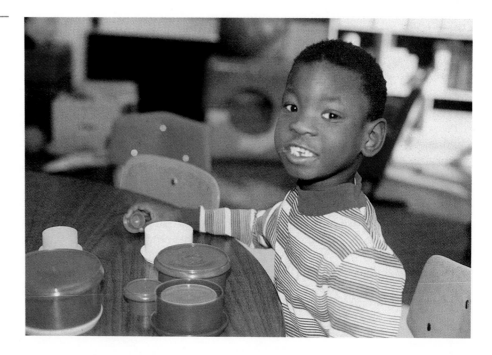

cabulary usage, and reasoning ability. Gradually, the multiple-ability approach became more popular than the unitary intelligence notion. Its proponents were convinced that the universe of intellectual functions was extensive. Moreover, they believed that the intelligence assessment instruments utilized at that time measured a very small portion of an individual's true intellectual capacities.

One of the key contributors to the multidimensional theory regarding intelligence was Guilford (1950; 1959). Guilford's work led many researchers to consider intelligence more than a broad, unitary ability. He saw intelligence as a diverse range of intellectual and creative abilities. His theoretical contributions prompted many researchers to focus their scientific efforts on the emerging field of creativity and its various subcomponents, such as divergent thinking, problem solving, and decision making. Gradually, tests or measures of creativity were developed, using the constructs drawn from models created by Guilford and others.

In summary, conceptions of giftedness during the early 1920s were closely tied to the score that one obtained on an intelligence test. Thus a single score, an IQ, was the index by which one was identified as being gifted. Commencing with the work of Guilford (1950; 1959) and Torrance (1961; 1965; 1968) notions regarding giftedness were greatly expanded. Giftedness began to refer not only to those with high IQs but also to those who demonstrated high aptitude on creativity measures. More recently the term *talented* has been added to the descriptors associated with giftedness. As a result, individuals who demonstrate remarkable skills in the visual or performing arts, or who excel in other areas of performance, may be designated as being among the gifted.

Currently, there is no federal mandate requiring state and local education agency personnel in the United States to provide educational services for students identified as gifted, as is the case with other exceptional conditions. The funding and provision of services are a state-by-state challenge, and as such there is tremendous variability in the quality and types of programs offered to students. Unfortunately, we are seriously neglecting the development of one of our most important natural resources, children who are gifted, talented, and creative.

DEFINITIONS AND CONCEPTS

Definitions of giftedness have been influenced by a variety of innovative and knowledgeable individuals. One definition characterizing the changes that have occurred over time is that provided by the Gifted and Talented Children's Act of 1978 (Purcell, 1978):

FOCUS 2
Briefly identify six major components of definitions that have been developed to describe giftedness.

> The term "gifted and talented" means children, and whenever applicable, youth who are identified at the preschool, elementary, or secondary level as possessing demonstrated or potential abilities that give evidence of high performance capability in areas such as intellectual, creative, specific academic or leadership ability, or in performing and visual arts and who by reason thereof require services or activities not ordinarily provided by the school (Section 902).

Capturing the essence of any human condition in a definition can be very perplexing. This is certainly the case in defining the human attributes, abilities, and potentialities that constitute giftedness. However, definitions serve a number of important purposes. For example, definitions may have a profound influence on the following: (1) the number of students that are ultimately selected; (2) the types of instruments and selection procedures utilized; (3) the scores one must obtain in order to qualify for specialized instruction; (4) the types of differentiated education provided; (5) the amount of funding required to provide services; and (6) the types of training individuals need to teach the gifted and talented. Thus definitions are important from both practical and theoretical perspectives (Kitano & Kirby, 1986).

Renzulli (1978) has also defined giftedness. His "three-ring conception" of giftedness has influenced the thinking and procedures employed by many practitioners. He pioneered the notion that giftedness was a combination of interacting clusters of behavior, and that one could not be identified as being gifted based on only one cluster of behavior. Renzulli's definition stated:

> Giftedness consists of an interaction among three basic clusters of human traits—these clusters being above-average general abilities, high levels of task commitment, and high levels of creativity. Gifted and talented children are those possessing or capable of developing this composite set of traits and applying them to any potentially valuable area of human performance. Children who manifest or are capable of developing an interaction among the three clusters require a wide variety of educational opportunities and services that are not ordinarily provided through regular instructional programs (1978, p. 261).

The clusters emphasized in this definition were drawn from research dealing with individuals who, as adults or youths, had distinguished themselves by their remarkable achievement and/or creative contributions. Renzulli (1978) claimed that his definition was an operational one because it met several important criteria. First, as noted earlier, he developed the definition based on research on gifted individuals and their characteristics. Second, Renzulli asserted that it provided direction for selecting or developing instruments and procedures that could be used to devise defensible identification plans. In addition, he believed that such a definition directed practitioners to focus their programs on the essential characteristics of giftedness that really lead to future achievements and contributions.

Each of the various definitions presented reveals the complexity associated with defining the nature of giftedness, a difficulty that is common to definitions in the behavioral sciences. In a multicultural, pluralistic country such as the United States, different abilities and capacities are encouraged and valued by different parents and teachers. Also, our definitions of giftedness are often a function of our educational, societal, and political priorities at a particular time. The problems of definition and description are not easily resolved, and yet such efforts are vital to both research and practice.

PREVALENCE

Determining the number of children who are gifted is a challenging task. The complexity of the task is directly related to problems inherent in determining who the gifted are and what constitutes giftedness. As we know, giftedness has been defined in several ways. Some definitions are quite restrictive in terms of the number of children to which they apply; others are very inclusive and broad. Consequently, there is tremendous variability in prevalence estimates.

Prevalence figures prior to the 1950s were primarily limited to the intellectually gifted—those identified for the most part by intelligence tests. At that time, 2 to 3 percent of the general population was considered gifted. During the 1950s, a number of writers advocated an expanded view of giftedness (Conant, 1959; DeHann & Havighurst, 1957). Such work had a substantial effect on the prevalence figures suggested for program planning. Terms such as *academically talented* were used to refer to the upper 15 to 20 percent of the general school population.

Thus prevalence estimates have fluctuated depending on the views of researchers and professionals during various periods of the twentieth century. Currently, 3 to 15 percent of the students in the school population may be identified as gifted. However, regulations governing the number of students that can be identified and served vary from state to state.

CHARACTERISTICS

FOCUS 3
Identify four problems inherent in accurately describing the characteristics of the gifted.

Accurately identifying the characteristics of the gifted is an enormous task. Many characteristics attributed to the gifted have been generated by different types of studies (MacKinnon, 1962; Terman, 1925). Frequently, these studies served as catalysts for the production of lists of distinctive characteristics. Gradually, what emerged from the studies was a stereotypical view of giftedness.

Unfortunately, much of the initial research relating to the characteristics of the gifted has been conducted with restricted population samples. Generally, the studies did not include adequate samples of females or individuals from various ethnic and cultural groups; nor did early researchers carefully control for factors directly related to socioeconomic status (Callahan, 1981). Therefore characteristics generated by these studies may not be representative of the gifted population as a whole, but rather a reflection of a select group of gifted individuals from advantaged environments (Olszewski-Kubilius, Kulieke & Krasney, 1988).

Given the present multifaceted definitions of giftedness, we must conclude, as Callahan (1981) did, that the gifted are members of a heterogeneous population of individuals. Consequently, research findings of the past and present must be interpreted with great caution by practitioners assessing a particular youth's behavior and attributes.

Shortly after the publication of the Stanford-Binet Individual Intelligence Scale, Terman (1925) was funded to inaugurate his intriguing *Genetic Studies of Genius*. His initial group of subjects included more than 1,500 students who had obtained IQ scores at or above 140 on the Stanford-Binet. The subjects were drawn from both elementary and secondary classroom settings. In conjunction with other associates, he investigated their physical characteristics, personality attributes, psychological and marital adjustment, educational attainment, and career achievement at the average ages of twenty, thirty-five, and so on (see Table 13–1). Terman's work provided the impetus for the systematic study of gifted individuals.

Since 1929, other researchers have sought to add to the knowledge base about the characteristics of gifted populations. Recent work completed by Adler, Mueller, and Ary (1987) suggests that elementary students who are gifted are

TABLE 13–1 Terman's Findings in the Study of the Gifted

Domains	Characteristics of the Gifted
Physical characteristics	• Robust and in good health. • Above average in physical stature.
Personality attributes and psychological adjustment	• Above average in willpower, popularity, perseverance, emotional maturity, aesthetic perceptivity, and moral reasoning. • Keen sense of humor and high levels of self-confidence. • Equal to their peers in marital adjustment. • Well adjusted as adults and had fewer problems with substance abuse, suicide, and mental health.
Educational attainment	• Generally read before school entrance. • Were frequently promoted. • Excelled in reading and mathematical reasoning. • Consistently scored in the top 10 percent on achievement tests.
Career achievement	• Mates were primarily involved in professional and managerial positions. • Women were teachers or homemakers (probably due to cultural expectations at the time). • Individuals by age forty had completed 67 books, 1400 scientific and professional papers, 700 short stories, and a variety of other creative and scholarly works. • Adult achievers came primarily from encouraging home environments.

frequently sought out as "helpmates." The "bookworm" or social loner image that frequently comes to mind when we think of children who are gifted is simply not true. They are sought out more frequently by their less able peers and play an important role in the learning and growth of others.

Clark (1988) has synthesized the work of past investigators and developed a comprehensive listing of differential characteristics of the gifted, their needs, and their possible problems. Provided in Table 13–2 is a representative listing of some of the characteristics of children and youth who are gifted, according to Clark's five domains: cognitive, affective, physical, intuitive, and societal. Again, remember that individuals who are gifted vary greatly in the extent that they exhibit any or all of the characteristics identified by researchers. One of the interesting features of Clark's listing is the delineation of possible concomitant problems that may surface as a result of the individual's characteristics.

ORIGINS OF GIFTEDNESS

FOCUS 4
What four factors appear to contribute significantly to the emergence of various forms of giftedness?

Scientists have long been interested in identifying the contributing sources of intelligence. Conclusions have varied greatly. For years, many scientists adhered to a hereditary explanation of intelligence—that people inherit their intellectual capacity at conception. Thus intelligence was viewed as an innate capacity that

TABLE 13–2 Representative Characteristics of the Gifted and Potential Concomitant Problems

Domains	Differentiating Characteristics	Problems
Cognitive (thinking)	Extraordinary quantity of information, unusual retentiveness	Boredom with regular curriculum; impatience with waiting for group
	High level of language development	Perceived as a showoff by children of the same age
	Persistent, goal-directed behavior	Perceived as stubborn, willful, uncooperative
	Unusual capacity for processing information	Resent being interrupted; perceived as too serious; dislike for routine and drill
Affective (feeling)	Unusual sensitivity to the expectations and feelings of others	Unusually vulnerable to criticism of others, high level of need for success and recognition
	Keen sense of humor—may be gentle or hostile	Use of humor for critical attack on others, resulting in damage to interpersonal relationships
	Unusual emotional depth and intensity	Unusual vulnerability; problem focusing on realistic goals for life's work
	Advanced levels of moral judgment	Intolerance of and lack of understanding from peer group, leading to rejection and possible isolation
Physical (sensation)	Unusual discrepancy between physical and intellectual development	Result in gifted adults who function with a mind/body dichotomy; gifted children who are comfortable expressing themselves only in mental activity, resulting in a limited development both physically and mentally
	Low tolerance for the lag between their standards and their athletic skills	Refusal to take part in any activities where they do not excel, limiting their experience with otherwise pleasurable, constructive physical activities
Intuitive	Early involvement and concern for intuitive knowing and metaphysical ideas and phenomena	Ridiculed by peers, not taken seriously by elders; considered weird or strange
	Creativity apparent in all areas of endeavor	Seen as deviant; become bored with mundane tasks; may be viewed as troublemaker
Societal	Strongly motivated by self-actualization needs	Frustration of not feeling challenged; loss of unrealized talents
	Leadership	Lack of opportunity to use this ability constructively may result in its disappearance from child's repertoire or its being turned into a negative characteristic, e.g., gang leadership
	Solutions to social and environmental problems	Loss to society if these traits are not allowed to develop with guidance and opportunity for meaningful involvement

Source: Adapted from Barbara Clark, *Growing Up Gifted* (2nd ed.), pp. 91–99. Copyright © 1983 Merrill Publishing Company, Columbus, Ohio. Used with permission.

remained relatively fixed during an individual's lifetime. The prevailing belief then was that little could be done to enhance one's intellectual ability.

During the 1920s and 1930s, scientists such as John Watson began to explore the new notion of behavioral psychology, or behaviorism. Like other behaviorists who followed him, Watson believed that the environment played an important role in the development of intelligence as well as personality traits. Initially, Watson largely discounted the role of heredity and its importance in intellectual development. Later, however, he moderated his views, moving somewhat toward a theoretical perspective in which both hereditary and environment contributed to an individual's intellectual ability.

During the 1930s, many investigators sought to determine the proportional influence of heredity and environment on intellectual development (Laycock, 1979). Some genetic proponents asserted that as much as 70 to 80 percent of an individual's capacity is determined by heredity, and the remainder by environmental influences. Environmentalists believed otherwise. The controversy regarding the respective contributions of heredity and environment to intelligence (known as the nature-nurture controversy) is likely to continue for some time—in part because of the complexity and breadth of the issues involved.

Thus far we have focused our attention on the origins of intelligence rather than giftedness per se. Many of the theories regarding the emergence or essence of giftedness have been derived from the study of general intelligence. Few authors have focused directly on the origins of giftedness (Callahan, 1981). Moreover, the ongoing changes in the definitions of giftedness have further complicated the precise investigation of its origins.

Research continues to provide a range of answers in terms of the inheritability of high intellectual capacity, creativity, and other exceptional talents. Davis and Rim (1989) concluded that, "heredity and environment, working together in some favorable combination, are obvious explanations for the origin of high talent" (p. 32).

The nature-nurture issue is also present in the literature pertaining to the origins of creativity. For example, Gowan, Khatena, and Torrance (1979) defined creativity as "an emergent characteristic of the escalation of developmental process when the requisite degrees of mental ability and environmental stimulation are present" (p. 276). The latter part of this definition illustrates the nature-nurture interactionist point of view; that is, that creativity cannot emerge without the requisite degrees of mental ability and environmental stimulation. In this regard, Gowan et al. (1979) have identified three major theories regarding the origins of creativity. The first is directly related to mental ability as conceptualized by Guilford (1959) in his "structure of intellect" model (see Figure 13–1). In particular, individuals endowed with unusually high levels of ability in the divergent production "slice" of Guilford's model have an excellent chance of becoming very creative. The second theory posits that creativity is an outcome of good mental health or progress toward self-actualization (full utilization of one's potential). The third theory is directly related to environmental aspects of an individual's upbringing. Individuals who are reared in democratic family environments that foster risk taking, openness, and spontaneity are more likely to be creative as youths and adults. Another source of creativity may lie in the

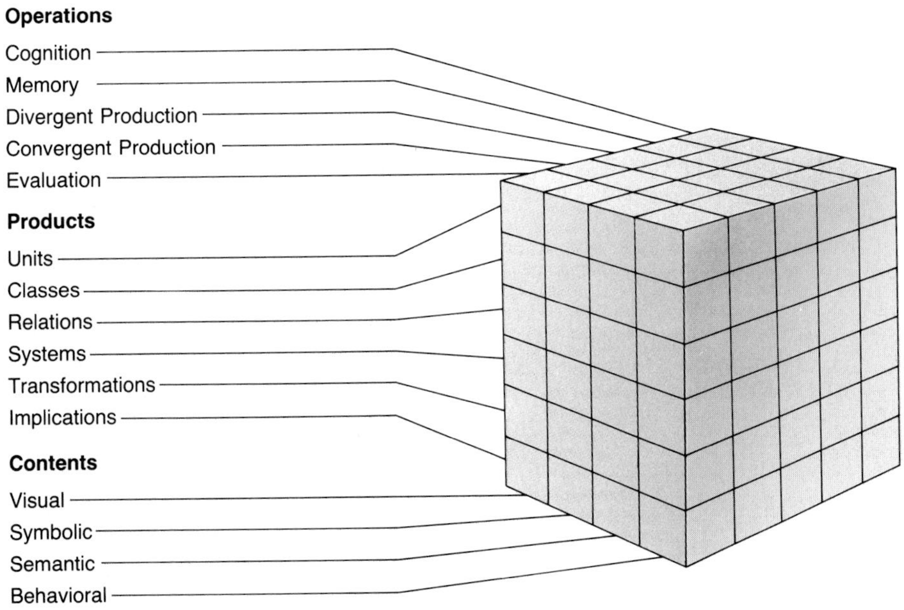

Operations

Cognition

Memory

Divergent Production

Convergent Production

Evaluation

Products

Units

Classes

Relations

Systems

Transformations

Implications

Contents

Visual

Symbolic

Semantic

Behavioral

Figure 13–1
Guilford's Structure of Intellect Model. Each little cube represents a unique combination of one kind of operation, one kind of content, and one kind of product, and hence a distinctly different intellectual ability or function. (*Source:* J. P. Guilford, *Way Beyond the IQ* [Buffalo, N.Y.: Creative Education Foundation, 1977], p. 151.)

encouragement of imagery through experiences designed to stimulate the functions of the right hemisphere of the brain (Khatena, 1982).

Research pertaining to the origins of exceptional talent is limited. This is in part a function of the imprecise definitions to date regarding the nature of remarkable talents. Bloom (1985) studied the development of talent in young people in five fields of talent development: music and art, athletics, and mathematics and science. Each of the 120 talented individuals were selected because they were considered to be among the top twenty-five individuals within their talent area in the United States. His summary of his and others' research regarding these extremely talented individuals is as follows:

> The majority of parents were strongly committed to the work ethic. . . . Typically the talented individuals that we studied tended to be good exemplars of the work ethic, and this was especially true in their talent field (p. 539).
>
> Our present findings point to the conclusion that exceptional levels of talent development require certain types of environmental support, special experiences, excellent teaching, and appropriate motivational encouragement at each stage of development. No matter what the quality of initial gifts, each of the individuals we have studied went through many years of special development under the care of attentive parents and the tutelage and supervision of a remarkable series of teachers and coaches . . . (p. 543).

Only rarely were the individuals in our study given their initial instruction in the talent field because parents or teachers saw in the child unusual gifts to be developed more fully. They were given the initial instruction and encouragement because their parents placed very high value on one of the areas—music and the arts, sports, or intellectual activities. The parents wanted all of their children to have a good opportunity to learn in the talent area that they preferred.

We speculated that if the talented individuals we studied had been reared in a very different home environment, it is probable that their initial instruction and encouragement to learn would have been very different. And it is not likely that they would have reached the level or type of talent for which they were included in this study (pp. 542–44).

It was the child's small successes and interests that resulted in early learning in a talent field that teachers and parents noted. . . . These early minor achievements, rather than evidence of unusual gifts and qualities, were the basis for providing the child with further opportunities to develop in the talent field (p. 544).*

Thus the precise origins of the various forms of giftedness are yet to be determined. Current thinking favors an interaction of natural endowment and appropriate environmental stimulation. As Laycock stated, "Neither heredity nor environment alone is sufficient [as an explanation]" (1979, p. 153). Consequently, all children who are capable of becoming gifted should have the opportunity to realize their creative and intellectual potential. Future research will enhance our abilities to provide this opportunity for all children, regardless of their ethnicity, social-class standing, or geographic location.

ASSESSMENT

FOCUS 5
Identify the range of assessment devices used to determine the various types of giftedness.

Young gifted children are identified using several approaches. The first task of parents and other care providers is to be aware of the behaviors that may signal giftedness in their child or children (Anderson, 1987). Given the heterogeneous nature of giftedness, this can be a challenging task. There are vast differences in the ways children identified as gifted develop. Some may read, walk, and talk quite early, while others may be slow in these areas. Aspects of giftedness may emerge early in a child's development, or later on, as the child matures. Consequently, the identification process is ongoing and continuous throughout a youth's developmental growth years.

Elementary and secondary students who are gifted are identified in a variety of ways. The first step in the identification process is generally screening. During the screening phase, teachers, psychologists, and other school personnel attempt to select all students who are potentially gifted. A number of procedures are employed in the screening process. Historically, information obtained from group intelligence tests and teacher nominations has been used to select the initial pool of students. However, many other measures and data-collection techniques have been instituted since the perspective of giftedness changed from a unidimensional

---

*From *Developing Talent in Young People*, by Benjamin Bloom. Copyright © 1985 by Benjamin Bloom. Reprinted by permission of Ballantine Books, a division of Random House.

to multidimensional approach (Irvine, 1987). They may include developmental inventories, achievement tests, creativity tests, newly developed information-processing tests, biographical inventories, motivation assessment, teacher nominations, and evaluation of student projects. However, the most commonly used instrument for identifying gifted learners continues to be one of the Wechsler scales, even though other instruments and approaches have been developed (Klausmeier, Mishra, & Maker, 1987). Let us briefly highlight some of the findings related to teacher nomination, intelligence testing, achievement testing, information-processing tests and assessment of creativity.

Teacher Nomination

Teacher nominations have been an integral part of many screening approaches. This approach is, however, fraught with a number of problems. Teachers often favor children who are well dressed, cooperative, and task-oriented. Bright underachievers as well as bright disruptive students may be passed over. Teachers are often given few if any specific criteria for nominating gifted students. Another problem is the restriction on the number of students teachers are allowed to nominate. Fortunately, some of these problems have been addressed. There are now several scales to aid teachers and others responsible for making nominations (Borland, 1978; Renzulli, Smith, White, Callahan, & Hartman, 1976; Renzulli, Reis, & Smith, 1981).

Intelligence and Achievement Tests

Intelligence testing has and continues to be a major approach to identifying intellectual giftedness. Research related to intelligence assessment, however, reveals some interesting findings. Wallach (1976) analyzed a series of studies on the relationship between future professional achievement and scores obtained earlier on academic aptitude tests or intelligence tests. He found that performance scores in the upper ranges, particularly those frequently used to screen and identify students who are gifted, served as poor criteria for predicting future creative and productive achievement. Other criticisms have been aimed at intelligence tests and their uses, some of which we discussed earlier in this chapter. One of the major criticisms relates to the restrictiveness of such instruments. Many of the higher mental processes that characterize the functioning of gifted individuals are not measured adequately, and some are not assessed at all. Another criticism involves the limitations inherent in using the typical intelligence tests with culturally different individuals. As noted earlier, few of the instruments currently available are suitably designed to assess the abilities of those who are substantially different from the core culture. The use of nonverbal intelligence tests as well as chronometric devices that monitor closely the speed with which students respond to various stimuli may prove useful in identifying minority children who are gifted (Baldwin, 1987).

Similar problems are inherent in achievement tests. For example, achievement tests are not generally designed to measure the true achievement of children who are academically gifted. Such youngsters are often prevented from demonstrating their unusual prowess because of the restricted range of the test items.

These ceiling effects, as they are known, prevent the children who are gifted from demonstrating their achievement at higher levels.

Information-Processing Tests

Researchers have recently become interested in the ways in which normal students and students identified as gifted process information, and the relationship of these processing skills to intellectual giftedness (Davidson & Sternberg, 1984; Sternberg, 1981; Sternberg, 1987). Sternberg (1981) developed a means for analyzing human problem solving and identified five elementary information processes or metacomponents: planning and decision-making procedures; acquisition; retention; and transfer of problem-solving approaches to other types of problems. From this perspective, individuals who are gifted are those who are identified as having superior skills in processing information for the purpose of problem solving. Kaufman and Kaufman (1983) have developed an assessment battery for children that purportedly measures the mental processing or problem-solving abilities of children. This battery and others that will be developed in the near future may provide us with an alternative and more accurate means of assessing giftedness in all children.

Creativity Tests

Because of the nature of creativity and the many forms in which it can be expressed, developing tests to assess its presence and magnitude is a formidable task (Davis & Rim, 1989). In spite of these challenges, a number of creativity tests have been formulated (Torrance, 1966; Williams, 1980). There are presently two main categories of creativity tests. They are (1) tests designed to assess divergent thinking, and (2) inventories that provide information about students' personalities and biographical traits. A typical question on a divergent-thinking test may read as follows: What would happen if your eyes could be adjusted to see things as small as germs?

Taylor and Ellison (1983) reported on their successful use of various biographical inventories in identifying children and adults who were gifted. These inventories encompass a wide range of questions about childhood activities, sources of satisfaction, descriptions of parents, self-descriptions, self-evaluations, and academic experiences (see Figure 13–2). The questions were derived from biographical research dealing with highly creative research scientists, effective leaders, and other very creative individuals. Thus children or youth whose inventory results compare favorably to the criteria established by gifted adults may, as both students and later in life, make significant contributions to their selected fields of endeavor.

Once the screening steps have been completed, the actual identification and selection of students is begun. During this phase, each of the previously screened students is carefully evaluated again, using more individualized procedures and assessment tools. Ideally these techniques should be closely related to the definition of giftedness used by the district or school system and the nature of the program envisioned for the students.

Historically, a single index or IQ score was used as the basis for placing

13. Do you make your own decisions when you can?
    A. Almost always
    B. Usually
    C. Sometimes
    D. Not very often
    E. Almost never

18. Compared to other students in your class, how often do you ask the teacher questions about the class subject?
    A. Much more often than the other students
    B. A little more than the other students
    C. About as often as the other students
    D. A little less often than others
    E. Much less often than others

34. How often do you, on your own, work math problems which have not been assigned to you in courses?
    A. Not very often
    B. About once or twice a month
    C. About once a week
    D. A few times a week

136. What is your ability to do assignments in new and different ways?
    A. Outstanding
    B. Excellent
    C. Somewhat above average
    D. About average
    E. Somewhat below average
    F. Once a day or more

Figure 13–2
Selected Items from the Biographical Inventory, Form U; Institute for Behavioral Research in Creativity, Salt Lake City, Utah, 1979

or serving young people in gifted programs. Now a variety of different types of measures and scores can be utilized to determine whether a student ought to be served or not. The Baldwin Identification Matrix 2 (Baldwin, 1984) is an example of an approach that allows assessment personnel to obtain a broad perspective regarding a student's overall capacities and talents. For example, a completed matrix for Dwight during the period that he was a sophomore in high school is shown in Figure 13–3. As you can see, he is gifted in a variety of areas and domains. The total score that Dwight or others may receive is used to determine whether they are eligible for participation in district or school programs.

INTERVENTION STRATEGIES

Mary is unusually artistic. Her paintings have been judged excellent by art teachers since elementary school. She contributes artwork to school newspapers and other publications, but she refuses to enter her work in

STUDENT <u>DWIGHT</u> BIRTHDATE <u>N.A.</u> AGE <u>17</u> SEX <u>M</u> GRADE <u>JR.</u> DATE <u>10/10</u>

Area	Assessment Items	Mode of Score	Data Card Info	5	4	3	2	1	B-NA	No. of Items	Raw Score	Area Score (RS + N)
1. Cognitive	1.1 General IQ	41.1	140	5								
	1.2 Learning	22.2	28		4							
	1.3											
	1.4											
	1.5											
	Total Cognitive			5	4	0	0	0		2	9	4.5
2. Psychosocial	2.1 Peer Nomination	56	5	5								
	2.2											
	2.3											
	2.4											
	2.5											
	Total Psychomotor											
3. Creative/ Products	3.1 Musical Perf.	42	10	5						1	5	5
	3.2											
	3.3											
	3.4											
	3.5											
	Total Creative Products											
4. Psychomotor	4.1 Sch. Assessm't.	50	30	5	0	3	0	0		1	5	5
	4.2											
	4.3											
	4.4											
	4.5											
	Total Psychomotor			0	0	3	0	0		1	3	3
5. Motivation	5.1 Motivation	37.2	48	5								
	5.2											
	5.3											
	5.4											
	5.5											
	Total Motivation			5	0	0	0	0		1	5	5
6. Creative Problem-Solving	6.1 Creativity	37.2	48	5								
	6.2											
	6.3											
	6.4											
	6.5											
	Total Creative Problem-Solving			5	0	0	0	0		1	5	5
Matrix Totals	Maximum Points For This Matrix											30
	STUDENT TOTALS											27.5

Figure 13–3

The Baldwin Identification Matrix 2 (*Source:* A. Baldwin [1984]. *The Baldwin Identification Matrix 2 for Identification of the Gifted and Talented: A Handbook for Its Use.* New York: Trillium Press.)

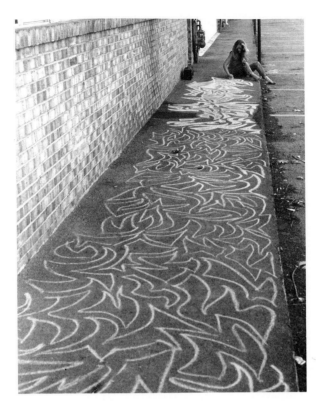

What is creativity? How can it be measured? (Mary Kate Stillings)

art contests. She is not interested in pursuing an art-related education or career after high school because she thinks, "My stuff isn't that good."

Marge is a uniquely creative and intellectually talented young lady. Her IQ is in the 150 range. Her poetry is mature and perceptive and has been accepted for publication in several English journals. Her grades are almost all *A*s, though she puts forth little effort. She is very pretty and appears very independent. Since tenth grade, her parents (upper middle class and very strict) have found her unmanageable. She drinks excessively and appears to be involved with several young men. She is presently a senior in high school but has no intention of going on to college. Her only goal is to get married.

Elizabeth is a shy fifth-grader. She has a high IQ and is a good student. Although her teacher finds her to be a delightful child, Elizabeth tells her mother that she really hates school. On further questioning, she shows her mother a secret drawer stuffed full of stories she has written. She shows her mom her favorite one, which has just been returned from her teacher. Written across the top of the page is the following: "Elizabeth, you have copied this story from a book and that is dishonest. Be sure never to do that again." Elizabeth has been sick frequently and says she likes staying in bed until she is "completely better."

David is a very active third-grader. His schoolwork is frequently incomplete and his handwriting is illegible. Kids like David, but teachers don't. His main problem seems to be his outspoken sense of humor. His jokes and comments, which always send the class into hysterics, usually appear at the most inappropriate times—during lessons, when guests are in the room, or in the middle of a serious class discussion. David seems to be a capable child, but his school activities are dominated by practical jokes, humorous remarks, and poorly done assignments. Parents and teachers are searching for a way to get David motivated to apply himself to schoolwork (Davis & Rimm, 1979, pp. 227–8).*

The vignettes above typify some of the problems children and youth identified as gifted experience in school and elsewhere. In some instances, the problems are family-related. In others, the school environment has caused the problems; and of course many of the problems are a result of both family and school factors. Can some of these problems be resolved with appropriate interventions or specialized programs? What can parents do to aid their children who are gifted? What types of school programs are available for students? Are they effective? Are they harmful to students socially or emotionally? Does specialized programming for the gifted make a difference?

Early Childhood

FOCUS 6
What eight interventions are utilized to foster the development of children and adolescents who are gifted?

Parents can promote the early learning and development of their children in a number of ways (Koopmans-Dayton & Feldhusen, 1987). During the first eighteen months of life, 90 percent of all social interactions with children take place during such activities as feeding, bathing, changing diapers, and dressing (Clark, 1988). Parents who are interested in advancing their child's mental and social development use these occasions for talking to their children; providing varied sensory experiences such as bare-skin cuddling, tickling, and smiling; and conveying a sense of trust. As children gradually progress through their infancy, toddler, and preschool periods, the experiences provided become more varied and uniquely suited to the child's emerging interests. Language and cognitive development are encouraged by means of stories read and told to them. Children are also urged to make up their own stories for telling. Brief periods are also reserved for discussions or spontaneous conversations that arise from events that have momentarily captured their attention. Requests for help in saying or printing a word are promptly fulfilled. Thus many children who are gifted learn to read before they enter kindergarten or first grade.

---

* G. A. Davis and S. Rimm (1979). Identification and counseling of the creatively gifted. In N. Colangelo and R. T. Zaffrann (Eds.), *New Voices in Counseling the Gifted.* Dubuque, Iowa: Kendall Hunt Publishing Company. Copyright © 1979. Reprinted by permission of Kendall/Hunt Publishing Company.

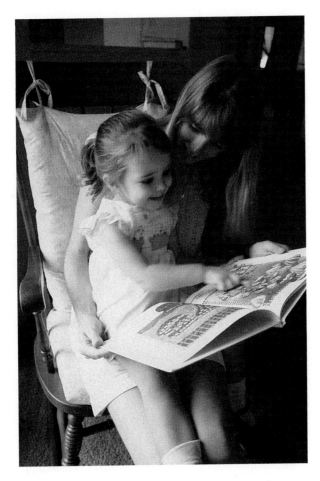

Parents can encourage their child's language and cognitive development by reading stories together. Many children who are gifted learn to read before they enter the school system. (Mary Kate Stillings)

During the school years, parents continue to advance their children's development by providing opportunities that correspond to their children's strengths and interests (Shaughnessy & Neely, 1987). The simple identification games played during the preschool period now become more complex. Discussions frequently take place with peers and other interesting adults in addition to parents. The nature of the discussions and the types of questions asked become more sophisticated. Parents assist their children in moving to higher levels of learning by asking questions that involve analysis (comparing and contrasting ideas), synthesis (integrating and combining ideas into new and novel forms), and evaluation (judging and disputing books, newspaper articles, etc.). Other ways parents can help include (1) furnishing books and reading materials on a broad range of topics; (2) providing appropriate equipment as various interests surface (microscopes, telescopes, chemistry sets, etc.); (3) encouraging regular trips to the public library and other learning-resource centers; (4) providing opportunities for participation in cultural events, lectures, and exhibits of various kinds; (5) encouraging participation in extracurricular and community activities outside the home; and (6) fostering relationships with potential mentors (Hendricks & Scott, 1987; Hanson, 1987) and other resource people in the community.

Preschool Programs. A variety of preschool programs have been developed for young children who are gifted (Gross & Kirsten, 1987; Roedell, Jackson, & Robinson, 1980). Some children are involved in traditional programs, which are characterized by activities and curricula devoted primarily to the development of academic skills. Many of the traditional programs emphasize affective and social development as well. The entry criteria for these programs is varied, but the primary consideration is usually the child's IQ and social maturity. Moreover, the child must be skilled in following directions, attending to tasks of some duration, and controlling impulsive behavior.

Creativity programs are designed to help children develop their natural endowments in a number of artistic or creative domains. Another purpose of such programs is to help the children discover their own areas of promise. Children in these programs are also prepared for eventual involvement in the traditional academic areas of schooling.

Preschool Programs for Children with Disabilities. Preschoolers with disabilities who are gifted are now served in several programs in the United States (Karnes, 1978, 1979; Blacher-Dixon, 1977; Blacher-Dixon & Turnbull, 1979). Each program pursues the education and development process in varied ways. Some programs use Bloom's (1969) *Taxonomy of Educational Objectives*, while others employ Guilford's (1956) Structure of Intellect Model as the basis for advancing the children's thinking processes. Individualization is a key component in the process. Programs also vary according to the amount of structure provided in the preschool environment. The RAPYHT Program (Retrieval and Acceleration of Promising Young Handicapped and Talented) provides children with open-classroom as well as structured-classroom experiences. The open-classroom experiences provide children with opportunities to initiate their own learning activities. The children also select the pace at which they will accomplish their goals. Teachers in this classroom environment serve as facilitators. In contrast, the structured classroom is teacher-directed. Learning activities are selected by the teacher and the sequence of learning experiences is tightly structured (Karnes & Bertschi, 1978).

Childhood and Adolescence

Giftedness in elementary and secondary students may be nurtured in a variety of ways (Van Tassel-Baska, 1988). A number of service-delivery systems and approaches are used in responding to the needs of the gifted. Frequently, the nurturing process has been referred to as **differentiated education;** that is, an education uniquely and predominately suited to the capacities and interests of individuals who are gifted.

Intervention Approaches. Selection of intervention approaches and organizational structures occurs as a function of a variety of factors (Van Tassel-

Baska, 1988; Williams, 1988). First, a school system must determine what types of giftedness it is capable of serving. It must also select identification criteria and measures that allow it to select qualified students fairly. If the system is primarily interested in advancing creativity, measures and indices of creativity should be utilized. If the focus of the program is devoted to accelerating math achievement and understanding, instruments measuring mathematical aptitude and achievement should be employed. With regard to identifying giftedness in the culturally different, progress in instrumentation and measurement development has been made (Khatena, 1982). A variety of formal and informal approaches have been developed that allow practitioners to measure potential giftedness in the culturally divergent (Meeker, 1978; Mercer & Lewis, 1978; Taylor & Ellison, 1966; Torrance, 1971, 1977). Second, the school system must select the organizational structures through which children who are gifted are to receive their differentiated educations. Third, school personnel must select the intervention approaches that are to be utilized within each program setting. Fourth, school personnel must select continuous evaluation procedures and techniques that help them assess the overall effectiveness of the program. Data generated from program evaluation-efforts can serve as a catalyst for making appropriate changes.

Service-Delivery Systems. Once the types of giftedness to be emphasized have been selected and appropriate identification procedures have been selected, planning must be directed at selecting suitable service-delivery systems. Organizational structures for students who are gifted are similar to those found in other areas of special education. Clark (1983) described a continuum model that has been used to develop services for students who are gifted (see Figure 13–4). Each of the learning environments in the model has its inherent advantages and disadvantages (Kramer, 1987a & 1987b). For example, students who are enrolled in a regular classroom and are given opportunities to spend time in a seminar, resource room, special class, and other novel learning circumstances profit from the experiences because they are allowed to work at their own level of ability (Parke, 1989). Furthermore, such pull-out activities provide a means for students to interact with each other and to pursue areas of interest that may not be a part of their usual school curriculum (Renzulli & Van Tassel-Baska, 1987). The disadvantages are many. The major part of the instructional week is spent doing things that may not be appropriate for the students, given their abilities and interests. Additionally, when they return to their regular school classes, they are frequently required to make up missed assignments.

Another example of Clark's continuum is the special class with opportunities for course work integrated with regular classes. It has many advantages. Students who are involved in this service-delivery pattern have the best of both worlds academically and socially. Directed independent studies, seminars, mentorships, and cooperative studies are types of involvement that are made possible through this arrangement. Students are able to interact in an intensive fashion with other able students, as well as with students in their integrated classes. The disadvantages are these: A special class requires a well-trained teacher, and many school systems simply do not have sufficient funds to secure the services of a specially trained teacher. Without a skilled teacher, the special-class instruction or other specialized

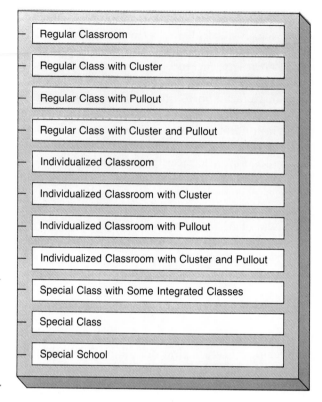

Regular Classroom

Regular Class with Cluster

Regular Class with Pullout

Regular Class with Cluster and Pullout

Individualized Classroom

Individualized Classroom with Cluster

Individualized Classroom with Pullout

Individualized Classroom with Cluster and Pullout

Special Class with Some Integrated Classes

Special Class

Special School

Figure 13–4
Clark's Continuum Model for Ability Grouping (*Source:* Adapted from Barbara Clark, *Growing Up Gifted* (2nd ed.), pp. 140–142. Copyright © 1983. Merrill Publishing Company, Columbus, Ohio. Used with permission.

learning activities may just be more of the regular curriculum. Unfortunately, many of the special classes that have been developed for students who are gifted emphasize quantity of assignments rather than quality.

The selection of the service-delivery systems is a function of the available financing and human resources (trained personnel, specialists in gifted education, mentors, etc.), as well as local community values and conditions. Optimally, the delivery systems should facilitate achievement of the program goals. Furthermore, the selection of delivery systems should correspond with the types of giftedness being nurtured.

Acceleration.   Traditionally, programs for students who are gifted have emphasized the practices of acceleration and enrichment. **Acceleration** allows students to achieve at a rate consonant with their capacities. Acceleration approaches provide for one or many of the following options: grade skipping, telescoped programs, rapid progress through subject matter, and early entry to college or advanced placement. Grade skipping used to be a common administrative practice in providing for the needs of learners of high abilities, but it takes place much less frequently now. The decline in this practice is attributed to the conviction of some individuals that grade skipping may heighten a student's likelihood of becoming socially maladjusted. Others believe that accelerated students would experience significant gaps in their learning because of grade skipping. Acceleration is generally limited to two years in the typical elementary school program.

Another practice, related to grade skipping, is telescoped or condensed schooling, which makes it possible for students to progress through the content of several grades in a significantly reduced time span. An allied practice is that of allowing students to progress rapidly through a particular course or content offering. Acceleration of this nature provides students with the sequential, basic learning at a pace commensurate with their abilities. School programs that are ungraded are particularly suitable for telescoping. Because of their very nature, students, regardless of their chronological ages, may progress through a learning or curriculum sequence that is not constricted by artificial grade boundaries.

Other forms of condensed programming occur at the high-school level. They may include earning credit by examination, enrolling in extra courses for early graduation, reducing or eliminating certain course work, enrolling in intensive summer programs, and completing university requirements while taking approved high-school courses. Many of these options make it possible for students to enter college early or to begin their bachelor's programs with other advanced students. Dwight, the talented musician and broadcasting entrepreneur described earlier in the chapter, was able to profit from honors courses in high school by earning college credit before his actual enrollment in a university. According to Solano & George (1976), many students who are gifted are ready for college-level course work at age fourteen, fifteen, or sixteen. Some students of unusually high abilities are prepared for college-level experiences prior to age fourteen.

Research on acceleration and its impact suggests that carefully selected students profit greatly from such experiences (Brody & Benbow, 1987; Stanley, 1977; Thomas, 1987). The major benefits of acceleration, as established by research and effective practice, include improved motivation, confidence, and scholarship. In addition, acceleration prevents the "habits of mental laziness" (Van Tassel-Baska, 1989a, p. 189).

Enrichment. Enrichment refers to experiences that extend or broaden a person's knowledge in a vertical or horizontal fashion (Aylward, 1987; Klausmeier, 1986). Horizontal enrichment refers to courses of study such as music appreciation, foreign languages instruction, or mythology that are added to a student's curriculum. These courses are usually not any more difficult than other classes in which the student is involved. By contrast, vertical enrichment involves experiences in which the student develops sophisticated thinking skills (synthesis, analysis, interpretation, and evaluation) or opportunities to develop and master advanced concepts in a particular subject area (McAuliff & Stoskin, 1987). Some forms of enrichment are actually types of acceleration. A student whose enrichment involves having an opportunity to fully pursue mathematical concepts that are well beyond his or her present grade level is experiencing a form of acceleration. Obviously the two approaches are interrelated.

The enrichment approach is the most common administrative provision utilized in serving students who are gifted. It is also the most abused approach, in that it is often applied in name only and in a sporadic fashion, without well-delineated objectives or rationale. There are also other problems with it. The enrichment approach is the least expensive service-delivery option; consequently, it is often utilized by school systems in a superficial fashion, as a token response to the demands of parents of children who are gifted. Enrichment activities are

Reflect on This 13–1

Eleven Years Old and . . .

John is just a few days away from being eleven years old. On the Washington Pre-College Test (WPC) he recently scored in the 80th percentile on the verbal portion of the test and in the 10th percentile on the quantitative portion. For the past two years, he has been enrolled at the California State University, Los Angeles (CSULA), taking math courses and other college-level classes. During this time period, he has endeavored to improve his math performance. By the way, John's junior high has an excellent program for highly gifted students, and he has been enrolled in that program, but he finds his university classes to be more challenging and varied.

John's initial experiences with his university course work were fraught with problems. His elementary school training has not provided him with any skill in taking notes. His parents, however, were and are very supportive. When they discovered that he was having difficulty in taking notes, his mother obtained permission to attend some of his courses with him. They both took notes and then made comparisons each day after class. Within three weeks, John had mastered the skill and was well on his way to becoming a competent note taker.

When he first began his university work, he viewed himself as being a "mathematical moron" because of his low entry scores on the WPC. The change in his self-perception as a mathematician came when he enrolled in a chemistry course at CSULA. It really captured his attention and interest. He soon discovered that an understanding of algebra was central to succeeding in the course. Motivated by this discovery, he soon became proficient in algebra. In his most recent test, he scored in the 70th percentile on the quantitative portion of the WPC.

John experienced a lot of fluctuations in his general feelings about himself and his capacity after his early entrance to college. Sometimes he felt overconfident and other times discouraged. Now he has a realistic view of his strengths and weaknesses and is pursuing his university course work with a balanced perspective on himself.

This fall he will enroll full-time as a college student. He is now fourteen and has a full year of college credit under his belt. By the time he is fifteen, he will be a junior. Today he is probably thinking about the graduate school he would like to attend at the conclusion of his bachelor's degree.

viewed by some professionals as periods devoted to educational trivia or instruction heavy in student assignments but light in content (Gallagher, 1975). Quality enrichment programs are characterized by carefully selected activities, modules, or units; challenging but not overwhelming assignments; and evaluations that are rigorous and yet fair.

There is a paucity of systematic experimental research regarding enrichment programs. Despite many of the limitations of current and past research, there is some evidence that supports the effectiveness of enrichment approaches (Callahan, 1981). Long-term experimental research addressing the effectiveness of enrichment programs is, however, particularly sparse (Klausmeier, 1986). Nonexperimental evaluations of enrichment programs indicate that students, teachers, and parents are generally satisfied with their nature and content. Enrichment activities do not appear to detract from the success students experience on regularly administered achievement tests. Sociometric data regarding students who are pulled out of their regular classrooms for enrichment activities are also positive. Students do not appear to suffer socially from the involvement in enrichment programs that take place outside normal classrooms.

Special Programs and Schools. Programs designed to advance the talents of individuals in nonacademic areas, such as the visual and performing arts, have grown rapidly in recent years. Students involved in these programs frequently spend half their school day working in academic subjects and the other half in arts studies. Often the arts instruction is provided by an independent institution, but some school systems maintain their own separate schools. Most programs provide training in the visual and performing arts, but a few emphasize instruction in creative writing, motion picture and television production, and/or photography.

"Governor's schools" and specialized residential or high schools in various states also provide valuable opportunities for students who are talented and academically gifted (Carpenter, 1987; Gold, 1980; Gold, Koch, Jordan, & Pendavis 1987; Taffel, 1987). Competitively selected students are provided with curricular experiences that are closely tailored to their individual aptitudes and interests. Faculties for these schools are meticulously selected for competence in various areas and for their ability to stimulate and motivate students. In Pennsylvania, the "governor's school" focuses solely on the visual and performing arts (Gold, 1980). Also, a number of universities offer exciting summer and year-round programs for high school students who are gifted (Clark & Zimmerman, 1987; Hollingsworth, 1987; Leroux & DeFazio, 1987; Olszewski-Kubilius, 1989).

Career Education. Career education and career guidance are essential components of a comprehensive program for students who are gifted (Van Tassel-Baska, 1989b). Ultimately, career education activities and experiences are designed to help students make educational and occupational decisions. Differentiated learning experiences provide elementary and middle school students with opportunities to investigate and explore. Many of these investigations and explorations are career related and designed to help students understand what it might be like to be a zoologist, a neurosurgeon, or a film maker. The students also become familiar with the training and effort necessary for work in these fields. In group meetings they may discuss the factors that influenced a scientist to pursue a given problem or experiments that led to his or her eminence. As gifted students grow and mature both cognitively and physically, the nature and scope of their career education activities become more sophisticated and varied. New programs for the gifted emphasize leadership development and prepare students for active involvement in all kinds of organizations (Addison, Oliver, & Cooper, 1987).

Mentoring. Some students are provided opportunities to work directly with research scientists or other professionals who are conducting studies and investigations. They may spend as many as two days a week, three or four working hours a day, in laboratory facilities. These students are mentored by the scientists and professionals with whom they work. Other students rely on intensive workshops or summer programs in which they are exposed to specialized careers through internships and individually tailored instruction.

FOCUS 7
What six problems complicate the selection of a career or professional pursuit for young people who are gifted?

Career Choices and Challenges. As one might surmise, there is a broad array of career choices and problems that students who are gifted must contend with in selecting a career. By virtue of their multifaceted abilities and interests, they are often perplexed about what direction they should take in pursuing their studies. The following statements exemplify the dilemmas they face:

I have found that if I apply myself I can do almost anything. I don't seem to have a serious lack of aptitude in any field. I find an English assignment equally as difficult as a physics problem. I find them also to be equally as challenging and equally as interesting. The same goes for math, social studies, music, speech, or any other subject area. . . . Nothing is so simple for me that I can do a perfect job without effort, but nothing is so hard that I cannot do it. That is why it is so difficult to decide my place in the future. Many people wouldn't consider this much of a problem; but to me, this lack of one area to stand out in is a very grave problem indeed.*

When I look for a career in my future, the clouds really thicken. There are so many things I'd like to do and be, and I'd like to try them all; where to start is the problem. Sometimes there is so much happiness and loneliness and passion and joy and despair in me that I practically take off over the trees, and when I get like that I love to write poetry. Sometimes I go for months without writing any, and then it kind of bursts out of me like spontaneous combustion. I'll probably always be like this, but I would also like to be able to discipline myself enough to write more short stories or novels. I'd like to be a physical therapist, a foreign correspondent, a psychiatrist, an anthropologist, a linguist, a folk singer, an espionage agent, and a social worker.†

Career guidance and other forms of counseling play an important role in helping people who are gifted utilize their remarkable abilities and talents. These students may have a difficult time making educational and career choices *because of* their multiple talents; may feel an inordinate amount of pressure to select a certain career or achieve in a certain manner because of the expectations of others; may experience social isolation as a result of their unique abilities and preferences; and may have problems selecting career options because of traditional cultural values and expectations. These problems can be addressed and perhaps solved if appropriate assistance is provided by skilled counselors and parents (Silverman, 1989).

The techniques used by counselors vary according to the nature of the problems and the student's characteristics. In some instances, students need help in resolving personal or social problems before they are able to address issues regarding career development and preparation. If the problem is one of social isolation, the counselor may help the student by involving him or her in a social skills group or group counseling program that emphasizes self-understanding

---

* Reprinted, by permission, from Bruce G. Milne (1979). Career Education. In A. H. Passow (Ed.), *The gifted and the talented: Their education and development, Seventy-eighth yearbook of the National Society for the Study of Education*, Part 2 (pp. 253–4). Chicago: University of Chicago Press.

† M. P. Sanborn (1979). Career development: Problems of gifted and talented students. In N. Colangelo and R. T. Zaffrann (Eds.), *New Voices in Counseling the Gifted*. Dubuque, Iowa: Kendall Hunt Publishing Co. Copyright © 1979. Reprinted by permission of Kendall/Hunt Publishing Company.

and positive peer feedback. Problems caused by excessive or inappropriate parental expectations may need to be addressed in a family context, wherein the counselor helps the parents develop realistic expectations that fit their child's abilities and true interests.

Problems and Challenges of Giftedness.   There are a number of problems with which students who are gifted must cope (Sanborn, 1979; Van Tassel-Baska, 1989b). One problem is the expectations they have of themselves and those that have been explicitly and implicitly imposed by parents, teachers, and others. Students who are gifted frequently feel an inordinate amount of pressure to achieve high grades or to select a particular profession. They often feel obligated or duty-bound to achieve and contribute with excellence in every area. Such pressure often fosters a kind of conformity, preventing students from selecting avenues of endeavor that truly fit them and their personal interests. A "survival" guide has been developed by Delisle and Galbraith (1987) that helps students eleven to eighteen years of age deal with the challenges and problems of being gifted.

Van Tassel-Baska (1989b) has identified several social-emotional needs of students who are gifted, which differentiate them from their same-age peers. They include a need to understand how they are different from and similar to their peers, to appreciate and value their own uniqueness and the individual differences in others, to understand and develop relationship skills, to develop and value their high-level sensitivity, to gain a realistic understanding of their own abilities and talents, to identify ways of nurturing and developing their abilities and talents, to adequately distinguish between "pursuits of excellence" and "pursuits of perfection," and to develop the behaviors associated with negotiation and compromise.

Students who are gifted often have access to adult role models who have interests and abilities that parallel theirs, and their importance cannot be underestimated (Haeger & Feldhusen, 1987; Seeley, 1985). Role models are particularly important for able students who grow up and receive their schooling in rural and remote areas. They often complete their public schooling without the benefit of having a mentor or professional person with whom they can talk or discuss various educational and career-related problems.

HISTORICALLY NEGLECTED GROUPS

Females Who Are Gifted

Silverman (1986, p. 43) posed the question, "What happens to the gifted girl?" The number of girls identified as gifted appears to decline with age. This phenomenon is peculiar when one realizes that girls tend to walk and talk earlier than their male counterparts; that girls, as a group, read earlier; that girls score higher than boys on IQ tests during the preschool years; and that the grade-point averages of girls during the elementary years are higher than those of boys (Silverman, 1986). Just exactly what happens to them? Is the decline related to their socialization over time? Is there some innate physiological or biological

Reflect on This 13–2

Encouraging Giftedness in Daughters

- Hold high expectations for daughters.
- Do not purchase sex-role stereotyped toys.
- Avoid overprotectiveness.
- Encourage high levels of activity.
- Allow them to get dirty.
- Instill beliefs in their capabilities.
- Support their interests.
- Get them identified as gifted during their preschool years.
- Find gifted playmates for them to identify with and emulate.
- Foster interest in mathematics outside of school.

- Consider early entrance and other opportunities to accelerate.
- Encourage them to take every mathematics course possible.
- Introduce them to professional women in many occupations.
- Encourage their mothers to acknowledge their own giftedness.
- Encourage their mothers to work at least part-time outside the home.
- Spend time alone with father in "masculine" activities.
- Share household duties equally between the parents.
- Assign chores to siblings on a nonsexist basis.

- Discourage the use of sexist language or teasing in the home.
- Monitor television programs for sexist stereotypes and discuss these with children of both sexes.
- Encourage siblings to treat each other equitably, rather than according to the traditional sex-role stereotypes they see outside the home.

Source: Adapted from L. K. Silverman (1986). "What Happens to the Gifted Girl?" In C. J. Maker (Ed.), *Critical Issues in Gifted Education Vol. 1: Defensible Programs for the Gifted.* (pp. 43–89). Austin, Tx: Pro-Ed. (Copyright owned by author.)

mechanism that accounts for this decline? The answers for these and other important questions are gradually emerging.

One of the explanations given for this decline is the sex-role socialization that girls receive. Behaviors associated with competitiveness, risk taking, and independence are not generally encouraged in girls. Behaviors that are generally fostered in girls include dependence, cooperation, and nurturing. The elimination of independent behaviors in girls is viewed by Silverman (1986) as being the most damaging aspect of their socialization. Without independence, the development of high levels of creativity, achievement, and leadership are severely limited. Research indicates that females who achieve with a high degree of excellence as adults combine the beliefs, values, expectations and behaviors that are a composite of both sexes (Silverman, 1986).

FOCUS 8
What are some of the problems that girls experience in using their giftedness in careers and other pursuits?

Females who are gifted and talented experience problems, in addition to those identified above, that are unique to them (Feldhusen, Van Tassel-Baska & Seeley, 1989; Silverman, 1986). These problems include fear of success, competition between marital and career aspirations, stress induced by traditional cultural and societal expectations, and self-imposed and/or culturally imposed restrictions related to educational and occupational choices (Buescher, Olszewski, & Higham, 1987; Kerr, 1985). Although many of the problems are far from being resolved at this point, some progress is being made (Fox & Tobin, 1988;

Reflect on This 13–3

Suggestions for Teachers and Counselors in Fostering Giftedness in Girls

- Believe in girls' logicomathematical abilities and provide many opportunities for them to practice mathematical reasoning within other subject areas.

- Accelerate girls through the science and mathematics curriculum whenever possible.

- Have special clubs in mathematics for high-achieving girls.

- Design co-educational career development classes in which both sexes learn about career potentialities for women.

- Expose boys and girls to role models of women in various careers.

- Discuss nontraditional careers for women, including salaries for men and women and schooling requirements.

- Help girls set long-term goals.

- Discuss underachievement among gifted females and ask how they can combat it in themselves and others.

- Have girls read biographies of famous women.

- Arrange opportunities for girls to "shadow" a female professional for a few days to see what her work entails.

- Discourage sexist remarks and attitudes in the classroom.

- Boycott sexist classroom materials and write to the publishers for their immediate correction.

- Discuss sexist messages in the media.

- Advocate special classes and after-school enrichment opportunities for the gifted.

- Form support groups for girls with similar interests.

Source: L. K. Silverman (1986). "What Happens to the Gifted Girl?" In C. J. Maker (Ed.), *Critical Issues in Gifted Education Vol. 1: Defensible Programs for the Gifted* (pp. 43–89). Austin, Tx: Pro-Ed. Copyright owned by author.)

Goldsmith, 1987; Hollinger & Fleming, 1988). Women in greater numbers are now choosing to enter professions traditionally pursued primarily by men.

Fortunately, multiple role assignments are emerging in many family units, wherein the usual tasks of mothers are shared by all members of the family or are completed by someone outside the family. Cultural expectations are changing and, as a result, options for women who are gifted are rapidly expanding.

Giftedness in Persons with Disabilities

For some time, intellectual giftedness has been largely associated with high IQs and high scores on aptitude tests. These tests, by their very nature and structure, measure a limited range of mental abilities. Because of their limitations, they have not been particularly helpful in identifying persons with disabilities who are intellectually gifted.

However, researchers and clinicians have discovered that persons with disabilities such as cerebral palsy, learning disabilities, and other disabling conditions can in fact be gifted (Whitmore & Maker, 1985). Helen Keller was a prime example of an individual who was disabled and also gifted.

A gifted person in this context is defined as "one who has exhibited exceptional potential for (a) learning, (b) achieving academic excellence in one or more

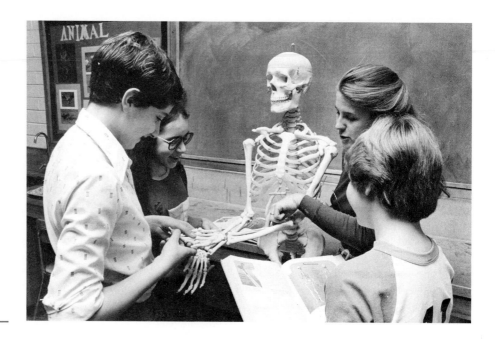

Today females in greater numbers are choosing to enter professions that have been traditionally dominated by males. (John Telford)

subject areas, and (c) manifesting superior abilities through language, problem solving and creative production" (Whitmore & Maker, 1985, p. 10). Although there are still many challenges associated with identifying individuals who are disabled and gifted, much headway is being made. Factors critical to successful identification of giftedness include environments that elicit signs of mental giftedness, and information about the individual's performance gathered from many sources. With regard to these eliciting environments, it is important that the child or youth be given opportunities to perform tasks that are not impeded by the disabling condition. Also, if and when tests of mental ability are used, they must be appropriately adapted both in their administration and scoring (Whitmore & Maker, 1985).

Differential education for children and youth who are disabled and gifted is still in its infancy. A great deal of progress has been made, particularly in the adaptive uses of computers and related technologies, but there is still much development work to be done. Additionally, a great deal is still unknown about the service-delivery systems and materials that are best suited for these children and youth.

Giftedness in Children and Youth Who Are Disadvantaged

Typical identification procedures often fail to identify children and youth as being gifted when they come from minority groups or disadvantaged environments. However, recent research conducted by Van Tassel-Baska & Chepko-Sade (1986) suggests that as many as 15.5 percent of the gifted population may be youth who are disadvantaged. In fact, the actual number of students who are disadvantaged and also gifted may be even greater, given the identification criteria used in this study. By definition, children and youth who are gifted and come from economically deprived or culturally different environments do not have the resources to "make it on their own" (Van Tassel-Baska, 1989c, p. 54).

Several procedures have been developed to more accurately identify children and youth who are disadvantaged and also gifted. They include employing nontraditional measures, using multiple criteria, considering broader ranges of scores for inclusion in gifted programs, peer nomination, parent nomination, assessments by persons other than educational personnel, and information provided by adaptive-behavior assessments. For example, if 60 percent of the students in a given school population come from a certain minority group and only 2 percent are identified as gifted using traditional measures, the screening committee may reexamine its identification procedures or adjust the cutoff scores for students who represent the minority group.

Intervention programs for children and youth who are disadvantaged and gifted have several key components. There is a general consensus that the programs should begin early. The programs should be tailored to the needs of these children. Often the emphasis in the early years is on reading instruction, language development, and foundation skills. Other key components include parental involvement in the educational program model, experiential education that provides children with many opportunities for hands-on learning, activities that foster self-expression, plentiful use of mentors and role models who represent the child's ethnic group, involvement of the community, and counseling, throughout the school years, that gives serious consideration to the cultural values of the family and the child who is gifted (Van Tassel-Baska, 1989c).

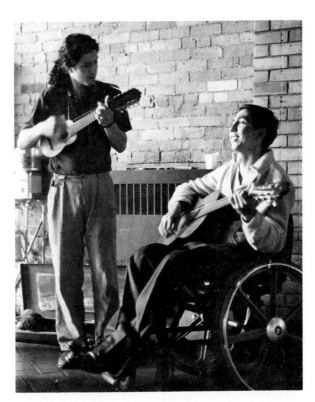

Society has only recently begun to recognize that people with disabilities can also be gifted. What kinds of programs can best encourage their talents? (Mary Kate Stillings)

Reflect on This 13–4

Specific Characteristics of Hispanic Students Who May Be Gifted

■ Rapidly acquires English language skills once exposed to the language and given an opportunity to use it expressively

■ Exhibits leadership ability, be it open or unobtrusive, with heavy emphasis on interpersonal skills

■ Has older playmates and easily engages adults in lively conversation

■ Enjoys intelligent (or effective) risk-taking behavior, often accompanied by a sense of drama

■ Is able to keep busy and entertained, especially by imaginative games and ingenious applications, such as getting the most out of a few simple toys and objects

■ Accepts responsibilities at home normally reserved for older children such as supervising younger siblings or helping others do their homework

■ Is "street-wise" and is recognized by others as a youngster who has the ability to "make

it" in the anglo-dominated society (Van Tassel-Baska, 1989, pp. 56–57)

Source: E. M. Bernal (1974), "Gifted Mexican-American Children: An Ethnoscientific Perspective," *California Journal of Educational Research 25* (5), 251–273; J. Van Tassel-Baska (1989), "The Disadvantaged Gifted." In J. Feldhusen, J. Van Tassel-Baska, & K. Seeley (Eds.), *Excellence in Educating the Gifted.* Denver: Love Publishing Co.

REVIEW

FOCUS 1: Briefly describe several historical developments directly related to the measurement of various types of giftedness.

□ Alfred Binet developed the first developmental scale for children during the early 1900s.

□ Gradually the notion of mental age emerged; that is, a representation of what the child was capable of doing compared to age-specific developmental tasks.

□ Lewis M. Terman translated the Binet scale and made modifications suitable for children in the United States.

□ Gradually the intelligence quotient or IQ (mental age/chronological age × 100 = IQ) came into use.

□ The intelligence quotient became the major gauge for determining giftedness.

□ Intelligence, for a long time, was viewed as being a unitary structure or underlying ability.

□ Gradually the view of the nature of intelligence changed, and researchers began to believe that intelligence was represented in a variety of distinct capacities and abilities.

□ Guilford and other social scientists began to develop a multidimensional theory of intelligence.

□ The multidimensional view of intelligence prompted

other researchers to develop models and assessment devices for examining creativity.

□ Programs were gradually developed to foster and develop creativity in young people.

FOCUS 2: Briefly identify six major components of definitions developed to describe giftedness.

□ Gifted individuals should be identified by qualified assessment personnel.

□ Gifted youngsters may demonstrate their extraordinary abilities in a variety of domains—general intellectual abilities, specific academic aptitude, creative or productive thinking, leadership abilities, visual or performing arts, or psychomotor ability.

□ Gifted children may be identified during the preschool, elementary- or secondary-school periods.

□ Gifted children exhibit high levels of task commitment and high levels of creativity.

□ Gifted children combine their high levels of intelligence, task commitment and creativity to eventually make lasting contributions in their fields of endeavor.

□ Gifted children need special educational opportunities

in order to realize their full intellectual and creative potential.

FOCUS 3: Identify four problems inherent in accurately describing the characteristics of the gifted.

☐ Gifted individuals vary significantly on a variety of characteristics; they are not a homogeneous group.

☐ Research regarding the characteristics of the gifted has been conducted with different population groups; therefore, the characteristics that have surfaced represent the population studied rather than the gifted population as a whole.

☐ Many early studies of gifted individuals led to a stereotypical view of giftedness.

☐ Historically, studies regarding the characteristics of the gifted have not included adequate samples of females, minority or ethnic groups, or socioeconomic groups.

FOCUS 4: What four factors appear to contribute significantly to the emergence of various forms of giftedness?

☐ Genetic endowment certainly contributes to manifestations of giftedness in all of its varieties.

☐ Environmental stimulation provided by parents, teachers, coaches, tutors, and other persons contributes significantly to the emergence of giftedness.

☐ It is the interaction of innate abilities with environmental influences and encouragement that fosters the development and expression of giftedness.

☐ The development of high levels of task commitment in gifted individuals determines the level and nature of contributions that they eventually make to themselves and their extended communities.

FOCUS 5: Identify the types of assessment devices used to identify the various types of giftedness.

☐ The multifaceted assessment process (screening and identification) is carried out with a variety of measures: developmental checklists or scales, parent inventories, teacher inventories, intelligence tests, problem-solving or information-processing tests, achievement tests, creativity tests, biographical inventories, and other observational measures.

FOCUS 6: What interventions are utilized to foster the development of children and adolescents who are gifted?

☐ Interventions include environmental stimulation provided by parents from infancy through adolescence, and differentiated education and specialized service-delivery systems that provide enrichment activities and/or possibilities for acceleration (grade skipping, early entrance to college, honors programs on the high-school and college levels, specialized schools in the performing and visual arts, mentor programs with university professors and other talented individuals, and specialized counseling facilities).

FOCUS 7: What six problems complicate the selection of a career or professional pursuit for young people who are gifted?

☐ Because gifted individuals are often talented, capable, and interested in a broad spectrum of areas, they find it difficult to make an appropriate choice relative to a career or profession.

☐ Gifted women may lack adequate models or mentors with whom to identify in pursuing various career and professional options.

☐ Women may be influenced by traditional cultural and societal expectations that are restrictive.

☐ Gifted young people may be unduly influenced by their parents' expectations, their own expectations for excellence, and their preconceived notions as to what gifted people ought to do professionally or academically.

☐ Some gifted youths are socially isolated, in the sense that they do not have access to other gifted persons of their own age with whom they can discuss their aspirations, interests, and problems.

☐ Rural or remote gifted youth may have few, if any, role models with whom they can relate or identify.

FOCUS 8: What are some of the problems that girls who are gifted experience in using their giftedness in careers and other pursuits?

☐ These problems include fear of success, competition between marital and career aspirations, stress induced by traditional cultural and societal expectations, and self-imposed or culturally imposed restrictions related to educational and occupational choices.

Debate Forum

What Would You Do with Jane?

Many gifted children are prevented from accelerating their growth and learning for fear that they will be hurt emotionally and socially. Parents' comments such as these are common: "She's so young." "Won't she miss a great deal if she doesn't go through the fourth- and fifth-grade experiences?" "What about her friends?" "Who will her friends be if she goes to college at such a young age?" "Will she have the social skills to interact with kids that are much older?" "If she skips these two grades, won't there be gaps in her learning and social development?"

On the other hand, the nature of the questions or comments by parents about acceleration may also be positive: "She is young in years only! She will adjust extremely well." "Maybe she is emotionally mature enough to handle this type of acceleration." "The increased opportunities provided through university training will give her greater chances to develop her talents and capacities." "Perhaps the older students with whom she will interact are better suited to her intellectual and social needs."

Let us consider Jane. She is a gifted child. In third grade, she thrived in school, and just about everything associated with her schooling at that time was positive. Her teacher was responsive and allowed her and others to explore well beyond the usual read-the-text-then-respond-to-the-ditto-sheet routine. A lot of self-pacing was possible. Materials galore were presented for both independent studies and queries.

In the fourth and fifth grades, however, things began to change radically. Jane's teachers were simply unable to provide enough interesting and hard work for her. It was during the latter part of the fourth grade that she began to view herself as being different. Not only did she know but her classmates knew that learning came exceptionally easily to her. At this same time, she was beginning to change dramatically in her cognitive capacity. Unfortunately, her teachers persisted in unnecessary drills and other mundane assignments. She gradually became bored and lapsed into a type of passive learning. Rather than attacking assignments with vigor, she performed them carelessly, often making many "stupid" errors. Gradually what ensued was a child who was very unhappy in school. Where she

most wanted to be before she entered fourth grade became a source of pain and boredom.

Jane's parents decided that they needed to know more about her capacities and talents. Although it was expensive and quite time consuming, they visited a nearby university center for psychological services. The results were very revealing. For the first time they had some objective information about her capacities. She was in fact an unusually bright and talented young lady. They then began to consider the educational alternatives available to them.

The counselor who provided the interpretation of the results at the university center strongly recommended that Jane be advanced to the seventh grade in a school that provided services to the talented and gifted. This meant that Jane would skip one year of elementary school and have an opportunity to move very rapidly through her junior high and high school studies. Furthermore, she would potentially be able to enter the university well in advance of her peers.

Her parents know that Jane's performance has diminished significantly in the last year. Moreover, her attitude and disposition about her schooling seem to be worsening. Should they allow her to participate in the acceleration programs that are available? If so, why? Or should they be primarily concerned with the social ramifications of her acceleration? Maybe the grade skipping and attendant acceleration programs would be socially and emotionally detrimental to her. What would you do as her parents? What factors would you consider important in making the decision? Is the decision Jane's and hers alone? What factors ought to be addressed by Jane and her parents in reaching a viable solution to her current situation in school?

Point Yes, Jane should be allowed to accelerate her educational pace. Moving to the seventh grade will benefit her greatly, intellectually and socially. Most girls develop more rapidly physically and socially than boys do. Skipping one grade will not hinder her social development at all. In fact, she will benefit from the interactions that she will have with other able students, some of whom will also have skipped a grade or two.

Additionally, the research regarding the impact of accelerating students is positive, particularly if the students are carefully selected. Jane has been carefully evaluated and deserves to have the opportunity to be excited about learning and achieving again.

Counterpoint   There are some inherent risks in having Jane skip her sixth-grade experience and move on to the seventh grade. Jane is neither socially nor emotionally prepared to deal with the junior-high environment. She may be very able intellectually and her achievement may be superior, but this is not the time to move her into a junior-high environment. Socially, she is still quite awkward for her age. This awkwardness would be intensified in the junior-high setting. Acceleration for Jane should be considered later on, when she has matured more socially.

She should be able to receive the acceleration that she needs in her present elementary school. Certainly there are other able students in her school who would benefit from joining together for various activities and learning experiences. The acceleration should take place in her own school, with other gifted students of her own age. Maybe all she needs is some released time to attend a class or two elsewhere. Using this approach, she could benefit from involvement with her same-age peers and still receive the stimulation that she so desperately needs. Allowing her to skip a grade now would hurt her emotionally and socially in the long run.

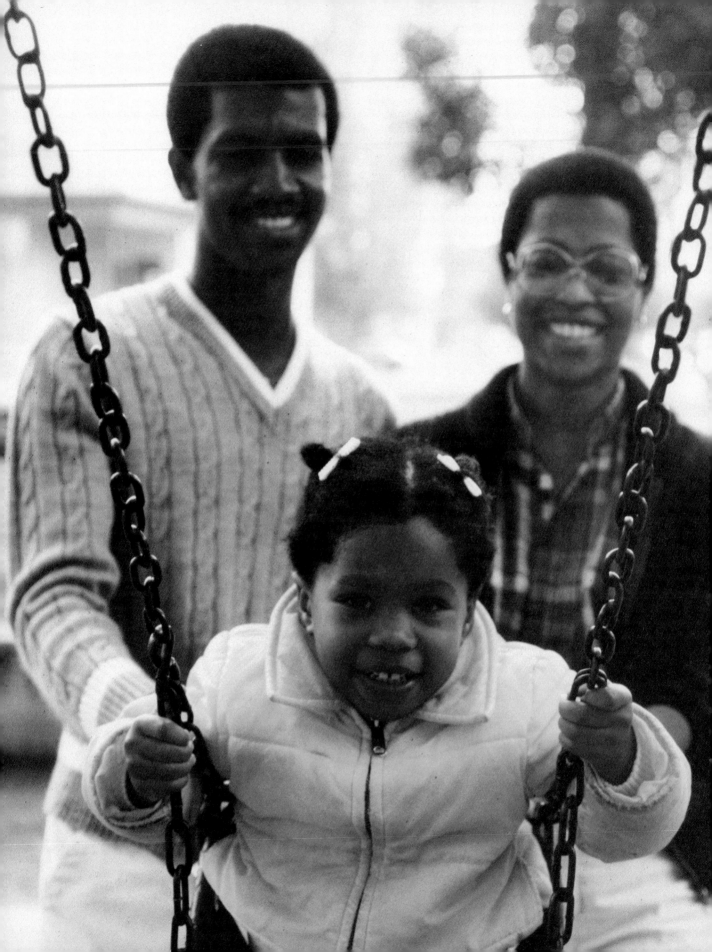

14 Family Impact

To Begin With . . .

- No one plans to have a handicapped child.

- For every one hundred babies born, three will have major defects. This statistic has remained stable since 1960 when researchers first began to collect these data (Adler, 1987).

- It can cost a family over $100,000 to raise a handicapped child to the age of 18. There is some feeling that costs of equipment, in particular, may be inflated. For example, in 1982 a motorized wheelchair cost $3,450. In comparison, a two-seated motorized golf cart cost $1,900, while a farm tractor cost $3,000 (Hutchinson, 1982).

- Since 1970, over 80% of the litigation for rights and services has been decided in favor of disabled children and their families. However, subsequent improvement in opportunities and programs has not matched the extent of the legal victories (Blatt, 1988).

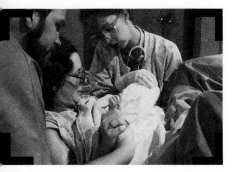

I had been looking forward to this event all my life. I was about to give birth to our first child and had done everything imaginable to prepare for this momentous day. I ate the right foods. I avoided taking any medication, as my obstetrician advised. I even maintained a regular fitness program. My husband was amazed at the diligence that I exhibited in pursuing my many regimens.

Finally, the day came. At the end of my regular appointment with the obstetrician, she told me that I should call my husband and prepare to enter the hospital that evening. Bill managed to get off work early, and we both left for the hospital with great expectations and a few normal fears. About 9:15 P.M., my labor pains intensified. Bill was excited about being able to join me in the delivery room. In a short time, we went in. The actual birth of our son proceeded normally—but then it happened. The atmosphere in the delivery room changed from one of joy to concern and then gloom. Sometime during that brief period, I was informed by the obstetrician that my new little infant boy had a serious birth defect known as spina bifida. It all happened so quickly. I saw my son only briefly before he was whisked away to the special neonatal unit.

A million thoughts raced through my groggy mind: Can I handle this? Why did this happen to us? What could I have done to have this happen to our family? Bill must be very disappointed in me! What are we going to do? Just then I felt Bill squeezing my hand and trying to get my attention. He said, "We'll get through it somehow." The next few days were like a series of nightmares—fleeting images of people in white coats, constant fear, and the terrifying feeling of despair. There were so many things to consider and decisions to make. I felt helpless, unable to think clearly. Maybe he'll die, I thought to myself, but then I felt guilty—so guilty. Bill was there most of the time, but we didn't talk much. Needless to say, this day changed our lives forever.

INTRODUCTION

FOCUS 1
Identify five factors that influence the ways in which families respond to an infant with a birth defect or disability.

Nowhere is the impact of an exceptional individual so strongly felt as in the family. The birth of an infant with disabilities may alter the family as a social unit in a variety of ways. Parents and siblings may react with shock, disappointment, anger, depression, guilt, and/or confusion. Relationships between family members often change, in either a positive manner or a negative one. The impact of such an event is great, and it is unlikely that the family unit will ever be the same.

A child with physical, intellectual, or behavioral problems presents unique and diverse challenges to the family unit (Chandler, 1987; Pueschel, 1986; Sherman, 1988). In one instance, the child may hurl the family into crisis, resulting in major conflicts among its members. Family relationships may be weakened by the added and unexpected physical, emotional, and financial stress imposed on them (Shelton, Jeppson, & Johnson, 1987). In another instance, family members may see this child as a source of unity that bonds them together and actually strengthens relationships. Many factors influence the reactions of family members: the emotional stability of each individual, religious values and beliefs, socioeconomic status, the severity of the child's disability, and the type of disability, to identify only a few.

In this chapter we discuss how rearing children with disabilities affects parents. We examine a broad array of family and parental issues directly related to rearing children with various types and degrees of exceptional conditions. We review the family as a social system defined by a set of purposes, roles, and expectations. Each family member fulfills various roles that are consistent with expectations established by discussion, tradition, or other means. Each member functions in an interdependent manner with other members to pursue family goals. Using a social-system framework, we can see how changes in one family member can have an effect on every other member and consequently the entire family system. If we accept the notions and concepts associated with this sociological view of a family, we can see how the birth and continued presence of a child with a disorder can significantly affect the family unit over time.

FAMILY CRISIS: THE INITIAL IMPACT

The birth of an infant with significant disabilities has a profound impact on the family. The "expected" or "fantasized" child whom the parents and other family members have anticipated does not arrive (Chinn, Winn, & Walter, 1978; Heward, Dardig, & Rossett, 1979). The birth of an infant with a conspicuous congenital defect or abnormality throws parents into a kind of emotional shock (Blacher, 1984; Crnic, Greenberg, Ragozin, Robinson, & Basham, 1983).

Some conditions, such as spina bifida or Down syndrome, are readily apparent at birth (Volpe & Koenigsberger, 1981), while others, such as hearing disorders and learning disabilities, are not detectable until later (Haynes, 1977; Tjossem, 1976). Even if attending physicians suspect the presence of a disabling condition, they may be unable to give a confirmed diagnosis without the passage of some time and further testing. When the parents also suspect that something may be wrong, waiting for a diagnosis can be agonizing.

The most immediate and predictable reaction to the birth of a child with a disorder is depression, often exhibited in the form of grief or mourning. Some parents describe the mourning as being very much like that suffered after the death of a loved one (Chinn, Winn, & Walter, 1978). Mothers whose abnormal babies survive frequently suffer more acute feelings of grief than mothers whose abnormal infants die. Mothers also tend to mourn for a longer period before they recover in this instance (D'Arcy, 1968). Recurrent sorrow and frequent feelings of inadequacy are persistent emotions that many parents experience as they gradually adjust to having an atypical infant (Peterson, 1987).

Other reactions on the part of family members include shock, uncertainty, disappointment, anger, frustration, guilt, denial, fear, withdrawal, and rejection (Blacher, 1984; Bristor, 1984; Crnic et al., 1983; Rose, 1987). The level of impact varies, but for most parents such an event creates a family crisis of considerable magnitude.

Shontz (1965) suggests that parental responses can be separated into four stages: shock, realization, defensive retreat, and acknowledgment. However,

FOCUS 2
What four statements can you safely make about the stages that parents may experience in responding to infants or young children with disabilities?

recent research completed by Blacher (1984) suggests that the stage approach used by many professionals to understand, predict, and help parents deal with their newborn children with disabilities needs further refinement and validation. What we can assume is that parents of children with disabilities experience common feelings and reactions that may occur during certain periods of time. However, the nature of the feelings, their intensity, their relationship to specific stages, and the eventual adjustments that are made personally and collectively by family members vary from one person to another. Stages associated with various kinds of emotions may overlap with one another. Emotions of one period may resurface again during another period. Some parents may go through distinct periods of adjustment, whereas others may adjust without passing through any sequence of stages. Further research will help us understand the very complex, multifaceted relationships that exist among these factors and the responses that parents and other family members make during a disabled child's lifetime. We can, however, say that the process of adjustment for parents is continuous and distinctively individual.

> When our son was born my husband and I were told that the parents of a handicapped child move through certain stages of reaction: shock, guilt, reaction, and anger, all terminating in the final, blissful stage of adjustment. I do not believe in this pattern. I now know too many parents of handicapped children to be a believer in any set pattern.
>
> I feel we do move through these emotions, and just because we have come to adjustment (which I prefer to call "acceptance" because we spend our whole lives adjusting, although we may at one point accept the situation), that does not mean we never return to other emotions. We may continue to feel any of these emotions at any time, in any order (West, 1981, p. S10).

In sum, mothers and fathers of handicapped children are affected in diverse ways. The range and sequence of emotions can be highly variable. Some parents move through distinct stages and phases while others seem to bounce around in their feelings. At this juncture we analyze some of the phases that parents may experience in responding to their handicapped child. This section helps you to understand the vast array of possible feelings parents may face.

Shock

The initial response to the birth of a disabled infant is generally shock. This phase may be distinguished by feelings of anxiety, guilt, numbness, confusion, helplessness, anger, disbelief, denial, and despair. Sometimes there are feelings of detachment, bewilderment, or bereavement. At this time, when many parents are most in need of assistance, the least amount of help may be available. The length of time it takes the parents to deal with these feelings or move through this period depends on their psychological makeup, the types of assistance rendered, and the seriousness of the handicapping condition.

During the initial shock period, parents may be unable to process or comprehend information provided by medical and other health-related personnel. For this reason, information given to the parents may need to be repeated on several occasions until they have fully grasped the concepts presented. It is also during this time that parents experience the greatest assaults on their self-worth and value systems. They may blame themselves for the disabilities present in their child. They may seriously question their positive perceptions of themselves. Likewise, they may be forced to reassess the meaning of life and the reasons for their present challenges. Blacher (1984) has referred to this stage as the period of emotional disorganization.

Buscaglia (1975) surveyed parents of disabled children in an attempt to assess the level of psychological support rendered by hospital staff at the time of the children's birth. He found that parents were generally given some knowledge of the child's special medical problems, but that the information was viewed as inadequate. Moreover, parents indicated that psychological counseling was insufficient during this period. Thus parents begin the child-rearing process with only a small amount of medical information and significant apprehensions about the future of the child and their family.

Realization

The stage of realization is characterized by several types of parental behavior. Parents may be anxious or fearful about their ability to cope with the demands of caring for a child with unique needs. They may be easily irritated or upset. Considerable time may be spent in self-accusation, self-pity, or self-hate. Information provided by health-care professionals during this period may still be rejected or denied. However, during this stage parents come to understand the actual demands and constraints that will come with raising their exceptional child. This realization frequently overwhelms couples, and as a result they may remove themselves from family and social activities for a period of time.

WINDOW 14–1

What Do I Do Now?

I learned of my son's condition when my wife telephoned me to come to the hospital soon after the birth of our fourth child. This was the third day of life for my son, and it was then that I learned he was mongoloid—a term I soon replaced with the description Down syndrome.

My first reaction was, "What do I do now? How do I take care of this person?" It was a feeling of helplessness and challenge. One of my wife's first comments was, "I don't even want to hold him!" This impulse to reject the new baby lasted only one or two days, but was replaced by a numbness. After that feeling of self-pity and wondering why this had happened to us came along, after we were tired of not doing anything, we decided to do something and began looking for help from people and organizations. My wife and I decided to treat him in the same manner as we did our other children as much as possible. Our expectations have been great, and in most cases our son has fulfilled them.

I wouldn't wish this traumatic experience on any family, but after eleven years my son has brought a whole new dimension of understanding, patience, and happiness to me and other members of our family.

Charles, *a father*

Defensive Retreat

The stage of defensive retreat is one in which the parents attempt to avoid dealing with the anxiety-producing realities of their child's condition. They may try to solve their dilemma by seeking placement for the child in a clinic, institution, or residential setting. Some parents respond by disappearing for a while or by retreating to a safer and less demanding environment. One mother, on returning home from the hospital with her infant with Down syndrome, quickly packed her suitcase and left with the infant in the family car, not knowing exactly what her destination would be. She simply did not want to face her immediate family or relatives. After driving around for several hours, she decided to return home. Within several months, she adapted very well to her daughter's needs and began to provide the stimulation necessary for gradual, persistent growth. Her daughter is now married and works full time in a day care center for young children.

Acknowledgement

Acknowledgement is a stage in which parents are able to mobilize their strengths to confront the conditions created by having an exceptional child. At this stage, parents become capable of involving themselves in the intervention and treatment process. They are also better able to comprehend information or directions provided by a specialist concerning their child's condition and treatment. At this time, some parents become interested in joining an organization that is suited to their child's condition and the needs of the family. During this stage, parents begin to accept the child with the disability as well as others and even themselves. It is during this stage that they become capable of directing their energies to tasks and problems outside of themselves.

Once parents come to acknowledge their child's condition, they can become more involved in the intervention and treatment process. (John Telford)

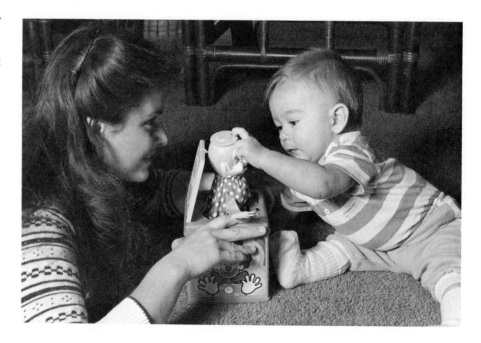

We must remember, however, that patterns of parental response are highly variable. Parents and families respond to the birth and ongoing development of children and siblings with disabilities in common and yet divergent ways. Furthermore, the time required for parents and others to make the various adjustments is extremely variable. The stage approach provides us with one frame of reference for understanding the ongoing reactions and adjustments parents make in rearing children with congenital or acquired disabilities. Further research will help us to understand the range, duration, and nature of these parental responses.

Parents of exceptional children have many other concerns. They especially want to know what their child's future educational and social needs will be (Shelton, 1972). They want to know what their child will be capable of doing as he or she grows older and becomes an adult. They want to know how the presence of the child will affect other family members. Most important, they want to know how to maintain normal family functioning and minimize the stress associated with having an exceptional child.

FOCUS 3
What are four major concerns of parents of exceptional children?

THE IMPACT OF EXCEPTIONALITIES ON THE FAMILY

The birth and continued presence of a child with disabilities strongly influence the manner in which family members respond to one another, particularly if the child is severely disabled or has multiple disabilities. In many families, it is often the mother who experiences the greatest amount of trauma and role strain in responding to conditions created by the presence of an exceptional child. In caring for the child, she may no longer be able to handle the other tasks she once performed, such as preparing meals, doing laundry, doing the weekly grocery shopping, and assisting with homework assignments. Her time with the family may also be greatly reduced because of time spent taking care of the child's unique needs. When the mother is drawn away from the tasks she used to perform, other family members must often assume more responsibility. It may be difficult for family members to adjust to the new strains and routines that result from having an exceptional child in the family. Each family member may need to alter his or her personal routine in order to assist the mother as she cares for the exceptional child. Initially, the demands and needs of the exceptional child may be numerous and time consuming. For families that are already experiencing serious emotional, financial, or other problems, the addition of an exceptional child may serve as the catalyst for dissolution.

As the child grows older, the mother is frequently faced with a unique dilemma. The dilemma revolves around striking a balance between the nurturing activities she associates with her role as care-giver and the activities associated with fostering independence. It can be difficult for mothers to see their exceptional children struggle at new tasks and suffer some of the natural consequences of trying new behaviors. For many mothers, overprotectiveness is extremely difficult to conquer, but it can be accomplished with help provided by others who have already experienced and mastered this problem. If the mother or other care providers continue to be overprotective, the results can be disastrous, particularly

FOCUS 4
Identify three ways in which a newborn child with moderate to severe disabilities influences the manner in which family members respond to each other.

when the child reaches late adolescence and is unprepared for entry into adulthood or semi-independent living.

Each family exhibits a characteristic pattern of conveying information to family members. The pattern and type of communication varies according to the size of the family, its cultural background, and members' ages. Generally, information conveyed to the family regarding the nature of a child's disorder is provided by the father, particularly if the exceptionality is diagnosed at birth. Once initial information regarding the child's condition has been conveyed to siblings, the older children frequently become responsible for providing additional clarification to younger ones.

At first, a new closeness may occur in families who discover that one of the children has a disorder. During this period, the mother frequently senses this closeness and it serves to support her. Over time, however, this support may wane, and family members may gradually move away from the family unit to associate more closely with peers or friends. Questions children may want to ask parents regarding family issues may be posed to older siblings, or they may not be asked at all. Such behavior is probably a function of the strain that the children sense in their parents. It is a natural outcome and one that is to be expected in families in which parents must direct a great deal of their attention to an exceptional child.

Mothers often develop a strong dyadic relationship with the exceptional child. Other dyadic relationships may also develop, between various other members of the family. Certain siblings may turn to each other for support and nurturing. Older siblings may take on the role of parent substitutes as a result of their new care-giving responsibilities. Younger children, who come to depend on older siblings for care, then tend to develop strong relationships with them.

Every family has a unique power structure. In some families, most of the power or control is held by the father. In other families, the governance of the family lies with the mother or the family at large. Power, in the context of this discussion, is defined as the amount of control or influence a family member or group of family members exerts in managing family decisions, assigning family tasks, and implementing family activities. Families vary greatly in their membership and their organization. Some families have both parents living at home, while others have only one. In a similar fashion, the power structure within each family varies according to the characteristics of each family member. Family power structure is often altered substantially by the arrival of an exceptional infant. It is not uncommon for older siblings to assume greater power than before, as they assume more responsibility.

FOCUS 5
What kind of a relationship may develop between the mother and her child with a disability?

Husband–Wife Relationships

We were just beginning to get our feet on the ground when it happened. We had been in our new home for about two years. My job had been demanding and yet fulfilling. Our daughter, Maria, was doing well in the fifth grade, and everything about our family life and marriage was almost ideal. Angela was pregnant, and we were excited about having our last child. I was hoping for a boy, and I think Angela was too.

Our boy, Juan, did arrive, but during the birth process he suffered extensive brain damage. From that point on, the tone of our marriage and family life went from optimism to pessimism and continual doubt. My wife spent so much time reading books about brain damage, keeping medical appointments, and caring for Juan that Maria and I have been forced to pursue other activities. We often avoid contact with my wife, since she has become demanding and domineering. I find it difficult to communicate with her. Somehow we have lost the affection and affinity we once had for each other.

According to Featherstone (1980), "A child's handicap attacks the fabric of a marriage in four ways. It excites powerful emotions in both parents. It acts as a dispiriting symbol of shared failure. It reshapes the organization of the family. It creates fertile ground for conflict" (p. 91). An infant with disorders may require more immediate and prolonged attention from the mother for feeding, treatment, and general care. Her attention becomes riveted on the life of the child. The balance that once existed between being a mother and a wife is now absent. The wife has become so involved with caring for the exceptional child that other relationships may lose their quality and intensity. Comments representative of some of these feelings are exemplified in the following statements: "Angela spends so much time with Juan that she has little energy left for me. It is as if she has become consumed with his care." "You ask me to pay attention to Juan, but you rarely spend any time with me. When am I going to be a part of your life again?" "I am developing a resentment toward you and Juan. Who wants to come home when all your time is spent waiting on him?" One can sense from these comments the types of feelings a husband might have regarding a wife's involvement with the exceptional child. Husbands may also become excessively involved with their children's lives, promoting the same kinds of feelings in their wives.

Marital partners also have other types of feelings. Fear, anger, guilt, resentment, and other related feelings often interfere with a couple's capacity to communicate and seek realistic solutions. Fatigue also has a profound effect on the ways in which couples function and communicate. All these feelings and conditions are exacerbated by the presence of an exceptional child in the home. Some parents are now joining together to create respite-care programs (Cobb, 1987). These programs give parents a chance to be away from the demands of child raising. Moreover, the respite care gives them the opportunity to relax and renew their relationship.

A number of other factors may also contribute to marital stress: unusually heavy financial burdens incurred by the family to provide medical treatment or therapy; frequent visits to treatment facilities; a reduction of time spent together in couple-related activities, decreased time for sleep, particularly in the early years of a disabled child's life; and social isolation from relatives and friends (Beckman-Bell, 1981; Blackard & Barsh, 1982; Fredericks, 1985; Gallagher, Beckman-Bell, & Cross, 1983). The factors identified above, and a host of others, account for the marital stress that many married couples experience in rearing an exceptional child.

FOCUS 6
What are the factors that contribute to marital stress?

Reflect on This 14-1

When I Think about Having Another Child, I . . .

When I think about having another child, I panic. In fact, I have consumed hours of psychological time thinking about my little boy and our response to him. Actually, my husband and I really haven't dealt successfully with the feelings that seem to be ever-present in our thinking. The problem is simply this. Two years ago I gave birth to a little boy who was severely deformed. At the time, I was about twenty-six years old and my husband was twenty-seven. We married later than most, and having this little boy was something that was neither planned nor unplanned. We did know that we wanted to have children, and so we let nature take its course.

We didn't know much about children, let alone handicapped children; nor did we ever think that we would have a child who would be seriously deformed. When the pediatrician suggested institutionalization for the child we just nodded our heads. Believe it or not, I had not even touched our son. I had merely looked at him through the observation windows once or twice.

After the baby's birth, I didn't return to work. In fact, within several days after the delivery and placement of the child, my husband and I decided to take a vacation to sort things out. Well, the "sorting" didn't really take place. Gradually since that time, I have become less and less interested in things. I sleep a lot more, and, to be honest with you, I don't really look forward to getting up each day. My old friends have stopped coming by, and my husband chooses to do less and less with me. He spends his free time with old friends because I have little energy for any activity outside our home.

Recently, my husband gave me an ultimatum: "Either you decide to have some children or I'm going to find someone who will." (There are of course other things that are bothering him.) But since the birth of this child I have been absolutely terrified of becoming pregnant again. As a result, my responses to my husband's needs for physical affection have been practically absent, or should I say nonexistent. I'm driving not only myself crazy, but also my husband. I guess you could say I really need some help.

Research related to marital stress and instability is limited. McAndrew (1976) studied 116 families with physically disabled children. He found that the majority of mothers surveyed reported a good marital relationship with their spouses. Of the remaining families, only seventeen wives believed that their marriages had worsened as a result of having a disabled child. However, more recent statistics reveal that divorce is three times more frequent in families with handicapped children (Schell, 1981).

Fowle (1968) assessed the level of marital integration in couples who chose to care for their retarded child at home, versus those who chose to have their child cared for in an institution. He found no significant differences between the two groups, as measured by Farber's Index of Marital Integration. It is important to note that children who did remain at home were served by a day-care center. Such services probably lessened the burden on the parents and other family members in caring for the retarded child. In a related study, Fotheringham, Skelton, and Hoddinott (1971) evaluated families of severely retarded children prior to placement of the child in a community or institutional setting. One to three months before the children were placed in their various settings, a comprehensive evaluation was made of each family. The evaluation procedures were implemented again after the children had lived for at least one year in their respective placements. Families whose children had been served in institutional settings showed greater improvement in family functioning than those whose children were served in community programs. However, there are many variables involved in analyzing the efficacy of community placement versus institutional placement, and it has been well over a decade since Fotheringham et al. conducted their investigations. The availability of community support systems, including mandated public education for exceptional children, direct client care, homemaker assistance, family counseling, day programming, and respite-care opportunities, has changed steadily during this period (Lipsky, 1987; Sherman, 1988). However, increases in funding for family and community referenced programs are necessary if realistic alternatives to residential and institutional care are to be provided (Gardner & Markowitz, 1986; Sherman, 1988).

Cleveland (1980) studied the adaptations made by seventeen families after a youngster in each family had experienced traumatic spinal cord injury. She examined the family's adaptation shortly after the accident and one year later. Changes in family functioning and specific intrafamilial relationships were the focus of the study. With regard to marital functioning, Cleveland identified several sources of spousal irritation and distress. As a rule, mothers in each of the families assumed the major role of caring for the injured youths. Husbands reported feeling angry toward their wives because of their involvement with the injured child. Conversely, wives expressed hostility toward their husbands for a lack of empathy and understanding about the care they provided. In addition, overprotectiveness by the mothers was identified as a major source of tension for couples. Most husbands felt that their spouses were overly solicitous and shielding in their care-giving activities. Generally, couples reported that their marriages had been made neither better nor worse as a function of the injury to their child. They were, however, concerned about the prolonged period of parenthood that they would have to provide. They also felt they would have to alter some of the plans they had made for the postparenthood phase of their lives.

Tew, Lawrence, Payne, and Townsley (1977) investigated the impact of having a child with spina bifida on marital stability. They concluded that the divorce rate for the couples whose children survived the condition was nine times higher than that for average families. For those parents whose children died as a result of the condition, the divorce rate was three times higher.

In a comprehensive review of the effects of having a child with learning disabilities, Scagliotta (1974) found that parents generally reacted to their child's problems in one of two distinct ways. Some parents worked as a cooperative team, perceiving the child's behaviors from similar points of view. They usually agreed on the types of child-management techniques that they used to handle their child's problems. Their expectations for the child's behavior were also compatible. Other parents responded to their child's learning and behavior difficulties in a disjointed fashion. They had problems reaching agreement in selecting and implementing various discipline strategies. For instance, a mother may be the only adult family member actively involved in assisting the child, whereas a father may purposely separate himself from the child's treatment process. He may participate only as an observer or occasional critic of the interventions.

Parent counseling and training can be extremely helpful in avoiding many of the problems encountered in coping with an exceptional child in the family (Abrams & Kaslow, 1977; Baker, 1970; Friedman, 1978; Hetrick, 1979). Counseling may help parents work through such feelings as anger, resentment, and discouragement. Parent training may help parents develop appropriate expectations for their child's current and future achievement. In addition, parents may acquire specific skills to help them respond more effectively and therapeutically to their child's difficulties.

Parent-Child Relationships

My initial response to Tyrone's birth was very negative. I didn't quite know what to do. My pediatrician came into my room right after the delivery and said something to the effect, "I think we have a problem." What he was trying to say was, "Your child has Down syndrome." The emotional surge of feelings I had then cannot be accurately described.

I can distinctively remember the first thoughts that I had as I spoke to my husband after I had my brief visit with the pediatrician. I wanted to throw my new son out the window . . . not literally, but somehow I didn't want to deal with this immensely new and complex problem. At least, that's how I viewed the situation at the time.

In retrospect, as I think about those earlier feelings regarding Tyrone, I am sorry I felt that way. But I think my thoughts at that time were really very typical. I didn't know a lot about Down syndrome and I wasn't sure what to expect, so I expected the worst.

The relationships between parents and their children are a function of many factors. Some of the more critical factors include the child's age, the child's sex, the socioeconomic status of the family, the family's coping strength, the nature and seriousness of the disability, and the composition of the family (one-parent family, two-parent family, or reconstituted family).

FOCUS 7
What are four general phases of the developmental cycle that parents go through in rearing a child with disabilities?

Seligman (1979) described a developmental cycle that families go through in responding to the needs and nuances of caring for an exceptional child. The cycle includes the following phases: (1) the time at which parents learn about or suspect a disability in their child, (2) the period in which the parents determine what action to take regarding the child's education, (3) the point at which the disabled individual has completed his or her education, and (4) the time when the parents become older and may be unable to care for their adult offspring. We do not review all of these periods here, but we highlight some of the more common relationship patterns that appear over time in the life of an individual with disabilities. Of course the nature and severity of the disability and the willingness of the parents to make adjustments and to educate themselves regarding their role in helping the child have an appreciable influence on the parent/child relationship that eventually emerges.

The Mother-Child Relationship.   If a child's impairment is congenital and readily apparent at birth, it is often the mother who becomes primarily responsible for relating to the child and his or her needs. If the infant is born prematurely or needs extensive, early medical assistance, the relationship that emerges may be slow in coming. There are many reasons for this delay. The mother may be prevented from engaging in typical feeding and care-giving activities that most mothers would perform with a new infant. The child may need to spend many weeks in an isolette supported by sophisticated medical equipment. Some mothers come to question whether they really had a baby because of the remoteness they experience in not being able to interact immediately with their infant in a personally satisfying manner (Jogis, 1975). Many mothers report that they are not given adequate direction as to how they could become involved with their disabled infants (Leigh, 1975). Without minimal levels of involvement and appropriate support from other adults or professionals, many mothers become estranged from their infants and find it difficult to begin the caring process. Physicians, nurses, and other health-related personnel responsible for providing parents with appropriate explanations, instruction, and expectations set the stage for the development of healthy and realistic parent/infant relationships. The mother's expectations are particularly important, for they shape the types of responses she later makes in caring and seeking assistance for her infant (Lavelle & Keogh, 1980).

In other cases, the mother may be virtually forced into a close physical and emotional relationship with her injured or disabled offspring. The bond that develops between mother and child is one that is strong and often impenetrable (Leigh, 1987). The mother becomes, according to Cleveland (1980), the "guardian of affective needs." She assumes primary responsibility for fostering the child's emotional adjustment. She also becomes the child's personal representative or interpreter. In this role, the mother has the responsibility of communicating the child's needs and desires to other family members. Because of the sheer weight of these responsibilities, other relationships often wane or even disappear. The mother who assumes this role and develops a very close relationship with her disabled offspring often walks a variety of tightropes. In her desire to protect her child, she often overprotects him or her, thus preventing the child from having optimal opportunities to practice the skills and participate in the activities that ultimately lead to independence. The mother may also underestimate her child's capacities. She may be reluctant to allow her child to engage in challenging or risky ventures. In this regard, the mother might be described as being overprotective. On the other hand, some mothers may neglect their exceptional child and not provide the stimulation so critical to his or her optimal development. Such neglect constitutes child abuse that should receive the prompt attention of appropriate child-care workers.

Several investigators (Ross, 1964; Seligman, 1979) have suggested that it is the youngsters with mild disabilities and their families who experience the most severe adjustment problems. Barsh (1968) found that parents of the blind and deaf showed the greatest ease in rearing their children, compared to parents whose children had other impairments. There could be many reasons for this. One reason may be that a diagnosis of blindness or deafness can occur earlier than that of other conditions, allowing the parents to begin the adjustment

FOCUS 8
What are four factors influencing the relationship that develops between infants with disabilities and their mothers?

process earlier. Likewise, the services for these children may be more fully developed, thus easing some of the burdens parents experience in raising a blind or deaf child.

Hackney (1981) identified several ways in which gifted children impact family functioning. He found that the gifted child can alter family roles. For example, gifted children's adultlike capacities may lead them to occasionally serve as the "third parent" in the family. Disciplining the child who is verbally and intellectually skilled also poses some challenges for parents. The usual pat answers provided by parents for choosing a particular discipline remedy may be logically and quickly challenged and repudiated. Furthermore, parents may feel greater pressure to provide additional learning experiences or talent-enhancement activities for their gifted children. Last, socially skilled, gifted children are often viewed by their parents as being highly manipulative. The tenacity and skill with which such children pursue their goals and desires can be a perplexing problem for mothers and fathers.

FOCUS 9
Identify three ways in which some fathers respond to their children with disabilities.

The Father-Child Relationship. There has not been much written about fathers and their relationships with children with disabilities. The information available is primarily anecdotal in nature or appears in the form of case studies. As indicated earlier, it is the father who is often responsible for conveying the news that the mother has given birth to an exceptional child, and for a time the father may well be responsible for keeping the family aware of the mother's status and the child's condition. The father's reactions to the birth of an injured or damaged child are generally more reserved than those of other family members (Lamb, 1983). Fathers are more prone to respond with such coping mechanisms as withdrawal, sublimation, and intellectualization. They are more likely to internalize their feelings than to express them openly. Fathers of children with mental retardation are typically more concerned than mothers about their children's capacity to develop socially adequate behavior, particularly their sons'. They are also more concerned about their children's eventual social and educational status. Likewise, they are more affected by the visibility of their children's retardation than are mothers (Lamb, 1983).

The relationships that emerge between fathers and their exceptional children are a function of the same factors reviewed above concerning mother/child relationships. One important factor may be the sex of the child. If the child is male and the father had idealized the role he would eventually assume in interacting with a son, the adjustment for the father can be very difficult. The father may have had hopes of playing football with the child, having him eventually become a business partner, or participating with his son in a variety of activities. Many of these hopes may never be realized with a disabled child.

Investigating the effect of traumatic spinal-cord injury, Cleveland (1980) found that the initial response of fathers to injured sons was one of an increased feeling of closeness. Sons described their fathers as being more nurturing and supporting. With the passage of time, however, the father/son relationship became clouded with problems related to the meaning of maleness and manliness. Fathers did not know how to respond to a son who was unable to participate in activities traditionally associated with being a man. Sons faced the same dilemma. They, too, were at a loss as to what their new roles and activities would be in light of their physical limitations. We can easily see how perplexing such an injury can be to both father and son who expected to play baseball, go camping, and water ski together.

Certainly adjustments and modifications can be made for those who are unable to walk on their own or utilize their arms and hands fully. Fathers and sons can eventually participate in a variety of activities, but the period of transition is almost always traumatic and difficult. Expectations and goals must be modified. In conjunction with a variety of professionals, fathers must find new ways to help their sons manifest their masculinity and strengths. There are now many activities in which physically injured individuals can participate, both competitively and noncompetitively.

Sibling Relationships

I found that I was purely fascinated by my brother. Why didn't he speak? How did he think if he didn't know words? As a sibling, I could be intrigued without the pains of reality and natural motherly awareness of a son's abnormalities. I could take him out shopping in supermarkets, which he loved, and not be bothered or embarrassed if he accidentally knocked down a huge display. My sister would have become nervous and distraught, while my mother would have been close to tears. Taking a walk around the beach with him was an education in people. I learned from their fearful expressions, their sympathy, their ignorance. Yet, some did not notice anything unusual, as he was so physically beautiful, except when he would flap his hands or do his little foot shuffle. Then they often noticed. . . .

I consider myself to have had a very special upbringing. I learned so much from my brother, indirectly. I enjoy being around people like him, although, of course, there is no one as special as my brother Ben. (Lettic, 1979, p. 294)

Siblings respond to an exceptional member of the family in a variety of ways. The titles of several recent articles in a popular publication for parents of exceptional children illustrate this point: "I'm Not Going to Be John's Baby Sitter Forever: Siblings, Planning, and the Disabled Child" (1987) and "When I Grow Up, I'm Never Coming Back! The Adolescent and the Family" (1988). The responses siblings make to their sister or brother with a handicap are subject to a number of variables. Farber (1962) identified several factors that may be predictive of family and sibling adjustment to a retarded brother or sister. These include the quality of the interpersonal relationship between the child's parents, the retarded child's sex, the social class of the family, and the interaction patterns of the family. Grossman (1972a; 1972b) found that families in the upper income brackets were capable of relieving their normal children of some burdens associated with caring for a retarded sibling. By contrast, lower-income families often placed much of the burden for the retarded child's care on young, female siblings.

Siblings who learn that they have an exceptional brother or sister are frequently encumbered with many different kinds of concerns. Such questions as "Why did this happen?" "Is my brother contagious? Can I catch what he has?" "What

FOCUS 10
Identify four ways in which siblings respond to their exceptional brothers or sisters.

am I going to say to my friends?" and "Am I going to have to take care of him all of my life?" are common. Like their parents, siblings want to know and understand as much as they can about the condition of their impaired sibling. They want to know how they should respond and how their lives might be different as a result of this event. If these concerns can be adequately addressed, the prognosis for positive sibling involvement with the impaired brother or sister is much better than otherwise. Lamb (1980) has reviewed a number of books that may be used therapeutically to help children accept their exceptional siblings. Through these stories, children may become vicariously involved with the problems of having an exceptional sister or brother.

We would be remiss in our discussion of this topic if we were to leave the impression that all sibling problems can be handled through appropriate orientation, education, and counseling programs. Even with excellent counseling support and assistance, having a disabled child in the family can be challenging and painful for both parents and siblings. In spite of assistance, many siblings may continue to disdain and resent their brother or sister.

An important factor affecting the attitudes of children toward an exceptional sibling is the attitude of the parents (Grossman, 1972a; Klein, 1972; Love, 1973), since children tend to mirror the attitudes and values of their parents. If parents are optimistic and realistic in their views toward the exceptional child, then their other children are likely to share these attitudes. If children are kindly disposed toward assisting the exceptional sibling, they can be a real source of support (Koch & Dobson, 1971; Murphy, 1979). Many siblings play a critical role in fostering the intellectual, social, and affective development of an exceptional brother or sister.

Anger is one of the many feelings that normal siblings may express or feel. Loneliness, anxiety, guilt, and envy are also common in normal siblings. Feelings of loneliness may surface in children who wanted a brother or sister with whom they could play. Anxiety may be present in a youth who wonders who will care for the impaired sibling when the parents are no longer capable or alive. Guilt may come from many sources. Normal siblings may feel that they are obligated to care for the disabled sibling. In their minds, failure to provide such care would make them bad or immoral. Similarly, they may feel guilty about the real thoughts and feelings they have about their sibling. These feelings may include frustration, resentment, and even hate. Realizing that many parents would not respond positively to the expression of such feelings, some siblings carry them inside for a long time, only to express them later.

Many siblings resent the time and attention parents must devote to their sister or brother. This resentment may also take the form of jealousy (Forbes, 1987). Some siblings feel as if they are emotionally neglected, that their parents are not responsive to their needs for attention and emotional support. For some siblings, the predominant feeling is one of bitter resentment or even rage. For others, the predominant attitude toward the family experience of growing up with a disabled brother or sister is a feeling of deprivation. They feel as if their social, educational, and recreational pursuits have been seriously limited because of the presence of the disabled sibling. The following statements are examples of such feelings: "We never went on a family vacation because of my brother,

Reflect on This 14–2

Letter from Aviva Rich

My Family and I

My name is Aviva Rich. I turned 11 years old in February. I have a sister named Tammy. She is 14. I have a brother named Richard. He is 12. Both my sister and brother are adopted. My sister is blind. My brother can't use his right hand. But they still act normal.

My sister came to my family when I was 4 and she was 9. For a while we didn't talk that much. She was going to a school for the blind for a while then changed to a public school called Rushmore. My sister has a lot of friends. Sometimes we play together. I like Tammy a lot.

My brother came to my family when I was eight. Lots of people used to make fun of his right hand. My brother has learning disabilities. He goes to a public school. He can't have sugar. But once in a while he is allowed to have it. He likes sports, food, games and music. But he hates going to bed and hates going to school. I like my brother.

I have always been with my family. I play the flute and the piano. I started school early, but I had to take a test. I am the youngest person in fifth grade. I like gymnastics, drawing, writing, playing the flute, chocolate, pizza and reading.

I share a room with my sister. I have over fifty dolls from around the world. I am half Jewish and half Christian. I go to temple. My favorite holidays are Purim, Chanuka, Christmas and my birthday.

I like my whole family, not just one part of it, my whole family.

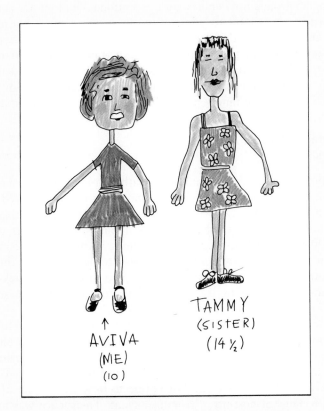

AVIVA
(ME)
(10)

TAMMY
(SISTER)
(14 ½)

Source: From "My Family and I" by Aviva Rich. Reprinted with the permission of *The Exceptional Parent*, 1170 Commonwealth Avenue, Boston, MA 02134.

Steven." "How could I invite a friend over? I never knew how my autistic brother would behave." "How do you explain to a date that you have a retarded sister?" "Many of my friends stopped coming to my house because they didn't know how to handle my deaf brother, Mike. They simply could not understand him." "I was always shackled with the responsibilities of tending my little sister. I didn't have time to have fun with my friends." "I want a real brother, not a retarded one." As mentioned earlier, Grossman found that older, female siblings from low-income families frequently have to assume responsibility for caring for the disabled family member. In these cases, many siblings resent having to assume the role of caregiver and feel deprived of some of the important opportunities most young people want to have in growing up.

Siblings of exceptional children may also feel as if they must compensate for their parents' disappointment about having a disabled child (Murphy, 1979). They may feel an undue amount of pressure to excel or to be successful in a particular academic or artistic pursuit. Such pressure can have a profound effect on the siblings' physical and mental health. Likewise, the expressed expectations of parents can serve as a source of pressure and emotional pain to siblings: "Why do I always feel as if I have to be the perfect child or the one who always does things right? I'm getting tired of constantly having to win my parents' admiration. Why can't I just be average for once?"

Sibling support groups for families with exceptional children are emerging and can be particularly helpful to adolescents. In these groups, children and youths can be introduced to the important aspects of having an exceptional sibling in their family (Atkins, 1987). Appropriate expectations can be established, and questions that children may be hesitant to ask in a family context may be freely discussed. These groups can also provide a therapeutic means by which these individuals can analyze family problems and identify practical solutions.

The Exceptional Individual and the Extended Family

> I can distinctly remember the tears of my father-in-law, and my mother-in-law's reluctance to visit me in the hospital when they discovered that I had given birth to a child with an open spine (spina bifida). During my mother-in-law's first visit, all she could talk about was the dinner party she had held the night before and her upcoming vacation. All I could think about was my baby and whether he was going to make it through the night. At the time I was extremely angry and upset by her lack of sympathy and understanding. I could not figure out why she was so insensitive to my feelings and my son's condition.
>
> Because of the seriousness of our son's defect, the consulting physicians recommended that Eric immediately undergo an operation. Shortly thereafter my mother-in-law asked me who had given permission for this operation, implying that it might have been better to have allowed Eric not to survive or die on his own. Attempting to be stoic in spite of my heightened feelings of hostility, I remained silent. The silence was broken with another hurtful comment: "My son will be burdened for life."

These and other similar comments were common during the first twenty-four months of Eric's life. It was as though I had burdened *her*.

As I reflect on this time period, I can see that I was simply too overwhelmed by my own feelings to give careful consideration to the comments made by my in-laws, neighbors, and friends. With the passage of time, however, I have come to understand my husband's parents and their responses to our exceptional son. They, in turn, have also developed an appreciation and understanding of our son and us. It took quite a bit of time, and we all had to adapt and change a great deal.

Eric is now ten. He loves both of his grandparents and looks forward to spending time with them on special weekend visits. It is during these weekends that my husband and I take time to renew our relationship and restore ourselves with recreational activities.

Extended family is a term frequently used to describe a household in which a nuclear family lives accompanied by a number of close relatives. For the purposes of this section, the term *extended family* is used to identify those individuals who are close relatives of the nuclear family and have regular and frequent contacts with it even though they do not live in the same household. These individuals may include the disabled child's grandparents, uncles, aunts, or cousins.

When a new child is born and becomes part of a family, he or she also becomes part of an extended family. Usually it is the grandparents who make the first official family visit or call to the hospital. This first visit from the grandparents can be extraordinarily taxing and difficult if it entails providing congratulations and support to a daughter who has given birth to a child with an exceptionality. In a very real fashion, grandparents perceive grandchildren as an extension of themselves (Berns, 1980). They look forward to babying, bragging about, and showing snapshots of their grandchildren, without worrying about the burdens of responsibility that parents must assume. When a grandchild is born with an impairment, the joy of the occasion may dissipate. Like parents, grandparents are hurled into a crisis that necessitates reevaluation and reorientation (Pieper, 1976). They must decide not only how they will respond to their child, who is now a parent, but also how they will relate to the new grandchild. Many grandparents grew up in a time when deviancy of almost any variety was barely tolerated, much less understood. Therefore they enter the crisis process without much understanding. In their day, such a birth may have signified the presence of "bad blood" within a family. As a result of this attitude and other similar perceptions, the mother or father of the newborn child may be selected as the scapegoat. But blaming only provides a temporary form of relief. It does little to promote the optimal family functioning that becomes so necessary in the weeks and months to come.

Little research is available regarding the impact of grandparents on the functioning of a family with an exceptional child. Davis (1967) contrasted the support maternal grandmothers gave their daughters who had given birth to a retarded child with the support provided by maternal grandmothers to daughters

Reflect on This 14–3

Help for Siblings

As you are discovering, children with a disabled brother or sister may experience a number of problems in dealing with their parents, their friends, and other situations both inside and outside the home. A new and innovative organization has been established for the siblings of disabled individuals. This organization is the Sibling Information Network. Its members enjoy the following resources: a quarterly newsletter with quality resource materials, a bibliography of children's literature related to handicapping conditions, a list of media on siblings, a list of all its members and persons who have organized sibling groups, a bibliography of journal articles on siblings, and a collection of articles from the newsletter on various programs and workshops. The headquarters for this new network are located at the University of Connecticut, Department of Educational Psychology, Storrs, Connecticut. Involvement with this network may be very helpful to children who are experiencing difficulties in relating to a new sibling who is disabled.

who gave birth to normal children. Less than half the families with a retarded child received "effective" support from maternal grandmothers. By contrast, the normal families received "effective" support from three-quarters of the maternal grandmothers. In a related study, McAndrew (1976) found that 33 percent of 116 parents interviewed believed that their relationships with grandparents and friends were adversely affected by the birth of a disabled child.

FOCUS 11
What are three types of assistance that grandparents can render to families with an exceptional child?

Grandparents and other family members can, however, contribute much help to the primary family unit (Howard, 1978). If they live near the family, they can become an integral part of the resource network. They may also be able to provide support before the energies of their children are so severely depleted that they need additional, costly help. In order to be of assistance they must be prepared and informed, which can be achieved in a variety of ways. They must have an opportunity to voice their questions, feelings, and concerns about the disorder and its complications. They must have means by which they can become informed. Parents can aid in this process by sharing with their parents and siblings the pamphlets, materials, and books suggested by health and educational personnel. They can also encourage their families to become involved in parent discussion groups. In such informal meetings, they learn about the struggles and feelings of their own children. These meetings are also catalysts for frank and open conversation. Extended family members need positive feedback regarding their efforts and support. When these conditions are met, they can be an important part of the total treatment process. Norma McPhee, grandmother of a child with cerebral palsy, shares some of her feelings in the following vignette:

I was determined to find ways to stimulate him and motivate him. I tried to verbalize for him his frustrations and to help him find outlets for expression. I became aware of things that I did that didn't require speaking, using my hands or my feet.

Story records went his way and he loved them. I scoured stores for cookie cutters to help him with holiday preparations. He could hold them and wait until they were needed.

We carried on one-way, long-distance telephone conversations. I cried the first time I heard his sounds in response on the other end of the line. We shared canoe rides and picnics on a camping trip. We visited an orchard and picked apples.

One day I stopped by his picture, saw the lopsided smile and realized what a very special magic there is between grandparents and grandchildren. I realize just how much I loved him—just as he was . . . (McPhee, 1982, p. 16).

According to Pieper (1976), grandparents can be helpful in several ways. They may be able to give parents a weekend reprieve from the pressures of maintaining the household, as did Norma McPhee. They may also assist with transportation or baby-sitting. Grandparents may often serve as third-party evaluators, providing solutions to seemingly unresolvable problems. The child with an impairment

---

WINDOW 14–2

We Decided to Educate Ourselves

When I discovered that our grandson was retarded, I wasn't sure how I should respond. You must remember that in my day, retarded children weren't talked about a lot. They were actually hidden or sent away to a state hospital or something like that. My husband was particularly perplexed by the birth of our new grandson. He really didn't know what to say or how to respond. Of course, I wasn't much better. We decided that we needed to educate ourselves. Our daughter was kind enough to give us a few pamphlets that helped us learn about our new grandson's condition. We also talked to some other friends of ours who have a mongoloid granddaughter. They didn't know a whole lot more than we did, but the talking did us both some good.

Since that time we've tried to be supportive of our daughter and her situation. We try to volunteer whatever assistance we can when she seems to be pressed or to need a reprieve for a couple of hours. We're glad that we live somewhat close to her.

I remember our first contacts with Richard. We weren't sure how different he would be. Actually, it took very little time for us to realize that Richard wasn't all that different. We found that he does things a little bit more slowly, but other than that he's pretty much normal.

We think our daughter and her husband, John, have handled this situation extremely well. In fact, we're very proud of them. And we realize that this could happen to anyone.

We enjoy Richard a lot. Yes, we worry a little about his future and what he'll do when he's older, but we've learned from John and Marilyn that sometimes it's better to take things one day at a time.

Betty, *a grandmother*

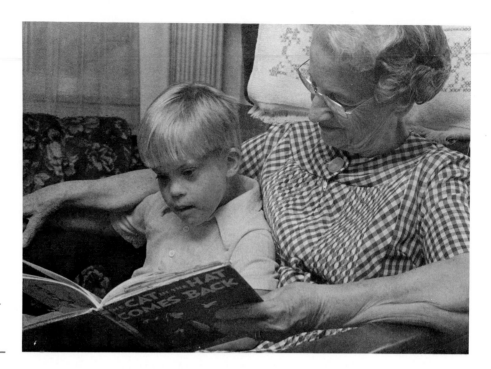

Grandparents can play an invaluable role in caring for a child with disabilities. (John Telford)

profits from the unique attention that only grandparents can provide. This attention can be a natural part of such special occasions as birthdays, vacations, fishing trips, or other traditional family activities.

We have highlighted the positive ways in which extended-family members may assist the primary family unit, but the types of assistance and support described may be difficult to arrange. For instance, few family members freely volunteer to tend a hyperactive child. Baby-sitting exchanges and other similar arrangements are also much more difficult to set up when the tending involves a difficult child. Such is the case with many family activities. The exceptional child is not as likely as others to be invited to participate in recreational activities such as sleeping overnight at a friend's or cousin's house, eating dinner with neighbors, or going with another family on a weekend camping trip.

WINDOW 14–3

My Parents Have Always Helped

Over the years, I have found it is better for Tammy if my husband and I are not the only people who take care of her. Our patience isn't strained and Tammy learns to interact and adjust to a variety of people.

My parents have always helped a great deal. My neighbors and friends are all supportive too. They are not apprehensive about having Tammy over or taking care of her because they are used to her. Tammy has grown up with her classmates. One special friend drives Tammy home on the days I work. She goes far out of her way to bring Tammy home, and insists that she enjoys it. I think it makes my friends feel good when they can really help me take care of Tammy. (Salkever, 1981, pp. 15–7)

Mary Salkever, *mother of Tammy, a young lady with cerebral palsy*

Reflect on This 14–4

Baby-sitters! We Need Just One!

Marcia's a pretty mature girl for her age, but she becomes almost terrified when she thinks that she might have to hold our new son, Jeremy. He is multihandicapped.

I don't dare leave him with our other two children, Amy and Mary Ann. They're much to young to handle Jeremy. But I need to get away from the demands that seem to be ever-present in caring for Jeremy. If I could just find one person who could help us, even just once a month, things would be a lot better for me and my family.

A dilemma faced by many parents of severely disabled or chronically ill children is finding a baby-sitter. The challenge is far greater than one might imagine: frequently the parents of such children never find someone who can provide them and their other children with the reprieve they so much need.

As you might guess, the more disabled the child is, the more difficult it is to find a person who can provide the needed care. Unfortunately, many parents discover all too late how much a good baby-sitter could have helped them. What are the reasons for endeavoring to find a baby-sitter?

We have learned that the presence of a disabled or seriously ill child in the family can produce a lot of strain, not only for the parents, but also for other members of the family. Having an opportunity to be away from the seriously disabled child provides the immediate care givers and siblings with a chance to have some of their own needs met. It also gives parents an opportunity to become recharged or revitalized for the demanding regimen they often have to follow in taking care of such a child. Too, respites in which nondisabled children are able to have the exclusive attention of their parents reaffirm their importance in the family and their value as individuals.

In some areas of the country, enterprising teenagers have developed baby-sitting businesses that specialize in tending children who are disabled or otherwise require unusual baby-sitting approaches. Frequently local disability associations can also be helpful in providing qualified assistance in the important area of baby-sitting.

In addition, relatives and neighbors may be critical of management procedures that parents have been encouraged to employ with their child. Procedures such as social isolation and various forms of punishment may be viewed as abusive parental behavior by close friends and relatives. Other types of treatment may also be viewed with a jaundiced eye, if they include the use of stimulant drugs, very controlled diets, or point systems. Parents who must administer these home-based interventions often feel that they are completely alone. On the other hand, the support provided by extended-family members, if properly applied, can have a positive effect on the physical and social/emotional well-being of the primary family.

THE FAMILY'S DILEMMA: LEARNING TO WORK WITH PROFESSIONALS

I waited eagerly for the news that our obstetrician was about to bring regarding the birth of our first child. My wife and I were new at this enterprise, but we felt as if we were ready for the new arrival. Many pleasant pictures passed through my mind as I waited, daydreaming about the future of our family. Dr. Stephens, our obstetrician, entered the small waiting-room area and immediately informed me that I had a new daughter and that my wife was fine. As he delivered this joyful news to me, his voice was flat. When we went to the viewing area to see my daughter, I sensed that the nurses and Dr. Stephens were much more interested in my responses to my daughter than I had expected. As we stood there, Dr. Stephens asked how she looked, to which I responded, "I think she looks just fine!" It was as though he thought my child's impairment would be readily apparent to me. I saw nothing different in my child's appearance.

After viewing my daughter for the first time, I immediately went to the recovery room, where my wife was waiting to be taken to her own hospital room. She was in good spirits and I could tell that she was excited about our new daughter. She asked, "How does she look? Is she okay? Do you like her?" Although her speech was slightly slurred, she asked the questions in rapid succession. Again I responded as I had to Dr. Stephens, "Yes, she looks just fine. I think her name should be Melinda."

In the days that followed, Melinda lost quite a bit of weight, and she seemed to be very sleepy and difficult to arouse. Our pediatrician was concerned, but not overly so, with the rapid weight loss. During this period, we felt as if we were in the dark. Little was said about Melinda except that she was making adequate progress. The nursing staff remained distant. They communicated only information that was essential. We began to sense that something might be wrong with our daughter. We felt that they knew something about our child that we were expected to discover by ourselves.

On the fourth day, after discussing the situation in some depth, we demanded a consultation with our pediatrician. Early the next morning we were told of the diagnosis: Down syndrome. We were simply told that Melinda would be retarded and that her condition was stable at the present time. Our pediatrician also briefly talked about one of his relatives who had a Down syndrome child. He described the child as being quite happy, but such comments failed to provide us with any comfort or hope for Melinda's future. Our discussion ended within fifteen minutes. We were still very much in the dark and wondering how we were to care for our new baby.

The interaction that occurs between professionals and parents is often marked by confusion, dissatisfaction, disappointment, and anger. Several writers have documented these and other negative feelings in parents (Buscaglia, 1975; Dougan, Isbell, & Vyas, 1979; Muir-Hutchinson, 1987; Fox, 1975; Turnbull & Turnbull, 1978). What are the sources of these feelings? Are they to be expected? A certain amount of dissatisfaction is present in even the best of relationships. However, the research information available has led many observers to believe that the relationship between parents and professionals could be significantly improved (Kotze, 1986; Kroth, 1987).

Many professionals are inadequately prepared to deal with the challenges of informing parents of their child's exceptionality. In a similar vein, many professionals do not have the counseling skills necessary for the development of satisfactory relationships with patients and their families. In examining these problems, Seligman and Seligman (1980) identified three types of professional understanding essential to establishing positive working relationships with families. First, professionals need to understand the impact they have on parents. Second, they need to understand the impact the exceptional individual has on the family over time. Third, they need to understand the impact the exceptional child and family have on the professional.

Medical and other health-related personnel have a profound impact on the ways parents respond to the birth or injury of a child. They cannot prevent the shock felt by parents as they learn of the child's impairment, but they can lessen its impact. They can also provide parents with perspective and direction as they attempt to adjust their lives and make room for the child.

Physicians set the stage and prepare the family for the first few days, weeks, and months. Unfortunately, some are not adequately prepared to counsel parents regarding the steps to take. In fact, many medical personnel are unaware of the resources and services available for exceptional infants and children (Gorham, 1975; Gorham, DesJardins, Page, Pettis, & Scheiber, 1975). They are also unprepared to deal with the parents' present situation and feelings. Therefore, parents frequently leave the hospital or clinic confused and disoriented, not knowing exactly what their options are or how they should proceed. Wunderlich (1977) aptly captured many parents' sentiments when he indicated that the physician's role includes more than just providing a diagnosis.

In a comprehensive review of research related to counseling the disabled and their parents, Leigh (1975) concluded:

1. Parents are often dissatisfied with the information, or lack of information, provided by professionals regarding their children's problems.

2. "Shopping" parents are generally seeking valid assistance regarding new problem behaviors of their children, rather than a new diagnosis.

3. The amount of meaningful information gained during the initial consultation is generally a function of the quality of the interactions that occur between the counselor and the parents.

4. Parents are much more likely to carry out the recommendations of the counselor or physician if they concur with the diagnosis.

5. Professionals often devalue the importance of the parents' attitudes in communicating with and attempting to assist them in caring for their children.

Gorham (1975), who is a parent of a profoundly retarded child, provided some helpful suggestions for professionals interested in enhancing the positive impact they have on parents. Her suggestions include such practices as using appropriate key language in report writing and informal conversations; providing realistic management plans for the family that outline procedures to be taken during the next several weeks and months; emphasizing the children's assets and abilities as well as their weaknesses and deficits; referring parents to appropriate community agencies and organizations; and helping parents to realize that their

FOCUS 12
What are three types of professional understanding that are essential to establishing positive relationships with parents and families?

exceptional child will provide them with a series of problem-solving opportunities that they will not have to meet alone.

Professional Burn-out

Little has been written about the impact the exceptional child and his or her family have on the lives of educational and health personnel. The information available is primarily anecdotal in nature. Like parents, professionals are subject to emotional exhaustion (Maslach, 1978). Emotional exhaustion may exhibit itself in numerous ways. Professionals may become apathetic, pessimistic, or cynical about their work and involvement with patients, students, or clients. They may focus on the negative aspects of their work and feel that their perceptions have become constricted. Depression is also a common characteristic of emotional exhaustion. Personnel affected this way may feel they have no power to enact meaningful changes in their work environments (Pagel & Price, 1980).

Emotional and physical exhaustion cannot be attributed entirely to the actions of families and children, but they do play an important role. As physicians, educators, and therapists interact with impaired children and their families, there are problems that frequently arise. Caring for an exceptional individual in a medical or educational setting can be very challenging. Progress may be exceedingly slow. Interventions may be unsuccessful. The exceptional individual may not be making the progress anticipated. Parents may be disappointed with the quality of services and may complain or even threaten to sue. Prescribed medication may be ineffective. These conditions can have an immense impact on the physical and mental well-being of the professionals who feel responsible for exceptional

---

WINDOW 14—4

My Students Are Incredibly Challenging

Actually, I really enjoy teaching and working with my students. Yes, they are at times incredibly challenging. For example, a third grader in my self-contained class recently climbed up on his desk and engaged in a little urine-sprinkling activity. At first, I couldn't believe what I was seeing, but nothing surprises me anymore.

The kids are the least of my problems, however. It's the paperwork, the legal requirements, regular teachers who are strongly opposed to mainstreaming, uncooperative parents who won't even sign a simple "end of the day report," and administrative personnel who provide little, if any, support that really bother me. Also, the teaching resources and materials I have are very meager. How can anyone expect me to do a good job of teaching when I don't even have the essential tools and materials?

By the way, when I do need some help dealing with serious student problems, I generally get it quite quickly. The assistance usually is provided by John, our school psychologist, or by Jane, the social worker. Each of them has really made a difference. John has helped me deal with some super-aggressive students. Jane has been helpful with some of my children's parents. I wish I had something good to say about my principal, but he's practically worthless when it comes to supporting special education. He has no idea what needs to be done.

Sarah, *a teacher of young children with behavior disorders*

individuals and their families. The recurring frustration, tedium, pressure, and dissatisfaction that characterize the work of helping professionals can at times be overwhelming and debilitating.

Because of the stress inherent in working with exceptional persons, many professionals experience a phenomenon known as burn-out (Freudenberger, 1977; Maslach, 1978). Child-care workers in a variety of settings leave their professional pursuits because of the excessive demands they confront. Smith and Cline (1980) evaluated the sources of stress for special education personnel. In order of importance, the following tasks were identified as causing stress in teachers: (1) completing individual educational programs and due-process paperwork, (2) coping with parents, (3) taking care of school-related work after the usual hours, (4) dealing with excessive student loads, (5) diagnosing and assessing, and (6) working with other teachers. It is interesting to note that the second most stressful item was dealing with parents. In a related study, Pagel and Price (1980) reported similar findings. They found that teachers were frequently bothered by "disruptive and unmotivated students" as well as "uncooperative parents" (p. 46).

Kraft and Snell (1980) have studied parent-teacher conflicts. In their discussion, they include the "blame-oriented parent" and the "pseudoexpert parent." Each type provides teachers, physicians, and other care providers with some unique challenges and problems. However, communication and understanding must prevail if parents and professionals are to share in the task of helping exceptional individuals achieve their fullest potential. There is still much work to be done. Both parents and professionals need to become more sensitive to one another and their respective needs. Schools that prepare people for the helping professions must provide better training for those who will be responsible for helping and counseling parents. Schools of education should also provide their students with healthy means for coping with the stresses inherent in working with exceptional individuals and their families.

Training for Professionals and Parents

Fortunately, professional and parent training programs are being developed to help teachers and parents communicate and work more effectively with each other (Chandler, Fowler, & Lubeck, 1985; Turnbull, Strickland, & Goldstein, 1978; Tynan and Fritsch, 1987). Many teachers and parents are truly unprepared to consult and work with one another (McKinney & Hocutt, 1982). Teachers have been prepared primarily to work with children, not with parents and families. Parents may have little understanding of the educational processes involved in evaluating, placing, and instructing children with disabilities. Therefore they may have difficulty responding knowledgeably and productively in the usual planning, placement, and annual evaluation meetings required by Public Law 94–142. However, as training programs for parents and teachers emerge, the problems should improve, particularly if parent training is individualized, a need stressed by Turnbull and Turnbull (1986). The outcomes of effective parental involvement are very positive (Bristol & Gallagher, 1982; Cartwright, 1981; Welch & Odum, 1981). The engagement and cooperation of parents can add greatly to the overall rate and quality of success that children and teachers experience in achieving academic, social, and vocational skills.

FOCUS 14
What has been done to help parents and professionals work more effectively with one another?

REVIEW

FOCUS 1: Identify five factors that influence the ways in which families respond to an infant with a birth defect or disability.

☐ The five factors are the emotional stability of each family member, their religious values and beliefs, socioeconomic status, the severity of the disability, and the type of disability.

FOCUS 2: What four statements can you safely make about the stages that parents may experience in responding to infants or young children with disabilities?

☐ The stage approach needs further refinement and validation before we can accurately use it to understand, predict, or help parents deal with young infants and children with disabilities.

☐ Parental responses are highly variable.

☐ The adjustment process, for most parents, is continuous and distinctively individual.

FOCUS 3: What are four major concerns of parents of exceptional children?

☐ What are our child's future educational and social needs?

☐ What will our child be capable of doing as an adult?

☐ How will our child influence our other children and our family as a whole? How can we maintain our normal family functioning with the presence of this child?

FOCUS 4: Identify three ways in which a newborn child with moderate to severe disabilities influences the manner in which family members respond to each other.

☐ The mother may have less time to relate to the other children in the family.

☐ The other members of the family may have to assume some of the roles and responsibilities that were once the mother's.

☐ The mother's need for support and assistance may bring the family closer together as a unit.

FOCUS 5: What kind of a relationship may develop between the mother and her child with a disability?

☐ A strong dyadic relationship may develop between the mother and the child.

FOCUS 6: What are three factors that contribute to marital stress?

☐ Factors include a decrease in the amount of time available for the couple's activities, sometimes heavy financial burdens, and fatigue.

FOCUS 7: What are four general phases of the developmental cycle that parents go through in rearing a child with disabilities?

☐ The first phase is the diagnostic period. Does the child truly have a disability?

☐ The second phase is the school period (elementary and secondary) with its inherent challenges (e.g., dealing with teasing and other peer-related behaviors; learning academic, social, and vocational skills). Included in this period are the challenges of adolescence.

☐ The third phase is the postschool period, when the child makes the transition from school to other educational or vocational activities.

☐ The fourth phase is the period when the parents are no longer able to provide direct care and guidance for their son or daughter.

FOCUS 8: What are four factors influencing the relationship that develops between infants with disabilities and their mothers?

☐ The mother may be unable to engage in the typical feeding and care-giving activities because of the intensive medical care being provided.

☐ Some mothers may have difficulty bonding to a child with whom they have little physical and social interaction.

☐ Some mothers are given little direction as to how they might become involved with their children. Without minimal involvement, some mothers become estranged from their children and find it difficult to begin the caring process.

☐ The expectations that mothers have about their children and their function in nurturing them play a significant role in the relationships that develop.

FOCUS 9: Identify three ways in which some fathers respond to their children with disabilities.

☐ Fathers are more likely to internalize their feelings than are mothers.

☐ Fathers often respond to sons with disabilities differently from how they respond to daughters.

☐ Fathers may resent the time their wives spend in caring for their children with disabilities.

FOCUS 10: Identify four ways in which siblings respond to their exceptional brothers or sisters.

☐ Siblings tend to mirror the attitudes and behaviors of their parents toward a child with disabilities.

☐ Some siblings play a critical role in fostering the intellectual, social, and affective development of the exceptional child.

☐ Some siblings respond by eventually becoming members

of helping professions that serve exceptional populations.

□ Some siblings respond with feelings of resentment or deprivation.

FOCUS 11: What are three types of assistance grandparents can render to families with an exceptional child?

□ They can provide their own children with a weekend reprieve from the pressures of the home environment.

□ They can assist occasionally with baby-sitting or transportation.

□ They can help their children in times of crisis by listening and helping them deal with a seemingly unresolvable problem.

FOCUS 12: What are three types of professional understanding that are essential to establishing positive relationships with parents and families?

□ Professionals need to understand the impact that they have on families over time.

□ Professionals need to understand the impact that the child with disabilities has on the family over time.

□ Professionals need to understand the impact that children with disabilities and their families have on them.

FOCUS 13: Identify the three ways in which children with disabilities and their families impact teachers and health-care workers.

□ Professionals may become emotionally exhausted from the pressures involved in educating or helping exceptional children.

□ They may become apathetic, pessimistic, or cynical about the work with patients, clients, or students.

□ They may feel powerless to enact meaningful changes in their work environments.

FOCUS 14: What has been done to help parents and professionals work more effectively with one another?

□ Professional and parent training programs are being developed to help teachers and parents communicate and work more effectively with each other.

Debate Forum

Interventions: Should This One Be Undertaken?

Parents of children with limited intellectual capacity often do quite well in responding to the needs of their children during the childhood years. However, with the passage of time, these same children become teenagers or young adults, and their parents can be faced with a variety of very difficult philosophical, moral, and practical questions. The most problematic of these questions concern such issues as marriage, parenthood, and sterilization.

Excerpted below is an article written by Nat Mills (1977), a father of a child with Down syndrome.

Our teenage daughter, who is mentally retarded, has long dreamed of having a husband and children on whom she could pour out her love. She is now 14, and although she is afflicted with Down's syndrome, her sexuality and procreative abilities are already fully developed. While we welcome her capacity for love and her emerging

sexuality as giant steps forward toward full maturity, we, her parents, believe that her ability to have children must be destroyed. We are saddened at the thought that our daughter will not be able to have children of her own, and it has not been easy for us to come to this decision. Nonetheless, we are urgently seeking such intervention because we are convinced that her ability to have children constitutes a pervasive threat to her future happiness (p. M2).

By making this decision for our daughter, are we overriding her superior right to give or withhold "informed consent"? Are we preventing her from assuming a mature responsibility for her own life? Should some professional intervene to prevent domination by insensitive parents?

If we have learned anything in the past 15 years, it is that we must continually weigh how much independence we can expect and encourage in our daughter against the reality of her limited comprehension and ability to cope. No abstract principles can point a straight path between the achieved growth and constant frustrations. At the same time that we nurture all signs of maturity in her, we are forced to recognize and accept a developmental plateau that requires life-long guardianship.

We are now seeking appropriate medical intervention that will guarantee our daughter's right to the full protection against pregnancy that she needs and can get in no other way. If someone feels that this right must not be granted, let him or her prove that such denial can in any way benefit our daughter. As her loving parents we have no doubt that sterilization is in her life-long best interest (p. M4).*

Here are some questions for you to ponder and discuss. Does this youth's child-bearing capacity represent an ever-present hazard that could disrupt whatever emotional or vocational stability she may develop? What if she were able to find a loving husband? Could they, with their combined strengths, care for children?

_____

* Nat Mills (1977). "Our Daughter's Happiness Depends on Her Being Sterile." *Exceptional Parent*, 7(2), M2–M5. Reprinted with the permission of *Exceptional Parent*, 1170 Commonwealth Avenue, Boston, MA 02134.

How much competence must one have to qualify for child bearing and rearing? Who has the right to decide if a person is fit to be a parent?

Point   The right to determine whether this young person should have children is not solely the right of the parents. The interests of the child who will eventually become an adult must also be served. A legally empowered, independent review board should be involved in assessing the merits of this child's case. Members of the review board should be persons who are professionally qualified to address the medical, legal, and social issues of each request for sterilization. If they determine that the child should be sterilized, after reviewing all of the pertinent information and if the parents concur, then the child may be sterilized.

Counterpoint   Parents have the right to determine what medical actions ought to be taken to ensure the well-being and eventual happiness of their child. They are the best judges of the child's adaptive and coping capacities. Because they bear the responsibility for partially or fully supporting the child during her lifetime, they have the right to determine what medical actions should be taken in preparing their child for the adulthood period. Parents should not have this right infringed on by a review board composed of well-meaning professionals.

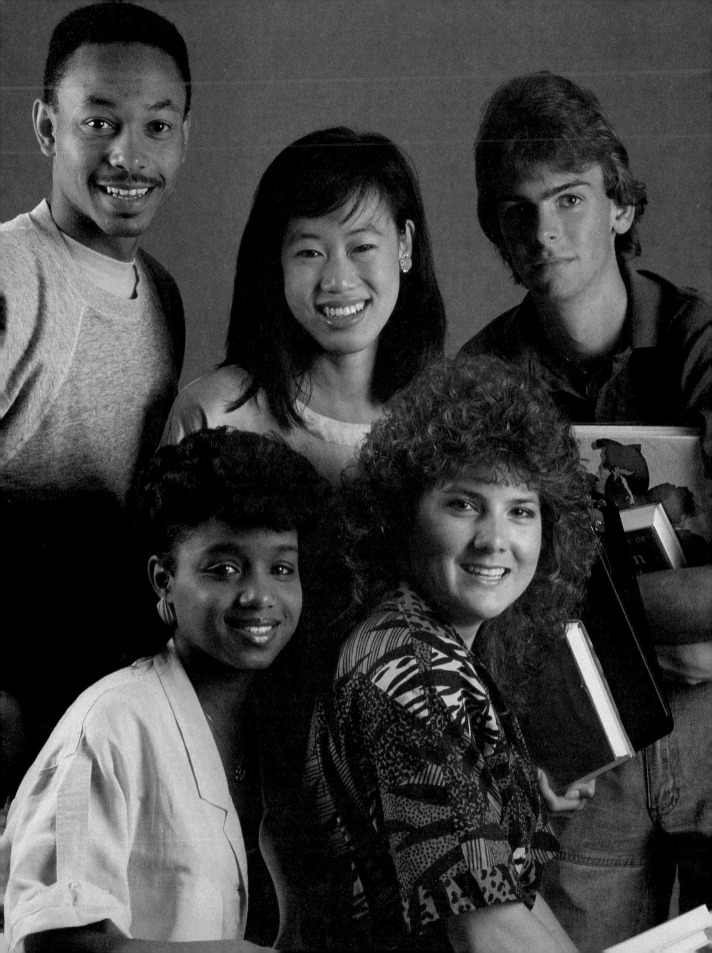

15 Multicultural Perspectives and Issues

To Begin With...

■ Between 1978 and 1984, the percentage of ethnic minority children in our schools increased from ¼ to over ⅓, yet few persons of ethnic minority are preparing to become teachers (Office of Civil Rights, 1986).

■ There are significant language minorities in every state, with seven states having more than a million language minority persons. There are approximately 10.6 million Spanish speaking persons, the majority in the Southwestern states. And there are almost 2 million speakers whose language background is Chinese, Filipino, Japanese, Korean or Vietnamese (Heath & Heath, 1989).

■ Although figures vary from state to state, there are disproportionately large percentages of black children in classes for the mentally retarded and the seriously emotionally disturbed. Hispanic and American Indian children are also highly disproportionately represented in classes for the mentally retarded (Chinn & Hughes, 1987).

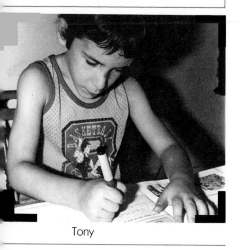

Tony

Tony had great difficulty understanding much of what went on in the world around him. In school, his classmates and teacher spoke a language he had heard now for a rather long time, but it was not the same one his mother and father spoke. When his teacher spoke, the sound seemed harsh and unpleasant to him; the words had none of the softness and pretty sound that he heard at home and in the fields when he was helping pick berries. At this school, he had two teachers and went to different classrooms at different times of the day. Tony couldn't understand why his classmates laughed at him when he went to the afternoon teacher. He felt like he must have done something wrong because their laughter wasn't a cheerful sound, but more like they were making fun of him.

Moving was something Tony was very accustomed to; his family moved two or three times a year. When the berries were all picked the family got in the truck and drove a long way, to another farm, where they worked on onions. Tony thought moving was fun because he and his sisters got to ride in the back of the truck.

Mary was in the fifth grade, sort of. She had been in school for eight years now, and the room she went to in the afternoon said Fifth Grade on the door. The class she attended in the morning had a longer sign on it that she couldn't read but she did know it started with an *R*. She thought she probably went there because her last name started with that letter. She had been given a test just before she started in the class. Mary thought she had done well on the test. Her mother told her she got a 64, and that was higher than she usually got in class. Mary's African ancestry was very evident from her facial features and skin color. She would have been considered a pretty girl except that she had lost most of her front teeth last year in a violent attack by three young men, who had raped and beaten her. She also had a large, diagonal scar across her chin and lower lip from that incident. Nothing happened to the boys afterward, because Mary was too frightened to identify them to the police. Her previous experience with law officers had been frightening, and she was afraid the three adolescents would hurt her more—they all lived within two blocks of her home.

INTRODUCTION

FOCUS 1
What are two ways the purposes of education in general differ from special education and multicultural education?

Special interests in education tend to emerge when a particular group's needs are not being adequately met by general system efforts. This is the case for both **multicultural education** and special education. Multicultural education arose from a belief that the needs of children with cultural backgrounds differing from the majority were not being appropriately met. Other societal unrest related to racial discrimination fueled and augmented this belief. Likewise, special education grew out of presumed failures of the general education system. Certain children were not learning in the same way or manner as their age-mates. With regard to both multicultural and special education, there was also a belief that children within their respective realms of interest were being *mis*treated, in one case because of their cultural or racial background, and in the other because of their learning or behavior problems.

Two basic factors need examination as we introduce the topic of multicultural perspectives and issues in this volume. Initially, it is important to explore the basic purposes and goals of education. These must then be compared and contrasted with the underlying purposes of both special and multicultural education. The second factor requiring attention is the linkage between multicultural and special education. With these points as background, we can logically proceed to examine multicultural perspectives and issues in the context of this book's major focus, human exceptionality in society, school, and family.

Purposes of Education

In general, education in the United States is intended for everyone. All children are presumably provided a free education to a certain level, usually the twelfth grade—the end of high school. The manner in which this is typically implemented involves collecting youngsters into groups, for the most part based on chronological age, and teaching those groups. They are taught what society generally accepts as appropriate for young people of each age. In most cases their performance level is evaluated based on what society expects children and youth of each age to achieve. Society uses as its yardstick for this expectation an average of what youngsters of each age learn. In other words, education in this country is aimed at the masses and performance is judged on an average. Through this system,

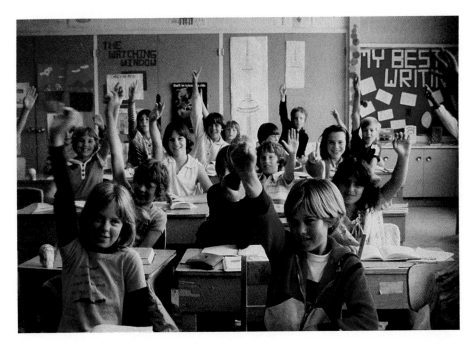

In the typical U.S. classroom, students are divided into groups according to age and taught what society expects children of that age to know. Education is aimed at the masses, and performance is judged on an average. (© Suzanne Szasz/Photo Researchers, Inc.)

there is an attempt to bring most young people to a similar point in knowledge level, at least on a minimal basis.

Most special education professionals would agree, at least in principle, that the fundamental purpose of special education in contemporary society is to provide an education to each person that maximizes the development of his or her potential. The current manner in which this is often implemented involves focusing on the individual and his or her strengths and limitations. Such an approach has been found to be important because the children and youth being served in special education seem unable to function well when instruction is broadly directed, at large groups.

Currently, multicultural education is viewed as education that values and promotes **cultural pluralism.** It is not intended to be limited to those of cultural or racial minorities, but more appropriately teaches all students about cultural diversity. Chinn and McCormick (1986) cite four elements included in ideal multicultural education as: "1) teaching values that support cultural diversity and individual uniqueness, 2) encouraging and accepting the qualitative expansion of existing ethnic cultures, 3) supporting exploration in alternative and emerging life styles, and 4) encouraging multiculturalism, multilinguism, and multidialectism" (p. 99). Adding to this description, Rodriguez notes that "multicultural education rejects the view that schools should seek to melt away cultural differences or the view that schools should merely tolerate cultural pluralism" (1982, p. 221).

Education, Special Education, and Multicultural Education. Certain differences emerge as we discuss the fundamental purposes of education, special education, and multicultural education. This is not terribly surprising since, as noted above, special-interest efforts emerge from broader efforts when the latter are unsuccessful. However, as we examine educational goals from these viewpoints, we will find that there are certain gaps, places where the jigsaw puzzle does not fit neatly together, either because of a lack of conceptual clarity or because of implementation shortfalls. These gaps create certain difficulties, often in areas where professionals are trying to collaborate and work together to fill them. In addition to gaps, there are certain conceptual inconsistencies evident *within* areas. These points of logic vacuum also create problems, within professional groups and between professionals and the lay public.

The main purpose of general education runs somewhat counter to both that of special education and that of multicultural education. As mentioned above, general education is aimed at serving the masses. In so doing, it creates a leveling effect to some extent—bringing everyone to more or less the same level and teaching similar topics in groups, with evaluation based on a norm or average. Special education tends to focus on the individual, presumably promoting growth to each person's maximum potential. Thus, rather than focusing on broad groups and broad topics, special education tends to emphasize individuals and specific skill levels. Evaluation, at least in part, is based on individual growth to a specified mastery level and only partly on **norm-based averages.**

Likewise, the contemporary view of multicultural education is one of promoting differences and diversity, which is in some measure at variance with general education's goal of bringing the population to a similar level of performance in similar areas of knowledge. Further, general education largely reflects a societal self-portrait of the United States as a "melting pot" for peoples of all backgrounds. The **melting pot** perspective, although perhaps outdated and from an earlier period of time, still has a great influence on many aspects of society. Contemporary multicultural education, on the other hand, sees education as a powerful tool for promoting diversity (Erickson & Walker, 1983). These differences in goals are more than just words and create at least surface difficulty as one faction (multicultural education) implements efforts within the broader confines of another (general education). While much of this would seem to create an adversarial or competitive situation, such a conclusion may be the result of inaccurate understandings, which may be diminished with thoughtful examination. Table 15–1 presents a summary of some apparent divergencies, in the form of myths and realities.

Cooperation, collaboration, and communication are essential but may also be troublesome between educational interests as conceptual inconsistencies emerge within such groups. (Pragmatic issues often enter the picture too, as all groups compete for funding.) Statements of purpose are often public relations tools, provided for others to see as well as within-group guides or missions. Consequently, they are usually stated in terms that are most honorable and polished in a fashion that removes rough edges. These public statements do not always reflect the missteps or less desirable actions that implementation has taken en route to our current status. Special and multicultural education are not without such blemishes.

The historic trajectory of services to exceptional populations has not always been as positive as the currently stated purpose sounds. There have been times when intervention approaches included institutional placements out of the societal mainstream that were essentially "dehumanizing warehouses with no adequate treatment" (Drew, Logan, & Hardman, 1988, p. 342). Other types of treatment have also emerged periodically that do not fit the notion of promoting individual growth and development of skills, such as involuntary sterilization. Some of these circumstances still exist or are not very far removed historically. They pose difficulties as the field aspires to become what the purpose states and as we work within the general field of education.

The view of multicultural education evident in its stated purpose is also somewhat different from that held by many outside the field. Likewise, it varies from the notion that special interests emerge from needs of children that are not being met. The multicultural education perspective described above emphasizes that all education should promote cultural pluralism, and promote it for everyone. This is a view that has evolved and changed over the years. Initial concerns revolved around issues of discrimination and inappropriate instruction for youngsters with different language and cultural backgrounds. Furthermore, many remnants of inappropriate education are still prominent in multicultural education. As we continue this chapter, we will see references to **test bias, stigma** from placements, and other criticisms. Further, it is still in circumstances where we find needs not being met that multicultural advocates most vociferously voice concerns. Thus the purpose of teaching all youngsters about cultural diversity remains a goal and somewhat out of line with what is often implemented. Goals

TABLE 15–1 Myths and Realities about Multicultural Education

Myth	Reality
Multi-ethnic education creates divisiveness by emphasizing ethnic differences. We should be emphasizing commonalities among groups.	Commonalities cannot be recognized unless differences are acknowledged. For too long we have ignored ethnic differences; we have treated ethnic differences as bad characteristics and thereby have not recognized commonalities or differences in American society.
Multi-ethnic education would shatter the melting pot.	A genuine melting pot society—one that molds its ethnic groups into one great society—has never existed in the U.S. Actually, this kind of society is an ideal that must be continually nurtured. When U.S. society truly interweaves the best of all its cultures, it will be a melting pot society.
Multi-ethnic education would not build a harmonious society.	One reason U.S. society is not harmonious is that certain groups have been denied their cultural rights. Multi-ethnic education would restore those rights by emphasizing cultural equality and respect.

and implementations are often inconsistent as the former is actually where the latter *wants* to be. This point is noted here because it is one that contributes to difficulties both within and beyond the education profession.

Multicultural–Special Education Linkages

The link between multicultural education and special education is not always a comfortable one, nor one that was intended. In fact, to a significant degree, much of the relationship between the two areas has been viewed with concern— a problem of both racial discrimination and inappropriate educational programming. Part of the link grew from the operational level of special education, which serves children who are essentially failing in the general education system. Unfortunately, many youngsters placed in special education are from minority backgrounds—a number disproportionately large, given the percentage of minority people in the population at large (Willig & Greenberg, 1986). Such circumstances seem to suggest that special education has been used as a tool of discrimination, a means of separating racial minorities from the majority. For obvious reasons, this is not widely viewed as a positive situation. We examine this issue further in the section entitled Contributing Factors.

There are other links between special and multicultural education. Some environmental influences that appear operative in special education also seem operative in multicultural education. In part, these influences are causes of school

Myth	Reality
Multi-ethnic education detracts from the basics in public schools. Students should be taught to read, write, and compute.	Multi-ethnic education need not detract from the basics of education. Students can be taught basic skills while also learning to respect cultures. A strong argument can be made for multi-ethnic education as a basic in education.
Multi-ethnic education is to enhance the self-concepts of ethnic minority students.	A half-true myth. Multi-ethnic education should enhance the self-concepts of all students because it provides a more balanced view of American society.
Teaching ethnic pride, such as black pride or Chicano pride, would also teach ethnic minority students to dislike white cultures and students.	Pride is the wrong word. Teaching ethnic respect, respect for oneself and one's group, would cause the opposite reaction. To engender respect, a student must learn to respect others.

Source: Garcia, R. L. (1978). *Fostering a pluralistic society through multiethnic education.* Bloomington, Ind.: Phi Delta Kappa Educational Foundation. (pp. 44–5)

or academic difficulties. They are also discussed in the section Contributing Factors. Additionally, certain instructional interventions in special and multicultural education may have common elements. They often surface when academic problems require specific or focused instructional approaches. As this chapter proceeds we attempt to identify common and different educational elements in multicultural education and special education.

CONTRIBUTING FACTORS

In discussing the various types of exceptionality in this book we have typically included a section on causation. Such an approach does not serve us well in this chapter; instead we deviate from that format and examine contributing factors. In some cases, contributing factors may be very similar to causation, but we explore a much broader view here. In this section, we discuss factors that contribute to serious concerns about the link between special and multicultural education. We also examine influences that contribute to the *placement* of youngsters from culturally diverse backgrounds in special education—whether such placements are appropriate or inappropriate. We examine such contributing factors as language, poverty, migrancy, and cultural-social mores. All of these interact in a complex fashion and become pertinent considerations in multicultural perspectives of exceptionality.

It should be noted that the topics we address are not separate entities; they are interrelated to a very high degree. It is not at all unusual to find poverty among culturally different groups or racial minorities, and likewise poverty often contributes to disadvantage (e.g., malnutrition, poor health care) in early life and academic disadvantage or deficiencies during the school years.

Conceptual Contributors

FOCUS 2
What are three conceptual factors that have contributed to heightened attention and concern regarding the placement of minority youngsters in special education?

There are certain conceptual factors that contribute to the link between special and multicultural education. Some of these elicit serious concern regarding the placement of minority youngsters in special education, while others pertain to how such placements might occur. We discuss these from a conceptual perspective and focus on the notion of interactions between differing cultures—cultural differences in a literal sense, rather than from an inferior–superior perspective (Gollnick & Chinn, 1986).

The basic purpose of special education stated above focuses on *differences*. If a young boy is encountering great academic difficulty, perhaps failing reading and math, then that youngster is singled out as being different. He is different in that his math and reading performances are far below that of his peers or what is expected. Because of this difference he may receive special help in reading and math in an attempt to improve his performances. Several questions emerge as we consider this example:

1. How do we determine that the youngster is doing poorly in reading and math?
2. Is the boy a candidate for special education?
3. What is the primary reason he might be a candidate for special education?
4. What if we find out the boy's name is Tony, the youngster in the opening vignette?

Certainly, one major point that arises in this case relates to the third question. Is Tony considered exceptional due to his performance, or is he in this situation due primarily to his cultural difference? This is not an easily answered question and, in fact, it may not have a clear answer (Chinn, 1979). Contributing factors may be so intertwined that they cannot be separated in any meaningful manner. Tony may be appropriately considered for special education as long as his performance is *not* preeminently a cultural matter; that is, just because he is from a background other than the majority's. Some might argue that it does not matter why Tony is receiving special help as long as he is being served— receiving extra instructional assistance. While this perspective has a certain degree of intuitive appeal, it is not a satisfactory position for professionals involved in multicultural education. If Tony is receiving special education because of his cultural background and not primarily because he is handicapped, he is being labeled and placed inappropriately.

Special education often carries with it a certain degree of stigma. For a child to receive special education has the connotation that he or she is somehow "less than" those children who do not require such extra or different instruction. This view remains despite all efforts by professionals to change it. Peers often ridicule children in special education. Furthermore, whether they would admit it or not, the parents of such youngsters would frequently be pleased if their children were among the faceless students in regular education classes. Even parents of children who are gifted and talented are often quick to point out that their children are in some type of accelerated class rather than special education. While this negative perspective should not be present in an ideal world, it is a double hazard for Tony if it arises from mislabeling, and multicultural advocates may correctly claim that it is nothing more than another means of discrimination, perhaps oppression, by the cultural majority (Hilliard, 1980). From this view, it is not difficult to see why multicultural education advocates are concerned, even angry, when culturally different children appear to be overrepresented in special education.

There may be an additional problem if Tony's special education placement is not one that is multiculturally sensitive and appropriate. Special education intervention alone does not often promote cultural pluralism. Furthermore, even the most effective math instruction available is ineffective if it is provided in English and Tony cannot understand English or only understands it poorly. Thus, just as the reason Tony is in special education may be in error, so may the intervention be in error.

Tony's placement in special education places a shadow of even further jeopardy over him to the degree that it becomes a self-fulfilling prophecy. The notion of self-fulfilling prophecy was introduced very early in this volume as we discussed the effects of labeling. Self-fulfilling prophecy, in a word, means you become what you are labeled. If Tony is labeled (as he probably would be in the process of receiving special services), his performance in reading and mathematics *may* meet the expectations of that label. Thus, if the initial assessment

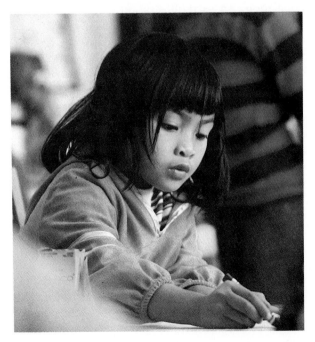

Even the most effective instruction will be ineffective if the student does not understand the language being used. (Eric A. Roth/The Picture Cube)

is inaccurate because of his cultural differences, Tony may be made a poor reader or math student by the system.

The self-fulfilling prophecy concept has been around for many years, first mentioned directly by Merton (1948) and catapulted into the center of attention by Rosenthal and Jacobson (1968a; 1968b; 1968c). The work of Rosenthal and Jacobson stimulated immediate controversy, which remains very much alive in the current literature (Rosenthal, 1987; Wineburg, 1987). There is still a great deal to be learned about the effects of expectations, specifically how and the degree to which they affect performance (Merton, 1987). However, there is sufficient concern regarding this factor to demand attention and caution, particularly as we consider multicultural and special education matters (Wineburg, 1987).

Language Contributors

FOCUS 3
What are two ways in which language may contribute to linkages between multicultural and special education?

Language differences derived from cultural diversity may represent substantial contributors to academic and social difficulties in school. If language is not considered during assessment and educational planning, such differences may result in an inappropriate special education placement for a culturally different child. There are a substantial number of children in the United States educational system who are non–English-speaking youngsters. Linguistically different children are found in the school systems of every state in the country, with several states having more than a million each (Baca & Cervantes, 1984).

The educational and psychological literature is replete with claims and empirical evidence indicating that bilingual and minority children are **overrepresented** in special education classes. Overrepresentation, in this context, means that there is a higher percentage of such youngsters in special education than would be projected from the proportion of their cultural group in the general population. An early illustration of this was found in Mercer's (1973) study, where Mexican-American youngsters were 10 times as likely to be in special education as their Caucasian peers. While Mercer's research focused on youngsters labeled as mentally retarded, other special education areas, such as learning disabilities and speech impairments, have also shown overrepresentations (Tucker, 1980; Willig & Greenberg, 1986; Wright & Santa Cruz, 1983).

Somewhat different from the situation described above is one where a youngster has a language difference (e.g., primarily speaks Japanese) contributing to learning problems, but also has a handicapping language deficiency such as delayed language development. This type of circumstance presents a very perplexing problem for the professional. It is extremely difficult to determine the degree to which each of the problems contributes to deficiency in academic achievement. The question arises whether such a child should be placed in special education and, if so, whether such placement occurs because he or she is linguistically different culturally or linguistically deficient developmentally.

Our illustrations thus far have focused on situations where the language difference arose in part from being descended from the culture of another country such as Spain or Japan. But language differences may also present difficulties if they represent what is termed *nonstandard language cultures*. Black English is an example. While such speaking may be nonstandard from some points of view, Black English is an illustration of a dialect that has its own grammatical style and pronunciation rules (Folb, 1980; White, 1984). However, it is not difficult to see how a youngster who cannot be understood by a teacher from the cultural majority might be viewed as having a language deficiency or disorder. Table 15–2 illustrates some linguistic characteristics of Black English. The several types of nonstandard English raise the question regarding the degree to which one's language style must conform to that of the cultural majority. This question, like many others in this chapter, presents a serious philosophic dilemma, but it also presents a very difficult practical problem for both teachers and children on a daily basis.

A major culprit in the contribution of language differences to special education placement has historically been assessment. Criticism has followed the reasoning that assessment of children who are linguistically different often represents a biased assessment, one that is inaccurate for special education placement. The literature has included substantial attention to assessment as a problem. On the other hand, there are others who see assessment as a much-maligned excuse for overrepresentation (Maheady, Towne, Algozzine, Mercer, & Ysseldyke, 1983).

Poverty Contributors

Perhaps the most evident example of how social and cultural factors interrelate is found in the social conditions pertaining to poverty. A youngster from an impoverished environment may be headed toward special education before he or she is even born. Gelfand, Jenson, and Drew (1988) cite statistical data and describe the prenatal development circumstances in this way: "Only 5 percent of white upper-class infants suffer complications at birth, compared with 15 percent of low-socioeconomic-status (low SES) whites and *51 percent* of all nonwhites (who have very low incomes as a group)" (p. 64, emphasis in the original). Youngsters beginning their lives with such problems are more likely to have difficulty later than those who do not. They may be frail, sick more often, and exhibit more neurological problems that later contribute to academic difficulties (Magrab, Sostek, & Powell, 1984).

As youngsters develop during the important early years, impoverished environments place them further at risk through malnutrition, toxic agents such as lead, and generally insufficient parental care. As with the statistics cited above, these conditions are found more often in minority family circumstances (Brooks-Gunn & Furstenberg, 1986; Field, 1980; National Center for Health Statistics, 1982). Furthermore, poverty is associated with ethnic minority status. In 1984, 33.8 percent of the Black population and 28.4 percent of the Hispanic population in the United States lived below the poverty level, compared to 11.5 percent of the White population (U.S. Bureau of the Census, 1985). The conditions of poverty often contribute to poor academic performance and special education referrals. Conditions of poverty are also often found in populations having multicultural education concerns, which contributes to the link between the two.

Migrancy Contributors

Our opening vignette about Tony suggested at least two circumstances that might contribute to his experiencing school-related difficulties: a language difference and the fact that his family moves often to follow harvest times where they can obtain employment. But migrancy may or may not be associated with

FOCUS 4
What are two ways that poverty may contribute to children from culturally different backgrounds experiencing academic difficulties and being referred to special education?

FOCUS 5
What are two ways that migrancy among culturally diverse populations is associated with academic difficulties?

TABLE 15–2 Some Characteristics of Black English

Linguistic Categories	Characteristics	Examples	
		Standard English	*Black English*
Phonological differences			
Initial position	Merging of /f/ with /th/	thigh	fie
	Merging of /v/ with /th/	Thou	vow
Medial position	Deletion of /r/	Carol	cal
	Merging of /i/ and /e/	pen	pin
	Merging of /v/ with /th/	mother	movver
	Merging of /f/ with /th/	birthday	birfday
Final position	Deletion of /r/	sore	saw
	Deletion of /l/	Saul	saw
	Simplification of consonant clusters:		
	/st/	past	pass
	/ft/	left	leff
	/nt/	went	wen
	/nd/	wind	wine
	/zd/	raised	raise*
	/md/	aimed	aim*
	/ks/	six	sick
	/ts/	it's	it*
	/lt/	salt	saught
Morphological differences			
Future	Loss of final /l/	you'll	you
Past tense	Simplification of final consonants such as:		
	/st/	passed	pass
	/nd/	loaned	loan

* These items also are morphological differences.

minority status and poverty. In a certain number of cases, neither poverty nor minority status is involved in situations where a student moves often. Frequent mobility can be found in families where there is considerable affluence, such as situations where mobility means moving from a summer home to a winter home on a schedule that suits parents rather than school schedules. Youngsters in these circumstances may also find themselves in and out of school due to extended intercontinental vacations or other trips, which the wealth of their parents permits. Likewise, children of military personnel may change schools more frequently than most youngsters, and on a schedule that is not determined by academic-year considerations. Regardless of the reason, forces that interrupt the continuity of schooling have an impact on learning, teacher and peer relationships, and general academic progress (Barresi, 1982). The migrancy or mobility of the wealthy and people subject to frequent reassignment, such as military personnel,

Linguistic Categories	Characteristics	Examples	
		Standard English	**Black English**
Plural	Deletion of final /s/ and /z/	50 cents 3 birds	50 cent 3 bird
Syntactical differences			
Auxiliary verb	Deletion of auxiliary	He is gone.	He goin.
Subject expression	Repetition of subject	John lives in NY.	John, he live in NY.
Verb form	Substitution of past participle for simple past form	I drank the milk.	I drunk the milk.
Verb agreement	Deletion of /s/ for third person singular present tense	He runs home.	He run home.
Future form	Substitution of a variation of present progressive tense	I will go home.	I'ma go home.
Negation	Use of double negative	I don't have any.	I don't got none.
Indefinite article	Deletion of /n/	I want an apple.	I want a apple.
Pronoun form	Substitution of objective for nominative case	We have to do it.	Us got to do it.
Preposition	Difference in preposition	He is over at his friend's house.	He is over to his friend house.
Copula ("be")	Use of durative *be* for *is*	He is here all the time.	He be here.

Source: From "Special Education and the Linguistically Different Child," by D. N. Bryen, *Exceptional Children, 40* (1974): 593. Copyright 1974 by The Council for Exceptional Children. Reprinted with permission.

has an impact but this is often offset by other circumstances that contribute to a child's general education. Although these children are mobile and migrant, they are not subject to the other risks of migrant youngsters from culturally different backgrounds.

In many cases, the circumstances of migrancy are associated with ethnic or cultural differences, as well as both economic disadvantage and language differences. Hunter (1982) cites figures indicating that 74.7 percent of the migrant farmworkers in H.E.W. Region X (Alaska, Oregon, Idaho, and Washington) were Hispanic and 20.2 percent were Black. While consistent data are not available for other regions of the country, migrancy is a situation that is widespread, affecting an estimated 15 percent of the American population (Barresi, 1982) and usually involving Hispanic backgrounds but also including Black, Asian, and Native American minority groups.

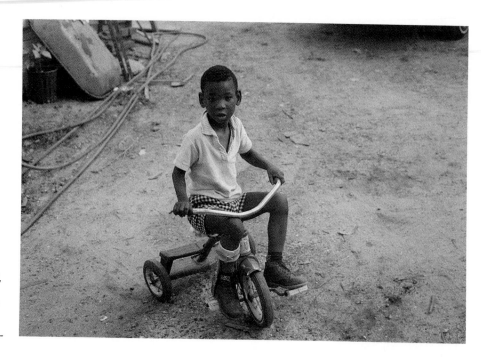

The conditions of poverty often contribute to poor academic performance and, consequently, special education referrals. (William Lupardo)

Migrancy presents a very difficult situation for a child's academic progress. As if poverty and language differences were not enough, the child may move three or four times each year (Salend, Michael, & Taylor, 1984). Such children have limited continuity and great inconsistency in their educational programming as they move about. They often have limited access to, or availability of, services because of their short-term enrollments or the schools' limited capabilities to deliver services (Frith, 1982; Hunter, 1982; Pyecha & Ward, 1982). While it is difficult to determine the singular effects of such mobility, the problem is a significant one.

Cultural-Social Mores as Contributors

FOCUS 6
What are two ways in which differing cultural-social mores may affect educational programming for youngsters having academic problems and/or handicapping conditions?

Education, as viewed from the mainstream perspective in America, predominantly reflects the philosophy of the cultural majority. This is not surprising since social institutions, in this instance formal schooling, are typically initiated and continued based on such views. However, in a situation where multiple cultures live together and those cultures reflect the broad diversity of beliefs evident in the United States, social mores in the many subcultures often emphasize different priorities. Table 15–3 illustrates some of the differences in cultural values between our dominant culture and Native American views. Activities thought to be of the utmost importance by one cultural group may be seen very differently or as less crucial by another, or may even be viewed with disdain. For example, although mental retardation is universally recognized among differing cultures, its conceptualization, social interpretation, and treatment are culturally specific (Manion

TABLE 15–3 Dominant Culture versus Native American Views

Native American	Dominant Culture
Wisdom of age and experience is respected. Elders are revered by their people.	Older people are made to feel incompetent and rejected.
Excellence is related to a contribution to the group—not to personal glory.	Competition and striving to win or to gain status is emphasized.
Cooperation is necessary for group survival.	Competition is necessary for individual status and prestige.
Children participate in adult activities.	Adults participate in children's activities.
Family life includes the extended family.	Family life includes the nuclear family.
Time is present oriented—this year, this week—NOW—a resistance to planning for the future.	Time is planning and saving for the future.
Clocktime is whenever people are ready—when everyone arrives.	Clocktime is exactly that.
Work is when necessary for the common good. Whatever Indian people have, they share. What is mine is ours.	Work is from 9–5 (specified time) and to obtain material possessions and to save for the future. What is mine, stays mine.
Good relationships and mutual respect are emphasized.	Success, progress, possession of property and rugged individualism is valued above mutual respect and maintaining good relationships.
People express their ideas and feelings through their actions.	People express themselves and attempt to impress others through speech.
People conform to nature.	People try to dominate and desecrate nature.
Early childhood and rearing practices are the responsibility of the kin group.	Early childhood and rearing practices are the responsibility of the nuclear family.
Native religion was never imposed or proselytized to other groups.	Religious groups proselytize, coerce and impose their beliefs on others.
Land gives the Indian his identity, his religion and his life. It is not to be sold, not owned, but used by all.	Land is for speculation, for prestige, to be owned, sold, or torn up.
Going to school is necessary to gain knowledge. Excelling for fame is looked down upon by the Indian.	Going to school is necessary to gain knowledge and to compete for grades.
Indians have a shorter childhood and the male is held to be a responsible person at the age of 16.	There is an extended childhood and the male is held to be a responsible person at the age of 21.
People are usually judged by what they do.	People are usually judged by their credentials.

Source: Pepper, F. C. (1976). Teaching the American Indian child in mainstream settings. In R. L. Jones (Ed.), *Mainstreaming and the minority child* (pp. 135–6). Reston, Va.: Council for Exceptional Children.

& Bersani, 1987). Table 15–4 compares some Western and non-Western cultural perspectives. Along a similar line of thinking, Collier and Hoover (1987) note that certain behaviors which might suggest a learning disability may in fact be a product of acculturation and considered normal in a child's cultural background. With these thoughts in mind, we briefly examine how social values or mores have an impact on general education, special education, and multicultural education.

Acceptance of a handicapping condition is not an easy task for any parent, and a family's attitude toward exceptionality can have a major influence on how a child's intervention proceeds. People with differing cultural backgrounds often have perspectives and beliefs regarding handicapping conditions that are different from the cultural majority—the main group that has designed, developed, and perpetuated our existing educational system. For example, Hispanic families often have great difficulty accepting handicaps such as visual impairments (Correa, 1987), and religious beliefs and superstitions tend to have a considerable impact on such acceptance (Smith, 1987). The extended-family structures common in Black and Hispanic cultures also result in differing beliefs regarding the provision of care from a larger community, as well as anxieties about adjusting to the new or alien cultural influences that may be represented by special education (Fishgrund, Cohen, & Clarkson, 1987; Turner, 1987; Yacobacci-Tam, 1987).

In addition to differences in acceptance of handicapping conditions, matters

TABLE 15–4 Some Western and Non-Western Cultural Perspectives

Polynesian Native American	Asian	Western
1. Individual valued as part of family	1. Individual valued as part of family	1. Individual held as supreme value
2. Self-control, humility	2. Self-control, humility	2. Self-expression, pride
3. Submit to family system	3. Submit to family rule	3. Negotiates within family
4. Spiritual harmony	4. Spiritual harmony	4. Spiritual duality
5. Reverence/respect for life	5. Partnership with nature	5. Master nature
6. Cooperation, mutual help	6. Cooperation, mutual help	6. Competition, self-reliance
7. Loyalty, obedience, shared responsibility	7. Obedience, duty, honor	7. Self-pride, honor, duty
8. Do what is necessary, play more	8. Hard work, little play	8. Work hard, then play

Source: Patton, J. R., Payne, J. S., Kauffman, J. M., Brown, G. B., & Payne, R. A. (1987). *Exceptional children in focus* (p. 189). Columbus, Ohio: Merrill Publishing Co.

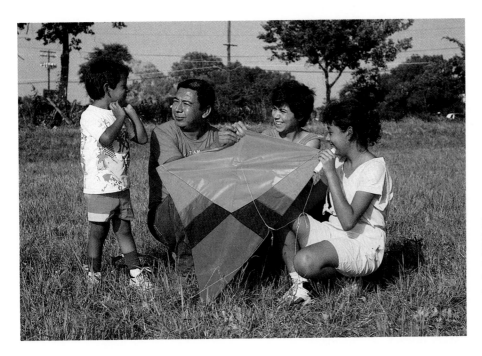

Each culture has its own perspectives and beliefs regarding handicapping conditions, which impact on how families cope with children who have special needs. (Bob Daemmrich/ Stock Boston)

pertaining to delivering service to children of culturally different families involves certain consideration. For example, the importance of manners and deference to others in traditional Hispanic families needs to be taken into account by professionals (Smith, 1987). Likewise, Asian families may be reluctant to receive assistance from outside the family, and interactions with professionals may be quite different than that of the cultural majority (Leung, 1987). Southeast Asian parents may feel great shame that their child is identified as handicapped, which influences not only acceptance but also service delivery (Morrow, 1987). And to make matters even more complex, professionals should also keep in mind that the immigration status of some families may influence the manner in which they react to education professionals attempting to obtain services for their children (Smith, 1987). Although immigration status is more of a pragmatic consideration for families than a belief difference, it certainly impacts the delivery of special education instruction in many cases.

ASSESSMENT

Assessment is a topic of central importance in all special education, and has been throughout its entire history. It is important because in special education we are usually measuring discrepancies from a standard that suggests extra or specialized intervention is necessary. Assessment of academic and behavioral deficiencies or differences represent the central bases on which we make referrals and plan instructional programs for special education.

FOCUS 7
What are two ways that assessment may contribute to the overrepresentation of culturally different youngsters in special education?

Assessment, or more correctly, assessment error, has been a major focal point of controversy and concern involving special and multicultural education. It is a problem that cannot be overlooked. Children from minority backgrounds represent a disproportionately large group in special education areas that involve labeling and placement decisions based on psychoeducational assessment, such as mental retardation (Prasse & Reschly, 1986). The major difficulty has been one of bias in the measurement instruments employed. **Measurement bias,** in this context, refers to an unfairness or inaccuracy of results that are due to cultural background, "artifacts of the test" rather than actual mental abilities or skills (Reynolds, 1987). Minority groups argue that cultural bias and prejudice are involved in both the construction/development phase and the use of assessment instruments (Roberts & DeBlassie, 1983; Slate, 1983). This has particularly been the case with standardized, norm-referenced instrumentation, where minority children's performances are often compared with norms developed from other populations. Under these conditions, minority children often appear at a disadvantage because of cultural differences (Wood, Johnson, & Jenkins, 1986). The unfairness of such assessment has been central in well-known court cases where lawsuits were filed on behalf of both Black students (*Larry P.* v. *Riles,* 1972, 1979) and Hispanic students (*Diana* v. *State Board of Education,* 1970, 1973). Although both of these cases were in the State of California, they have had an impact nationwide.

Bias in psychological assessment has been recognized as a problem for many years (Burt, 1921), and attention in the literature continues to date (Lopez, 1988; Malgady, Rogler, & Constantino, 1987; Miller-Jones, 1989). Some assessment procedures simply do not result in the same level of performance by individuals with differing backgrounds, even if they have similar abilities. For many years such circumstances were referred to as *test bias,* and considerable effort was expended in attempts to develop culture-free or culture-fair instruments (Cattell, 1940; Cattell, Feingold, & Sarason, 1941; Raven, 1938). This approach was based on the belief that the test itself was the major element contributing to bias or unfairness. Such a single-minded perspective was fundamentally flawed, although over the years improvements were made that minimized "blatantly obvious cultural effects by eliminating or decreasing the degree of culture-specific language required, as well as the cultural content contained in test items" (Luftig, 1989, p. 227). However, even these refinements are limited in their effectiveness in the absence of appropriate and conceptually sound utilization (Drew, 1973; Kaufman, 1979). More recent attention has focused on minimizing assessment bias in procedures as well as instrumentation (Reynolds & Brown, 1984), with an emphasis on the need for improved professional preparation (Elbert, 1984). Personal impressions are formed, *sometimes based on a single cue,* which trigger biased categorization, even in the face of evidence to the contrary (Skowronski & Carlston, 1989). Professionals involved in psychoeducational assessment, particularly with ethnic minority children, must be properly trained to minimize the formation of such impressions which may bias their procedures. Additionally, assessment professionals must be constantly alert to potential bias due to language differences as well as other contributing factors, which may mask abilities and be reflected in evaluation results. In many cases, interviews with parents, guardians, or others who are involved in a child's home life can provide valuable insight that is helpful in both assessment administration and interpretation of results. Figure 15–1 summarizes illustrative guidelines and topics for such interviews.

Assessment is one of several important tools in education, a particularly important one in both special and multicultural education. For assessment to be a properly functioning part of the process, and not a source of concern, it needs to be correctly constructed and used. Furthermore, the purposes of the assessment must be considered from the outset for an instrument or procedure to be correctly designed and used. Are we attempting to bring the bulk of our citizenry to a similar point in education or knowledge? In so doing, are we thereby creating a leveling effect, attempting to make us all look alike to some degree? Or are we promoting individual growth and development and encouraging cultural diversity and individual differences?

We are probably both leveling and promoting differences to some degree. We must, however, be very clear in our thinking about what we are undertaking regarding both assessment and education. The whole notion of individualized

---

After talking with community members about the general cultural characteristics of the community, it is still necessary to discover what experiences each child has had. The following set of questions can be used to find out about the direct cultural and environmental experiences of the child so that appropriate educational programs can be planned.

1. What language(s) do the parents speak to each other?
2. What language(s) do the parents speak to the child?
3. What language(s) do the children use with each other?
4. What language does the referred child prefer to use when playing with friends?
5. Who takes care of the child after school? What language is used?
6. Who lives in the home (parents, grandparents, etc.)?
7. How much time does each parent have to interact with the child?
8. With whom does the child play when at home?
9. What television programs are seen in each language?
10. Are stories read to the child? In what language is the reading material written?
11. What language is used in church services, if attended?
12. What does the child do after school and on weekends?
13. What responsibilities does the child have in the home?
14. How is the child expected to act toward parents, teachers, and other adults?
15. In what cultural activities does the family participate?
16. How do the parents expect adults to act toward the child?
17. Are there any specific prohibitions in the everyday interactions between adults and children, for example, do not look adults in the eye when talking to them, do not pat children on the top of the head, do not ask children questions?
18. How long has the family been in this country?
19. How long has the family been in the local community?
20. How much contact does the family have with the homeland? What kind of contact?

Figure 15–1
Guidelines for Interviewing Parents about Cultural and Environmental Influences (*Source:* Reprinted with permission from Mattes, L. J., & Omark, D. R. (1984). *Speech and Language Assessment for the Bilingual Handicapped.* Boston: College-Hill Press, Appendix A, pp.111–112.

instruction in special education runs somewhat counter to basic pedagogy as practiced in the United States, where we educate everyone. The pressure of surviving in today's educational system often leads us to continue implementing our effort in a manner that is not in line with current thinking or knowledge. Such circumstances were clearly evident to one of the authors when he encountered the use of what was claimed to be a culture-fair test with minority students—without consideration for how it was administered—during the 1988 school year. Perhaps even more alarming, this assessment was conducted in a bilingual program and under the direction of a trained school psychologist who is a member of an ethnic minority.

It is essential that we achieve clear conceptual knowledge of what we are doing and not claim to do one thing while actually accomplishing another. Such circumstances lead to (and certainly have in multicultural education) a feeling that those in the larger educational system are less than truthful about what is intended and what is done. This in turn creates a situation of mistrust that inhibits the communication and cooperative efforts so essential to successful service delivery.

PREVALENCE

FOCUS 8
What are the population status and trends among culturally diverse groups in the United States and how do these impact our educational system?

The issue of prevalence in this chapter is even more difficult to nail down than in the earlier chapters addressing the traditional areas of exceptionality. Prevalence figures obviously differ depending on whether one is speaking only of the linguistically different or those served by multicultural special education through poverty programs. As emphasized earlier, counting the occurrences of a phenomenon depends greatly on the definition of that phenomenon.

However, we can describe what we know to be the case even if actual prevalence figures are elusive. A very high percentage—perhaps as high as 41 percent—of all special education students are from culturally divergent backgrounds (Bedell, 1989). This is true in general education but even more so in special education (Salend, Michael, & Taylor, 1984; Willig & Greenberg, 1986). Many minority youngsters in special education drop out of school: Recent figures indicate that 36 percent of those dropping out of school are Black and 44 percent are Hispanic (U.S. Department of Education, 1989).

Several populations from culturally or ethnically diverse backgrounds are growing rapidly, due to both birth rates and immigration levels. An example is Black Americans, who represented approximately 11.5 percent of the total population in the United States in 1980 (McDavis, 1980) and are increasing at a rate twice that of the Caucasian population (Schildroth, 1986). Hispanic-Americans also represent a large and rapidly growing group in special education. Growth in these groups will continue to place an increased load on the educational systems as diverse needs for appropriate services are addressed.

From purely a language standpoint, Baca and Certantes (1984) indicate that there were approximately 5 million children of school age that spoke languages other than English in 1976. This represented 10 percent of the school-age population in the United States at that time. Immigration levels since the Vietnam conflict suggest that the Vietnamese constitute a continually growing population. The general non–English-speaking population has a projected growth of 24 percent from 1976 to 1990, and 43 percent (to 40 million people) by the year 2000 (Baca & Cervantes, 1984). If the ratio of school-age children remains stable relative to the general population, this would result in approximately 7.2 million youngsters between the ages of six and eighteen who are language minorities in the year 2000. This places an obvious demand and need for linguistically appropriate instruction on the school systems in the United States; it also emphasizes the increasing need for vigilance and caution in assessment.

The figures above represent mainly the number of students who are either bilingual or linguistically different. Certainly, a portion of these youngsters come from backgrounds that permit them to achieve academically in a school system that is based primarily on the English language. However, the National Foundation for the Improvement of Education estimates that approximately 3.5 million children in the United States could benefit from bilingual programs (NFIE, 1982). While this estimate is certainly not as high as the 1976 5-million prevalence figure, it suggests a considerable need for appropriate bilingual services. With this level of need, magnified considerably when one considers other multicultural factors, it is clear why a careful examination of educational purpose(s) must accompany services provided, particularly when striving for appropriate educational service.

Fiscal resources have become increasingly strained during the past few years. Every special educator is sensitive to the fact that special programs are often viewed as luxuries when funding is limited. Both multicultural and special education must find negotiable positions of compromise with such a heavy load on the general educational system, or place themselves in jeopardy of being unable to serve the populations that need them.

INTERVENTION

FOCUS 9
What are three general factors necessary to achieve appropriate multicultural special education?

Addressing intervention in this chapter once again deviates from the approach in earlier chapters because intervention here is not the same as treatment. We are not discussing a type or even a limited constellation of learning difficulties. We are addressing, in some measure, the social fabric of many different cultures and the manner in which that impacts on educating exceptional children.

Some authors suggest that *appropriate* instruction is the pivotal concept in multicultural special education, and that considerations beyond this are of lesser importance. Hilliard notes that, "It should be clear that cultural diversity requires no unusual special education" (1980, p. 587). Similarly, Heward and Orlansky state that "effective instructional procedures apply to children of all cultural backgrounds" (1988, p. 469). These are fundamentally sound statements when based on the premise of instructional appropriateness. What are problematic are some of the steps, approaches, and process elements necessary to achieve appropriateness. Some of these important components require changes in both how service delivery is implemented and how professionals undertaking the task are trained.

Appropriate education for culturally diverse populations must emanate from purpose(s) that are moving toward common goals on a systemwide basis. A careful examination of educational purposes, by those driving the general system and those involved in multicultural and special education, must be undertaken. Where there are important gaps in effort, there may have to be additional plans laid to prevent segments of the clientele from "slipping through the cracks." Where there are goals or objectives that seem at variance or perhaps adversarial among the three interests, negotiation, compromise, or possibly only greater mutual understanding must be reached. At any rate, divergence in purpose, particularly when it may detract from service, needs to be reconciled or minimized to enhance the potency of joint efforts. This should not be interpreted as a call for only single goals; that is not our intent. But it is most important to have purposes in the form of guiding principles that are working toward common ends.

Beyond the broad-system level, youngsters who enter special education for extra instructional help do so on the basis of assessment of some type, a topic examined earlier. For students of culturally diverse backgrounds it is vital that assessment be undertaken in an appropriate manner. Here it is essential that evaluation of performance or ability is a primary focus, with attempts made *not* to unfairly represent these because of race or cultural heritage.

Assessment is (or should be) part of instruction, in both the general education system and specialized service areas. Students are referred for initial evaluations based on judgments made by their teachers, which occur before they ever reach the school psychologist. As teachers make these referrals they need to be alert to some of the reasons why their students are not performing at the desired level, whether that level is based on a classwide average or some normative data. Youngsters from culturally different backgrounds do not always act in the same way or perform in a similar fashion as their peers from the cultural majority. Since part of this may be due to differences in perspectives about life, academics, and interpersonal interaction that flow from their native culture (Patton, Payne, Kauffman, Brown, & Payne, 1987; Pepper, 1976), awareness and vigilence on the part of the regular-class teacher regarding these issues may change the manner in which classroom performance is evaluated. It may either change the nature of a referral for testing, or even eliminate it in favor of some other options that might be undertaken without moving the youngster from the classroom. If this occurs, then the first step in assessment has been altered.

Assessment after a referral has occurred must also be considered as an area where particular care is necessary with culturally diverse youngsters. Initially, evaluation needs to be undertaken with a clear idea of what its purpose is and how it fits with educational goals and objectives. Without such consideration, assessment represents testing for the sake of testing, which is not defensible (Drew, Logan, & Hardman, 1988). Additionally, the selection of an assessment instrument by the person administering it (e.g., a school psychologist) should involve care with respect to avoidance of culturally biased construction and development. In some cases efforts to eliminate or minimize cultural unfairness due to language differences and specific knowledge biases have already been accomplished. Assessment personnel should use such instrumentation. Furthermore, the manner in which assessment is undertaken should be unbiased, and individuals administering evaluations should guard against formation of biased judgments. Lastly, as part of interpreting results, the assessment specialist should incorporate as much other information as possible regarding family status, cultural background, and other relevant factors (Mattes & Omark, 1984). The assessment process must include attention to cultural perspectives that may influence both formal test responses and interactions and reactions of the youngster to the evaluation itself.

We now turn to appropriate instructional intervention. If a youngster from a culturally different background is appropriately placed in special education, the personnel involved must be familiar with a great deal of information about him or her. Cultural background can greatly influence how the family reacts to their child receiving special assistance (Correa, 1987; Manion & Bersani, 1987; Smith, 1987). This is likely to have an impact on the child's perception and may influence the success of the program considerably. If a language difference exists, care must be taken to provide instruction that takes that into account.

We have only taken a brief glimpse at intervention because what must be taken into account, if education is to be truly appropriate, are all the contributing factors discussed earlier in the chapter—language, migrancy, and cultural mores. Each has an impact on a youngster as he or she interacts with the educational system, and that influence must receive attention in the educational process. What has not yet been mentioned is the heart of how this is accomplished— through people, those who are the professionals in the system delivering the service. The success or limitation of a multicultural special education effort probably hinges more on the people involved than on any other single factor. This is easily stated, but it is the most difficult to address. Teachers and other professionals interacting with culturally diverse students and their parents must be aware of the broad dimensions of cultural perspectives. They must also be knowledgeable about details and nuances that are not evident on the surface

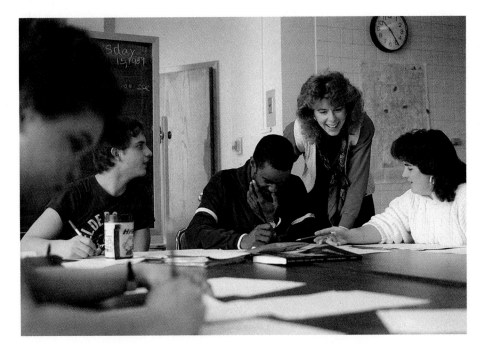

The success of multicultural special education probably depends more on the teacher than on any other single factor. (Michael McGovern/The Picture Cube)

but have a substantial influence on their pupils' actions and performance. Professionals must employ this knowledge with a clear understanding of their own cultural background and how that influences the interpersonal exchanges they encounter. They must know about language differences and, in some cases, be fluent in languages other than English when the circumstances so dictate. What are required of professionals in multicultural special education are more than competencies, but they all lead to competence.

The system, process, and personnel all require attention for an appropriate multicultural special education program to be delivered. All three aspects have implications for professional preparation, which means that there is a need for greater awareness and sensitivity by higher education institutions that prepare administrators, psychologists, and teachers for work of this kind. Progress has occurred over the past twenty years, but there remains much to be accomplished.

REVIEW

FOCUS 1: What are two ways the purposes of general education differ from special education and multicultural education?

- ☐ A major purpose of general education is to provide education for everyone and to bring all students to a similar level of performance.
- ☐ Special education focuses on individual differences and often evaluates performance on an individually set or prescribed performance level.
- ☐ Multicultural education promotes cultural pluralism and therefore differences.

FOCUS 2: What are three conceptual factors that have contributed to heightened attention and concern regarding the placement of minority youngsters in special education?

- ☐ There is a stigma attached to special education.
- ☐ Special education placement for cultural minority children may not be educationally effective in meeting their academic problems.
- ☐ A self-fulfilling prophecy may be operative, resulting in youngsters' becoming what they are labeled.

FOCUS 3: What are two ways in which language may link multicultural and special education?

- ☐ Non–English-speaking youngsters may be seen as having speech or language disorders and be referred to special education.
- ☐ Youngsters' language may be nonstandard, in the sense that it does not conform to the style of the cultural majority, which may result in a special education referral.
- ☐ A child's academic or psychological assessment may be an inaccurate portrayal of ability due to his or her language differences.

FOCUS 4: What are two ways that poverty may contribute

to children from culturally different backgrounds experiencing academic difficulties and being referred to special education?

- ☐ Circumstances resulting in disadvantaged prenatal development and birth complications occur much more frequently among those of low-SES status and nonwhite populations.
- ☐ Environmental circumstances, such as malnutrition and toxic agents, placing youngsters at risk are found most frequently in impoverished households, and poverty is most frequently evident among ethnic minority populations.

FOCUS 5: What are two ways that migrancy among culturally diverse populations may contribute to academic difficulties?

- ☐ In many cases, migrancy is found among circumstances of economic disadvantage and language differences.
- ☐ Children in migrant households may move and change educational placements several times a year, contributing to limited continuity and inconsistent educational programming.

FOCUS 6: What are two ways in which differing cultural-social mores may affect educational programming for youngsters having academic problems and/or handicapping conditions?

- ☐ Certain behaviors that may suggest a handicapping condition needing special education assistance are viewed as normal in some cultural environments.
- ☐ People from some cultural backgrounds view special assistance from educational institutions with disdain or shame and are reluctant to accept assistance from sources outside the family unit.

FOCUS 7: What are two ways that assessment has potentially contributed to overrepresentation of culturally different youngsters in special education?

☐ Through assessment instruments that are designed and constructed with specific language and content favoring the cultural majority.

☐ Through assessment procedures, and perhaps personnel, that are negatively biased, either implicitly or explicitly, toward culturally different youngsters.

FOCUS 8: What are the population status and trends among culturally diverse groups in the United States and how do these impact our educational system?

☐ Ethnically and culturally diverse groups, such as Hispanic Americans, Black Americans, and others, represent substantial proportions of the United States population; some individual groups over 11 percent and collectively much higher.

☐ Population growth in ethnically and culturally different groups is increasing at a phenomenal rate; in some cases, twice that of the Caucasian group. Both immigration and birth rate contribute to this growth.

☐ Culturally diverse populations not currently receiving appropriate education plus the significant growth rates are placing increased demands for services on the educational system.

FOCUS 9: What are three general factors necessary to achieve appropriate multicultural special education?

☐ A systemwide examination of purposes must be undertaken to minimize adversarial perspectives and maximize efforts toward effective collaboration.

☐ Referral and assessment must include attention to cultural differences and avoidance of biased instrumentation and processes.

☐ Instructional programming is effective only to the degree that professional personnel are competent and knowledgeable about the many dimensions of cultural diversity.

Debate Forum

Bilingual Education—Yes or No?

Students from culturally diverse backgrounds represent a very large portion of the school enrollment population in the United States. This places a considerable burden on the educational system's ability to provide specialized educational services to meet students' needs. Choose a position and defend it.

Point Children from different cultures are going to be required to survive in the world of the cultural majority. They should be taught in English and taught the knowledge base of the cultural majority for their own good. It will better prepare them for success and more efficiently utilize the limited funds available, since specialized culturally sensitive services will not be required.

Counterpoint Children from cultures different from the majority must have an equal advantage to learn in the most effective manner possible. This often means teaching them in their native language, at least for some of the time. To do otherwise is a waste of talent, which can ultimately affect the overall progress of our country and is also a means of discrimination on the part of the cultural majority.

Glossary

AAMR Adaptive Behavior Scale. A scale developed by the American Association on Mental Retardation to assess the ability of a person to interact appropriately with his or her environment.

Aberration. Deviation from what is common or normal.

ABIC. The Adaptive Behavior Inventory for Children, a part of SOMPA.

Abnormal behavior. A general term referring to behavior that is unusual to the degree that it exceeds the boundaries of what society views as normal.

Academic achievement. Refers to the level of proficiency in academic subjects such as math and reading.

Acceleration. A process whereby students are allowed to achieve at a rate that is consonant with their capacity, faster than average students.

Achievement discrepancy. A difference between a child's performance and his or her measured potential. The term is used in learning disabilities and generally refers to academic performance lower than expected.

Acoustic aids. Any means of assisting a person to hear.

Activity group therapy. A group-oriented approach used for treatment of youngsters with behavior disorders.

Acute lymphocytic leukemia (ALL). A disorder of blood-cell production in which abnormal white blood cells accumulate in the blood and bone marrow.

Adaptive behavior. A parameter of classification that refers to one's ability to be socially appropriate and personally responsible.

Adaptive fit. Compatibility between demands of a task or setting and a person's needs and abilities.

Adaptive Learning Environments Program (ALEM). A program for students with learning and behavior disorders that is based on the concept of adaptive fitting. See **Adaptive fit.**

Adaptive physical education. Physical education that has been modified (adapted) to meet the needs and disabilities of exceptional youngsters.

Adult service agencies. Agencies whose major focus is on providing the necessary services to assist individuals with disabilities to become more independent.

Akinetic seizure. A seizure that is evidenced by an absence or poverty of repetitive or clonic movements.

Amblyopia. Loss of vision due to an imbalance of eye muscles.

Amendments to the Education of the Handicapped Act, 1986. Public Law 99–457, which extended the authority of P.L. 94–142 to ages three through five and established an early-intervention program for infants and toddlers ages birth through two.

American Association on Mental Retardation (AAMR). An organization of professionals from many disciplines involved in the study and treatment of mental retardation. Previously this organization was named the American Association on Mental Deficiency (AAMD).

American Sign Language. A type of sign language commonly used by people with hearing disorders.

Ameslan. The nickname for American Sign Language.

Amniocentesis. A prenatal assessment of a fetus which involves analysis of amniotic fluid.

Amputations. The absence of a limb, either congenitally or acquired after birth.

Anemia. A condition in which the blood is deficient in red blood cells.

Anencephaly. A condition in which the person has a partial or complete absence of cerebral tissue.

Anopthalmos. An absence of the eyeball.

Anorexia nervosa. A condition of self-inflicted starvation, most often found in adolescent females, wherein body weight is at least 15 percent below that which is expected.

Anoxia. A lack of oxygen.

Antibodies. Proteins formed in the bloodstream to fight infection.

Anticonvulsants. Medication prescribed to control convulsions.

Antigens. Any of a class of biochemical substances that stimulate the production of antibodies.

Antiretroviral agents. An agent that inhibits the activity of a retrovirus, which is a particular virus characterized by a reversing of the transfer of genetic code information from one type to another.

Anti-Rh gamma globulin. A medication used to combat incompatibility in blood type between a mother and her fetus (RhoGAM).

Anxiety disorders. A condition that is characterized by excessive fears or anxiety about persons, places, or events.

Anxiety-withdrawal. A category of behavior disorder involving overanxiety, social withdrawal, seclusiveness, shyness, sensitivity, and other behaviors implying a retreat from the environment.

Apgar scoring. An evaluation of a newborn that assesses heart rate, respiratory condition, muscle tone, reflexes, and color.

Aphasia. An acquired language disorder, caused by brain damage, that is characterized by complete or partial impairment of language comprehension, formulation, and use.

Aqueous humor. A fluid that lies between the lens and cornea of the eye.

Arteriographic examination. A visual examination of an artery or arteries, after injection of dyes and other matter, that can be seen by x-rays.

Arthritis. A disease involving inflammation of the joints due to infections, metabolic, or constitutional (genetic) causes.

Articulation disabilities. Speech problems such as omissions, substitutions, additions, and distortions.

Articulation disorder. An abnormality in the speech-sound production process resulting in inaccurate or otherwise inappropriate execution of speaking.

Asphyxia. An impaired or absent exchange of oxygen and carbon dioxide.

Asthma. A condition, often of allergic origin, characterized by continuous labored breathing accompanied by wheezing, a sense of constriction in the chest, and attacks of coughing and gasping.

Astigmatism. A refractive problem that occurs when the surface of the cornea is uneven or structurally defective, preventing the light rays from converging at one point.

Ataxia. A condition wherein the individual experiences extreme difficulties in controlling fine and gross motor movements.

Athetosis. A condition characterized by constant, contorted twisting motions in the wrists and fingers.

Atonia. A condition evidenced by lack of muscle tone.

Atresia. The absence of a normal opening.

Atropinization. A treatment for cataracts that involves washing the eye with atropine, which permanently dilates the pupil.

Attention deficit disorder (ADD). See **Attention-deficit hyperactivity disorder (ADHD).**

Attention-deficit hyperactivity disorder (ADHD). A diagnostic label used by the American Psychiatric Association to signify a condition in which a child exhibits signs of developmentally inappropriate hyperactivity, impulsivity, and inattention.

Audiogram. A record obtained from an audiometer, which graphs an individual's threshold of hearing at various sound frequencies.

Audiologist. A specialist in the assessment of a person's hearing ability.

Audiometer. An electronic device used to detect a person's response to sound stimuli.

Audition. The act or sense of hearing.

Auditory association. The ability to associate verbally presented ideas or information.

Auditory blending. The act of blending the parts of a word into an integrated whole when speaking.

Auditory cortex. That portion of the brain that is associated with hearing.

Auditory discrimination. The act of distinguishing between different sounds.

Auditory global method. A general term describing an approach to teaching deaf people communication where the main channel for speech and language development is auditory (although not always exclusive) and fluent; connected speech is the means of input.

Auditory memory. The ability to recall verbally presented material.

Auditory-oral. An approach to teaching deaf people communication skills that includes a combination of the oral and auditory methods, also termed *aural-oral*.

Aura. A subjective sensation experienced by some individuals before the onset of a grand mal seizure.

Aural-oral. An approach to teaching deaf people communication skills that includes a combination of the oral and auditory methods, also termed *auditory-oral*.

Autism. A severe behavior disorder, with onset in early childhood, that is characterized by extreme withdrawal and self-stimulation.

Autosomal recessive trait. A characteristic that originates from a chromosome other than the sex chromosome. To be seen or expressed, such a trait would require the combining of two recessive genes; if paired with a dominant gene, the recessive trait would not appear. (For example, blue eyes result from the two recessive genes, but brown eyes may

occur from one dominant (brown) and one recessive (blue) or two dominant genes.)

Bacterial meningitis. An inflammation of the membranes in the brain or spinal cord caused by bacterial infection.

Barrier-free facility. A building or other structure that is designed and constructed so that people with mobility disabilities (such as those in wheelchairs) can move freely throughout and access all areas without encountering architectural obstructions.

Basic-skills approach. Pertaining to instruction that lays the groundwork for further development and higher levels of functioning.

Behavior disordered. A term applied to people who cannot care for themselves, are unable to function in society, and/or are a threat to themselves or others because of behavioral excesses or deficits.

Behavior checklists. Objective protocols that permit an observer to count or check for the existence or absence of a given behavior or set of behaviors through direct observation of the individual being evaluated.

Behavioral contract. An agreement, written or verbal, between two people stating that if one behaves in a certain manner (such as completing a homework assignment), the other (teacher, parent, etc.) will give him or her a specific reward.

Behavioral manifestations. A parameter of classification that focuses on a description of behavior.

Behavior shaping. A general term referring to the process of changing a person's behavior, often developing new behaviors that have not yet been evident, using one of the several procedures involved in behavior therapy.

Binet-Simon Scales. An individual test of intelligence developed by Alfred Binet and Theodore Simon in 1905 in France. Later translated into English (1908), and revised and standardized by Lewis Terman. See also **Stanford-Binet Intelligence Scale.**

Biographical inventory. An individual history of a person that includes information about a wide range of activities and achievements of the individual being studied.

Blind. According to the American Medical Association, a term to describe a person whose central visual acuity does not exceed 20/200 in the better eye with correcting lenses, or whose visual acuity, if better than 20/200, has a limit in the central field of vision.

Braille. A system of writing used by many people who are blind, involving combinations of six raised dots punched into paper, which can be read with the fingertips.

Breech presentation. A situation in which the fetus is positioned with buttocks toward the cervix at delivery.

Bulimia nervosa. An eating disorder in which there are frequent episodes of uncontrolled binge eating followed by self-induced vomiting or other extreme measures to prevent weight gain.

Bupthalmos. An abnormal distention and enlargement of the eyeball.

Burn-out. A concept that describes professionals (or others) who become exhausted on a long-term basis because of physical, emotional, and other demands that exceed their tolerance.

Cardiac disorders. Diseases of the heart that affect its functioning and output.

Case management. The planning, implementation, and monitoring of a person's program from diagnosis through treatment.

Cataract. A clouding of the eye lens, which becomes opaque, resulting in visual problems.

Categorical descriptors. Labels that divide disabilities into the traditional categories of mental retardation, behavior disorders, and learning disabilities.

CAT scan. An x-ray of the brain taken to determine the presence of a structural abnormality such as a tumor. CAT is an abbreviation for Computerized Axial Tomography.

Ceiling effects. A restricted range of test questions or problems that does not permit students to demonstrate their true capacity of achievement.

Central nervous system disorders. Diseases and/or conditions that affect the brain and/or spinal cord.

Cerebral palsy. A neurological disorder characterized by motor problems, general physical weakness, lack of coordination, and perceptual difficulties.

Chest physiotherapy. Physical therapy applied to the chest.

Child abuse. Inflicted, nonaccidental, sexual, physical, and/or psychological trauma and/or injury to a child.

Child neglect. A lack of interaction with a child on the part of other family members, which deprives that youngster of vital opportunities for development.

Choroid. A vascular membrane in the eye containing pigment cells, which lies between the retina and sclera.

Choroidoretinal degeneration. Deterioration of the choroid and retina of the eye.

Chromosomes. Threadlike material that carry the genes and therefore play a central role in inherited characteristics.

Chromosomal abnormalities. Defects or damage in the chromosomes of an individual.

Cleft palate. A gap in the soft palate and roof of the mouth, sometimes extending through the upper lip.

Closed-caption. A process by which people with hearing disorders are provided translated dialogue from television programs in the form of subtitles. Also called the line-21 system, since the caption is inserted into blank line 21 of the picture.

Cluttering. A speech disorder characterized by excessively rapid, disorganized speaking, often including words or phrases unrelated to the topic.

Cochlea. A structure in the inner ear that converts sound coming from the middle ear into electrical signals that are transmitted to the brain.

Cochlear implant. A surgical implanting of electronic prosthetic components, which provide stimulation of the auditory nerve and restore hearing.

Cognition. The act of thinking, knowing, or processing information.

Cognitive functioning. Refers to the level of proficiency in thinking, processing information, and knowledge.

Communication. The process of transmitting or receiving messages and their meaning.

Community mental health centers. Local agencies that provide mental health assistance to a given community or surrounding area.

Computer-assisted instruction. The use of computers to provide instruction, rehearsal, and testing.

Conditioning. The process in which new objects or situations elicit responses that were previously elicited by other stimuli.

Conduct disorder. A condition characterized by overt physical aggression, disruptiveness, negativism, irresponsibility, and defiance of authority.

Conductive hearing loss. A hearing loss resulting from poor conduction of sound along the passages leading to the sense organ.

Congenital. A condition existing at birth.

Congenital aural atresia. A condition where the external auditory canal is either malformed or absent at birth.

Congenital heart diseases. Conditions that ensue for inborn anomalies in heart structure or functioning.

Congenital rubella. German measles contracted by a mother during pregnancy, which causes a variety of problems, including mental retardation, deafness, blindness, and other neurological problems.

Congenital syphilis. Syphilis transmitted from a pregnant mother to her unborn child, which may cause spontaneous abortion, stillbirth, or other problems in the child.

Congestive heart failure. Heart failure or improper functioning because of an unnatural accumulation of fluids around the organ.

Consultive services. Assistance provided by specialists to improve the quality of education or other intervention for a person with a disability.

Consulting teacher. Teachers who support regular classroom teachers and their students, through specialized training and assistance in modifying the regular education curriculum and environment to accommodate exceptional students.

Contingency contracting. A procedure in which treatment or education personnel write specific agreements with students or clients that specify the amount and kind of behavior necessary to obtain a reward.

Cornea. The external covering of the eye.

Corti's organ. A structure in the cochlea; highly specialized cells that translate vibration into nerve impulses that are sent to the brain.

Criterion-referenced assessment. Referring to assessment that compares a person's performance to some specific established level (the criterion); his or her performance is not compared with that of other people.

Crosscategorical definitions. An approach to grouping individuals with learning and behavior disorders on the basis of the severity of the problem rather than traditional categorical labels.

Cued speech. A communication method used by people with hearing disorders, which combines hand signals with speech-reading. Gestures provide additional information regarding sounds not identifiable by lip reading.

Cultural-familial. A term applied to people with mental retardation whose condition may be attributable to both sociocultural and genetic factors.

Cultural labeling approach. An approach to labeling that defines normalcy relative to standards established by a particular social structure.

Cultural pluralism. A view of multiple cultural subgroups living together in a manner that maintains subsocietal differences, thereby continuing each group's cultural or ethnic traditions.

Curriculum specialist. A professional who provides consultive support services to classroom teachers in the areas of curriculum design and implementation strategies.

Custodial. A level of mental retardation, based on educability expectation, which involves measured intelligence below 40. Often unable to achieve sufficient skills even to care for basic needs and usually require significant care and supervision during the person's lifetime.

Cystic fibrosis. A hereditary disease that usually appears during early childhood. It involves a generalized disorder of exocrine glands and is evidenced by respiratory problems and excessive loss of salt in perspiration.

Cytomegalic inclusion. A condition in newborns due to infection by cytomegalovirus (CMV).

Deaf. A term used to categorize individuals who have hearing losses greater than 75 to 80 dB, have vision as their primary input, and cannot understand speech through the ear.

Deaf-blindness. A disorder involving simultaneous vision and hearing deficiencies.

Decibel (dB). A unit used to measure sound intensity.

Delayed speech. A deficit in speaking proficiency where the individual performs like someone much younger.

Denasality. A voice resonance problem that occurs when too little air passes through the nasal cavity.

Developmental aphasia. A language disorder in children, caused by brain damage, that is characterized by complete or partial impairment of language comprehension, formulation, and use.

Developmental labeling approach. An approach to labeling that is based on deviations in the course of development from what is considered normal.

Developmental period. Specifically, as stated in the AAMR definition of mental retardation, the period of time between birth and the eighteenth birthday.

Deviant. A term used to describe the behavior of individuals who are unable to adapt to social roles or to establish appropriate interpersonal relationships.

Diabetes mellitus. A familial constitutional disease characterized by inadequate utilization of insulin, resulting in disordered metabolism of carbohydrates, fats, and proteins.

Differentiated education. Instruction and learning activities that are uniquely and predominantly suited to the capacities and interests of gifted students.

Disability. More specific than a disorder. Results from a loss of physical functioning or difficulties in learning and social adjustment that significantly interfere with normal growth and development.

Disabled. One who has a disability. See also **Disability**.

Disorder. A disturbance in normal functioning (mental, physical, or psychological).

Disordered. One who has a disorder. See also **Disorder**.

Disorders associated with immaturity and inadequacy. Behavioral disorders in which an individual may be exceptionally clumsy, socially inadequate, or easily flustered.

Diplegia. Paralysis that affects the legs more than the arms.

Double hemiplegia. Paralysis that involves both sides of the body, with one side being more greatly affected.

Down syndrome. Sometimes called mongolism. A condition resulting from a chromosomal abnormality that results in varying degrees of mental retardation.

Due process. A legal term referring to the regular administration of the law wherein no person may be denied his or her legal rights.

Dyadic relationship. A relationship between two people; a two-part relationship.

Dyslexia. A severe impairment of the ability to read.

Eating disorders. Conditions that include abnormal fears regarding eating; significant weight loss from either not eating or regurgitating food; disturbed body image; binge eating; and eating nonnutritive substances.

Echolalia. A meaningless repetition or imitation of words that are heard.

Educable. A level of mental retardation, based on educability expectation, which involves measured intelligence of 55 to about 70, with academic achievement at the second- to fifth-grade level. Social adjustment often permits some degree of independence in the community and occupational sufficiency permits partial or total self-support.

Educability expectation. A parameter of classification that represents a prediction of expected educational achievement.

Educational blindness. Refers to whether a student must use Braille when reading.

Education of All Handicapped Children Act. Public Law 94–142, federal legislation passed in 1975, which makes available a free and appropriate public education for all handicapped children in the United States.

EEG. See **Electroencephalogram**.

Ego. A term based on psychoanalytic theory that refers to the reality component of one's subconscious.

Elective mutism. A disorder of childhood where the youngster has speaking abilities but chooses not to use them; a persistent refusal to talk.

Electroacoustic aids. A general term referring to electronic devices that assist a person to hear.

Electroencephalogram (EEG). A record of brain wave patterns made with an instrument known as an electroencephalograph.

Emotionally disturbed. See **Behavior disordered**.

Emphysema. A condition where the lungs are unable to perform properly, causing shortness of breath.

Encephalitis. An inflammation of brain tissue.

Encopresis. Lack of bowel control.

Enrichment. Educational experiences for gifted students that enhance their thinking skills and extend their knowledge in various areas.

Enuresis. Lack of bladder control.

Environmental bias. A subjective point of view based on the environment (culture and social structure).

Epilepsy. A syndrome characterized by differing types of recurrent seizures.

Epileptic. One who has epilepsy.

Epiphora. An overflow of tears from obstruction of the lacrimal ducts of the eye.

Ethnocentrism. The belief that one's own group or culture is superior.

Etiology. The cause(s) of a condition. Also used as a parameter of classification.

Eugenics. The science of improving offspring through careful selection of parents.

Eustachian tube. A structure that extends from the throat to the middle-ear cavity and controls air flow between the two.

Exceptional. Refers to any individual whose physical, mental, or behavioral performance deviates so substantially (higher or lower) from the average that additional services are necessary to meet the individual's needs.

Exchange transfusion. Replacing blood with that which is fresh and has normal characteristics.

Expressive language disorders. Difficulties in language production.

Extended family. Close relatives of a family who visit or interact with the family on a regular basis.

Federal mandate. An order by the federal government.

Feebleminded. A term appearing in the early literature on mental retardation that is now outdated; roughly meaning "of weak mind."

Fenestration. Refers to the surgical creation of a new opening in the labyrinth of the ear to restore hearing.

Fetal alcohol syndrome. Damage caused to the fetus by maternal consumption of alcohol.

Fetoscopy. A procedure for examining the unborn baby using a needlelike camera, which is inserted into the womb to videoscan the fetus for visible abnormalities.

Field of vision. Refers to the breadth or degree of angle that a person can see without turning his or her head or moving the eyes; includes the limits of peripheral sight or that which lies to the sides of straight ahead.

Figure–ground discrimination. The process of distinguishing an object from its background.

Fine motor development. Development of precise and delicate abilities such as reaching, grasping, and the manipulation of small objects.

Finger spelling. A sign system of communication that incorporates all letters of the alphabet, signed independently on one hand, to form words.

Finger stick. Drawing blood from one's finger with one of several spring-loaded devices available for home use by diabetics.

Fluency disabilities. Speech problems such as repetitions, prolongation of sound, hesitations, and impediments in speech flow.

Fluency disorder. A type of speech disorder where the natural flow and rhythm of speaking is excessively interrupted, often by frequent pauses, prolongation of sounds, repetitions, or unrelated sounds.

Focal motor seizure. A seizure emanating from a particular area of the brain that governs or controls various motor functions.

Focal seizures. Seizures that affect specific motor, sensory, and psychomotor functions.

Fraternal twins. Twins that develop from two fertilized eggs and develop in two placentas. Many times such twins do not resemble one another closely.

Free and appropriate public education (FAPE). One of the basic intents of Public Law 94–142, to ensure a free and appropriate education be made available to all handicapped children.

Functional academic curriculum. Curriculum that teaches academic material (reading, math, etc.) with content that is the most commonly relevant and necessary for a person's daily living.

Functional age. An individual's level of ability to perform various tasks relative to the average age of others who can perform the same tasks.

Functional articulation disorders. Refers to articulation problems that are not due to structural defects or neurological problems, but are more likely the result of environmental or psychological influences.

Functional life/compensatory curriculum. An instructional approach that teaches only those practical skills that facilitate a student's accommodation to society; for example, self-care, social skills, and occupational/vocational skills. See also **Functional academic curriculum.**

Galactosemia. A metabolic disorder where an infant has difficulty processing lactose. May cause mental retardation and other problems.

Genealogical. Refers to a record or account of a person's family and ancestry.

Generalization. The ability to apply a set of skills or knowledge learned under one set of conditions to other conditions or environments.

Genetic counseling. A process of informing parents concerning decisions they have to make regarding having children; often done where there is some reason to believe that a genetic abnormality may result.

Genetic counselor. A specially trained professional who counsels people considering having a child regarding their chances of producing a handicapped baby based on their genetic history.

Geneticist. A person who specializes in the study of heredity.

Genetic screening. A search in a population for persons possessing certain genotypes (genes transmitted from parents to offspring) that are (1) already associated with disease or predisposed to disease, (2) may lead to disease in their descendants, or (3) produce other variations not known to be associated with disease.

Genetics specialist. See **Geneticist.**

Gifted, creative, and talented. Terms applied to those with extraordinary abilities in one or more areas and capable of superior performance.

Glaucoma. A disorder in the eye characterized by high pressure inside the eyeball.

Glucose. A sugar.

Glycosuria. An increased concentration of glucose in the urine.

Grand mal seizures. Seizures that involve a sudden loss of consciousness followed immediately by a generalized convulsion.

Gross motor development. Development of head and neck control, righting of the body, sitting, standing, and general mobility.

Habilitation. The process of making fit; often refers to training.

Handicap. A limitation imposed on an individual by the environment and the person's capacity to cope with that limitation.

Haptic. Refers to touch sensation and information transmitted through body movement and/or position.

Hard-of-hearing. A term used to categorize individuals with a sense of hearing that is defective but somewhat functional.

Health disorders. Conditions or diseases that interfere with an individual's functioning but do not necessarily or initially have an impact on their ability to move about independently in various settings.

Hearing disorder. Pertaining to the loss of hearing, the term includes both persons who are hard-of-hearing and persons who are deaf.

Hearing impaired. Any individual who has a hearing loss that requires special assistance (such as a hearing aid) or educational adaptation.

Heart attack. A sudden inability of the heart to function properly.

Hertz (Hz). A unit used to measure the frequency of sound in terms of the number of cycles that vibrating molecules complete per second.

Hemiplegia. Paralysis that involves one side of the body in a lateral fashion.

Histamines. Substances transmitted in a number of fashions (such as foods and odors), which cause a constriction or swelling of bronchial muscles.

Hormone. An internally secreted compound formed in endocrine organs.

Human Immunodeficiency Virus (HIV). A virus that reduces the immune-system functioning in affected individuals and has been linked to AIDS.

Hydrocephalus. An excess of cerebrospinal fluid, often resulting in enlargement of the head with pressure on the brain, which may cause mental retardation.

Hyperactivity. See **Hyperkinetic.**

Hyperglycemia. An increased concentration of glucose in the blood.

Hyperkinetic. Refers to an excess of behavior in inappropriate circumstances.

Hypernasality. A voice resonance disorder that occurs when excessive air passes through the nasal cavity, often resulting in an unpleasant twanging sound.

Hyperopia. Farsightedness. A refractive problem wherein the eyeball is excessively short, focusing light rays behind the retina.

Hypoglycemia. A condition characterized by an abnormal decrease of sugar in the blood.

Hyponasality. A voice disorder involving resonance, where too little air passes through the nasal cavity; denasality.

Hypotonia. Poor muscle tone.

Id. A term, based on psychoanalytic theory, that refers to the drives component of one's subconscious.

Identical twins. Twins that develop from a single fertilized egg in a single placental sack. Such twins are the same sex and usually resemble one another closely.

IEP. See **Individualized education program.**

Idiot. A very early classification used in mental retardation, now considered derogatory, which involved individuals with measured IQs of about 29 and below.

Imbecility. A very early classification used in mental retardation, now considered derogatory, which involved individuals with measured IQs of about 25 or 30 to 49.

Immaturity. Pertaining to behavior disorders, a category involving preoccupation, short attention span, passivity, daydreaming, sluggishness, and other behavior not in accord with developmental expectations.

Immune system. The normally functioning system within a person's body that protects from disease.

Immunosuppressive drugs. Medication that discourages the body from rejecting implanted organs.

Impairment. A physical deviation or defect that is either acquired or congenital (e.g., spina bifida, cerebral palsy, or spinal-cord injury).

Incidence. The number of new cases of a condition that have been identified within a specific period of time (e.g., one year).

Individual labeling approach. Labeling that occurs when an individual imposes a label on himself or herself.

Individualized education program (IEP). An educational plan tailored to an individual student's needs. Required by Public Law 94–142 for exceptional students.

Individualized family service plan (IFSP). A plan of intervention, similar in content to the IEP, which includes statements regarding the child's present development level, the family's strengths and needs, the major outcomes of the plan, a delineation of the specific interventions and delivery systems to accomplish outcomes, dates of initiation and duration of services, and a transition plan.

Individualized language plan (ILP). A language-training program tailored to an individual's needs in terms of strengths and limitations.

Infant stimulation. Refers to early intervention procedures that emphasize providing an infant with an array of visual, auditory, and physical stimuli to promote development.

Infantile perseveration. The articulation part of delayed speech where a youngster relies on speech as his or her main means of communication and attempts words, phrases, and sentences, but does so immaturely because of sound omissions and substitutions.

Infantile spasms. Seizures that infants (three months to two years of age) experience, characterized by flexor spasms of the arms, legs, and head. Also known as jackknife seizures.

Information processing. A model used to study the way people acquire, remember, and manipulate information.

Insane. An outdated term that referred to serious mental illness.

Institution. An establishment or facility governed by a collection of fundamental rules.

Insulin. A secretion of the pancreas, which assists the body by allowing glucose to enter cells.

Insulin infusion pump. Battery-operated devices that dispense insulin to diabetic patients on a continuous basis.

Intelligence quotient (IQ). A score obtained from an intelligence test that provides a measure of mental ability in relation to age.

Interindividual. Refers to comparisons of an individual's performance with that of others.

Intoxication. Refers to an excessive level of some toxic agent in the mother–fetus system, which may cause cerebral damage.

Intraindividual. Refers to comparisons of an individual's different areas of performance.

Introspection. Looking into oneself to analyze experiences.

in utero. A term pertaining to child development in the uterus, or before birth; may refer to abnormalities or accidents that occur during this developmental period, such as in utero infection.

Iris. The colored portion of the eye.

Itinerant teacher. A teacher who regularly visits an incapacitated student in his or her home or in a hospital setting to provide tutorial instruction.

Juvenile rheumatoid arthritis. A childhood viral disease characterized by inflammation and swelling of joint structures.

Ketoacidosis. A diabetic condition that results in dehydration, vomiting, drowsiness, labored breathing, and frequent urination.

Kinesthetic. Pertaining to sensations derived from muscles or movement.

Kurzweil reading machine. A reading device for people who are blind that converts printed matter into synthetic speech.

Labeling. The process of naming a category of exceptionality.

Language. The intended messages contained in a speaker's utterances.

Language delay. A term used when the normal rate of language development is interrupted but the developmental sequence remains intact.

Language disorder. A term used when the sequence of language development is seriously disrupted.

Laryngeal. Pertaining to the larynx.

Larynx. The portion of the throat that contains the vocal mechanism.

Laser cane. A mobility device for people who are blind that converts infrared light into sound as light beams strike objects.

Learning disabled. See **Learning disability.**

Learning disability. A disorder in one or more of the basic psychological processes in understanding or using language.

Learning disordered. A term applied to people who are significantly below average in learning performance when compared to others of a comparable chronological age.

Learning set. Refers to learning how to learn and the ability to apply what is learned to new experiences.

Least restrictive environment (LRE). The most normal environment possible for instruction, treatment, and/or living. Also referred to as the least restrictive alternative.

Lens. The clear structure in the eye that focuses light rays on the retina.

Leukemia. A type of blood cancer which has an impact primarily on the blood-forming organs.

Line-21 system. See **Closed-caption.**

Low birth weight. A term applied to babies that weigh 5½ pounds (2,500 grams) or less at birth.

LRE. See **Least restrictive environment.**

Lymphoma. A type of blood-related cancer that is localized in lymph nodes.

Mainstreaming. The temporal, instructional, and social integration of exceptional children and youth with their regular-education peers in the school setting.

Malocclusion. Refers to an abnormal fit of the upper and lower dental structures.

Manual communication. Communication that involves sign language.

Master teacher. A highly trained and skilled teacher who serves on a supervisory and consultive basis, assisting classroom teachers primarily with implementation problems.

Maternal infection. Infection in a mother during pregnancy, usually concerned with potential injury to the unborn child.

Maternal malnutrition. Refers to nutritional inadequacy in a pregnant mother.

Maternal rubella. German measles contracted by a mother during pregnancy.

Maturation philosophy. A view that early childhood services do not remedy problems (and perhaps create difficulties) because young children may not be mature enough to cope with the pressures of structured learning.

MBD. See **Minimal brain dysfunction.**

Measurement bias. Refers to an unfairness or inaccuracy of results due to cultural background, sex, or race. See also **Test bias.**

Melting pot. A view, often associated with the United States, that many cultures blend together into one, losing their distinctive and diverse elements.

Meningitis. An inflammation of the membranes covering the brain and spinal cord.

Mental age. A concept used in psychological assessment that relates to the general mental ability possessed by the average child of a given chronological age.

Mental illness. A general term referring to any of the various forms of mental disorders; not widely used in professional circles, where such general terminology has been replaced by more specific, descriptive language.

Mental retardation. Significantly subaverage general intellectual functioning existing concurrently with deficits in adaptive behavior and manifested during the developmental period. (Grossman, 1977, p. 11)

Mentally retarded. See **Mental retardation.**

Metabolic. Refers to the body's ability to process (metabolize) substances.

Metabolic errors. Defects in the body's ability to process substances normally.

Micropthalmos. An abnormally small eyeball.

Mild learning and behavior disorders. A generic classification of disorders involving academic and/or social-interpersonal performance deficits that generally become evident in a school-related setting and make it necessary for the individual to receive additional support services beyond those typically offered in a regular education setting. However, it is assumed mildly disordered students remain in the regular education setting for the majority of the school day. The severity of the performance deficits for this population ranges from one to two standard deviations below the interindividual and/or intraindividual mean on the measure(s) being recorded.

Minor motor seizures. Seizures that have been identified as myoclonic (shocklike contractions in muscles or muscle groups), akinetic (sudden loss of muscle tone), and infantile spasms (jackknife seizures).

Minimal brain dysfunction. The condition in which an individual exhibits behavioral and sensorineural problems.

Mirror writing. Writing backwards from right to left, the letters appearing like ordinary writing seen in a mirror.

Mixed hearing loss. A hearing loss resulting from a combination of conductive and sensorineural problems.

Modeling. A teaching process wherein the instructor demonstrates the appropriate behavior or skill to be learned as a means of teaching.

Moderate learning and behavior disorders. A generic classification of disorders involving intellectual, academic, and/or social-interpersonal performance deficits that range between two and three standard deviations below the interindividual and/or intraindividual mean on the measure(s) being recorded. These performance deficits are not limited to any given setting but are typically evident in the broad spectrum of environmental settings. Etiology of the problem(s) may be identified in some cases but typically cannot be precisely pinpointed. Individuals with functional disorders at this level require substantially altered patterns of service and treatment and may need modified environmental accommodations.

Mongoloid. A term that used to be employed in referring to those with Down syndrome, now outdated.

Monoplegia. Paralysis that involves one limb.

Moron. A very early classification used in mental retardation, now considered derogatory, which involved individuals with measured IQs of about 50 to 69.

Morphology. The form and internal structure of words. The transformation of words in such ways as tense and number.

Mosaicism. A type of Down syndrome in which the chromosomal accident occurs after fertilization.

Motokinesthetic. Refers to a type of speech training used with hearing-disordered people, involving the feeling of an individual's face and reproducing breath and voice patterns.

Mowat sensor. A hand-held travel aid approximately the size of a flashlight, used by people who are blind. An alternative to the cane for warning of obstacles in front of the individual.

Multicultural education. Education that promotes learning about multiple cultures and their values.

Multidisciplinary. Refers to several disciplines (like educators, psychologists, and others) in a joint venture, such as the multidisciplinary team required for assessment by Public Law 94–142.

Muscular dystrophy. A group of inherited, chronic disorders that are characterized by gradual wasting and weakening of the voluntary skeletal muscles.

Myoclonic seizure. A seizure that is characterized by shocklike contractions involving parts of a muscle, an entire muscle, or groups of related muscles.

Myopia. Nearsightedness. A refractive problem wherein the eyeball is excessively long, focusing light in front of the retina.

Myringoplasty. A surgical reconstruction of a perforated eardrum.

Nature vs. nurture. The issue of determining how much of a person's ability is related to sociocultural influences (nurture) as opposed to genetic factors (nature).

Negativism. Refers to circumstances when the demands on a young child exceed his or her performance level, which results in withdrawal and refusing to speak.

Neonatal period. The time immediately following birth.

Neonatal seizures. Seizures in newborns evidenced by alternating contractions of various muscle groups.

Neonates. Newborn children or children of less than one month of age.

Neurofibromatosis. An inherited disorder resulting in tumors of the skin and other tissue (e.g., the brain).

Neurological. Pertaining to the nervous system.

Neuroses. Behavior that involves a partial disorganization, characterized by combinations of anxieties, compulsions, obsessions, and phobias.

Neurotic disorders. See **Neuroses.**

Noncompliance. Pertaining to children who exhibit troublesome behaviors, this term refers to refusal to follow directions. Pertaining to service delivery, this term refers to an agency's not meeting the requirements of the law or regulations.

Nondiscriminatory and multidisciplinary assessment. One of the provisions of Public Law 94–142. This component requires that testing be in a child's native or primary language; procedures are selected and administered to prevent cultural or racial discrimination; assessment tools used are validated for the purpose they are being used; and that assessment is conducted by a multidisciplinary team using several pieces of information to formulate a placement decision.

Nondisjunction. A type of Down syndrome in which the chromosomal pairs do not separate properly as the sperm or egg cells are formed; also known as Trisomy 21.

Normal. A general term applied to behavior or abilities that fall within the average range; that which is considered acceptable, not exceptional.

Normality. See **Normal.**

Normalization. Making an individual's life and surroundings as culturally normal as possible.

Norm-based. See **Norm-referenced.**

Norm-referenced assessment. Refers to assessment where a person's performance is compared with the average of a larger group.

Nystagmus. Uncontrolled, rapid eye movements.

Occlusion. The closing and fitting together of dental structures.

Occupational therapist. A professional who specializes in designing and delivering instruction concerning potential work-related activities.

Occupational therapy. Intervention related to potential work-related activities. See also **Occupational therapist.**

Open classroom. Programs and experiences used for instructional settings wherein the children are provided opportunities to initiate their own learning activities.

Opportunistic infection. An infection caused by germs that are not usually capable of causing infection in normal people, but can do so given certain changes in the immune system (opportunity).

Optacon. A tactile scanner for reading, by people who are blind, that does not use the Braille system. The Optacon "reads" printed material and reproduces it on a finger pad through a series of vibrating pins.

Optic atrophy. A degenerative disease that results from deteriorating nerve fibers connecting the retina to the brain.

Optic nerve. The nerve that connects the eye to the visual center of the brain.

Ossicular chain. The three small bones (malleus, incus, and stapes, or hammer, anvil, and stirrup) that transmit vibrations through the middle ear cavity to the inner ear.

Otitis media. An inflammation of the middle ear.

Otologist. One who is involved in the study of the ear and its diseases.

Otosclerosis. A condition associated with disease of the inner ear, characterized by destruction of the capsular bone in the middle ear and growth of a weblike bone that attaches to the stapes. May result in hearing disorders.

Ototoxic drugs. Drugs that can be poisonous to or have a deleterious effect on the eighth nerve or on the organs of hearing and balance.

Outcome-based. Refers to selection of an intervention based on its results.

Overrepresented. Pertaining to multicultural issues, this term refers to circumstances where a group has a higher percentage of youngsters in special education than would be projected based on the proportion of their cultural group in the general population.

Paperless brailler. A device for writing in Braille where the information is recorded and retrieved in some manner not using paper such as a standard magnetic-tape cassette.

Parameters of classification. The basis used for classification.

Paraplegia. Paralysis that involves the legs only.

Partially sighted. According to the National Society for the Prevention of Blindness, refers to persons with a visual acuity greater than 20/200 but not greater than 20/70 in the better eye after correction.

Pathology. Alterations in an organism caused by disease.

Perceptual abnormality. An abnormality in one's ability to interpret the stimuli around him or her.

Perceptual disorders. Disorders related to an inability to use one or more of the senses.

Perceptual-motor. Pertaining to an individual's ability to interpret stimuli and then perform appropriate actions in response to those stimuli.

Performance feedback. Information given to students by teachers or therapists regarding how well they performed.

Personality. The characteristic way in which individuals behave and respond to various environments.

Personality disorders. Behavior disorders in which an individual is overly anxious, extremely shy, or unusually sad much of the time.

Petit mal seizures. Seizures characterized by brief periods of inattention, with rapid eye-blinking or head-twitching.

Phenylalanine. A substance found in foods such as milk, which, when not processed, can cause damage to the central nervous system.

Phenylketonuria (PKU). A genetic disorder that may cause mental retardation if left untreated.

Phonic generalization. Refers to the ability to generalize information related to sounds from one word or configuration to another, predicting that which might follow, in order to approximate proper spelling.

Phonology. The system of speech sounds that an individual utters.

Physical disorders. Bodily impairments that interfere with an individual's mobility, coordination, communication, learning, and/or personal adjustment.

Physical therapy. The treatment of a physical deficiency by stretching, exercise, or massage.

PKU. See **Phenylketonuria.**

Platelet transfusion. A blood transfusion in which the red blood cells are removed and the remaining blood is rich with platelets, which prevent bleeding.

Pneumocystis carinii pneumonia (PCP). A rare form of pneumonia involving a tiny parasite.

Postural drainage. Refers to the draining of fluids through changing the posture of an individual such as is done with cystic fibrosis.

Postlingual disorders. Pertaining to hearing disorders, those occurring at any age following speech development.

Postpartum period. Pertaining to the period of time shortly after childbirth.

Pragmatics. A component of language that is concerned with the use of language in social contexts, including rules that govern language functions and forms of messages when communicating.

Precipitous birth. A delivery wherein the time between the onset of labor and birth is unusually short, generally less than two hours.

Precision teaching. An instructional approach that specifically pinpoints the skills to be taught, measures the initial level of those skills, specifies goals and objectives for improvement, and measures on a daily basis in order to alter the program design if progress is not sufficient.

Prematurity. Refers to infants delivered before 37 weeks from the first day of the last menstrual period.

Prenatal. The time before birth, while a baby is developing during pregnancy.

Prevalence. The number of persons in any given population who exhibit a condition or problem at a specific point in time.

Prelingual disorders. Pertaining to hearing disorders, those occurring prior to the age of two, the time of speech development.

Prenatal rubella. See **Maternal rubella.**

Primary-care physician. A physician who has principal responsibility for an individual's care, perhaps a family physician.

Profoundly handicapped. An extreme level of limitation imposed on an individual by the environment and the person's capacity to cope with that limitation.

Profound/multiple disorders. See **Severe and profound/multiple disorders.**

Proprioceptive. Pertaining to stimuli receptors located in tissue that is under the skin, such as muscles.

Prosthetic. A device that replaces a missing or malfunctioning part of the body, such as an arm, a joint, or teeth.

Project Head Start. A prevention program that attempts to identify and teach high-risk children before they enter public school.

Pseudoglioma. A nonmalignant intraocular disturbance resulting from the detachment of the retina.

Psychometrist. A professional who specializes in the administration of psychological tests, differentiated from a school psychologist in most areas by the fact that psychometrists emphasize collaboration in interventions to a lesser degree.

Psychomotor retardation. A slowed development of abilities to perform acts involving cognitive and physical processes.

Psychomotor seizure. A seizure evidenced by inappropriate, purposeless behavior such as lip smacking, chewing, or other automatic reactions.

Psychosis. A general term referring to a serious behavior disorder resulting in loss of contact with reality; characterized by delusions, hallucinations, or illusions.

Psychotic disorders. See **Psychosis.**

Public Law 94–142. See **Education of All Handicapped Children Act.**

Public Law 99–457. See **Amendments to the Education of the Handicapped Act, 1986.**

Pull-out. A term applied to interventions that remove a student with a disability from the regular classroom to a separate class for at least part of the school day.

Pupil. The opening in the iris of the eye that expands and contracts to control the amount of light entering the eye.

Pure tone audiometry. Audiometric evaluation using tones that are free of external noise.

Quadriplegia. Paralysis that involves all four limbs.

Receptive eye problems. Disorders associated with the receiving structures of the eye, that is, the retina or the optic nerve.

Receptive language disorders. Difficulties in comprehending what others say.

Refractive problems. Visual problems that occur when the refractive structures of the eye fail to properly focus light rays on the retina.

Regular education initiative. A perspective that places a major portion of the responsibility for educating all mildly and some moderately disabled students with general education.

Rehabilitation. Refers to the process (or programs) aimed at teaching individuals who are recently handicapped the fundamental skills for independence.

Rehearsal strategies. Refers to plans or tactics for practicing material to be learned.

Related services. Services not usually defined as educational, including such matters as transportation, audiology, physical and occupational therapy, medical treatment, and counseling.

Remedial readers. Youngsters who need particular assistance in reading instruction; a term that was used earlier for youngsters who might now be known as learning disabled.

Remediation approach. Pertaining to instruction that focuses on the gaps or deficiencies in a student's repertoire of skills.

Replicate. To repeat. In research, to duplicate an experiment.

Research design. The procedural plan for undertaking a research study.

Resource room. A placement option for children with disabilities which involves a variable amount of time per day, depending on the student's needs, with the remainder of time being spent in his or her regular classroom. The specialized assistance provided in the resource room reinforces and supplements regular class instruction while allowing the student to remain in the same school.

Resource-room teacher. A teacher providing instruction in a resource room. See also **Resource room.**

Retina. The light-sensitive cells in the eye that transmit images to the brain via the optic nerve.

Retinal detachment. A condition that occurs when the retina is separated from the choroid and sclera.

Retinitis pigmentosa. A hereditary condition resulting from a break in the choroid.

Retinoblastoma. A malignant tumor in the retina.

Retrolental fibroplasia (RLF). Scar-tissue formation behind the lens of the eye, preventing light rays from reaching the retina. The result of administering excessive oxygen to premature infants.

Retropathy of prematurity. A term now used for retrolental fibroplasia. See also **Retrolental fibroplasia (RLF).**

Rh incompatibility. A situation in which the mother has Rh-negative blood and the fetus has Rh-positive blood. May result in birth defects.

Rheumatic heart disease. A condition that ensues from rheumatic fever wherein the muscles, valves, or lining of the heart may become inflamed and then permanently damaged.

RhoGAM. An anti-Rh gamma globulin medication used to combat incompatibility in blood type between a mother and her fetus.

Rigidity. A condition that is characterized by continuous and diffuse tension as the limbs are extended.

Role playing. The process of letting students rehearse and practice behaviors they are to learn, often pertaining to social behaviors.

Scales of independent behavior. A formal, standardized assessment instrument for evaluating adaptive behavior.

Schizophrenia. A severe behavior disorder involving a misconception or loss of contact with reality and distorted thought processes.

School phobia. An extreme fear of school and matters related to school.

Scientific method. A method of investigating questions that systematically approaches their study in order to obtain objective results.

Screening. A general term for any rapid, preliminary identification of children who are potentially handicapped and need further examination.

Segregated educational facilities. Educational facilities that are separate from the mainstream placements of nonhandicapped youngsters, often termed *special schools.*

Selective attention. Attention that often does not focus on centrally important tasks or information.

Self-care skills. Skills related to hygiene, feeding, and generally taking care of oneself.

Self-contained special education classroom. A separate classroom where special students spend the majority of their school day, while often being integrated with their nondisabled peers whenever possible, such as in nonacademically-oriented classes and on the playground.

Self-fulfilling prophecy. Refers to the theory that people become what they are labeled.

Seizure. A cluster of behaviors (altered consciousness, characteristic motor patterns, etc.) that occurs in response to abnormal neurochemical activity in the brain.

Seizure disorders (epilepsy). A cluster of brain disorders that result in a sudden altering of the individual's consciousness, accompanied by apparently uncontrolled jerking and motor activity.

Semantics. The component of language most concerned with the meaning and understanding of language.

Sensorineural hearing loss. A hearing loss resulting from an abnormal sense organ (inner ear) and a damaged auditory nerve.

Sensory disorders. Differences in vision and hearing affecting performance.

Sensory seizure. A seizure that is characterized primarily by visual, auditory, gustatory, olfactory, or emotional sensations.

Severe and profound multiple disorders. A generic classification of disorders that involve physical, sensory, intellectual, and/or social-interpersonal performance deficits beyond three standard deviations below the interindividual and/or intraindividual mean on the measures being recorded. These deficits are not limited to any given setting but are evident in all environmental settings and often involve deficits in several areas of performance. Etiologies are more identifiable at this level of functioning, but exact cause(s) may be unknown in a large number of cases. Individuals with functional disorders at this level require significantly altered environments with regard to care, treatment, and accommodation.

Severely handicapped. See **Severe and profound multiple disorders.**

Severely multiply handicapped. See **Severe and profound multiple disorders.**

Sexual abuse. A form of mistreatment involving sexual mistreatment, such as incest, assault, or sexual exploitation.

Shared responsibility. The concept that regular education and special education both have responsibilities, in a partnership manner, for the best education of students with disabilities.

Short attention span. An inability to focus attention on a task for a sustained period, often for more than a few seconds or minutes.

Sickle-cell anemia (SCA). An inherited disease that has a profound effect on the function and structure of red blood cells.

Sickle-cell trait (SCT). Refers to a person who is a carrier of sickle-cell anemia but does not actually suffer the disease effects.

Sight conservation. A point of view advocating restricted use of the eye to save remaining vision.

Sign language. An approach to communication that involves a systematic and complex combination of hand movements that communicate whole words and complete thoughts rather than letters of the alphabet.

Sign systems. Approaches to communication that are different from sign languages in that they attempt to produce equivalents to oral language through manual and visual means.

Six-hour retardate. A term arising from observations that certain youngsters appear retarded only during the six hours per day that they were in school.

Snellen test. A test of visual acuity.

Sonicguide. An electronic mobility device for people who are blind, which is worn on the head, emits ultrasound, and converts reflections from objects into audible noise.

Spasticity. A condition that involves involuntary contractions of various muscle groups.

Special children. A general term used to label children who do not meet educational expectations and require services and resources that are different from those needed by "normal" youngsters.

Special education classroom. See **Self-contained special education classroom.**

Special day schools. See **Special schools.**

Special schools. A general term applied to segregated educational placements that only handicapped youngsters attend.

Speech. The audible production of language.

Speech and language disorders. Difficulties in communicating effectively.

Social system. A grouping of people with a defined set of purposes, roles, and expectations.

Sociopathic. A severe behavior disorder in which the individual is aggressively antisocial and shows no remorse.

SOMPA. The System of Multicultural Pluralistic Assessment developed by Mercer and Lewis (1977).

Specific learning disability. See **Learning disability.**

Speech. The audible production of language.

Speech audiometry. The audiometric evaluation of spoken words.

Speech disorders. Speech behavior that is sufficiently deviant from normal or accepted speaking patterns to attract attention, interfere with communication, and adversely affect communication for either the speaker or the listener.

Spina bifida. A developmental defect of the spinal column.

Spina bifida cystica. A malformation of the spinal column in which a tumorlike sack is produced on the infant's back.

Spina bifida meningocele. A cystic swelling or tumorlike sack that contains spinal fluid but no nerve tissue.

Spina bifida myelomeningocele. A cystic swelling or tumorlike sack that contains both spinal fluid and nerve tissue.

Spina bifida occulta. A very mild condition of spina bifida in which an oblique slit is present in one or several of the vertebral structures.

Spinal-cord injury. An injury in which the spinal cord is traumatized or transected.

Spinal meningitis. An inflammation of the membranes of the spinal cord.

Spondylitis of adolescence. A form of rheumatoid arthritis that affects the entire body rather than isolated joints or areas.

Standard deviation. A statistical measure of the amount an individual score deviates from the average.

Standardized. A term applied to assessment, meaning that during its design and development the procedure or instrument has been field-tested and that administration and scoring have been refined into a specified, prescribed routine to assure that the process is consistent.

Stanford-Binet Intelligence Scale. A standardized, individual intelligence test, originally the Binet-Simon Scales, which were revised and standardized by Lewis Terman at Stanford University.

Stapedectomy. A surgical process that replaces defective stapes in the ear with a prosthetic device.

Statistical relativity. A method of labeling that defines deviance based on the frequency of a behavior or characteristic. An average frequency is calculated, and a person's status is compared with that average.

Stereotyped movement disorders. Conditions that are characterized by abnormal gross motor behaviors (tics).

Sterilization. The process of making an individual unable to reproduce, usually accomplished surgically.

Stigma. An unflattering view of someone associated with the label given to that individual.

Strabismus. Crossed eyes (internal) or eyes that look outward (external).

Stuttering. A speech disorder involving abnormal repetitions, prolongations, and hesitations as one speaks.

Substance abuse. The use of any such agents as alcohol or drugs to the degree that they become significantly detrimental to one's life and health.

Suicide. The intentional taking of one's own life.

Superego. A term, based on psychoanalytic theory, that refers to the conscience component of one's subconscious.

Symptom severity. A parameter of classification that refers to the degree of deviation from the norm.

Synapses. The region of contact between one neuron and another through which nerve impulses are transmitted.

Syndrome description. A parameter of classification that often describes exceptionalities in technical or medical terms.

Syntax. The order and way in which words and sequences of words are combined into phrases, clauses, and sentences.

System of Multicultural Pluralistic Assessment. See SOMPA.

Telecommunication devices for the deaf (TDD). Devices that send, receive, and print messages between stations at distant locations.

Teletypewriter (TTY). A typewriter that converts typed letters into electric signals, which are then sent through telephone lines and printed on another typewriter connected to a phone on the other end. This device is used by people with hearing disorders.

Teratogen. A drug or other agent that causes abnormal development.

Test bias. Unfairness in a testing procedure or instrument that gives one group a particular advantage or another a disadvantage, which may be due to matters unrelated to ability, such as culture, sex, or race. See also **Measurement bias**.

Therapeutic abortion. Termination of a pregnancy when a defect is found in the fetus during prenatal evaluation.

Therapeutic play school. A type of therapy used in cases of child abuse, which removes them from the circumstances of daily life and serves as a temporary island of reprieve.

Tinnitus. High-pitched throbbing or ringing sounds in the ear, associated with disease of the inner ear.

T lymphocytes. A type of white blood cell that attacks infections.

Token economy. See **Token reinforcement systems**.

Token reinforcement systems. A system in which students may earn plastic chips, marbles, "checkmarks" or other tangible items that may be exchanged for activities, food items, special privileges, or other rewards for positive behavior changes.

Tonic. The phase of a grand mal seizure that is marked by prolonged muscular contraction (rigidity).

Total communication. A communication philosophy/approach, used by people with hearing disorders, which employs various combinations of elements from manual, oral, and any other technique available to facilitate understanding.

Toxoplasmosis. An infection caused by protozoa carried in raw meat and fecal material.

Trainable. A level of mental retardation, based on educability expectation, which involves measured intelligence of 40 to 55, with learning primarily in self-help skill areas; some academic achievement; social adjustment often limited to home and closely surrounding area; vocational proficiencies include supported work in a community job or sheltered workshop.

Transducer. A device that receives energy from one system and retransmits it to another, often in a different form. Transducers are used in cochlear implants to alter sound into electric nerve-stimulating signals.

Transfer of training. The process of generalizing behaviors or skills learned in one setting to other settings or circumstances.

Transfusion. A general term referring to the transfer of blood from one person to another.

Transition from school to adult life. The process of bridging the time and environments between school and the adult world, which is being addressed by instructional programs in many areas.

Transition plan. A designed program delineating the transition of a person from school to adult life, by identifying the services needed for that specific individual, the activities that must occur during the school years, and the timelines and responsibilities for completion of these activities.

Translocation. A type of Down syndrome in which a portion of the twenty-first chromosome pair breaks off and fuses with another pair.

Transverse presentation. A situation in which the fetus lies across the birth canal.

Tremor. A motion or movement, which occurs in a limb, that is constant, involuntary, and uncontrollable.

Triplegia. Paralysis that involves three appendages, usually both legs and one arm.

Trisomy 21. A type of Down syndrome in which the chromosomal pairs do not separate properly as the sperm or egg cells are formed, resulting in an extra chromosome on the twenty-first pair. Also called *nondisjunction*.

Tuberous sclerosis. A birth defect that does not appear until late childhood, is related to mental retardation in about 66 percent of the cases, and is characterized by tumors on many organs.

Ultrasound. A prenatal evaluation procedure which employs high-frequency sound waves that are bounced through the mother's abdomen to record tissue densities.

Unspecified mental retardation. Refers to individuals with mental retardation whose condition has no known cause.

Verbalisms. The excessive use of speech (wordiness) in which individuals use words that have little meaning to them.

Vestibular mechanism. A structure in the inner ear containing three semicircular canals filled with fluid. It is sensitive to movement and assists the body in maintaining equilibrium.

Videodisc. A recordlike platter that stores information and combines usage of a television with computer-assisted systems.

Vineland Social Maturity Scale. A standardized assessment procedure for evaluating adaptive behavior.

Visual acuity. The sharpness or clearness of vision.

Visual discrimination. The act of distinguishing one visual stimulus from another.

Visual disorder. Pertaining to the loss of seeing or sight, the term includes both persons who are partially sighted and those who are blind.

Vitreous fluid. A jellylike substance that fills most of the interior of the eye.

Vocational rehabilitation specialist. The professional who specializes in designing and implementing programs to help people with disabilities obtain and hold employment.

Voice disorder. A condition in which an individual habitually speaks with a voice that differs in pitch, loudness, or quality from the voices of others of the same sex and age in a cultural group.

Wechsler Intelligence Scales. A battery of standardized intelligence scales that can be used from preschool levels, through childhood, to adulthood.

References

Chapter 1

Aloia, G. F., & MacMillan, D. L. (1983). Influence of the EMR label on initial expectations of regular-classroom teachers. *American Journal of Mental Deficiency, 88*(3), 255–62.

Avoiding handicapist stereotypes. (1977). *Interracial Books for Children Bulletin, 8*(6,7), 1.

Bak, J. J., Cooper, E. M., Dobroth, K. M., & Siperstein, G. N. (1987). Special class placements as labels: Effects on children's attitudes toward learning handicapped peers. *Exceptional Children, 54*(2), 151–55.

Baron, R. A., & Byrne, D. (1987). *Social psychology: Understanding human interaction* (5th ed.). Boston: Allyn and Bacon.

Becker, H. S. (1974). Labeling theory reconsidered. In P. Rock & M. McIntosh (Eds.), *Deviance and social control.* London: Tavistock Publications (distributed in the U.S. by Harper & Row).

Benedict, R. (1934). *Patterns of culture.* Boston: Houghton Mifflin.

Bertalanffy, L. von (1960). Some biological considerations of the problem of mental illness. In L. Appleby, J. Scher & J. Cumming (Eds.), *Chronic schizophrenia.* Glencoe, Ill.: The Free Press.

Bogdan, R. (1986). The sociology of special education. In R. J. Morris & B. Blatt (Eds.), *Special education: Research and trends* (pp. 344–59). New York: Pergamon Press.

Carlson, N. R. (1987). *Psychology: The science of behavior.* Boston: Allyn and Bacon.

Clark, R. S. (1977). *Edison: The man who made the future.* New York: G. P. Putnam's Sons.

Collins, J. J. (1975). *Anthropology: Culture, society, and evolution.* Englewood Cliffs, N.J.: Prentice-Hall.

Cowen, E. (1973). Social and community interventions. In P. H. Mussen & M. R. Rosenzweig (Eds.), *Annual review of psychology* (Vol. 24). Palo Alto, Calif.: Annual Reviews.

Dinitz, S., Dynes, R. R., & Clarke, A. C. (1975). *Deviance: Studies in definition, management, and treatment* (2nd ed.). New York: Oxford University Press.

Edgerton, R. B. (1976). *Deviance: A cross-cultural perspective.* Menlo Park, Calif.: Cummings Publishing Co.

Fiedler, C. R., & Simpson, R. L. (1987). Modifying the attitudes of nonhandicapped high school students toward handicapped peers. *Exceptional Children, 53*(4), 342–49.

Foster, G. G., Ysseldyke, J. E., & Reese, J. H. (1975). I wouldn't have seen it if I hadn't believed it. *Exceptional Children, 41*(7), 469–73.

Freeman, S., & Algozzine, B. (1980). Social acceptability as a function of labels and assigned attributes. *American Journal of Mental Deficiency, 84*(6), 589–95.

Frost, L. A. (1969). *The Thomas Edison album.* Seattle: Superior Publishing Co.

Goldenberg, H. (1977). *Abnormal psychology: A social/community approach.* Monterey, Calif.: Brooks/Cole Publishing Co.

Graham, S., & Dwyer, A. (1987). Effects of the learning disability label, quality of writing performance, and examiner's level of expertise on the evaluation of written products. *Journal of Learning Disabilities, 20*(5), 317–18.

Keogh, B. K., & Levitt, M. L. (1976). Special education in the mainstream: A confrontation of limitations. *Focus on Exceptional Children, 8*, 1–11.

Laing, R. D. (1967). *The politics of experience.* New York: Pantheon Books.

Leitch, D., & Sodhi, S. S. (1986). 'Specialness' of special education. *British Columbia Journal of Special Education, 10*(4), 349–58.

MacMillan, D. L., & Becker, L. D. (1977). Mainstreaming the mildly handicapped learner. In R. D. Kneedler & S. G. Tarver (Eds.), *Changing perspectives in special education.* Columbus, Ohio: Charles E. Merrill Publishing Co.

Merton, R. K. (1948). The self-fulfilling prophecy. *Antioch Review, 8*, 193–210.

Myrdal, A. (1971). *Towards equality: The Alva Myrdal report* (p. 17). Stockholm: Bokforlaget, Prisma.

Palmer, D. J. (1980). The effect of educable mental retardation descriptive information on regular classroom teachers' attribution and instructional prescription. *Mental Retardation, 18*, 171–75.

Reynolds, M. C., Wang, M. C., & Walberg, H. J. (1987). The necessary restructuring of special and regular education. *Exceptional Children, 53*(5), 391–98.

Roos, P. (1982). Special trends and issues. In P. T. Cegelka & H. J. Prehm (Eds.), *Mental retardation: From categories to people.* Columbus, Ohio: Charles E. Merrill Publishing Co.

Rosenhan, D. L. (1973). On being sane in insane places. *Science, 179*, 250–58.

Rosenthal, R. (1987). Pygmalion effects: Existence, magnitude, and social importance. *Educational Researcher, 16*(9), 37–41.

Rosenthal, R., & Jacobsen, L. (1968). *Pygmalion in the classroom.* New York: Holt, Rinehart & Winston.

Szasz, T. S. (1961). *The myth of mental illness.* New York: Hoeber-Harper.

Teltsch, K. (1989, June 22). Shrinking labor pool opens doors to millions of disabled. *New York Times, 1*, 9.

U.S. Bureau of the Census (1984–85). *Disability, functional limitation, and health insurance coverage* (p. 144). Washington, D. C.: U.S. Government Printing Office.

Van Bourgondien, M. E. (1987). Children's responses to retarded peers as a function of social behaviors, labeling and age. *Exceptional Children, 53*(5), 432–9.

Wineburg, S. S. (1987). The self-fulfillment of the self-fulfilling prophecy. *Educational Researcher, 16*(9), 28–37.

Ysseldyke, J. E., & Foster, G. G. (1978). Bias in teachers' observations of emotionally disturbed and learning disabled children. *Exceptional Children, 44*(8), 613–15.

Chapter 2

Abeson, A., & Weintraub, F. (1980). Understanding the individualized education program. In S. Torres (Ed.), *A primer on individualized education programs for handicapped children.* Reston, Va.: Council for Exceptional Children.

Ainsworth, S. H. (1959). *An exploratory study of educational, social, and emotional factors in the education of mentally retarded children in Georgia Public Schools.* Athens: University of Georgia.

Bachrach, L. L. (1985). Deinstitutionalization: The meaning of the least restrictive environment. In R. H. Bruininks & K. C. Lakin (Eds.), *Living and Learning in the Least Restrictive Environment.* Baltimore: Paul H. Brookes Publishing Co.

Baird, J. L., & Workman, D. S. (1986). *Towards Solomon's mountain.* Philadelphia, Pa.: Temple University Press.

Baldwin, W. K. (1958). The social position of mentally handicapped children in the regular classes in the public school. *Exceptional Children, 25,* 106–8.

Balla, D. (1976). Relationship of institution size to quality of care: A review of the literature. *American Journal of Mental Deficiency, 81,* 117–24.

Barr, M. W. (1915). The prevention of mental defect, the duty of the hour. *Proceedings of the National Conference on Charities and Corrections* 361–67.

Binet, A., & Simon, T. (1905). Methodes nouvelles pour le diagnostic du niveau ellectual des anormaux. *L'Annee Psychologique, 11,* 191–244.

Blatt, B., & Kaplan, F. (1966). *Christmas in purgatory: A photographic essay on mental retardation.* Boston: Allyn and Bacon.

Blatt, B., Ozolins, A., & McNally, J. (1979). *The Family papers: A return to purgatory.* New York: Longman.

Braddock, D., Hemp, R., & Howes, R. (1984). *Public expenditures for mental retardation and developmental disabilities in the United States.* Chicago: Institute for the Study of Developmental Disabilities.

Brown v. Topeka, Kansas, Board of Education (1954). 347 U.S. 483.

Butterfield, E. C. (1967). The role of environmental factors in the treatment of institutionalized mental retardates. In A. A. Baumeister (Ed.), *Mental retardation: Appraisal, education, and rehabilitation.* Chicago: Aldine Publishing Co.

Cassidy, V. M., & Stanton, J. E. (1959). *An investigation of factors involved in the educational placement of mentally retarded children: A study of differences between children in special and regular classes in Ohio.* U.S. Office of Education Cooperative Research Program, Project no. 043. Columbus: Ohio State University.

Cavalier, A. R., & McCarver, R. B. (1981). *Wyatt v. Stickney* and mentally retarded individuals. *Mental Retardation, 19*(5), 209–14.

Danielsen, L. C., & Bellamy, G. T. (1989). State variation in placement of children with handicaps in segregated environments. *Exceptional Children, 55*(5), 448–55.

Drew, C. J., Logan, D. R., & Hardman, M. L. (1988). *Mental Retardation: Life Cycle Approach* (4th ed.). St. Louis: C. V. Mosby Co.

Dunn, L. M. (1968). Special education for the mildly retarded—Is much of it justifiable? *Exceptional Children, 35,* 5–22.

Fernald, C. D. (1984). Too little too late: Deinstitutionalization and the development of community services for mentally retarded people. Chapel Hill: Bush Institute for Child and Family Policy, University of North Carolina.

Fernald, W. E. (1915). What is practical in the way of prevention of mental defect? Proceedings of the National Conference on Charities and Correction, 289–97.

Gearheart, B. R. (1980). *Special education for the '80s.* St. Louis: C. V. Mosby Co.

Goddard, H. H. (1912). *The Kallikak family: A study in the heredity of feeblemindedness.* New York: Macmillan Co.

Goddard, H. H. (1914). *Feeblemindedness: Its causes and consequences.* New York: Macmillan Co.

Goffman, E. (1975). Characteristics of total institutions. In S. Dinitz, R. R. Dynes, & A. C. Clarke (Eds.), *Deviance: Studies in definition, management, and treatment.* New York: Oxford University Press.

Goldenberg, H. (1977). *Abnormal psychology: A social/community approach.* Monterey, Ca.: Brooks/Cole Publishing Co.

Guralnick, M. J., Richardson, H. B., & Heiser, K. E. (1982). A curriculum in handicapping conditions for pediatric residents. *Exceptional Children, 48*(4), 338–46.

Halderman v. Pennhurst State School and Hospital (1974). No. 74–1345 (U. S. Dist. Ct., E. D. Pa.), filed May 30.

Hardman, M. L., & Drew, C. J. (1980). Parent consent and the withholding

of treatment from the severely defective newborn. *Mental Retardation, 18*(4), 165–69.

Hoffman, E. (1972). *The treatment of deviance by the education system.* Ann Arbor, Mich.: Institute for the Study of Mental Retardation and Related Disabilities.

International Center for the Disabled (1986). *The ICD survey of disabled Americans: Bringing disabled Americans into the mainstream.* New York: Author.

Itard, J. (1962). *The wild boy of Aveyron.* G. Humphrey & Muriel Humphrey, Eds. and trans. Englewood Cliffs, N.J.: Prentice-Hall. (Originally published 1801.)

Johnson, A. (1908). Custodial care. *Proceedings of the National Conference on Charities and Corrections,* 333–36.

Johnson, G. O. (1961). *A comparative study of the personal and social adjustment of mentally handicapped children placed in special classes with mentally handicapped children who remain in regular classes.* Syracuse: Syracuse University Research Institute, Office of Research in Special Education and Rehabilitation.

Johnson, G. O. (1962). Special education for the mentally handicapped— A paradox. *Exceptional Children, 29,* 62–69.

Jordan, A. M. (1959). Personal-social traits of mentally handicapped children. In T. G. Thurstone (Ed.), *An evaluation of educating mentally handicapped children in special classes and regular classes.* Chapel Hill: School of Education, University of North Carolina.

Karier, C. J. (1973). Testing for order and control in the corporate liberal state. In C. J. Karier, P. Violas, & J. Spring (Eds.), *Roots of crisis: American education in the twentieth century.* Chicago: Rand McNally & Co.

Lakin, K. C., & Bruininks, R. H. (1985). Contemporary services for handicapped children and youth. In R. H. Bruininks & K. C. Lakin (Eds.), *Living and Learning in the Least Restrictive Environment.* Baltimore: Paul H. Brookes Publishing.

Lakin, K. C., Bruininks, R. H., & Sigford, R. R. (1981). Early perspectives on the community adjustment of mentally retarded people. In R. H. Bruininks, C. E. Meyers, B. B. Sigford, & K. C. Lakin (Eds.), *Deinstitutionalization and community adjustment of mentally retarded people,* 28–50. Washington, D. C.: American Association on Mental Retardation.

Levine, M. (1982). The child with school problems: An analysis of physician participation. *Exceptional Children, 48*(4), 296–304.

MacMillan, D. L., & Becker, L. D. (1977). Mainstreaming the mildly handicapped learner. In R. D. Kneedler & S. G. Tarver (Eds.), *Changing perspectives in special education.* Columbus, Ohio: Charles E. Merrill Publishing Co.

McCarver, R. B., & Cavalier, A. R. (1983). Philosophical concepts and attitudes underlying programming for the mentally retarded. In J. L. Matson & F. Andrasik (Eds.), *Treatment issues and innovations in mental retardation,* 1–3. New York: Plenum.

McCleary, I. D., Hardman, M. L., & Thomas, D. (1989). International special education. In T. Husen & T. N. Postleware (Eds.), *International encyclopedia of education: Research and studies.* New York: Pergamon Press.

Menolascino, F. J., McGee, J. J., & Casey, K. (1982). Affirmation of the rights of institutionalized retarded citizens (Implications of *Youngberg v. Romeo). TASH Journal, 8,* 63–72.

Mills v. District of Columbia Board of Education (1972). 348 F. Supp. 866 (D. D. C.).

National Association for Retarded Citizens (1976). *Residential services: Position statements of the National Association for Retarded Citizens.* Austin, Tex.

The Organization for Economic Cooperation and Development (1986). *Young people with handicaps: The Road to Adulthood.* Paris, France: Author.

Pennhurst State School and Hospital v. *Halderman* (1981). 451 U. S. 1.

Pennsylvania Association for Retarded Citizens v. *Commonwealth of Pennsylvania* (1971). 334 F. Supp. 1257 (E. D. Pa. 1971).

Polloway, E. A. (1984). The integration of mildly retarded students in the schools: A historical review. *Remedial and Special Education, 5*(4), 18–28.

Rotegard, L. L., Hill, B. K., & Bruininks, R. H. (1983). Environmental characteristics of residential facilities for mentally retarded persons in the United States. *American Journal of Mental Deficiency, 88*, 49–56.

Robinson, N. M., & Robinson, H. B. (1976). *The mentally retarded child.* (2nd ed.). New York: McGraw-Hill Book Co.

Rothman, D. J., & Rothman, S. M. (1984). *The Willowbrook wars.* New York: Harper & Row.

Thurstone, T. G. (1959). *An evaluation of educating mentally handicapped children in special classes and regular classes.* U.S. Office of Education, Cooperative Research Project No. OE-SAE 6452. Chapel Hill: University of North Carolina.

U.S. Congress (1975). Education of All Handicapped Children Act, Public Law 94–142.

United States Senate Subcommittee on the Handicapped, Committee on Labor and Human Resources (1985). *Staff report on the institutionalized mentally disabled.* Washington, D.C.

Watson, J. B., & Rayner, R. (1920). Conditioned emotional reactions. *Journal of Experimental Psychology, 3*, 1–14.

Weiner, R., & Hume, M. (1987). *And education for all: Public policy and handicapped children.* Alexandria, Va.: Capitol Publications.

Westling, D. L. (1986). *Introduction to mental retardation.* Englewood Cliffs, N.J.: Prentice-Hall.

Wolfensberger, W. (1975). *The origin and nature of our institutional models.* Syracuse, N. Y.: Human Policy Press.

Wolfensberger, W. (1977). The principle of normalization. In B. Blatt (Ed.), *An alternative textbook in special education.* Denver: Love Publishing Co.

Wyatt v. *Stickney* (1972). 344 F. Supp. 387, 344 F. Supp. 373 (M. D. Ala. 1972).

Wyne, M. D., & O'Connor, P. D. (1979). *Exceptional children: A developmental view.* Lexington, Mass.: D. C. Heath & Co.

Youngberg v. *Romeo* (1982). No. 80–1429 U. S.

Zigler, E. (1973). The retarded child as a whole person. In D. K. Routh (Ed.), *The experimental psychology of mental retardation.* Chicago: Aldine Publishing Co.

Chapter 3

Akers, M. (1972). Prologue: The why of early childhood education. In J. J. Gordon (Ed.), *Early childhood education.* Chicago: University of Chicago Press. (Reprinted from Seventy-First Yearbook of the National Society for the Study of Education.)

Allington, R., & McGill-Franzen, A. (1989). Different programs, indifferent instruction. In D. K. Lipksky & A. Gartner (Eds.), *Beyond separate education: Quality education for all.* Baltimore: Paul H. Brookes Publishing Co.

Antely, T. R., & Dubose, R. F. (1981). A case for early intervention: Summary of program findings, longitudinal data, and cost-effectiveness. Unpublished manuscript. Seattle: University of Washington, Experimental Education Unit.

Bloom, B. S. (1964). *Stability and change in human characteristics.* New York: John Wiley & Sons.

Bricker, D. D., & Iacino, R. (1977). Early intervention with severely/profoundly handicapped children. In E. Sontag (Ed.), *Educational programming for the severely/profoundly handicapped.* Reston, Va.: Council for Exceptional Children.

Brinker, R. P. (1985). Interactions between severely mentally retarded students and other students in integrated and segregated public school settings. *American Journal of Mental Deficiency, 89*(6), 587–94.

Brodsky, M. (1983). Post–high school experiences of graduates with severe handicaps. Doctoral dissertation. Eugene: University of Oregon.

Brolin, D. E. (1977). Career development: A national priority. *Educating and Training of the Mentally Retarded, 12*(3), 154–56.

Brolin, D. E. (1982). *Vocational preparation of persons with handicaps* (2nd ed.). Columbus, Ohio: Charles E. Merrill Co.

Buchanan, M., & Wolf, J. (1981). Academic strategies. In M. L. Hardman,

M. W. Egan, & E. D. Landau (Eds.), *The exceptional student in the regular classroom.* Dubuque, Iowa: William C. Brown Co.

Cassell, T. Z. (1976). A social-ecological model of adaptive functioning: A contextual developmental perspective. In N. A. Carson (Ed.), *Final report: The contexts of life: A socioecological model of adaptive behavior and functioning.* East Lansing, Mich.: Institute for Family and Child Study, Michigan State University.

Casto, G., & Mastropieri, M. A. (1985). *The efficacy of early intervention programs for handicapped children: A meta-analysis.* Logan, Utah: Early Intervention Research Institute.

Casto, G., & White, K. R. (1984). The efficacy of early intervention programs with environmentally at-risk infants. *Journal of Children in Contemporary Society, 17*, 37–48.

Clark, G. M. (1979). *Career education for the handicapped child in the elementary classroom.* Denver: Love Publishing Co.

Fowler, W. (1975). A developmental learning approach to infant care in a group setting. In B. Z. Friedlander, G. M. Sterritt, & G. E. Kirk (Eds.), *Exceptional Infant Assessment and Intervention* (Vol. 3) (pp. 341–73). New York: Brunner/Mazel.

Gartner, A., & Lipsky, D. K. (1987). Beyond special education: Toward a quality system for all students. *Harvard Educational Review, 57*(4), 367–95.

Gartner, A., & Lipsky, D. K. (1989). New conceptualizations for special education. *European Journal of Special Needs Education, 4*(1), 16–21.

Hamre-Nietupski, S. (1980). Sensitizing nonhandicapped persons to severely handicapped students in regular public school settings. Paper presented at the National Conference of the Association for the Severely Handicapped, Los Angeles.

Hansen, C. L., & Eaton, M. D. (1978). Reading. In N. G. Haring, T. C. Lovitt, M. D. Eaton, & C. L. Hansen (Eds.), *The fourth R: Research in the classroom.* Columbus, Ohio: Charles E. Merrill Publishing Co.

Hasazi, S. B., Gordon, L. R., & Roe, C. A. (1985). Factors associated with the employment status of handicapped youth exiting high school from 1975 to 1983. *Exceptional Children, 51*, 455–69.

Hunt, J. M. (1961). *Intelligence and experience.* New York: Ronald Press.

Janrchi, M. P., & Wishiewski, H. M. (1985). *Aging and developmental disabilities: Issues and approaches.* Baltimore: Paul H. Brooks.

Marsh, G. E., Gearheart, C. K., & Gearheart, B. R. (1978). *The learning-disabled adolescent: Program alternatives in the secondary school.* St. Louis: The C. V. Mosby Co.

McDonnell, J., & Hardman, M. L. (1985). Planning the transition of severely handicapped youth from school to adult services: A framework for high school programs. *Education and Training of the Mentally Retarded, 20*(4), 275–286.

McDonnell, J., Wilcox, B., & Boles, S. M. (1985). Do we know enough to plan for transition? A national survey of state agencies responsible for service to persons with severe handicaps. Unpublished manuscript. Eugene: University of Oregon.

Meisels, S. J. (1985). The efficacy of early intervention: Why are we still asking this question? *Topics in Early Childhood Special Education, 5*(2), 1–11.

National Advisory Council on Education Professions Development (1976). *Mainstreaming: Helping teachers meet the challenge.* Washington, D.C.: Author.

Palmer, F. H., & Siegel, R. J. (1977). Minimal intervention at ages two to three and subsequent intellectual changes. In C. Day and R. K. Parker (Eds.), *The preschool in action: Exploring early childhood programs.* Boston: Allyn and Bacon, Inc.

Peterson, N. L. (1987). *Early intervention for handicapped and at-risk children.* Denver: Love Publishing Company.

Piaget, J. (1970). Piaget's theory. In P. H. Mussen (Ed.), *Carmichael's manual of child psychology* (3rd ed., Vol. 1). New York: John Wiley & Sons.

Ramey, C. T., & Baker-Ward, L. (1982). Psychosocial retardation and the early experience paradigm. In D. D. Bricker (Ed.), *Intervention with at-risk and handicapped infants: From research to application.* Baltimore: University Park Press.

Ramey, C. T., & MacPhee, D. (1985). Development retardation among the poor: A system theory perspective on risk and prevention. In D. C. Farran & J. D. McKinney (Eds.), *Risk in intellectual and psychosocial development*. New York: Academic Press.

Reaves, J., & Burns, J. (1982). An analysis of the impact of the handicapped children's early education program (Final Report No. 2 for Special Education Programs, U.S. Department of Education, Contract No. 300–81–0661). Washington, D. C.: Roy Littlejohn Associates.

Reynolds, M. C., & Birch, J. W. (1982). *Teaching exceptional children in all America's schools*. Reston, Va.: Council for Exceptional Children.

Reynolds, M. C., & Birch, J. W. (1987). Noncategorical special education: Models for research and practice. In M. C. Wang, M. C. Reynolds, & H. J. Walberg (Eds.), *Handbook of special education research and practice: Vol. 1, Learner characteristics and adaptive education* (pp. 331–56). New York: Pergamon Press.

Siegel, J. S. (1980). On the demography of aging. *Demography, 17*, 345–64.

Stainback, S., & Stainback, W. (1985). *Integration of students with severe handicaps*. Reston, Va.: Council for Exceptional Children.

Swanson, D. M., & Willis, D. J. (1979). *Understanding exceptional children and youth*. Chicago: Rand McNally Co.

U. S. Department of Education (1986). *To assure the free appropriate public education to all handicapped children, Eighth annual report to congress on the implementation of the education of the handicapped act, vol. 1*. Washington, D. C.: U.S. Government Printing Office.

Wang, M. C. (1981). Mainstreaming exceptional children: Some instructional design and implementation considerations. *Elementary School Journal, 81*(4), 195–221.

Wehman, P., & Hill, J. W. (1982). Preparing severely handicapped youth for less restrictive environments. *The Journal of the Association for the Severely Handicapped, 7*(1), 33–39.

Wehman, P., Kregel, J., & Barcus, J. M. (1985). From school to work: A vocational transition model for handicapped students. *Exceptional Children, 52*(1), 25–37.

White, B. L. (1975). *The first three years of life*. Englewood Cliffs, N.J.: Prentice-Hall.

White, K. R., Mastropieri, M. A., & Casto, G. (1984). An analysis of special education early-childhood education projects approved by the joint dissemination review panel. *Journal of the Division for Early Childhood Education, 9*, 11–26.

Wilcox, B., & Bellamy, T. (1982). *Design of high school programs for severely handicapped students*. Baltimore: Paul H. Brookes Publishing Co.

Will, M. (1986). Educating children with learning problems: A shared responsibility. *Exceptional Children, 52*, 411–15.

Will, M. (1984). *OSERS programming for the transition of youth with disabilities: Bridges from school to work life*. Washington, D.C.: Position Paper from the Office of Special Education and Rehabilitative Services.

Chapter 4

Abroms, K. I., & Bennett, J. W. (1983). Current findings in Down's syndrome. *Exceptional Children, 49*, 449–50.

Agran, M., Salzberg, C. L., & Stowitchek, J. (1987). An analysis of the effects of a social-skills training program using self-instructions on the acquisition and generalization of two social behaviors in a work setting. *Journal of the Association for Persons with Severe Handicaps, 12*(2), 131–39.

Bailey, D. B., & Wolery, M. (1989). *Assessing infants and preschoolers with handicaps*. Columbus, Ohio: Charles E. Merrill Co.

Batshaw, M. L., & Perret, Y. M. (1986). *Children with handicaps: A medical primer* (2nd ed.). Baltimore: Paul Brookes Publishing Co.

Bellamy, G. T., and Wilcox, B. (1981). Secondary education for severely handicapped students: Guidelines for quality services. In B. Wilcox and A. Thompson (Eds.), *Critical issues in the education of autistic children and youth*. Washington, D. C.: Office of Special Education.

Bensberg, G., and Siegelman, C. (1976). Definitions and prevalence. In

L. Lloyd (Ed.), *Communication, assessment, and intervention strategies*. Baltimore: University Park Press.

Best, J. W., & Kahn, J. V. (1989). *Research in education*. Englewood Cliffs, N.J.: Prentice-Hall, Inc.

Blatt, B. (1987). *The conquest of mental retardation*. Austin, Tex.: Pro-Ed.

Borkowski, J., & Day, J. (1987). *Cognition in special children: Comparative approaches to retardation, learning disabilities, and giftedness*. Norwood, N.J.: Ablex.

Borkowski, J., Peck, V. A., & Damberg, P. R. (1983). Attention, memory, and cognition. In J. L. Matson & J. A. Mulick (Eds.), *Handbook of mental retardation*. New York: Pergamon Press.

Brickey, M. P., Campbell, K. M., & Browning, L. J. (1985). A five-year follow-up of sheltered workshop employees placed in competitive jobs. *Mental Retardation, 20*(2), 52–57.

Brinker, R. P., & Thorpe, M. E. (1977). *Evaluation of severely handicapped students in regular education and community settings*. Princeton, N.J.: Educational Testing Service.

Browder, D. M., & Snell, M. E. (1987). Functional academics. In M. E. Snell (Ed.), *Systematic instruction of persons with severe handicaps* (pp. 436–68), Columbus, Ohio: Charles E. Merrill Co.

Bruininks, R. H. (1977). *Manual for Bruininks-Ostertsky Test of Motor Proficiency*. Circle Pines, Minn.: American Guidance Service, Inc.

Bruininks, R. H., & McGrew, K. (1987). *Exploring the structure of adaptive behavior*. Minneapolis: University Affiliated Program on Developmental Disabilities, University of Minnesota.

Burt, R. A. (1976). Authorizing death for anomalous newborns. In A. Milunsky & G. J. Annas (Eds.), *Genetics and the law*. New York: Plenum Publishing Corporation.

Cromer, R. F. (1974). Receptive language in the mentally retarded: Processes and diagnostic distinctions. In R. L. Schiefelbusch & L. L. Lloyd (Eds.), *Language perspectives—Retardation, acquisition, and intervention*. Baltimore: University Park Press.

Diagnostic and statistical manual of mental disorders, Third Edition Revised (DSM-III-R) (1987). Washington, D.C.: American Psychiatric Association.

Diamond, E. F. (1977). The deformed child's right to life. In D. J. Horan & D. Mall (Eds.), *Death, dying, and euthanasia*. Washington, D. C.: University Publications of America.

Drew, C. J., Logan, D. R., & Hardman, M. L. (1988). *Mental retardation: Life cycle approach* (4th ed.). St. Louis: C. V. Mosby Co.

Duff, R., & Campbell, A. (1973). Moral and ethical dilemmas in the special-care nursery. *New England Journal of Medicine, 289*, 890–94.

Fink, W. (1981). The distribution of clients and their characteristics in programs for the mentally retarded and other developmentally disabled throughout Oregon. Eugene: Oregon Mental Health Division.

Fletcher, G. P. (1968). Legal aspects of the decision not to prolong life. *Journal of the American Medical Association, 203*, 119–22.

Fletcher, J. (1975). Abortion, euthanasia, and care of defective newborns. *New England Journal of Medicine, 292*, 75–78.

Frank, H. S., and Rabinovitch, M. S. (1974). Auditory short-term memory: Developmental changes in rehearsal. *Child Development, 45*, 397–407.

Gentry, D., & Olson, J. (1985). Severely mentally retarded young children. In D. Bricker & J. Filler (Eds.), *Severe mental retardation: From theory to practice* (pp. 50–75). Lancaster, Pa.: Division on Mental Retardation of the Council for Exceptional Children.

Gold, M. W. (1975). Vocational training. In J. Wortis (Ed.), *Mental retardation and developmental disabilities: An annual review* (vol. 7). New York: Brunner/Mazel.

Grossman, H. J. (Ed.) (1973, 1977, 1983, eds.). *Manual on terminology and classification in mental retardation*. Washington, D.C.: American Association on Mental Deficiency.

Hallahan, D. P., & Reeve, R. E. (1980). Selective attention and distractibility. In B. K. Keogh (Ed.), *Advances in special education, Volume 1. Basic constructs and theoretical orientations*. Greenwich, Conn.: JAI Press.

Hardman, M. L., & Drew, C. J. (1978). Life management practices with the profoundly retarded: Issues of euthanasia and withholding treatment. *Mental Retardation, 16*(6), 390–96.

Hardman, M. L. (1984). The role of Congress in decisions related to the withholding of medical treatment from seriously ill newborns. *The Journal of the Association for Persons with Severe Handicaps, 9*(1), 3–7.

Hardman, M. L., and Drew, C. J. (1977). The physically handicapped retarded: A review. *Mental Retardation, 15*(5), 43–48.

Hardman, M. L., and Drew, C. J. (1975). Incidental learning in the mentally retarded: A review. *Education and Training of the Mentally Retarded, 1975, 10*(1), 3–9.

Hardman, M. L., & Drew, C. J. (1980). Parent consent and the practice of withholding treatment from the severely defective newborn. *Mental Retardation, 18,* 165–69.

Hetherington, E. M., & Parke, R. D. (1986). *Child psychology: A contemporary viewpoint* (3rd ed.). New York: McGraw-Hill.

Heber, R. (1961). A manual on terminology and classification in mental retardation (2nd ed.). *American Journal of Mental Deficiency, Monograph Supplement.*

Horan, D. J., & Mall, D. (Eds.) (1977). *Death, dying, and euthanasia.* Washington, D. C.: University Publications of America.

Information about Down's syndrome. (1984). Chicago, Ill.: National Down's Syndrome Congress.

Kaiser, A. P., Alpert, C. L., & Warren, S. (1987). Teaching functional language: Strategies for language intervention. In M. E. Snell (Ed.), *Systematic instruction of persons with severe handicaps* (pp. 247–72). Columbus, Ohio: Charles E. Merrill Co.

Kantrowitz, B., King, P. & Witherspoon, D. (1986, June 22). Help for retarded parents. *Newsweek,* 62.

Kirk, S. A. (1940). *Teaching reading to slow-learning children.* Boston: Houghton Mifflin Co.

Lenneberg, E. H. (1967). *Biological foundations of language.* New York: Wiley.

Lloyd, L. L. (1970). Audiologic aspects of mental retardation. In N. R. Ellis (Ed.), *International review of research in mental retardation* (vol. 4). New York: Academic Press, Inc.

MacMillan, D. L. (1982). *Mental retardation in school and society* (2nd ed.). Boston: Little, Brown & Co.

McDonald, A. C., Carson, K. L., Palmer, D. J., & Slay, T. (1982). Physician's diagnostic information to parents of handicapped neonates. *Mental Retardation, 20*(1), 12–14.

McDonnell, A., & Hardman, M. L. (1989). The desegregation of America's special schools: Strategies for change. *Journal of the Association for Persons with Severe Handicaps, 14*(1) 68–74.

McDonnell, A., & Hardman, M. L. (1988). A synthesis of "best practice" guidelines for early childhood services. *Journal of the Division for Early Childhood, 12*(4), 328–41.

Mercer, C. D., and Snell, M. E. (1977). *Learning-theory research in mental retardation: Implications for teaching.* Columbus, Ohio: Charles E. Merrill Publishing Co.

Miller, J. F. (1981). Early psycholinguistic acquisition. In R. L. Schiefelbusch & D. D. Bricker (Eds.), *Early language: Acquisition and intervention* (pp. 331–37). Baltimore: University Park Press.

Moon, M. S., & Bunker, L. (1987). Recreation and motor skills programming. In M. E. Snell (Ed.), *Systematic instruction of persons with severe handicaps* (3rd ed.) (pp. 214–44). Columbus, Ohio: Charles E. Merrill Co.

Mori, A. A., & Masters, L. F. (1980). *Teaching the severely mentally retarded.* Rockville, Md.: Aspen Systems Corporation.

National Academy of Sciences (1975). *Genetic screening: Programs, principles, and research.* Washington, D. C.: National Academy of Sciences.

Nirje, B. (1970). The normalization principle and its human management implications. *Journal of Mental Subnormality, 16,* 62–70.

Payne, J. S., Polloway, E. A., Smith, J. E., & Payne, R. A. (1981). *Strategies for teaching the mentally retarded* (2nd ed.). Columbus, Ohio: Charles E. Merrill Publishing Co.

Peck, C. A., Apolloni, T., & Cooke, T. P. (1981). Rehabilitation services for Americans with mental retardation: A summary of accomplishments in research and program development. In E. L. Pan, T. E. Backer, & C. L. Vash (Eds.), *Annual Review of Rehabilitation* (vol. 2). New York: Springer-Verlag.

Peterson, N. L. (1987). *Early intervention for handicapped and at-risk children: An introduction to early childhood-special education.* Denver: Love Publishing Co.

Polloway, E. A. (1984). The integration of mildly retarded students in the schools: A historical overview. *Remedial and Special Education, 5*(4), 18–28.

Pomerantz, D., & Marholin, D. (1977). Vocational habilitation: A time for change. In E. Sontag (Ed.), *Educational programming for the severely and profoundly handicapped.* Reston, Va.: Council for Exceptional Children, Division on Mental Retardation.

President's Commission for the Study of Ethical Problems in Medicine and Biomedical and Behavioral Research (1983a). *Securing access to health care.* Washington, D.C.: U.S. Government Printing Office.

President's Commission for the Study of Ethical Problems in Medicine and Biomedical and Behavioral Research (1983b). *Screening and counseling for genetic conditions.* Washington, D.C.: U.S. Government Printing Office.

Ramsey, P. (1973). Abortion. *Thomist, 37,* 174–226.

Rantakallio, P., & von Wendt, L. (1986). Mental retardation and subnormality in a birth cohort of 12,000 children in Northern Finland. *American Journal of Mental Deficiency, 90,* 380–87.

Robertson, J. A. (1975). Involuntary euthanasia of defective newborns: A legal analysis. *Stanford Law Review, 27,* 213–69.

Robinson, N. M., & Robinson, H. B. (1976). *The mentally retarded child: A psychological approach* (2nd ed.). New York: McGraw-Hill Book Co.

Schutz, R. P., Williams, W., Iverson, G. S., & Duncan, D. (1984). Social integration of severely handicapped students. In N. Certo, N. Haring, & R. York (Eds.), *Public school integration of severely handicapped students: Rational issues and progressive alternatives* (pp. 15–42). Baltimore, Md.: Paul H. Brookes Publishing Co.

Shaw, A. (1977). Dilemmas of "informed consent" in children. In D. J. Horan & D. Mall (Eds.), *Death, dying, and euthanasia.* Washington, D. C.: University Publications of America.

Stainback, S., and Stainback, W. (1982). Influencing the attitudes of regular class teachers about the education of severely retarded students. *Education and Training of the Mentally Retarded, 17*(2), 88–92.

Stainback, S., & Stainback, W. (1985). *Integration of students with severe handicaps into regular schools.* Reston, Va.: Council for Exceptional Children.

State of Iowa Department of Public Instruction (1981). *Assessment, documentation, and programming for adaptive behavior: An Iowa Task Force Report.* Des Moines: The Department.

Stroud, M., & Sutton, E. (1988). *Expanding options for older adults with developmental disabilities.* Baltimore: Paul H. Brooks.

U.S. Congress (1975). Education of All Handicapped Children Act, Public Law 94–142.

U.S. Department of Education (1989). To assure the free appropriate public education of all handicapped children. *Eleventh Annual Report to Congress on the Implementation of the Education of the Handicapped Act.* Washington, D.C.: U.S. Government Printing Office.

Van Riper, C. (1972). *Speech corrections: Principles and methods* (5th ed.). Englewood Cliffs, N.J.: Prentice-Hall, Inc.

Voeltz, L. M. (1982). Effects of structured interactions with severely handicapped peers on children's attitudes. *American Journal on Mental Deficiency, 86,* 380–90.

Wehman, P., & Hill, J. W. (1985). *Competitive employment for persons with mental retardation: From research to practice* (vol. 1). Richmond, Va.: Rehabilitation Research and Training Center, Virginia Commonwealth University.

Wehman, P., & Hill, J. (1982). Preparing severely handicapped youth for less restrictive environments. *The Journal of the Association for the Severely Handicapped, 7*(1), 33–39.

Westling, D. (1986). *Introduction to mental retardation.* Englewood Cliffs, N.J.: Prentice-Hall, Inc.

Wilcox, B., & Bellamy, T. (1982). *Design of high school programs for severely handicapped students.* Baltimore: Paul H. Brookes Publishers.

Williams, G. L. (1966). Euthanasia and abortion. *University of Colorado Law Review, 38,* 181–87.

Zigler, E., & Balla, D. (1981). Issues in personality and motivation of mentally retarded persons. In M. J. Begab, H. C. Haywood, & H. L.

Garber (Eds.), *Psychosocial influences in retarded performance: Vol. 1, Issues and theories in development*. Baltimore: University Park Press.

Chapter 5

Achenbach, T. M. (1966). The classification of children's psychiatric symptoms: A factor analytic study. *Psychological Monographs: General and Applied, 615,* 1–37.

Achenbach, T. M. (1980). The DSM-II classification of psychiatric disorders of infancy, childhood, and adolescence. *Journal of the American Academy of Child Psychiatry, 19,* 395–412.

Achenbach, T. M., & Edelbrock, C. S. (1980). *Child behavior checklist—Teacher's report form*. Burlington: University of Vermont, Center of Children, Youth, and Families.

Achenbach, T. M., & Edelbrock, C. S. (1981). Behavioral problems and competencies reported by parents of normal and disturbed children aged 4 through 16. *Monographs of the Society for Research in Child Development, 46* (Serial No. 188).

Achenbach, T. M., & Edelbrock, C. S. (1981). *Child behavior checklist for ages 4–16*. Burlington: University of Vermont.

Ackerson, L. (1942). *Children's behavior problems*. Chicago: University of Chicago Press.

American Psychiatric Association (1980). *Diagnostic and Statistical Manual of Mental Disorders* (3rd Ed.). Washington, D.C.: The Association.

American Psychiatric Association (1987). *Diagnostic and Statistical Manual of Mental Disorders (3rd Ed. Revised)*. Washington, D.C.: The Association.

Amish, P. L., Gesten, E. L., Smith, J. K., Clark, H. B., & Stark, C. (1988). Social problem-solving training for severely emotionally disturbed and behaviorally disordered children. *Behavior Disorders, 13*(3), 175–86.

Associated Press News Service (1989, June 11). Children and mental illness.

Barkley, R. A. (1985). Attention deficit disorder. In P. H. Bornstein & A. E. Kazdin (Eds.), *Handbook of clinical behavior therapy with children*. Homewood, Ill.: Dorsey Press.

Begley, S., & Fitzgerald, K. (1986, September 1). Freud should have tried barking. *Newsweek,* 65.

Benson, D., Edwards, L., Roseel, J., & White, M. (1986). Inclusion of socially maladjusted children and youth in legal definition of the behaviorally disordered population: A debate. *Behavior Disorders, 11*(3), 213–22.

Bower, E. M. (1959). The emotionally handicapped child and the school. *Exceptional Children, 26,* 6–11.

Bower, E. M. (1981). *Early Identification of emotionally handicapped children in the school* (3rd Ed.). Springfield, Ill.: Charles C. Thomas.

Bower, E. M. (1982). Defining emotional disturbance: Public policy and research. *Psychology in the Schools, 19,* 55–60.

Bower, E. M., & Lambert, N. M. (1962). *A process for in-school screening of children with emotional handicaps*. Princeton, N.J.: Educational Testing Service.

Bower, E. M. (1982). Defining emotional disturbance: Public policy and research. *Psychology in the Schools, 19,* 55–60.

Brown, G., McDowell, R. L., & Smith, J. (1981). *Educating adolescents with behavior disorders*. Columbus, Ohio: Charles E. Merrill Publishing Company.

Brown, R. T., Wynne, M. E., & Medenis, R. (1985). Methylphenidate and cognitive therapy: A comparison of treatment approaches with hyperactive boys. *Journal of Abnormal Child Psychology, 13,* 69–87.

Browne, A., & Finkelhor, D. (1986). Impact of child sexual abuse: A review of research. *Psychological Bulletin, 99,* 66–77.

Burks, H. F. (1977). *Burk's behavior rating scales, preschool and kindergarten edition, administration booklet*. Los Angeles: Western Psychological Services.

Center, D. B. (1986). Educational programming for children and youth with behavior disorders. *Behavior Disorders, 11*(3), 208–11.

Children's Defense Fund (1989). *A vision for America's future: An agenda for the 1990s*. Washington, D.C.: The Fund.

Clarizio, H. F., & McCoy, G. (1976). *Behavior disorders in children* (2nd Ed.). New York: Thomas Y. Crowell Co.

Coleman, M. C. (1986). *Behavior disorders: Theory and Practice*. Englewood Cliffs, N.J.: Prentice-Hall.

Coutinho, M. (1986). Reading achievement of students identified as behaviorally disordered at the secondary level. *Behavior Disorders, 11*(3), 200–207.

Cullinan, D., & Epstein, M. H. (1986). Behavior disorders. In N. Haring (Ed.), *Exceptional Children and Youth* (4th Ed.). Columbus, Ohio: Merrill.

D'Alonzo, B. J. (Ed.) (1983). *Educating adolescents with learning and behavioral problems*. Rockville, Md.: Aspen Systems Corporation.

Dick, M. (1987). Translating vocational assessment information into transition objectives and instruction. *Career development for exceptional individuals, 10*(2), 76–84.

Douglas, V. I., Barr, R. G., O'Neill, M. E., Britton, B. G. (1986). Short-term effects of methylphenidate on the cognitive, learning, and academic performance of children with attention deficit disorder in the laboratory and the classroom. *Journal of Child Psychology and Psychiatry, 27,* 191–211.

Emery, R. E., Hetherington, E. M., & DiLalla, L. F. (1984). Divorce, children, and social policy. In H. W. Stevenson & A. E. Siegel (Eds.), *Child development research and social policy* (Vol. 1). Chicago: University of Chicago Press.

Epstein, M. H., & Olinger, E. (1987). Use of medication in school programs for behaviorally disordered pupils. *Behavior Disorders, 12*(2), 138–45.

Executive committee for the Council for Children with Behavior Disorders (1987). Position paper on definition and identification of students with behavior disorders. *Behavior Disorders, 13*(1), 9–19.

Fiedler, J. F., & Knight, R. P. (1986). Congruence between assessed needs and IEP goals of identified behaviorally disabled students. *Behavior Disorders, 12*(1), 22–27.

Forness, S. R. (1988). Planning for the needs of children with serious emotional disturbance: The national special education and mental health coalition. *Behavior Disorders, 13*(2), 127–33.

Freeman, B. M., & Ritvo, E. R. (1984). The syndrome of autism: Establishing the diagnosis and principles of management. *Pediatric Annals, 13,* 284–96.

Gelfand, D. M., Jenson, W. R., & Drew, C. J. (1982). *Understanding child behavior disorders*. New York: Holt, Rinehart, & Winston.

Gelfand, D. M., Jenson, W. R., & Drew, C. J. (1988). *Understanding child behavior disorders*. (2nd ed.). New York: Holt, Rinehart, and Winston.

Gittelman-Klien, R., & Klein, D. F. (1987). Pharmacotherapy of childhood hyperactivity: An update. In H. Y. Meltzer (Ed.), *Psychopharmacology: The third generation of progress*. New York: Raven.

Greenan, J. P. (1985). Networking needs in vocational/special education. *Interchange, Office of Career Development for Special Populations*. Champaign, Ill.: National Network for Professional Development in Vocational Special Education, College of Education, University of Illinois at Urbana-Champaign.

Greenhill, L., Puig-Antich, J., Novacenko, H. H., Solomon, M., Anghern, C., Floreas, J., Goetz, R., Fiscina, B., & Sachar, E. (1984). Prolactin, growth hormone, and growth responses in boys with attention deficit disorder. *Journal of the American Academy of Child Psychiatry, 23,* 58–67.

Gropper, G., Kress, G., Hughes, R., & Pekich, J. (1968). Training teachers to recognize and manage social and emotional problems in the classroom. *Journal of Teacher Education, 19,* 477–85.

Gualtieri, C., Wargin, W., Kanoy, F., Patrick, K., Shen, C., Youngblood, W., Mueller, R., & Breese, G. (1982). Clinical studies of methylphenidate serum levels in children and adults. *Journal of the American Academy of Child Psychiatry, 21,* 19–26.

Guidubaldi, J., Perry, J. D., & Cleminshaw, H. K. (1984). The legacy of parental divorce: A nationwide study of family status and selected mediating variables on children's academic and social competencies. In B. B. Lahey & A. E. Kazdin (Eds.), *Advances in clinical child psychology* (Vol. 7). New York: Plenum.

Haley, J. (1963). Marriage therapy. *Archives of General Psychiatry, 8,* 213–24.

Harris, S. L. (1979). DSM-III—Its implications for children. *Child behavior therapy, 1,* 37–48.

Hechtman, L., Weiss, G., & Perlman, T. (1984). Young adult outcome of hyperactive children who received long-term stimulant treatment. *Journal of the American Academy of Child Psychiatry, 23,* 261–69.

Hewitt, L. E., & Jenkins, R. L. (1946). *Fundamental patterns of maladjustment: The dynamics of their origin.* Springfield: State of Illinois.

Hobbs, N. (1965). How the Re-ED plan developed. In N. J. Long, W. C. Morse, & R. G. Newman (Eds.), *Conflict in the classroom.* Belmont, Cal.: Wadsworth.

Jones, V. F. (1980). *Adolescents with behavior problems: Strategies for teaching, counseling, and parent involvement* (Abridged Ed.). Boston: Allyn and Bacon.

Karnes, M. B., & Zehrbach, R. R. (1979). Alternative models for delivering services to young handicapped children. In J. B. Jordan, A. H. Hayden, M. B. Karnes, & M. M. Wood (Eds.), *Early childhood education for exceptional children* (pp. 20–65). Reston, Va.: The Council for Exceptional Children.

Kauffman, J. M. (1977). *Characteristics of children's behavior disorders.* Columbus, Ohio: Charles E. Merrill Publishing Co.

Kauffman, J. M. (1982). Social policy issues in special education and related services for emotionally disturbed children and youth. In M. M. Noel & N. G. Haring (Eds.), *Progress or change: Issues in educating the emotionally disturbed,* Vol. 1, *Identification and program planning.* Seattle: University of Washington.

Kauffman, J. M. (1985). *Characteristics of children's behavior disorders* (3rd Ed.). Columbus, Ohio: Charles E. Merrill Publishing Co.

Kauffman, J. M. (1987). Strategies for the nonrecognition of social deviance. *Journal of Special Education, 11*(3), 201–14.

Kavale, K. A., Forness, S. R., & Alper, A. E. (1986). Research in behavioral disorders/emotional disturbance: A survey of subject indentification criteria. *Behavior Disorders, 11*(3), 159–67.

Kazdin, A. E. (1985). *Treatment of antisocial behavior in children and adolescents.* Homewood, Ill.: Dorsey Press.

Kelly, T. K., Bullock, L. M., & Dykes, M. K. (1977). Behavioral disorders: Teachers' perceptions. *Exceptional Children, 43*(5), 316–17.

Klein, D., Gittelman, R., Quitkin, F., & Rifkin, A. (1980). Diagnosis and treatment of childhood disorders. In D. S. Kleine; J. M. Davis (Eds.), *Diagnosis and drug treatment of psychiatric disorders (2nd ed.).* Baltimore, Md.: Williams and Wilkins.

Long, N. J., Fagen, S., & Stevens, D. (1971). *Psychoeducational screening system for identifying resourceful, marginal, and vulnerable pupils in the primary grades.* Washington, D. C.: Psychoeducational Resources.

Mattes, J., & Gittelman, R. (1983). Growth of hyperactive children on a maintenance regimen of methylphenidate. *Archives of General Psychiatry, 40,* 317–21.

McGinnis, E., Goldstein, A. P., Sprafkin, R. P., & Gershaw, N. J. (1984). *Skill-streaming the elementary school child: A guide for teaching prosocial skills.* Champaign, Ill.: Research Press Company.

McLeMore, C. W., & Benjamin, L. S. (1979). What ever happened in interpersonal diagnosis? A psychosocial alternative to the DSM-III. *American Psychologist, 17,* 17–34.

Miller, S. R. (1978). Career and vocational education: The necessity for a planned future. In D. A. Sabatino & A. J. Mauser (Eds.), *Intervention strategies for specialized secondary education.* Boston: Allyn and Bacon, Inc.

Miller, S. R., Sabatino, D. A., & Larsen, R. P. (1980). Issues in the professional preparation of secondary school special educators. *Exceptional Children, 46,* 344–50.

Minuchin, S. (1974). *Families and family therapy.* Cambridge, Mass.: Harvard University Press.

Morgan, D. P., & Jenson, W. R. (1988). *Teaching behaviorally disordered students.* Columbus, Ohio: Merrill Publishing Company.

Morse, W. C., Cutler, R. L., & Fink, A. H. (1964). *Public school classes for the emotionally handicapped: A research analysis.* Washington, D.C.: Council for Exceptional Children.

Newcomer, P. L. (1980). *Understanding and teaching emotionally disturbed children.* Boston: Allyn and Bacon, Inc.

O'Donnel, L. (1980). Intraindividual discrepancy in diagnosing specific learning disabilities. *Learning Disability Quarterly, 3*(1), 10–18.

Olson, J., Algozzine, B., & Schmid, R. E. (1980). Mild, moderate, and severe: An empty distinction. *Behavior Disorders, 5*(2), 96–101.

Patterson, G. R. (1982). *Coercive family process.* Eugene, Ore.: Castalia.

Patterson, G. R., & Bank, L. (1986). Bootstrapping your way in the nomological thicket. *Behavioral Assessment, 8,* 49–73.

Peterson, D. R. (1961). Behavior problems of middle childhood. *Journal of consulting psychology, 25,* 205–9.

Peterson, N. L. (1987). *Early intervention for handicapped and at-risk children: An introduction to early childhood special education.* Denver: Love Publishing Company.

Pollard, S., Ward, E. M., & Barkley, R. A. (1984). The effects of parent training and Ritalin on the parent–child interactions of hyperactive boys. *Child and Family Behavior Therapy, 5*(4), 51–69.

Polsgrove, L. (1977). Self-control: An overview of concepts and methods for child training. Paper delivered at the Advanced Training Institute for Teacher Trainers of Seriously Emotionally Disturbed Children, Minneapolis, Minn.

Porrino, L., Rapoport, J., Behar, D., Ismond, D., & Bunney, W. (1983). A naturalistic assessment of the motor activity of hyperactive boys, II, Stimulant drug effects. *Archives of General Psychiatry, 40,* 688–93.

Quay, H. C. (1972). Patterns of aggression, withdrawal, and immaturity. In H. C. Quay & J. S. Werry (Eds.), *Psychopathological disorders of childhood.* New York: John Wiley & Sons.

Quay, H. C. (1975). Classification in the treatment of delinquency and antisocial behavior. In N. Hobbs (Ed.), *Issues in the classification of children.* Vol. 1. San Francisco: Jossey-Bass.

Quay, H. C. (1979). Classification. In H. C. Quay & J. S. Werry (Eds.), *Psychopathological disorders of childhood* (2nd Ed.). New York: Wiley.

Quay, H. C., Morse, W. C., & Cutler, R. L. (1966). Personality patterns of pupils in special classes for the emotionally disturbed. *Exceptional Children, 32,* 297–301.

Radl, S. (1976). Why you are shy and hope to cope with it. *Glamour,* 64–84.

Ramsey, E., & Walker, H. M. (1988). Family management correlates of antisocial behavior among middle school boys. *Behavior Disorders, 13*(3), 187–201.

Redick, R. (1973). *Utilization of psychiatric facilities by persons under 18 years of age.* Washington, D. C.: U.S. Department of Health, Education, and Welfare.

Rubin, R. A., & Balow, B. (1978). Prevalence of teacher identified behavior problems: A longitudinal study. *Exceptional Children, 45,* 102–11.

Rizzo, J. V., & Zabel, R. H. (1988). *Educating children and adolescents with behavior disorders.* Boston: Allyn and Bacon, Inc.

Rosenburg, S. R. (1986). Maximizing the effectiveness of structured classroom management programs: Implementing rule-review procedures with disruptive and distractible students. *Behavior Disorders, 11*(4), 239–48.

Ross, D. M., & Ross, S. A. (1982). *Hyperactivity: Current issues, research, and theory.* New York: Wiley.

Safer, D. J., & Heaton, R. C. (1982). Characteristics, school pattern, and behavioral outcome of seriously disruptive junior high school students. In D. J. Safer (Ed.), *School programs for disruptive adolescents.* Baltimore: University Park Press.

Sandler, A. G., Arnold, L. B., Gable, R. A., & Strain, P. S. (1987). Effects of peer pressure on disruptive behavior of behaviorally disordered classmates. *Behavior Disorders, 12*(2), 104–10.

Satir, V. (1967). *Conjoint family therapy: A guide.* Palo Alto, Cal.: Science and Behavior Books.

Schacht, T., & Nathan, P. E. (1977). But is it good for psychologists? Appraisal and status of the DSM-III. *American Psychologist, 32,* 1017–25.

Schloss, P. J., Schloss, C. N., Wood, C. E., & Kiehl, W. S. (1986). A critical review of social skills with behaviorally disordered students. *Behavior Disorders, 12*(1), 1–14.

Schultz, E. W., Hirshoren, A., Manton, A. B., & Henderson, R. A. (1971). Special education for the emotionally disturbed. *Exceptional Children, 38,* 313–19.

Schultz, E., Salvia, J., & Feinn, J. (1974). Prevalence of behavior symptoms in rural elementary school children. *Journal of Abnormal Child Psychology, 1,* 17–24.

Scruggs, T. E., Mastropieri, M. A., Cook, S. B., & Escobar, C. (1986). Early intervention for children with conduct disorders: A qualitative synthesis of single-subject research. *Behavior Disorders, 11*(4), 260–71.

Shea, T. M., & Bauer, A. M. (1987). *Teaching children and youth with behavior disorders.* Englewood Cliffs, N.J.: Prentice-Hall.

Simpson, R. L. (1987). Social interaction of behaviorally disordered children and youth: Where are we and where do we need to go? *Behavior Disorders, 12*(4), 292–98.

Slate, J. R., & Saudargas, R. A. (1986). Differences in the classroom behaviors of behaviorally disordered and regular class children. *Behavior Disorders, 12*(1), 45–53.

Slavson, S. R., & Shiffer, M. (1975). *Group psychotherapies for children: A textbook.* New York: International Universities Press.

Smith, C. R. (1985). Identification of handicapped children and youth: A state agency perspective on behavior disorders. *Remedial and special education, 6*(4), 34–41.

Spivack, G., & Spotts, J. (1966). *Devereaux Child Behavior (DCB) Rating Scale.* Devon, Pa.: Devereaux Foundation.

Spivack, G., & Swift, M. (1967). *Devereaux Elementary School Behavior Rating Scale.* Devon, Pa.: Devereaux Foundation.

Spivack, G., Spotts, J., & Haimes, P. E. (1967). *Devereaux Adolescent Behavior (DAB) Rating Scale.* Devon Pa.: Devereaux Foundation.

Stainback, S., & Stainback, W. (1980). *Educating children with severe maladaptive behaviors.* New York: Grune & Stratton.

Stone, F., & Rowley, V. N. (1964). Educational disability in emotionally disturbed children. *Exceptional Children, 30,* 423–26.

Stroufe, L. A. (1975). Drug treatment with children with behavior problems. In F. Horowitz (Ed.), *Review of child development research Vol. 4.* Chicago: University of Chicago Press.

Sullivan, R. C. (1979). Siblings of autistic children. *Journal of autism and developmental disorders, 9*(3), 287–97.

Swartz, S. L., Mosley, W. J., Koenig-Jerz, G. (1987). *Diagnosing behavior disorders: An analysis of eligibility criteria and recommended procedures.* Paper presented at the Annual Convention of the Council for Exceptional Children, Chicago, Ill.

Swift, M. S., & Spivack, G. (1973). Academic success and classroom behavior in secondary schools. *Exceptional children, 30,* 392–99.

Tamkin, A. S. (1960). A survey of educational disability in emotionally disturbed children. *Journal of educational research, 53,* 313–15.

Towns, P. (1981). *Educating disturbed adolescents: Theory and practice.* New York: Grune & Stratton.

U.S. Office of Education (1975). *Estimated number of handicapped children in the United States, 1974–75.* Washington, D. C.: Office.

U.S. Department of Education (1989). To assure the free appropriate public education of all handicapped children. *Eleventh Annual Report to Congress on the Implementation of The Education of the Handicapped Act.* Washington, D. C.: Division of Educational Services, Special Education Programs.

U.S. Department of Health, Education, and Welfare (1977). Education of Handicapped Children (Implementation of Part B of the Education of the Handicapped Act). *Federal Register,* August 23, 1977, 42478.

Von Isser, A., Quay, H. C., and Love, C. T. (1980). Interrelationships among three measures of deviant behavior. *Exceptional Children, 46,* 272–76.

Vorrath, H., & Brendtro, L. K. (1974). *Positive peer culture.* Chicago: Aldine Press.

Walker, H. M. (1983). *Walker problem behavior identification checklist, revised 1983.* Los Angeles: Western Psychological Services.

Weinstein, L. (1969). Project Re-ED schools for emotionally disturbed children: Effectiveness as viewed by referring agencies, parents, and teachers. *Exceptional Children, 35,* 703–11.

Weiss, G. (1979). Controlled studies of efficacy of long-term treatment with stimulants of hyperactive children. In E. Denhoff & L. Stern (Eds.), *Minimal brain dysfunction.* New York: Masson Publishing.

Whalen, C., Henker, B., & Dotemoto, S. (1981). Teacher response to the methylphenidate (Ritalin) versus placebo status of hyperactive boys in the classroom. *Child Development, 52,* 1005–14.

Whalen, C., Henker, B., & Fink, D. (1980). Medication effects in the classroom: Three naturalistic indicators. *Journal of Abnormal Child Psychology, 9,* 419–33.

Whalen, C. K. (1983). Hyperactivity, learning problems, and attention deficit disorders. In T. H. Ollendick & M. Herson (Eds.), *Handbook of child psychopathology.* New York: Plenum.

Whalen, C. K., & Henker, B. (1976). Psychostimulants and children. *Psychological Bulletin, 83,* 1113–30.

Whelan, R. J. (1981). Prologue. In G. Brown, R. L. McDowell, & J. Smith (Eds.), *Educating adolescents with behavior disorders.* Columbus, Ohio: Charles E. Merrill Publishing Company.

Wicks-Nelson, R., & Israel, A. C. (1984). *Behavior disorders of childhood.* Englewood Cliffs, N.J.: Prentice-Hall, Inc.

Chapter 6

Achenbach, T. M. (1986). How is a parent rating scale used in the diagnosis of attention deficit disorder? *Journal of Children in Contemporary Society, 19,* 19–31.

Ackerman, P. T., Anhalt, B. S., & Dykman, R. A. (1986). Arithmetic automation failure in children with attention and reading disorders. *Journal of Learning Disabilities, 19,* 222–32.

Agrawal, R., & Kaushal, K. (1987). Attention and short-term memory in normal children, aggressive children, and nonaggressive children with attention deficit disorder. *Journal of General Psychology, 114,* 335–44.

Aman, M. G., & Turbott, S. H. (1986). Incidental learning, distraction, and sustained attention in hyperactive and control subjects. *Journal of Abnormal Child Psychology, 14,* 441–55.

American Psychiatric Association, *Diagnostic and statistical manual of mental disorders* (Third Edition Revised) (1987). Washington, D.C.: The Association.

Anderson, R. C., Hiebert, E. H., Scott, J. A., & Wilkinson, I. A. G. (1985). *Becoming a nation of readers.* Washington, D.C.: National Institute of Education.

Associated Press News Service (1989, June 3). 750,000 children take stimulants researchers say.

August, G. J. (1987). Production deficiencies in free recall: A comparison of hyperactive, learning-disabled, and normal children. *Journal of Abnormal Child Psychology, 15,* 429–40.

Bateman, B. D. (1965). An educator's view of a diagnostic approach to learning disorders. In J. Hellmuth (Ed.), *Learning disorders* (Vol. 1). Seattle: Special Child Publications.

Baxley, G. B., & LeBlanc, J. M. (1976). The hyperactive child: Characteristics, treatment, and evaluation of research design. In H. Reese (Ed.), *Advances in child development and behavior* (Vol. 11). New York: Academic Press.

Benton, A. L., & Pearl, D. (Eds.) (1978). *Dyslexia: An appraisal of current knowledge.* New York: Oxford University Press.

Bos, C. S., & Filip, D. (1984). Comprehension monitoring in learning-disabled and average students. *Journal of Learning Disabilities, 17,* 229–33.

Bransford, J. D., Stein, B. S., Nye, M. J., Franks, J. F., Auble, P. M., Mezynski, K. J., & Perfetto, G. A. (1982). Differences in approach to learning: An overview. *Journal of Experimental Psychology: General, 3,* 390–98.

Brown, L. (1986). Assessing socioemotional development. In D. D. Hammill (Ed.), *Assessing the abilities and instructional needs of students* (pp. 502–609). Austin, Tex.: Pro-Ed.

Choate, J. S., & Rakes, T. A. (1989). *Reading: Detecting and correcting special needs.* Boston: Allyn and Bacon, Inc.

Conners, C. K. (1986). How is a teacher rating scale used in the diagnosis of attention deficit disorder? *Journal of Children in Contemporary Society, 19,* 33–52.

Connolly, A. J. (1985). *KeyMath teach and practice.* Circle Pines, Minn.: American Guidance Service.

Coons, H. W., Klorman, R., & Borgstedt, A. D. (1987). Effects of methylphenidate on adolescents with a childhood history of attention deficit disorder. *Journal of the American Academy of Child & Adolescent Psychiatry, 26,* 368–74.

Cotugno, A. J. (1987). Cognitive control functioning in hyperactive and nonhyperactive learning-disabled children. *Journal of Learning Disabilities, 20,* 563–7.

Cruickshank, W. M. (1972). Some issues facing the field of learning disability. *Journal of Learning Disabilities, 5,* 380–88.

Davidson, J. (1969). *Using the Cuisenaire rods.* New Rochelle, N.Y.: Cuisenaire.

deHaas, P. A. (1986). Attention styles and peer relationships of hyperactive and normal boys and girls. *Journal of Abnormal Child Psychology*, 14, 457–67.

Deloach, T. F., Earl, J. M., Brown, B. S., Poplin, M. S., & Warner, M. M. (1981). LD teachers' perceptions of severely learning-disabled students. *Learning Disability Quarterly*, 4(4), 343–58.

Deshler, D. D., & Schumaker, J. B. (1983). Social skills of learning-disabled adolescents: Characteristics and interventions. *Topics in Learning and Learning Disabilities*, 3(2), 15–23.

Deshler, D. D., Schumaker, J. B., & Lenz, B. K. (1984). Academic and cognitive interventions for LD adolescents: Part I. *Journal of Learning Disabilities*, 17, 108–17.

Deshler, D. D., Schumaker, J. B., Lenz, B. K., & Ellis, E. (1984). Academic and cognitive interventions for LD adolescents: Part II. *Journal of Learning Disabilities*, 17, 170–79.

Draeger, S., Prior, M., & Sanson, A. (1986). Visual and auditory attention performance in hyperactive children: Competence or compliance. *Journal of Abnormal Child Psychology*, 14, 411–24.

Drew, C. J., Logan, D. R., & Hardman, M. L. (1988). *Mental retardation: A life cycle approach* (4th ed.). Columbus, Ohio: Merrill Publishing Co.

Dudley-Marling, C., & Edmiaston, R. (1985). Social status of learning-disabled children and adolescents: A review. *Learning Disability Quarterly*, 8, 189–204.

Dudley-Marling, C., & Searle, D. (1988). Enriching language learning environments for students with learning disabilities. *Journal of Learning Disabilities*, 21, 140–43.

Engelmann, S., & Carnine, D. (1972). *DISTAR arithmetic*. Chicago: Science Research Associates.

Engelmann, S., & Carnine, D. (1982). *Corrective mathematics program*. Chicago: Science Research Associates.

Englert, C. S., & Palincsar, A. S. (1988). The reading process. In D. K. Reid (Ed.), *Teaching the learning disabled: A cognitive developmental approach* (pp. 162–89). Boston: Allyn and Bacon, Inc.

Englert, C. S., & Thomas, C. C. (1987). Sensitivity to text structure in reading and writing: A comparison of learning-disabled and nondisabled students. *Learning Disabilities Quarterly*, 10, 93–105.

Enright, B. E. (1989). *Basic mathematics: Detecting and correcting special needs*. Boston: Allyn and Bacon, Inc.

Fair, G. W. (1988). Mathematics instruction in junior and senior high school. In D. K. Reid (Ed.), *Teaching the learning disabled: A cognitive developmental approach* (pp. 378–415). Boston: Allyn and Bacon, Inc.

Finch, A. J., Jr., & Spirito, A. (1980). Use of cognitive training to change cognitive processes. *Exceptional Education Quarterly*, 1, 31–39.

Fleener, F. T. (1987). Learning disabilities and other attributes as factors in delinquent activities among adolescents in a nonurban area. *Psychological Reports*, 60, 327–34.

Fuchs, D., & Fuchs, L. S. (1986). Test procedure bias: A meta-analysis of examiner familiarity effects. *Review of Educational Research*, 56, 243–62.

Gaddes, W. H. (1985). *Learning disabilities and brain function: A neuropsychological approach* (2nd ed.). New York: Springer-Verlag.

Gartner, A., & Lipsky, D. K. (1989). Equity and excellence for all students. *The education of students with disabilities: Where do we stand?* Briefing paper for testimony given at hearings conducted by the National Council on the Handicapped, June 7 and 8, 1989, Washington, D. C.

Gelfand, D. M., Jenson, W. R., & Drew, C. J. (1988). *Understanding child behavior disorders* (2nd ed.) New York: Holt, Rinehart, and Winston.

Gerber, M. M. (1985). Spelling as concept-driven problem solving. In B. Hutson (Ed.), *Advances in reading/language research* (Vol. 3, pp. 39–75). Greenwich, Conn.: JAI Press.

Gerber, M. M. (1986). Generalization of spelling strategies by LD students as a result of contingent imitation/modeling and mastery criteria. *Journal of Learning Disabilities*, 19, 530–37.

Goldstein, D., & Myers, B. (1980). Cognitive lag and group differences in intelligence. *Child Study Journal*, 10(2), 119–32.

Gordon, M. (1986). How is a computerized attention test used in the diagnosis of attention deficit disorder? *Journal of Children in Contemporary Society*, 19, 53–64.

Gottfredson, L. S., Finucci, J. M., & Childs, B. (1984). Explaining the adult careers of dyslexic boys. *Journal of Vocational Behavior*, 24, 355–73.

Griffith, P. L., Ripich, D. N., & Dastoli, S. L. (1986). Story structure, cohesion, and propositions in story recall by learning-disabled and nondisabled children. *Journal of Psycholinguistic Research*, 15, 539–55.

Grinnell, P. C. (1988). Teaching handwriting and spelling. In D. K. Reid (Ed.), *Teaching the learning disabled: A cognitive developmental approach* (pp. 245–78). Boston: Allyn and Bacon, Inc.

Gronlund, N. E. (1985). *Measurement and evaluation in teaching* (5th ed.) New York: Macmillan Publishing Co., Inc.

Hall, R. J. (1980). Cognitive behavior modification and information-processing skills of exceptional children. *Exceptional Education Quarterly*, 1, 9–15.

Hallahan, D. P., & Kauffman, J. M. (1976). *Introduction to learning disabilities: A psychobehavioral approach*. Englewood Cliffs, N.J.: Prentice-Hall, Inc.

Hallahan, D. P., Kauffman, J. M., & Lloyd, J. W. (1985). *Introduction to learning disabilities* (2nd ed.). Englewood Cliffs, N.J.: Prentice-Hall, Inc.

Hallgren, B. (1950). Specific dyslexia ("congenital word blindness"): A clinical and genetic study. *Acta Psychiatrica et Neurologica*, 65, 1–279.

Hamlett, K. W., Pellegrini, D. S., & Conners, C. K. (1987). An investigation of executive processes in the problem solving of attention deficit disorder-hyperactive children. *Journal of Pediatric Psychology*, 12, 227–40.

Hammill, D. D., Leigh, J. E., McNutt, G., & Larsen, S. C. (1981). A new definition of learning disabilities. *Learning Disability Quarterly*, 4(4), 336–42.

Harste, J. C., Burke, C. L., & Woodward, V. A. (1981). *Children, their language and world: Initial encounters with print*. Bloomington: Indiana University.

Healy, J. M., & Aram, D. M. (1986). Hyperlexia and dyslexia: A family study. *Annals of Dyslexia*, 36, 237–52.

Hermann, K. (1959). *Reading disability: A medical study of word-blindness and related handicaps*. Springfield, Ill.: Charles C. Thomas.

Houck, C. K. (1984). *Learning disabilities: Understanding concepts, characteristics, and issues*. Englewood Cliffs, N.J.: Prentice-Hall, Inc.

Idol, L. (Ed.) (1988). *Grace Fernald's remedial techniques in basic school subjects*. Austin, Tex.: Pro-Ed.

Idol-Maestas, L., Lloyd, S., & Lilly, S. (1981). A noncategorical approach to direct service and teacher education. *Exceptional Children*, 48, 213–20.

Johnston, R. B. (1987). *Learning disabilities, medicine, and myth: A guide to understanding the child and the physician*. Boston: Little, Brown and Co.

Kavale, K., & Nye, C. (1981). Identification criteria for learning disabilities: A survey of the research literature. *Learning Disability Quarterly*, 4(4), 383–88.

Kaluger, G., & Kolson, C. J. (1978). *Reading and learning disabilities* (2nd ed.). Columbus, Ohio: Charles E. Merrill.

Kelman, J. (1983, April). Can't read, write, or add. *Glamour*, 142–46.

Kirk, S. A. (1963). Behavioral diagnosis and remediation of learning disabilities. *Proceedings, Conference on Exploration into the Problems of the Perceptually Handicapped* (Vol. 1). First Annual Meeting, Chicago.

Kirk, S. A., & Chalfant, J. C. (1984). *Academic and developmental learning disabilities*. Denver: Love Publishing Co.

Kramer, J. R. (1986). Where are hyperactive children as young adults? *Journal of Children in Contemporary Society*, 19, 89–98.

la Greca, A. M. (1987). Children with learning disabilities: Interpersonal skills and social competence. *Journal of Reading, Writing, & Learning Disabilities International*, 3, 167–85.

Larsen, S. (1978). Learning disabilities and the professional educator. *Learning Disability Quarterly*, 1(1), 5–12.

Lerner, J. (1985). *Children with learning disabilities: Theories, diagnosis, and teaching strategies* (4th ed.). Boston: Houghton Mifflin.

Lindsey, J. D. (1987). *Computers and exceptional individuals*. Columbus, Ohio: Merrill Publishing Co.

Lloyd, J. (1980). Academic instruction and cognitive behavior modification: The need for attack-strategy training. *Exceptional Education Quarterly, 1,* 53–63.

Loper, A. B. (1980). Metacognitive development: Implications for cognitive training. *Exceptional Education Quarterly, 1,* 1–8.

Lynn, R., Gluckin, N. D., & Kripke, B. (1979). *Learning disabilities: An overview of theories, approaches, and politics.* New York: Free Press.

Matheny, A., Dolan, A., & Wilson, R. (1976). Twins with academic learning problems: Antecedent characteristics. *American Journal of Orthopsychiatry, 46,* 464–69.

McCue, P. M., Shelly, C., & Goldstein, G. (1986). Intellectual, academic, and neuropsychological performance levels in learning-disabled adults. *Journal of Learning Disabilities, 19,* 233–36.

McKinney, J. D., & Haskins, R. (1980). Cognitive training and the development of problem-solving strategies. *Exceptional Education Quarterly, 1,* 41–51.

McLoughlin, J. A., Clark, F., Mauck, A. R., & Petrosko, J. (1987). A comparison of parent–child perceptions of student learning disabilities. *Journal of Special Education Technology, 4,* 50–58.

McLoughlin, J. A., & Netick, A. (1983). Defining learning disabilities: A new and cooperative direction. *Annual Review of Learning Disabilities, 1,* 18–20.

Meier, J. H. (1971). Prevalence and characteristics found in second-grade children. *Journal of Learning Disabilities, 4,* 6–21.

Morris, R. J. (1985). *Behavior modification with exceptional children: Principles and practices.* Glenview, Ill.: Scott, Foresman.

Myklebust, H. R. (1968). Learning disabilities: Definition and overview. In H. R. Myklebust (Ed.), *Progress in learning disabilities* (Vol. 2). New York: Grune & Stratton.

Myklebust, H. R., Bannochie, M. N., & Killen, J. R. (1971). Learning disabilities and cognitive processes. In H. R. Myklebust (Ed.), *Progress in learning disabilities* (Vol. 2). New York: Grune & Stratton.

Myklebust, H. R., & Boshes, B. (1969). *Minimal brain damage in children* (Final report, Contract 108-65-142, Neurological and Sensory Disease Control Program). Washington, D.C.: U.S. Department of Health, Education, and Welfare.

National Advisory Committee on Handicapped Children (1968). *Special education for handicapped children: First annual report.* Washington, D.C.: Department of Health, Education, and Welfare.

National Center for Education Statistics (1988). *Condition of education* (p. 54). Washington, D. C.: U.S. Government Printing Office.

Nelson, H. E. (1980). Analysis of spelling errors in normal and dyslexic children. In U. Frith (Ed.), *Cognitive processes in spelling* (pp. 475–93). London: Academic Press.

Nix, G. W., & Shapiro, J. (1986). Auditory perceptual processing in learning-assistance children: A preliminary report. *Journal of Research in Reading, 9*(2), 92–102.

Osman, B. R. (1987). Promoting social acceptance of children with learning disabilities: An educational responsibility. *Journal of Reading, Writing, & Learning Disabilities International, 3,* 111–118.

Patberg, J., Dewitz, P., & Samuels, S. J. (1981). The effect of context on the size of the perceptual unit used in word recognition. *Journal of Reading Behavior, 13,* 33–48.

Pelham, W. E. (1983). The effects of psychostimulants on academic achievement in hyperactive and learning-disabled children. *Thalamus, 3*(1), 2–48. (Newsletter of the International Academy for Research in Learning Disabilities.)

Pelham, W. E. (1986). What do we know about the use and effects of CNS stimulants in the treatment of ADD? *Journal of Children in Contemporary Society, 19,* 99–110.

Pelham, W. E., & Ross, A. O. (1977). Selective attention in children with reading problems: A developmental study of incidental learning. *Journal of Abnormal Child Psychology, 5,* 1–8.

Perlmutter, B. F. (1987). Delinquency and learning disabilities: Evidence for compensatory behaviors and adaptation. *Journal of Youth & Adolescence, 16,* 89–95.

Polloway, E. A., & Smith, J. E. (1982). *Teaching language skills to exceptional learners.* Denver: Love Publishing Co.

Rakes, T. A., & Choate, J. S. (1989). *Language arts: Detecting and correcting special needs.* Boston: Allyn and Bacon, Inc.

Reid, D. K. (1988). Learning disabilities and the cognitive developmental approach. In D. K. Reid (Ed.), *Teaching the learning disabled: A cognitive developmental approach* (pp. 29–46). Boston: Allyn and Bacon, Inc.

Richardson, S. (1978). Careers of mentally retarded young persons: Services, jobs, and interpersonal relations. *American Journal of Mental Deficiency, 82,* 349–58.

Rosenberg, M. S. (1987). Psychopharmacological interventions with young hyperactive children. *Topics in Early Childhood Special Education, 6*(4), 62–74.

Rosenthal, R. H., & Allen, T. W. (1978). An examination of attention, arousal, and learning dysfunctions of hyperkinetic children. *Psychological Bulletin, 85,* 689–715.

Rourke, B. P. (1987). Syndrome of nonverbal learning disabilities: The final common pathway of white-matter disease/function. *Clinical Neuropsychologist, 1*(3), 209–234.

Samuels, S. J., & Kamil, M. L. (1984). Models of the reading process. In P. D. Pearson (Ed.), *Handbook of reading research* (pp. 185–229). New York: Longman.

Skinner, B. F. (1953). *Science and human behavior.* New York: Free Press.

Skinner, B. F. (1957). *Verbal behavior.* New York: Appleton-Century-Crofts.

Skinner, B. F. (1971). *Beyond freedom and dignity.* New York: Knopf.

Smith, D. D., & Lovitt, T. C. (1982). *The computational arithmetic program.* Austin, Tex.: Pro-Ed.

Stanford Research Institute (1989). National longitudinal transition study of special education students. *The education of students with disabilities: Where do we stand?* Briefing paper for testimony given at hearings conducted by the National Council on the Handicapped, June 7 and 8, 1989, Washington, D. C.

Swanson, H. L. (1979). Developmental recall lag in learning-disabled children: Perceptual deficit or verbal mediation deficiency? *Journal of Abnormal Child Psychology, 7,* 199–210.

Swanson, H. L. (1987). What learning-disabled readers fail to retrieve on verbal dichotic tests: A problem of encoding, retrieval, or storage? *Journal of Abnormal Child Psychology, 15,* 339–60.

Swanson, H. L. (1988). Toward a metatheory of learning disabilities. *Journal of Learning Disabilities, 21,* 196–209.

Swanson, H. L., & Watson, B. L. (1982). *Educational and psychological assessment of exceptional children.* St. Louis: C. V. Mosby.

Tansley, P., & Panckhurst, J. (1981). *Children with specific learning difficulties.* Windsor, Eng.: NFER-Nelson Publishing.

Tarver, S. G., Hallahan, D. P., Kauffman, J. M., & Ball, D. W. (1976). Verbal rehearsal and selective attention in children with learning disabilities: A developmental lag. *Journal of Experimental Child Psychology, 22,* 375–85.

Torgesen, J., & Dice, C. (1980). Characteristics of research on learning disabilities. *Journal of Learning Disabilities, 13*(10), 531–35.

U.S. Department of Education (1989). *Eleventh Annual Report to Congress on the Implementation of The Education of the Handicapped Act.* Washington, D.C.: Division of Educational Services, Special Education Programs.

Vogel, S. A. (1982). On developing LD college programs. *Journal of Learning Disabilities, 15,* 518–28.

Wallace, G., & McLoughlin, J. A. (1988). *Learning disabilities: Concepts and characteristics* (3rd ed.). Columbus, Ohio: Charles E. Merrill Publishing Co.

Wallander, J. L. (1988). The relationship between attention problems in childhood and antisocial behavior eight years later. *Journal of Child Psychology & Psychiatry & Allied Disciplines, 29,* 53–61.

Warner, M. M., Schumaker, J. B., Alley, G. R., & Deshler, D. D. (1980). Learning-disabled adolescents in the public schools: Are they different from other low achievers? *Exceptional Education Quarterly, 1,* 27–36.

Weiss, G., & Hechtman, L. T. (1986). *Hyperactive children grown up: Empirical findings and theoretical considerations.* New York: Guilford Press.

Weller, C., Strawser, S., & Buchanan, M. (1985). Adaptive behavior: Designator of a continuum of severity of learning-disabled individuals. *Journal of Learning Disabilities, 18*(4), 201–4.

Weller, C., & Strawser, S. (1987). Adaptive behavior of subtypes of learning-disabled individuals. *Journal of Special Education, 21,* 101–15.

Whalen, C. K. (1987). High risk, but also high potential: The plight and the promise of children with attention deficit disorders. Paper presented at the National Conference on Learning Disabilities, Washington, D. C.

Whalen, C. K., & Henker, B. (1976). Psychostimulants and children: A review and analysis. *Psychological Bulletin, 83,* 1113–30.

Whalen, C. K., & Henker, B. (1986). Cognitive behavior therapy for hyperactive children: What do we know? *Journal of Children in Contemporary Society, 19,* 123–41.

White, W. J., Deshler, D. D., Schumaker, J. B., Warner, M. M., Alley, G. R., & Clark, F. L. (1983). The effects of learning disabilities on postschool adjustment. *Journal of Rehabilitation, 49,* 46–50.

Wilson, L. R. (1985). Large-scale learning-disability identification: The reprieve of a concept. *Exceptional Children, 52,* 44–51.

Wong, B. Y. L. (1980). Activating the inactive learner: Use of question/prompts to enhance comprehension and retention of implied information in disabled children. *Learning Disability Quarterly, 3,* 29–37.

Wong, B. Y. L., & Sawatsky, D. (1984). Sentence elaboration and retention of good, average, and poor readers. *Learning Disability Quarterly, 7,* 229–36.

Zentall, S. S., & Kruczek, T. (1988). The attraction of color for active attention-problem children. *Exceptional Children, 54,* 357–62.

Chapter 7

Bellamy, G. T. (1985). Severe disability in adulthood. *Newsletter of the Association for Persons with Severe Handicaps, 11,* 1 & 6.

Becker, L. D. (1978). Learning characteristics of educationally handicapped and retarded children. *Exceptional Children, 44,* 502–11.

Binet, A., & Simon, T. (1905). New methods for the diagnosis of the intellectual level of subnormals. *L'Année Psychologique.* Translated and reprinted in A. Binet & T. Simon (1916), *The development of intelligence in children.* Baltimore: Williams & Wilkins.

Braaten, S., Kauffman, J. M., Braaten, B., Polsgrove, L., & Nelson, C. M. (1988). The regular education initiative: Patent medicine for behavioral disorders. *Exceptional Children, 55*(1), 21–278.

Dickie, R. F. (1982). Categorical vs. noncategorical conceptions of children: An issue revisited. *Education and Treatment of Children, 5,* 355–65.

Drew, C. J., Logan, D. R., & Hardman, M. L. (1988). *Mental retardation: Life cycle approach* (4th ed.). Columbus, Ohio: Charles E. Merrill Co.

Engelmann, S. E. (1977). Sequencing cognitive and academic tasks. In R. D. Kneedler & S. G. Tarver (Eds.), *Changing perspectives in special education.* Columbus, Ohio: Charles E. Merrill Publishing Co.

Eysenck, H. J., Wakefield, J. A., Jr., & Friedman, A. F. (1983). Diagnosis and clinical assessment: The DSM-II. *Annual Review of Psychology, 4,* 167–93.

Falvey, M. A. (1986). *Community-based curriculum: Instructional strategies for students with severe handicaps.* Baltimore: Paul H. Brookes.

Forness, S. R., & Kavale, K. A. (1984). Education of the mentally retarded: A note on policy. *Education and Training of the Mentally Retarded, 19*(4), 239–45.

Gartner, A., & Lipsky, D. (1987). Beyond special education: Toward a quality system for all students. *Harvard Educational Review, 57*(4), 367–95.

Gartner, A., & Lipsky, D. (1989, June). *Equity and excellence for all students.* Testimony presented before the National Council on Disability, Washington, D.C.

Goldman, J., & Gardner, H. (1989). Multiple paths to educational effectiveness. In D. K. Lipsky & A. Gartner (Eds.), *Beyond separate education: Quality education for all* (pp. 121–140). Baltimore: Paul H. Brookes.

Granger, L., & Granger, B. (1986). *The magic feather.* New York: E. P. Dutton.

Hallahan, D. P., & Kauffman, J. M. (1976). *Introduction to learning disabilities: A psychobehavioral approach.* Englewood Cliffs, N.J.: Prentice-Hall.

Hammill, D. D. (1976). Defining learning disabilities for programmatic purposes. *Academic Therapy, 12,* 29–37.

Hardman, M. L. (1981). Learner characteristics of students with mild learning and behavior differences. In M. L. Hardman, M. W. Egan, & E. D. Landau, *The exceptional student in the regular classroom.* Dubuque, Iowa: William C. Brown Co.

Jenkins, J. R., Pious, C. G., & Peterson, D. L. (1988). Categorical programs for remedial and handicapped students: Issues of validity. *Exceptional Children, 55*(2), 147–58.

Keogh, B., Becker, L., Kukic, S., & Kukic, M. (1972). *Programs for EH and EMR pupils: Review and recommendations.* Technical report. Los Angeles: University of California.

Larrivee, B. (1986). Effective teaching of mainstreamed students is effective teaching of all students. *Teacher Education and Special Education, 9*(4), 173–79.

Laycock, V. P. (1980). Environmental alternatives for mildly and moderately handicapped. In J. W. Schifani, R. M. Anderson, & S. J. Odle (Eds.), *Implementing learning in the least restrictive environment.* Baltimore: Paul H. Brookes.

Lilly, M. S. (1987). Lack of focus on special education in literature on educational reform. *Exceptional Children, 53*(4), 325–26.

Lovitt, T. C. (1977). *In spite of my resistance . . . I've learned from children.* Columbus, Ohio: Charles E. Merrill Co.

MacMillan, D. L., Meyers, C. E., & Morrison, G. M. (1980). System-identification of mildly mentally retarded children: Implications for interpreting and conducting research. *American Journal of Mental Deficiency, 85,* 108–15.

Marston, D. (1987). Does categorical teacher certification benefit the mildly handicapped child? *Exceptional Children, 53*(5), 423–31.

Mercer, J. R., & Lewis, J. F. (1979). *System of multicultural pluralistic assessment.* New York: The Psychological Corporation.

Mori, A. A., & Masters, L. F. (1980). *Teaching the severely mentally retarded.* Rockville, Md.: Aspen Systems Corp.

Reynolds, M. C., & Birch, J. W. (1988). *Adaptive mainstreaming.* New York: Longman.

Reynolds, M. C., Wang, M. C., & Walberg, H. J. (1987). The necessary restructuring of special and regular education. *Exceptional Children, 53*(5), 391–98.

Snell, M. E. (1987). What does an "appropriate" education mean? In M. E. Snell (Ed.), *Systematic instruction of persons with severe handicaps* (pp. 1–6). Columbus, Ohio: Charles E. Merrill Co.

Wang, M. C. (1989). Testimony before the National Council on Disability. *Education of students with disabilities: Where do we stand?* Washington, D.C.: National Council on Disability.

Wang, M. C., & Walberg, H. J. (1987). Four fallacies of segregation. *Exceptional Children, 55*(2), 128–37.

Wilcox, B. (1979). Severe/profound handicapping conditions: Administrative considerations. In M. S. Lilly (Ed.), *Children with exceptional needs.* New York: Holt, Rinehart, & Winston.

Ysseldyke, J. E. (1987). Classification of handicapped students. In M. C. Wang, M. C. Reynolds, & H. J. Walberg (Eds.), *Handbook of special education: Research and practice: Vol. 1 Learner characteristics and adaptive eduction.* New York: Pergamon Press.

Ysseldyke, J. E., Algozzine, B., Shinn, M., & McGue, M. (1982). Similarities and differences between low achievers and students classified as handicapped. *Journal of Special Education, 16,* 73–85.

Chapter 8

Allen, D. V., & Bliss, L. S. (1987). Concurrent validity of two language screening tests. *Journal of Communication Disorders, 20,* 305–17.

Ausubel, D. P., Sullivan, E. V., & Ives, S. W. (1980). *Theory and problems of child development* (3rd ed.). New York: Grune & Stratton.

Azrin, N. H., & Nunn, R. G. (1974). A rapid method of eliminating stuttering by a regulated breathing approach. *Behaviour Research and Therapy, 12,* 279–86.

Bernstein, D. K. (1985). The nature of language and its disorders. In D. K. Bernstein and E. Tiegerman (Eds.), *Language and communication disorders in children* (1–19). Columbus, Ohio: Charles E. Merrill Publishing Co.

Bishop, D. V. M., & Edmundson, A. (1987). Specific language impairment as a maturational lag: Evidence from longitudinal data on language and motor development. *Developmental Medicine and Child Neurology, 29,* 442–59.

Burrough, B. (1986, November 10). Second chances: A wave of communications services brings renewed sense of hope to handicapped. *Wall Street Journal,* p. 29d.

Chapman, K. L., & Terrell, B. Y. (1988). "Verb-alizing": Facilitating action word usage in young language-impaired children. *Topics in Language Disorders, 8*(2), 1–13.

Cole, M. L., & Cole, J. T. (1981). *Effective intervention with the language impaired child.* Rockville, Md.: Aspen Systems Corporation.

Cole, K. N., & Dale, P. S. (1986). Direct language instruction and interactive language instruction with language-delayed preschool children: A comparison study. *Journal of Speech and Hearing Research, 29,* 206–17.

Cooper, J. A., & Flowers, C. R. (1987). Children with a history of acquired aphasia: Residual language and academic impairments. *Journal of Speech and Hearing Disorders, 52,* 251–62.

Cooper, J. M., & Griffiths, P. (1978). Treatment and prognosis. In M. A. Wyke (Ed.), *Developmental dysphasia.* New York: Academic Press.

Crestwood Company (1987–88). Communication aids for children and adults, Catalog. Milwaukee, Wis.: The Company.

Cromer, R. F. (1981). Reconceptualizing language acquisition and cognitive development. In R. L. Schiefelbusch & D. D. Bricker (Eds.), *Early language acquisition and intervention.* Baltimore: University Park Press.

Cruz, M. delC., & Ayala, M. (1987). Developmental variables and speech–language in a special education intervention model. Paper presented at the 68th National American Educational Research Association Convention, Washington, D.C.

Education Daily (1983, June 2). Technology helps handicapped live independently, 6.

Eisenson, J. (1971a). Aphasia in adults: Basic considerations. In L. E. Travis (Ed.), *Handbook of speech pathology and audiology.* New York: Appleton-Century-Crofts.

Eisenson, J. (1971b). Therapeutic problems and approaches with aphasic adults. In L. E. Travis (Ed.), *Handbook of speech pathology and audiology.* New York: Appleton-Century-Crofts.

Emerick, L. L., & Haynes, W. O. (1986). *Diagnosis and evaluation in speech pathology* (3rd ed.). Englewood Cliffs, N.J.: Prentice-Hall.

Ewing-Cobbs, L. (1987). Language functions following closed-head injury in children and adolescents. *Journal of Clinical and Experimental Neuropsychology, 9,* 575–92.

Fitzgerald, M. T., & Karnes, D. E. (1987). A parent-implemented language model for at-risk and developmentally delayed preschool children. *Topics in Language Disorders, 7*(3), 31–46.

Gelfand, D. M., Jenson, W. R., & Drew, C. J. (1988). *Understanding children's behavior disorders* (2nd ed.) New York: Holt, Rinehart, & Winston.

Geschwind, N. (1968). Human brain: Left–right asymmetrics in temporal speech region. *Science, 161,* 186–87.

Groshong, C. C. (1987). Assessing oral language comprehension: Are picture-vocabulary tests enough? *Learning Disabilities Focus, 2,* 108–15.

Gruber, L., & Powell, R. L. (1974). Responses of stuttering and non-stuttering children to a dichotic listening task. *Perceptual and Motor Skills, 38,* 263–64.

Harlan, N. T., & Tschiderer, P. A. (1987). A primary prevention program: Teaching Models I and II. Paper presented at the Annual Convention of the American Speech-Language-Hearing Association, Detroit, Mich.

Hasbrouck, J. M., Doherty, J., Mehlmann, M. A., Nelson, R., Randle,

B., & Whitaker, R. (1987). Intensive stuttering therapy in a public school setting. *Language, Speech, and Hearing Services in Schools, 18,* 330–43.

Healey, E. C., & Howe, S. W. (1987). Speech shadowing characteristics of stutterers under diotic and dichotic conditions. *Journal of Communication Disorders, 20,* 493–506.

Hornby, G., & Jensen-Proctor, G. (1984). Parental speech to language-delayed children: A home intervention study. *British Journal of Disorders of Communication, 19,* 97–103.

Hurt, H. T., Scott, M. D., & McCrosky, J. C. (1978). *Communication in the classroom.* Reading, Mass.: Addison-Wesley Publishing Co.

Hutchinson, B. B., Hanson, M. L., & Mecham, M. J. (1979). *Diagnostic handbook of speech pathology.* Baltimore: Williams & Wilkins.

Klinger, H. (1987). Effects of pseudostuttering on normal speakers' self-ratings of beauty. *Journal of Communication Disorders, 20,* 353–58.

Knepflar, K. J. (1976). *Report writing in the field of communication disorders.* Danville, Ill.: Interstate Printers & Publishers.

Kraaimaat, F., Janssen, P., & Brutten, G. J. (1988). The relationship between stutterers' cognitive and autonomic anxiety and therapy outcome. *Journal of Fluency Disorders, 13,* 107–13.

Kretschmer, R. R., & Kretschmer, L. W. (1978). *Language development and intervention with the hearing impaired.* Baltimore: University Park Press.

Lucas, E. V. (1980). *Semantic and pragmatic language disorders: Assessment and remediation.* Rockville, Md.: Aspen Systems Corporation.

MacDonald, J. D., & Gillette, Y. (1986). Communicating with persons with severe handicaps: Roles of parents and professionals. *Journal of the Association for Persons with Severe Handicaps, 11,* 255–65.

Mecham, M. J., & Willbrand, M. L. (1985). *Treatment approaches to language disorders in children: Psycholinguistic and neurolinguistic approaches.* Springfield, Ill.: Charles C. Thomas.

Morris, A., & Greulich, R. (1968). Dental research: The past two decades. *Science, 160,* 1081–88.

Mowrer, D. E., & Conley, D. (1987). Effects of peer-administered consequences upon articulation responses of speech-defective children. *Journal of Communication Disorders, 20,* 319–26.

Perkins, W., Rudas, J., Johnson, L., & Bell, J. (1976). Stuttering: Discoordination of phonation with articulation and respiration. *Journal of Speech and Hearing Research, 19,* 509–22.

Pindzola, R. H. (1987). Durational characteristics of the fluent speech of stutterers and nonstutterers. *Folia Phonetica, 39,* 90–97.

Powers, M. H. (1971). Functional disorders of articulation—Symptomology and etiology. In L. E. Travis (Ed.), *Handbook of speech pathology and audiology.* New York: Appleton-Century-Crofts.

Prosek, R. A., et al. (1987). Formant frequencies of stuttered and fluent vowels. *Journal of Speech and Hearing Research, 30,* 301–05.

Rastatter, M. P., & Dell, C. (1987). Vocal reaction times of stuttering subjects to tachistoscopically presented concrete and abstract words: A closer look at cerebral dominance and language processing. *Journal of Speech and Hearing Research, 30,* 306–10.

Rastatter, M. P., & Loren, C. A. (1988). Visual coding dominance in stuttering: Some evidence from central tachistoscopic stimulation (tachistoscopic viewing and stuttering). *Journal of Fluency Disorders, 13,* 89–95.

Raver, S. A. (1987). Practical procedures for increasing spontaneous language in language-delayed preschoolers. *Journal of the Division for Early Childhood, 11,* 226–32.

Richard, N. B. (1986). Interaction between mothers and infants with Down syndrome: Infant characteristics. *Topics in Early Childhood Special Education, 6*(3), 54–71.

Sheehan, J. G., & Costly, M. S. (1977). A reexamination of the role of heredity in stuttering. *Journal of Speech and Hearing Disorders, 42,* 47–59.

Slorach, N., & Noeher, B. (1973). Dichotic listening in stuttering and dyslalic children. *Cortex, 9,* 295–300.

Tiegerman, E. (1985). The social bases of language acquisition. In D. K. Bernstein and E. Tiegerman (Eds.), *Language and communication disorders in children* (20–30). Columbus, Ohio: Charles E. Merrill Publishing Co.

U.S. Department of Education (1989). *To assure the free appropriate public education of all handicapped children.* Eleventh Annual Report to Congress on the Implementation of The Education of the Handicapped Act. Washington, D. C.: The Department of Education.

Van Riper, C., & Emerick, L. (1984). *Speech correction: An introduction to speech pathology and audiology* (7th ed.). Englewood Cliffs, N.J.: Prentice-Hall.

Waldo, A. L. (1984). *Sacajawea* (rev. exp. ed.). New York: Avon Books.

Webster, W. G. (1988). Neural mechanisms underlying stuttering: Evidence from bimanual handwriting performance. *Brain and Language, 33,* 226–44.

Wiig, E. H., & Semel, E. M. (1984). *Language assessment and intervention for the learning disabled* (2nd ed.). Columbus, Ohio: Charles E. Merrill Publishing Co.

Wnuk, L. (1987). A review of the Bzoch-League Receptive-Expressive Emergent Language Scale and the Test for Auditory Comprehension Language. *Canadian Journal for Exceptional Children, 3,* 95–98.

Wohl, M. T. (1968). The electric metronome—An evaluative study. *British Journal of Disorders of Communication, 3,* 89–98.

Wood, K. S. (1971). Terminology and nomenclature. In L. E. Travis (Ed.), *Handbook of speech pathology and audiology.* New York: Appleton-Century-Crofts.

Ylvisaker, M. (1986). Language and communication disorders following pediatric head injury. *Journal of Head Trauma Rehabilitation, 1*(4), 48–56.

Chapter 9

Abroms, I. F. (1977). Nongenetic hearing loss. In B. F. Jaffe (Ed.), *Hearing loss in children.* Baltimore: University Park Press.

Allen, T. (1986). A study of the achievement pattern of hearing-impaired students: 1974–1983. In A. Schildroth & M. Karchmer (Eds.), *Deaf children in America* (pp. 161–206). San Diego: College-Hill Press.

Altshuler, K. Z. (1964). Personality traits and depressive symptoms in the deaf. In J. Wortis (Ed.), *Recent advances in biological psychiatry* (Vol. 6). New York: Plenum Press.

American Speech-Language-Hearing Association (1982). Joint Committee on Infant Hearing: Position statement. *Asha, 24,* 1017–18. *Annual survey of hearing impaired children and youth (1977–1978).* Washington, D. C.: Office of Demographic Studies, Gallaudet College.

Bess, F. H. (1977). Condition of hearing aids worn by children in a public school setting. In *The condition of hearing aids worn by children in a public school program* (pp. 13–23). HEW Publication No. 77–05002 (OE). Washington, D.C.: U.S. Government Printing Office.

Bitter, G. B. (1981). Identification and educational management of hearing loss. In *Utah skills project.* Salt Lake City: Utah State Board of Education.

Boothroyd, A. (1971). *Some aspects of language function in a group of lower-school children* (Sensory Aids Research Project Report No. 6). Northampton, Mass.: C. V. Hudgins Diagnostic and Research Center, Clarke School for the Deaf.

Boulton, B., Cull, J. G., & Hardy, R. E. (1974). Psychological adjustment to hearing loss and deafness. In R. E. Hardy & J. G. Cull (Eds.), *Educational and psychological aspects of deafness.* Springfield, Ill.: Charles C. Thomas Publishing Co.

Brill, R. G., MacNeil, B., & Newman, I. R. (1986). Framework for appropriate programs for deaf children. *American Annals of the Deaf, 131*(2), 65–77.

Brooks, P. H. (1978). Some speculations concerning deafness and learning to read. In L. S. Liben (Ed.), *Deaf children: Developmental perspectives.* New York: Academic Press.

Butler, M. J. (1981). Teaching students with a hearing impairment. In M. L. Hardman, M. W. Egan, & E. D. Landau (Eds.), *What will we do in the morning? The exceptional student in the regular classroom.* Dubuque, Iowa: William C. Brown Co.

Caldwell, D. C. (1981). Closed-captioned television: Educational and sociological implications for hearing-impaired learners. *American Annals of the Deaf,* September, 627–30.

Chial, M. R. (1987). Electroacoustic assessment of children's hearing aids. In *The condition of hearing aids worn by children in a public school program* (pp. 25–51). HEW Publication No. 77–05002 (OE). Washington, D.C.: U.S. Government Printing Office.

Cole, P. R. (1987). Recognizing language disorders. In F. N. Martin (Ed.), *Hearing disorders in children* (pp. 113–50). Austin, Tex.: Pro-Ed.

Craig, W., & Craig, H. (Eds.) (1975). Directory of services for the deaf. *American Annals of the Deaf,* April, 120.

Davis, H. (1978). Abnormal hearing and deafness. In H. Davis and S. R. Silverman (Eds.), *Hearing and deafness* (4th ed.). New York: Holt, Rinehart, & Winston.

Davis, J. (1977). Personnel and services. In J. Davis (Ed.), *Our forgotten children: Hard-of-hearing pupils in the schools.* Minneapolis: University of Minnesota.

Did you know? (1983, Fall). *Caption.* Falls Church, Va.: National Captioning Institute.

Dipietro, L. J., Knight, C. H., & Sams, J. S. (1981). Health care delivery for deaf patients: The provider's role. *American Annals of the Deaf,* April, 106–12.

Fant, L. J. (1972). *Ameslan: An introduction to the American Sign Language.* Silver Spring, Md.: National Association of the Deaf.

Federal Register (1977). Education of Handicapped Children Act. Washington, D. C.: U.S. Department of Health, Education, and Welfare, August 23.

Garwood, V. P. (1987). Public school audiology. In F. N. Martin (Ed.), *Hearing disorders in children* (pp. 427–67). Austin, Tex.: Pro-Ed.

Gentile, A., & McCarthy, B. (1973). *Additional handicapping conditions among hearing-impaired students, United States: 1971–72.* Series D, No. 14. Washington, D. C.: Office of Demographic Studies, Gallaudet College.

Good Housekeeping (1985, December). A very special Santa, p. 136.

Heider, F., & Heider, G. M. (1940). Studies in the psychology of the deaf, no. 1. *Psychological Monographs, 52,* no. 242, Psychology Division, Clarke School for the Deaf.

Hicks, D. E. (1970). Comparison profiles of rubella and nonrubella children. *American Annals of the Deaf, 115,* 86–92.

Higgins, P. C. (1980). *Outsiders in a hearing world: A sociology of deafness.* Beverly Hills, Cal.: Sage Publications.

Hodgson, W. R. (1987). Test of hearing—The infant. In F. N. Martin (Ed.), *Hearing disorders in children* (pp. 185–216). Austin, Tex.: Pro-Ed.

Hoemann, H. W., & Briga, J. S. (1981). Hearing impairments. In J. M. Kauffman & D. P. Hallahan (Eds.), *Handbook of special education.* Englewood Cliffs, N.J.: Prentice-Hall.

Home video scores smash hit. (1984, Fall). *Caption.* Falls Church, Va.: National Captioning Institute.

Jaffe, B. F. (1977). History and physical examination for evaluating hearing loss in children. In B. F. Jaffe (Ed.), *Hearing loss in children.* Baltimore: University Park Press.

Jensema, C. J., Karchmer, M. A., & Trybus, R. J. (1978). *The rated speech intelligibility of hearing-impaired children: Basic relationships and a detailed analysis,* Series R, no. 6. Washington, D. C.: Office of Demographic Studies, Gallaudet College.

Karchmer, M., & Kirwin, L. (1977). *The use of hearing aids by hearing-impaired children in the United States,* Series S. no. 2. Washington, D. C.: Office of Demographic Studies, Gallaudet College.

Kodman, F. (1963). Educational status of hard-of-hearing children in the classroom. *Journal of Speech and Hearing Disorder, 28,* 297–9.

LaSasso, C. (1985). *National survey of materials and procedures used to teach reading to hearing-impaired students: Preliminary results.* Paper presented at the Conference on Reading Instruction for the Hearing Impaired, June. South Carolina State Department of Education: The Office of Programs for the Handicapped.

Lim, D. J. (1977). Histology of the developing inner ear: Normal anatomy and development anomalies. In B. F. Jaffe (Ed.), *Hearing loss in children.* Baltimore: University Park Press.

Ling, D. (1984a). Early total communication intervention: An introduction. In D. Ling (Ed.), *Early intervention for hearing-impaired children: Total communication options.* San Diego: College Hill Press.

Ling, D. (1984b). Early oral intervention: An introduction. In D. Ling (Ed.), *Early intervention for hearing-impaired children: Oral options.* San Diego: College Hill Press.

Ling, D. (1972). Rehabilitation of cases with deafness secondary to Otitis Media. In A. Glorig & K. S. Gerwin (Eds.), *Otitis Media*. Springfield, Ill.: Charles C. Thomas Publishing Co.

Ling, D., & Ling, A. H. (1978). *Aural rehabilitation: Foundations of verbal learning in hearing-impaired children*. Washington, D. C.: Alexander Graham Bell Association for the Deaf.

Lovrinic, J. H. (1980). Pure tone and speech audiometry. In R. W. Keith (Ed.), *Audiology for the physician*. Baltimore: Williams & Wilkins.

Mandell, C. J., & Fiscus, E. (1981). *Understanding exceptional people*. St. Paul, Minn.: West Publishing Co.

Maxon, A. B. (1987). Pediatric amplification. In F. N. Martin (Ed.), *Hearing disorders in children* (pp. 361–93). Austin, Tex.: Pro-Ed.

Mayberry, R. I. (1978). Manual communication. In H. Davis & S. R. Silverman (Eds.), *Hearing and deafness*. New York: Holt, Rinehart, & Winston.

McAnally, P. L., Rose, S., & Quigley, S. P. (1987). *Language learning practices with deaf children*. San Diego: College Hill Press.

McConnell, F. (1973). Children with hearing disabilities. In L. M. Dunn (Ed.), *Exceptional children in the school* (2nd Ed.). New York: Holt, Rinehart, & Winston.

Meadow, K. P. (1976). Personality and social development for deaf persons. In B. Bolton (Ed.), *Psychology of deafness for rehabilitation counselors*. Baltimore: University Park Press.

Meadow, K. P. (1980). *Deafness and child development*. Berkeley: University of California Press.

Mental Health Needs of Deaf Americans: Task panel reports submitted to the President's Commission on Mental Health, Vol. 3. (1978). Washington, D. C.: U.S. Government Printing Office.

Moores, D. (1987). *Educating the deaf: Psychology, principles, and practices* (3rd ed.). Boston: Houghton Mifflin.

Morgan, A. B. (1987). Causes and treatment. In F. N. Martin (Ed.), *Hearing disorders in children* (pp. 5–48). Austin, Tex.: Pro-Ed.

Myklebust, H. (1960). *The psychology of deafness*. New York: Grune & Stratton.

National Captioning Institute, Inc. (n.d.). *Reading TV in the classroom: Suggestions for using captioned TV in the teaching of reading*. Falls Church, Va.: The Institute.

Newton, L. (1987). The educational management of hearing-impaired children. In F. N. Martin (Ed.), *Hearing disorders in children* (pp. 321–60). Austin, Tex.: Pro-Ed.

Olmstead, R. W., Alvarez, M. C., Moroney, J. D., & Eversden, M. (1964). The pattern of hearing following acute Otitis Media. *Journal of Pediatrics, 65*, 252–55.

Oyers, H. J., & Frankmann, J. P. (1975). *The aural rehabilitation process: A conceptual framework analysis*. New York: Holt, Rinehart, & Winston.

Pahz, J. A., & Pahz, C. S. (1978). *Total communication*. Springfield, Ill.: Charles C. Thomas Publishing Co.

Patrick, P. E. (1987). Identification audiometry. In F. N. Martin (Ed.), *Hearing disorders in children* (pp. 402–25). Austin, Tex.: Pro-Ed.

Perkins, W. H., & Kent, R. D. (1986). *Functional anatomy of speech, language, and hearing*. San Diego: College Hill Press.

Pinter, R., Eisenson, J., & Stanton, M. (1941). *The psychology of the physically handicapped*. New York: F. S. Crofts & Co.

Quigley, S., and King, C. (Eds.) (1984). *Reading milestones*. Beaverton, Ore.: Dormac.

Rose, S., & Waldron, M. (1984). Microcomputer use in programs for hearing-impaired children: A national survey. *American Annals of the Deaf, 129*, 338–42.

Ross, M. (1977). Definitions and descriptions. In J. David (Ed.), *Our forgotten children: Hard-of-hearing pupils in the schools*. Minneapolis: Audiovisual Library Service, University of Minnesota.

Ross, M., & Calvert, D. R. (1984). Semantics of deafness revisited: Total communication and the use and misuse of residual hearing. *Audiology, 9*(9), 127–45.

Sanders, D. A. (1980). Psychological implications of hearing impairment. In W. M. Cruickshank (Ed.), *Psychology of exceptional children* (4th ed.). Englewood Cliffs, N.J.: Prentice-Hall.

Schein, J. D., & Delk, M. T. (1974). *The deaf population in the United States*. Silver Spring, Md.: National Association of the Deaf.

Schlesinger, H. S. (1978). The effects of deafness on childhood development: An Eriksonian perspective. In L. S. Liben (Ed.), *Deaf children: Developmental perspectives*. New York: Academic Press.

Schlesinger, H. S., & Meadow, K. P. (1976). Emotional support for parents. In D. L. Lillie, P. L. Trohanis, & K. W. Goin (Eds.), *Teaching parents to teach*. New York: Walker & Co.

Schreiber, F. C. (1979). *National Association of the Deaf*. In L. J. Bradford & W. G. Hardy (Eds.), *Hearing and hearing impairment*. New York: Grune & Stratton.

Scouten, E. L. (1983). *Turning points in the education of deaf people*. Danville, Ill.: Interstate.

Silverman, S. R., Lane, H. S., & Clavert, D. R. (1978). Early and elementary education. In H. Davis & S. R. Silverman (Eds.), *Hearing and deafness* (4th ed.). New York: Holt, Rinehart, & Winston.

Stepp, R. (1982). Microcomputers: Macro-learning for the hearing impaired. *American Annals of the Deaf, 127*, 472–75.

Sullivan, M. B., & Bourke, L. (1980). *Show of hands*. Reading, Mass.: Addison-Wesley.

Trybus, R. J. (1985). *Today's hearing-impaired children and youth: A demographic profile*. Washington, D.C.: Gallaudet Research Institute.

Trybus, R. J., & Karchmer, M. A. (1977). School achievement scores of hearing-impaired children: National data on achievement status and growth patterns. *American Annals of the Deaf, 122*, 62–69.

Tucker, B. P. (1981, May). Mental health services for hearing-impaired persons. *The Volta Review*, 223–35.

U.S. Department of Education (1989). Eleventh Annual Report to Congress on the Implementation of the Education of the Handicapped Act. Washington, D.C.: United States Department of Education.

Vernon, M. (1969). Sociological and psychological factors associated with hearing loss. *Journal of Speech and Hearing Research, 12*, 541–63.

Vernon, M., & Brown, B. (1964). A guide to psychological tests and testing procedures in the evaluation of deaf and hard-of-hearing children. *Journal of Speech and Hearing Disorders, 29*, 414–23.

Woodward, J. (1982). *How you gonna get to heaven if you can't talk to Jesus?* Silver Spring, Md.: T. J. Publishers.

Chapter 10

American Printing House for the Blind (1979). *Distribution of January 6, 1979, quota registrations by school, grades, and reading media*. Washington, D.C.

Anderson, E., Dunlea, A., & Kekalis, L. (1984). Blind children's language: Resolving some differences. *Journal of Child Language, 11*(3), 645–64.

Ashcroft, S. C. (1966). Delineating the possible for the multihandicapped adult with visual impairment. *Sight-Saving Review, 36*, 90–94.

Barraga, N. C. (1974). Utilization of sensory-perceptual abilities. In B. Lowenfeld (Ed.). *The visually handicapped child in school*. London: Constable.

Barraga, N. C. (1983). *Visual handicaps and learning*. Austin, Tex.: Exceptional Resources.

Barraga, N. C. (1986). Sensory perceptual development. In G. Scholl (Ed.), *Foundations of education for blind and visually handicapped children and youth*. New York: American Foundation for the Blind.

Bishop, V. E. (1987). Religion and blindness: From inheritance to opportunity. *Journal of Visual Impairment and Blindness, 81*(6), 256–59.

Braille: An overview—History, problems, technology, and future prospects (1982). Baltimore: National Federation of the Blind.

Chapman, E. K. (1978). *Visually handicapped children and young people*. London: Routledge & Kegan Paul.

Connor, F. P., Hoover, R., Horton, K., Sands, H., Sternfeld, L., & Wolinsky, G. F. (1975). Physical and sensory handicaps. In N. Hobbs (Ed.), *Issues in the classification of children* (Vol. 1). San Francisco: Jossey-Bass.

Craig, R. H., & Howard, C. (1981). Teaching students with visual impairments. In M. L. Hardman, M. W. Egan, & E. D. Landau (Eds.), *What will we do in the morning? The exceptional student in the regular classroom.* Dubuque, Iowa: William C. Brown Co.

Frisby, J. P. (1979). *Seeing: Illusion, brain, and mind.* New York: Oxford University Press.

Getman, G. N. (1965). The visuomotor complex in the acquisition of learning skills. In J. Hellmuth (Ed.), *Learning disorders* (Vol. 1). Seattle: Special Child Publications.

Ginsberg, E. (1973–1974). Preventive health: No easy answers. *Sight-Saving Review, 43,* 187–95.

Glass, P., et al. (1985). Effect of bright light in the hospital nursery on the incidence of retinopathy of prematurity. *New England Journal of Medicine, 313*(7), 401–4.

Gregg, J. R., & Heath, G. G. (1964). *The eye.* Lexington, Mass.: D. C. Heath & Co.

Halliday, C., & Kurzhals, I. W. (1976). *Stimulating environments for children who are visually impaired.* Springfield, Ill.: Charles C. Thomas Publishing Co.

Harley, R. K., Henderson, F. M., & Truan, M. B. (1976). *The teaching of Braille reading.* Springfield, Ill.: Charles C. Thomas Publishing Co.

Hatlen, P., & Curry, S. (1987). In support of specialized programs for blind and visually impaired children: The impact of vision loss on learning. *Journal of Visual Impairment and Blindness, 81,* 7–13.

Jernigan, K. (1982). Braille: Changing attitudes, changing technology. In *Braille: An overview—History, problems, technology, and future prospects* (pp. 163–9). Baltimore: National Federation of the Blind.

Kilpatrick, J. J. (1986, September 8). "Right" of the blind to read *Playboy. Indianapolis Star,* 32.

Kirtley, D. D. (1975). *The psychology of blindness.* Chicago: Nelson-Hall.

Lowenfeld, B. (1974). Psychological considerations. In B. Lowenfeld (Ed.), *The visually handicapped child in school.* London: Constable.

Lowenfeld, B. (1975). *The changing status of the blind: From separation to integration.* Springfield, Ill.: Charles C. Thomas Publishing Co.

Lowenfeld, B. (1980). Psychological problems of children with severely impaired vision. In W. M. Cruickshank (Ed.), *Psychology of exceptional children and youth* (4th ed.). Englewood Cliffs, N.J.: Prentice-Hall.

National Society for the Prevention of Blindness (1966). *Estimated statistics on blindness and vision problems.* New York: The National Society.

National Society to Prevent Blindness (1980). *Vision problems in the U.S.* New York: The National Society.

Parsons, A. S., & Sabornie, E. J. (1987). Language skills of young low-vision children: Performance on the preschool language scale. *Journal of the Division for Early Childhood, 11*(3), 217–25.

Raikes, A. (1979). Preliminary visual screening. In V. Smith & J. Keen (Eds.), *Visual handicap in children.* London: William Heinemann Medical Books.

Reynolds, M. C., & Birch, J. W. (1982). *Teaching exceptional children in all American's schools.* Reston, Va.: Council for Exceptional Children.

Rogers, M. (1989, April 24). More than wheelchairs. *Newsweek,* 66–67.

Schlaegel, T. F. (1953). The dominant method of imagery in blind as compared to sighted adolescents. *Journal of Genetic Psychology, 83,* 265–77.

Scholl, G. T. (1974). Understanding and meeting development needs. In B. Lowenfeld (Ed.), *The visually handicapped child in school.* London: Constable.

Schrock, R. E. (1978). Research relating to vision and learning. In R. M. Wold (Ed.), *Vision: Its impact on learning.* Seattle: Special Child Publications.

Suran, B. G., & Rizzo, J. V. (1979). *Special children: An integrative approach.* Glenview, Ill.: Scott, Foresman & Co.

Susan, age 27, who has been blind since birth, personal communication to one of the authors.

Telford, C. W., & Sawrey, J. M. (1981). *The exceptional individual* (4th ed.). Englewood Cliffs, N.J.: Prentice-Hall.

U.S. Department of Education (1989). *Eleventh Annual Report to Congress on the Implementation of the Education of the Handicapped Act.* Washington, D.C.: The Department.

Tobin, M. J., & James, R. K. (1974). Evaluating the Optacon: General reflections on reading machines for the blind. *Research Bulletin: American Foundation for the Blind, 28,* 145–57.

Toth, Z. (1983). *Die vorstellunswelt der blinden.* Leipzig: Johann Ambrosius Barth.

Tuttle, D. (1984). *Self-esteem and adjusting to blindness.* Springfield, Ill.: Charles C. Thomas Publishing Co.

Ward, M. (1986). The visual system. In G. Scholl (Ed.), *Foundations of education for blind and visually handicapped children and youth.* New York: American Foundation for the Blind.

Warren, D. H. (1984). *Blindness and early childhood development.* New York: American Foundation for the Blind.

Willis, D. J., Groves, C., & Fuhrman, W. (1979). Visually disabled children and youth. In B. M. Swanson & D. J. Willis (Eds.), *Understanding exceptional children and youth: An introduction to special education.* Chicago: Rand McNally & Co.

Chapter 11

Albrecht, G. L. (1976). Socialization and the disability process. In G. L. Albrecht (Ed.), *The sociology of physical disability and rehabilitation.* Pittsburgh: University of Pittsburgh Press.

Anderson, K. M. (1986). The nervous system. In G. M. Scipien, M. U. Barnard, M. A. Chard, J. Howe, & P. J. Phillips (Eds.), *Comprehensive pediatric nursing.* New York: McGraw-Hill Book Company.

Armstrong, R. W., Rosenbaum, P. L., & King, S. M. (1987). A randomized, controlled trial of a "buddy" programme to improve children's attitudes toward the disabled. *Developmental Medicine and Child Neurology, 29*(3), 327–36.

Arnold, J. H., & Gemma, P. B. (1983). *A child dies: A portrait of family grief.* Rockville, Md.: Aspen Systems Corporation.

Athreya, B. H., & Ingall, C. G. (1984). Juvenile rheumatoid arthritis. In J. Fithian (Ed.), *Understanding the child with chronic illness in the classroom.* Phoenix: The Oryx Press.

Backer, B. A., Hannon, N. H., & Russell, N. A. (1982). *Death and dying: Individuals and institutions.* New York: John Wiley & Sons.

Batshaw, M. L., and Perret, Y. M. (1981). *Children with handicaps: A medical primer.* Baltimore: P. H. Brookes.

Bechdol, B. (1985). Consumer organizations facilitate access to computers. *Exceptional Parent, 17*(6), 45–47.

Brown, S. E., Connors, D., & Stern, N. (1985). *With the power of each breath.* Pittsburgh, Pa.: Cleiss Press.

Buckingham, R. W. (1983). *A special kind of love.* New York: Continuum Publishing Company.

Cruickshank, W. M. (1976). The problem and its scope. In W. M. Cruickshank (Ed.), *Cerebral palsy: A developmental disability* (3rd ed.). Syracuse, N.Y.: Syracuse University Press.

Cunningham, P., & Gose, J. (1986, Oct.). Telecommunication for the physically handicapped. *Proceedings of the Conference on Computer Technology and Persons with Disabilities,* Northridge, Cal.

Cunningham, P., & Gose, J. (1986, Oct.). Telecommunications: A new horizon for the handicapped. *Proceedings of the Computer Technology/Special Education Rehabilitation,* Northridge, Cal.

Dickey, R., & Shealey, S. H. (1987). Using technology to control the environment. *The American Journal of Occupational Therapy, 41*(11), 717–21.

Dobling, J. (1983). *Prevention of spina bifida and other neural tube disorders.* London: Academic Press.

Dreifuss, F. E. (1988). What is epilepsy? In H. Reisner (Ed.), *Children with epilepsy.* Kensington, Md.: Woodbine House.

Dutton, D. H. (1986). Strategies to promote integration and acceptance of students with disabilities among their nondisabled peers, using microcomputers. *Proceedings of the Conference on Computer Technology and Persons with Disabilities,* Northridge, Cal.

Education Daily (1984, November 30). New Keyboard Allows Disabled to Type with Their Eyes, 2.

Education Development Center (1975). *No two alike: Helping children with special needs.* Cambridge, Mass.: The Center.

Foulds, R. (1986). *Interactive robotic aids—One option for independent living: An international perspective, 37* (Monograph). New York: World Rehabilitation Fund, Inc.

Freeman, J. M. (1973). To treat or not to treat: Ethical dilemmas of treating the infant with myelomeningocele. *Clinical Neurosurgery, 20,* 134–46.

Friedman, L. W. (1978a). *The psychological rehabilitation of the amputee.* Springfield, Ill.: Charles C. Thomas.

Friedman, L. W. (1978b). *The surgical rehabilitation of the amputee.* Springfield, Ill.: Charles C. Thomas.

Haeussermann, E. (1952). *Evaluating the developmental level of preschool children handicapped by cerebral palsy.* New York: United Cerebral Palsy Association.

Heilman, A. (1952). Intelligence in cerebral palsy. *The Crippled Child, 30,* 11–13.

Jones, L. E. (1988). The free limb scheme and the limb-deficient child in Australia. *Australain Paediatric Journal, 24*(5), 290–94.

Kadish, R. A. (1985). *Death, grief, and caring relationships* (2nd ed.). Monterey, Cal.: Brooks/Cole Publishing Company.

Kamenetz, H. L. (1986). Wheelchairs and other indoor vehicles for the disabled. In J. B. Reford (Ed.), *Orthotics et cetera.* Baltimore: Williams & Wilkins.

Krulik, T., Holaday, B., & Martinson, I. M. (1987). *The child and family facing life-threatening illness.* Philadelphia: J. B. Lippincott Company.

Leerhsen, C., & Padgett, C. (1989). The complete Jim Abbott. *Newsweek,* June 12, 1989, 60.

Lewandowski, L. J., & Cruickshank, W. M. (1980). Psychological development of crippled children and youth. In W. M. Cruickshank (Ed.), *Psychology of exceptional children and youth.* Englewood Cliffs, N.J.: Prentice-Hall.

Lotz, H. W. (1986). *Cerebral palsy not necessary: Maxi-move. Do-it-yourself for parents with movement-delayed children under eight.* Linthicum Heights, Md.: Willyshe Publishing Co.

Magill, J., & Hurlbut, N. (1986). The self-esteem of adolescents with cerebral palsy. *American Journal of Occupational Therapy, 40*(6), 402–7.

Mensch, G., & Ellis, P. M. (1986). *Physical therapy management of lower extremity amputations.* Rockville, Md.: Aspen Publishers, Inc.

Morfee, P., & Morfee, T. (1987). Julie goes to college. *Exceptional Parent, 17*(3), 36–38.

Northern Electric Company (1988). The Dental Care System. Sunbeam Dental Care Products, Northern Electric Company, Hattiesburg, Miss.

Olson, D. L. (1986, April). The education of disabled girls: Personal experiences and reflections. *Paper presented at the 70th Annual Meeting of the American Educational Research Association,* San Francisco, Cal.

Peters, D. M. (1964). Developmental and conceptual components of the normal child: A comparative study with the cerebral palsy child. *Cerebral Palsy Review, 25,* 3–7.

Poss, S. (1981). *Toward death with dignity: Caring for dying people.* Boston: George Allen & Unwin.

Petty, R. E. (1982). Epidemiology and genetics of the rheumatic diseases of childhood. In J. T. Cassidy (Ed.), *Textbook of pediatric rheumatology.* New York: John Wiley & Sons.

Pollingue, A. (1987). Adaptive behavior and low-incidence handicaps: Use of adaptive behavior instruments for persons with physical handicaps. *Journal of Special Education, 21*(1), 170–81.

Robison, A. Q. (1987). An open letter to Lynn's teacher. *Exceptional Parent, 17*(4), 13–14.

Romich, B. A., & Vagnini, C. B. (1985). *Integrating communications, computer access, environmental control & mobility.* Paper presented at the Technology for Disabled Persons, Discovery '84, Chicago, Ill.

Sanders, G. (1986). Lower limb amputations: A guide to rehabilitation. Philadelphia: F. A. Davis Company.

Schaeffler, C. (1988). Making toys accessible for children with cerebral palsy. *Teaching Exceptional Children, 20*(3), 26–28.

Schock, N. (1985). *The child with muscular dystrophy in school* (rev. ed.). Lexington, Mass.: Appalachian Satellite Program Resource Center.

Schumacker, H. R., Klippel, J. H., & Robinson, D. R. (Eds.) (1988). Primer on the rheumatic diseases, 9th ed. Atlanta, Ga.: Arthritis Foundation.

Scott, B. H. (1985). *Book of renovations: A compilation of drawings depicting the most common problems and solutions to renovating existing buildings and facilities to make them accessible to and usable by people with physical disabilities.* Jefferson City: Missouri Governor's Committee on Employment of the Handicapped.

Shurtleff, D., Lemire, R., & Warkany, J. (1986). Embryology, etiology, and epidemiology. In D. B. Shurtleff (Ed.), *Myelodysplasias and extrophies.* Orlando, Fla.: Grune and Stratton, Inc.

Stroud, M., & Sutton, E. (1988). *Expanding options for older adults with developmental disabilities.* Baltimore: Paul H. Brookes.

Tarnowski, K. J., & Drabman, R. S. (1986). Increasing the communicator usage skills of a cerebral palsied adolescent. *Journal of Pediatric Psychology, 11*(4), 573–81.

Turek, S. L. (1984). *Orthopaedics: Principles and their application.* Philadelphia: J. B. Lippincott Company.

U.S. Department of Health and Human Services (1980). *Muscular dystrophy and other neuromuscular disorders.* Bethesda, Md.: Office of Scientific and Health Reports, National Institute of Neurological and Communicative Disorders and Stroke, National Institute of Health (NIH Publication No. 80–1615).

Uniform federal accessibility standards (1985). Washington, D. C.: General Services Administration.

Van Biervlier, A. (1987, April). Instructional uses of bar-code technology. *Paper presented at the Annual Convention of the Council for Exceptional Children (65th),* Chicago, Ill.

Wass, H., & Corr, C. A. (1982). *Helping children cope with death: Guidelines and resources.* Washington, D.C.: Hemisphere Publishing Corporation.

Whaley, F. F., & Wong, D. L. (1985). Essentials of pediatric nursing. St. Louis: The C. V. Mosby Company.

Williams, S. E., & Matesi, D. V. (1988). Therapeutic intervention with an adapted toy. *The American Journal of Occupational Therapy, 42*(10), 673–76.

Williamson, G. G., & Szczepanshi, M. (1987). *Children with spina bifida: Early intervention and preschool programming.* Baltimore: P. H. Brookes Company.

Yashon, D. (1986). *Spinal injury (2nd ed.).* New York: Appleton-Century-Crofts.

Chapter 12

Aaronson, D. W., & Rosenberg, M. (1985). Asthma: General concepts. In R. Paterson (Ed.), *Allergic diseases.* Philadelphia: J. B. Lippincott Company.

Aggleton, P., & Homan, H. (1988). Introduction. In P. Aggleton & H. Homans (Eds.), *Social aspects of AIDS.* London: The Falmer Press.

Ambrosini, P. J., Rabinovich, H., & Puig-Antich, J. (1984). Biological factors and the pharmacologic treatment in major depressive disorder in children and adolescents. In H. S. Sudak, A. B. Ford, & N. B. Rushforth (Eds.), *Suicide in the young.* Boston: John Wright, PSG, Inc.

American Cancer Society (1984). *When your brother or sister has cancer.* New York: American Cancer Society.

American Diabetes Association (1988). Your child has diabetes . . . What you should know. Alexandria, Va.: American Diabetes Association.

Armington, C. S., & Creighton, H. (1971). *Nursing of people with cardiovascular problems.* Boston: Little, Brown & Company.

Batavia, A. I., DeJong, G., Smith, L. S., & Quenton, W. (1988). Primary medical services for people with disabilities. *American Rehabilitation, 14*(4), 9–12, 26–27.

Behrman, R. E., & Vaughn, V. C., III (1987). *Nelson textbook of pediatrics* (13th ed.). Philadelphia: W. B. Saunders.

Boat, T. F., & Dearborn, D. G. (1984). Etiology and pathogenesis. In L. N. Taussig (Ed.), *Cystic fibrosis.* New York: Thieme-Stratton, Inc.

Boyd, M. R. (1985). Strategies for the identification of new agents for the treatment of AIDS: A national program to facilitate the discovery and preclinical development of new drug candidates for clinical evaluation. In V. T. Devita, Jr., S. Hellman, & S. A. Rosenberg (Eds.), *AIDS: Diagnosis, treatment, and prevention*. Philadelphia: J. B. Lippincott Company.

Braasard, M. R., & McNeill, L. E. (1987). Child sexual abuse. In M. R. Brassard, R. Germain, & S. N. Hart (Eds.), *Psychological maltreatment of children and youth*. New York: Pergamon Press.

Buchwald, M., & Tusi, L. (1987). Current status of the genetics of cystic fibrosis. In J. R. Riordan & M. Buchwald (Eds.), *Genetics and epithelial cell dysfunction in cystic fibrosis*. New York: Alan R. Liss, Inc.

Bunn, H. F., & Forget, B. G. (1986). *Hemoglobin: Molecular, genetic and clinical aspects*. Philadelphia: W. B. Saunders Company.

Cheney, C., & Harwood, I. R. (1985). Cystic fibrosis. In R. B. Conn (Ed.), *Current diagnosis*. Philadelphia: W. B. Saunders Company.

Christi, G. H., Siegel, K., & Moynihan, R. T. (1988). Psychosocial issues: Prevention and treatment. In V. T. Devita, Jr., S. Hellman, & S. A. Rosenberg (Eds.), *AIDS: Diagnosis, treatment and prevention*. Philadelphia: J. B. Lippincott Company.

Clark, B. A. (1983). Improving adolescent parenting through participant modeling and self-evaluation. *Nursing Clinics of North America, 18*(2), 303–311.

Conley, C. L. (1980). Sickle-cell anemia: The first molecular disease. In M. W. Wintrobe (Ed.), *Blood, pure and eloquent*. New York: McGraw-Hill Book Co.

Curran, D. K. (1987). *Adolescent suicidal behavior*. Washington, D.C.: Hemisphere Publishing Corporation.

Cystic Fibrosis Foundation (1980). *Guidelines for health personnel: Cystic fibrosis*. Rockville, Md.: The Foundation.

Cystic Fibrosis Foundation (1987, Summer). CF heart–lung transplant gaining national attention. *Commitment,* 1–2.

Cystic Fibrosis Foundation (1988). *Living with cystic fibrosis*. A guide for adolescents. Rockville, Md.: Consumer Focus Committee and the Profession Education Committee.

Davidson, M. B. (1981). *Diabetes mellitus: Diagnosis and Treatment* (Vol. 2). New York: John Wiley & Sons.

deGruchy, G. C. (1978). Disorders of hemoglobin structure and synthesis. In D. Penington, B. Rush, & P. Castaldi (Eds.), *Clinical hematology in medical practice*. Oxford: Blackwell Scientific Publications.

Delano, C. (1986). Potential risks and hazards of adolescent pregnancies and implication for nursing practice. In J. Ouimette (Ed.), *Perinatal nursing: Care of the high-risk mother and infant*. Boston: Jones and Barllett Publishers.

Doershuk, C. F., & Boat, T. F. (1987). In R. E. Behrman & V. C. Vaughan, III (Eds.), *Nelson textbook of pediatrics* (13th ed.). Philadelphia: W. B. Saunders.

Falloon, J., Eddy, J., Roper, M., & Pizzo, P. (1988). AIDS in the pediatric population. In V. T. Devita, Jr., S. Hellman, & S. A. Rosenberg (Eds.), *AIDS: Diagnosis, treatment, and prevention*. Philadelphia: J. B. Lippincott Company.

Finkelhor, D. (1984). *Child sexual abuse*. New York: The Free Press.

Fischinger, P. J. (1988). Strategies for the development of vaccines to prevent AIDS. In V. T. Devita, Jr., S. Hellman, & S. A. Rosenberg (Eds.), *AIDS: Diagnosis, treatment, and prevention*. Philadelphia: J. B. Lippincott Company.

Ford, A. B., Rushford, N. B., & Sudak, H. S. (1984). The causes of suicide. In H. S. Sudak, A. B. Ford, & N. B. Rushforth (Eds.), *Suicide in the young*. Boston: John Wright, PSG, Inc.

Freeman, A. I., & Brecher, M. L. (1985). Diagnosis and treatment of childhood acute lymphocytic leukemia. In P. H. Wiernik, G. P. Canellos, R. A. Kyle, & C. A. Shiffer (Eds.), *Neoplastic diseases of the blood* (Vol. 1). New York: Churchill Livingstone.

Fuchs, V. R. (1983). *How we live*. Cambridge, Mass.: Harvard University Press.

Furstenburg, F. F. (1976). *Unplanned parenthood: The social consequences of teenage child bearing*. New York: Free Press.

Goedert, J. J., & Blattner, W. A. (1988). The epidemiology and natural history of human immunodeficiency. In V. T. Devita, Jr., S. Hellman, & S. A. Rosenberg (Eds.), *AIDS: Diagnosis, treatment, and prevention*. Philadelphia: J. B. Lippincott Company.

Gotta, A. W. (1989). The Anesthesiologist and AIDS. In A. W. Gotts (Ed.), *1989 Review of Course Lectures*. Cleveland, Ohio: International Anesthesia Research Society.

Greenberg, R. E. (1987). Diabetes mellitus. In R. A. Hoekelman, S. Blatman, N. M. Nelson, & H. M. Seidel (Eds.), *Primary pediatric care*. St. Louis: The C. V. Mosby Company.

Grunz, F. W. (1980). The dread leukemias and lymphomas: Their nature and their prospects. In M. W. Wintrobe (Ed.), *Blood, pure and eloquent*. New York: McGraw-Hill Book Co.

Hayes, E. (Ed.) (1987). *Risking the future: Adolescent sexuality, pregnancy, and childbearing* (Vol. 1). Washington, D.C.: National Academy Press.

Helfer, R. E. (1987). The developmental basis of child abuse and neglect: An epidemiological approach. In R. E. Helfer & R. S. Kempe (Eds.), *The battered child* (4th ed.). Chicago: The University of Chicago Press.

Herald Times (1987, July 17). AIDS creating orphans (National Briefs, p. A3, Bloomington, Ind.)

Hobbs, N., Perrin, J. M., & Ireys, H. T. (1985). *Chronically ill children and their families*. San Francisco: Jossey-Bass.

Homans, H., & Aggleton, P. (1988). Health education, HIV infection, and AIDS. In P. Aggleton & H. Homans (Eds.), *Social aspects of AIDS*. London: The Falmer Press.

Huntsman, R. G. (1987). *Sickle-cell anemia and thalassemia: A primer for health care professionals*. Ontario, Canada: The Canadian Sickle Cell Society.

Kaufman, J., & Zigler, E. (1987). Do abused children become abusive parents? *American Journal of Orthopsychiatry, 57*(2), 186–92.

Kempe, C. H., & Helfer, R. E. (1972). *Helping the battered child and his family*. Philadelphia: J. B. Lippincott Co.

Kempe, R. S. (1987). A developmental approach to treatment of the abused child. In R. E. Helfer & R. S. Kempe (Eds.), *The battered child* (4th ed.). Chicago: The University of Chicago Press.

Kempe, R. S., & Kempe, C. H. (1978). *Child abuse*. Cambridge, Mass.: Harvard University Press.

Kety, S. S. (1985). Genetic factors in suicide. In A. Roy (Ed.), *Suicide*. Baltimore: Williams and Wilkins.

Klemperer, M. R., Rubins, J. M., & Lichtman, M. A. (1978). Lymphocytosis. In M. A. Lichtman (Ed.), *Hematology for practitioners*. Boston: Little, Brown & Co.

Krolewski, A. S., & Warram, J. H. (1985). Epidemiology of diabetes mellitus. In A. Marble, L. R. Krall, R. F. Bradley, A. R. Christlieb, & J. S. Soeldner (Eds.), *Joslin's diabetes mellitus*. Philadelphia: Lea & Febiger.

Kuzemko, J. A. (1980). Incidence, prognosis, and mortality. In J. A. Kuzemko (Ed.), *Asthma in children* (2nd ed.). Baltimore, Md.: University Park Press.

Lawrence, R. A., & Merritt, T. A. (1983). Infants of adolescent mothers: Perinatal, neonatal, and infancy outcome. In E. R. McAnarney (Ed.), *Premature adolescent pregnancy and parenthood*. New York: Grune and Stratton.

Lerner, E. A. (1987). *Understanding AIDS*. Minneapolis: Learner Publications Company.

Lifson, A. R. (1988). Do alternate modes for transmission of human immunodeficiency virus exist? *Journal of the American Medical Association, 259*(9), 1353–56.

McKusick, L., Horstman, W., & Coates, T. J. (1985). AIDS and sexual behavior reported by gay men in San Francisco. *American Journal of Public Health, 75*(5), 493–96.

Mecklenburg, M., & Thompson, P. (1983). Adolescent family life program as a preventative measure. *Public Health Reports, 98* (1), 21–29.

Meier, J. H. (1985). *Assault against children*. San Diego: College-Hill Press.

National Cancer Institute (1987). *Help yourself*. Washington, D. C.: U.S. Government Printing Office.

Novick, J. (1984). Attempted suicide in adolescence: The suicide sequence. In H. S. Sudak, A. B. Ford, & N. B. Rushforth (Eds.), *Suicide in the young*. Boston: John Wright, PSG, Inc.

O'Connell, P., Leppert, P., Nakamura, Y., Dean, M., Park, M., Woude, G. V., Farrall, M., Wainwright, B., Williamson, R., Lathrop, G. M., Lalouel, J., and White, R. (1987). DNA markers for the cystic fibrosis locus. In J. R. Riordan & M. Buchwald (Eds.), *Genetics and epithelial cell dysfunction in cystic fibrosis*. New York: Alan R. Liss, Inc.

Patterson, J. M. (1988). Chronic illness in children and the impact on families. In C. Chilman, E. Nunnally, and F. Cox (Eds.), *Chronic illness and disability: Families in Trouble* (Vol. 2.) (pp. 69–107). Newbury Park, Cal.: Sage Publications.

Pfeffer, C. R. (1986). *The suicidal child.* New York: The Guilford Press.

Pless, I. B., & Perrin, J. M. (1985). *Issues common to a variety of illnesses.* In N. Hobbs and J. M. Perrin (Eds.), *Issues in the care of children with chronic illness* (pp. 41–60). San Francisco: Jossey-Bass.

Podolsky, S., Krall, L. P., & Bradley, R. F. (1980). Treatment of diabetes with oral hypoglycemic agents. In S. Podolsky (Ed.), *Clinical diabetes: Modern management.* New York: Appleton-Century-Crofts.

Polsky, B., & Armstrong, D. (1988). Other agents in the treatment of AIDS. In V. T. Devita, Jr., S. Hellman, & S. A. Rosenberg (Eds.), *AIDS: Diagnosis, treatment, and prevention.* Philadelphia: J. B. Lippincott Company.

Radbill, S. X. (1987). Children in a world of violence. In R. E. Helfer & R. S. Kempe (Eds.), *The battered child* (4th ed.). Chicago: The University of Chicago Press.

Raskin, P. (1983). Open and closed insulin infusion systems: Newer methods of insulin delivery. In M. Ellenberg & H. Rifkin (Eds.), *Diabetes mellitus: Theory and practice* (3rd ed.). New Hyde Park, N.Y.: Medical Examination Publishing Company, Inc.

Roberts, L. (1988). Race for cystic fibrosis gene nears end. *Science, 240,* 282–85.

Ross, H., Bernstein, G., & Rifkin, H. (1983). Relationship of metabolic control of diabetes mellitus to long-term complications. In M. Ellenberg & H. Rifkin (Eds.), *Diabetes mellitus: Theory and practice* (3rd ed.). New Hyde Park, N.Y.: Medical Examination Publishing Company, Inc.

Sadler, L. S., Corbett, M. A., Meyer, J. H. (1987). Setting up an adolescent health care program. In M. A. Corbett & J. H. Meyer (Eds.), *The adolescent and pregnancy.* Boston: Blackwell Scientific Publications.

Serjeant, G. R. (1985). *Sickle cell disease.* Oxford: Oxford University Press.

Silber, E. N. (1987). *Heart disease.* New York: Macmillan Publishing Company.

Silverman, M. (1986). What have we learned? In L. McKusick (Ed.), *What to do about AIDS.* Los Angeles: University of California Press.

Spinetta, J. J., & Deasy-Spinetta, P. (1981). *Living with childhood cancer.* St. Louis: The C. V. Mosby Company.

Stern, R. S. (1989). The primary care physician and the patient with cystic fibrosis. *The Journal of Pediatrics, 114*(1), 31–36.

Summit, R. (1985). Causes, consequences, treatment, and prevention of sexual assault against children. In J. H. Meier (Ed.), *Assault against children.* San Diego: College-Hill Press.

Tauer, K. (1983). Promoting effective decision making in sexually active adolescents. *Nursing Clinics of North America, 18* (2), 275–92.

U.S. Department of Health and Human Services (1987). *Talking with your child about cancer.* Bethesda, Md.: National Cancer Institute.

U.S. Department of Health and Human Services (1987). *Help yourself.* Bethesda, Md.: National Cancer Institute.

U.S. Department of Health and Human Services (1987). *The student with cancer: A resource for the educator.* Bethesda, Md.: National Cancer Institute.

U.S. Department of Health and Human Services (1988). *Young people with cancer.* Bethesda, Md.: National Cancer Institute.

U.S. Department of Health and Human Services (1988). *Young people with cancer: A handbook for parents* (NIH Publication No. 88–2378). Bethesda, Md.: National Cancer Institute.

U.S. Department of Health and Human Services (1982). *Monthly Vital Statistics Report, 31*(8), 1–40.

U.S. Department of Health, Education, and Welfare (1978). *Cystic fibrosis: State of the art and directions for future research efforts* DHEW No. NIH 78–1642. Bethesda, Md.: National Institutes of Health.

Williamson, R., Wanwright, B., Cooper, C., Scambler, P., Farrall, M. Estivill, X., & Pedersen, P. (1987). The cystic fibrosis locus. *Enzyme, 38*(1–4), 8–13.

Wintrobe, M. M., Lee, G. R., Boggs, D. R., Bithell, T. C., Foerster, J., Athens, J. W., & Lukens, J. N. (1981). *Clinical hematology* (8th ed.). Philadelphia: Lea & Febiger.

Chapter 13

Addison, L., Oliver, A. I., & Cooper, C. R. (1987). *Developing leadership potential in gifted children and youth, An ERIC exceptional child education report.* Reston, Va.: ERIC Clearinghouse on Handicapped and Gifted Children.

Adler, J., Lubenow, G. C., & Malone, M. (1988, June 13). Reading God's mind. *Newsweek,* 56–59.

Adler, J. C., Mueller, R. J., & Ary, D. (1987). *Nongifted elementary and middle-school children's sociometric choices of gifted vs. nongifted helpers.* Paper presented at the annual meeting of the American Education Research Association, Washington, D.C.

Anderson, M. A. (1987). Facilitating parental understanding of the "gifted" label. *Techniques, 3*(3), 236–44.

Aylward, M. (1987). Enriched-students' program: Nova Scotia, Canada. *Gifted Child Today, 10*(4), 46–47.

Baldwin, A. Y. (1984). *The Baldwin Identification Matrix 2 for identification of the gifted and talented: A handbook for its use.* New York: Trillium Press.

Baldwin, A. Y. (1987). Undiscovered diamonds: The minority gifted child. *Journal for the Education of the Gifted, 10*(4), 271–85.

Bernal, E. M. (1974). Gifted Mexican-American children: An ethnoscientific perspective. *California Journal of Educational Research, 25*(5), 261–73.

Binet, A., & Simon, T. (1905). Methodes nouvelles pour le diagnostique du nivea intellectuel des anomaux. *L'Anée Psychologique, 11,* 196–98.

Binet, A., & Simon, T. (1908). Le development de intelligence chez les enfants. *L'Anée Psychologique, 14,* 1–94.

Blacher-Dixon, J. (1977). *Preschool for the gifted-handicapped: Is it untimely, or about time?* Paper presented at the 55th Annual International Convention of the Council for Exceptional Children, Atlanta, April 11–15.

Blacher-Dixon, J., & Turnbull, A. P. A. (1979). A preschool program for gifted-handicapped children. *Journal of Education for the Gifted, 1*(2), 15–23.

Bloom, B. (1969). *Taxonomy of educational objectives.* New York: David McKay Co.

Bloom, B. (1985). *Developing talent in young people.* New York: Ballantine Books.

Borland, J. (1978). Teacher identification of the gifted. *Journal for the Education of the Gifted, 2,* 22–31.

Brody, L. E., & Benvow, C. P. (1987). Accelerative strategies: How effective are they for the gifted? *Gifted Child Quarterly, 31*(3), 105–10.

Buescher, T. M., Olszewski, P., & Higham, S. J. (1987). Influences on strategies adolescents use to cope with their own recognized talents. Paper presented at the biennial meeting of the Society for Research in Child Development, Baltimore Md.

Callahan, C. M. (1981). Superior abilities. In J. M. Kauffman & D. P. Hallahan (Eds.), *Handbook of special education.* Englewood Cliffs, N.J.: Prentice-Hall.

Carpenter, M. (1987). North Carolina school of the arts: ". . . infinitely the best school in America." *Gifted Child Today, 10*(5), 30–35.

Cattell, R. B. (1971). *Abilities: Their structure, growth, and action.* Boston: Houghton Mifflin Co.

Clark, B. (1983). *Growing up gifted* (2nd ed.). Columbus Ohio: Charles E. Merrill Publishing Co.

Clark, B. (1988). *Growing up gifted* (3rd ed.). Columbus Ohio: Charles E. Merrill Publishing Co.

Clark, G., & Zimmerman, E. (1987). More than meets the eye: Indiana University Summer Arts Institute. *Gifted Child Today, 10*(5), 42–44.

Conant, J. B. (1959). *The American high school today.* New York: McGraw-Hill Book Co.

Davidson, J. E., & Sternberg, R. J. (1984). The role of insight in intellectual giftedness. *Gifted Child Quarterly, 28,* 58–64.

Davis, G. A., & Rimm, S. B. (1989). *Education of the gifted and talented.* Englewood Cliffs, N.J.: Prentice-Hall.

Davis, G. A., & Rimm, S. (1979). Identification and counseling of the creatively gifted. In N. Colangelo & R. T. Zaffrann (Eds.), *New voices in counseling the gifted.* Dubuque, Iowa: Kendall Hunt Publishing Co.

Dehann, R., & Havighurst, R. J. (1957). *Educating gifted children.* Chicago: University of Chicago Press.

Delisle, J. R., & Galbraith, J. (1987). The gifted kids survival guide II: A sequel to the original. Minneapolis, Minn.: Free Spirit Publishing Co.

Feldhusen, J., VanTassel-Baska, J., & Seeley, K. (1989). *Excellence in educating the gifted.* Denver: Love Publishing Company.

Ford, B. G., & Ford, R. D. (1981). Identifying creative potential in handicapped children. *Exceptional Children, 48,* 115–22.

Fox, L., & Tobin, D. (1988). Broadening career horizons for gifted girls. *Gifted Child Today, 11*(1), 9–13.

Gallagher, J. J. (1985). *Teaching the gifted child* (3rd ed.). Boston: Allyn and Bacon.

Gold, M. J. (1980). Secondary level programs for the gifted and talented. In J. Morgan, C. G. Tennant, & M. J. Gold (Eds.), *Elementary and secondary level programs for the gifted and talented.* New York: Teachers College Press.

Gold, M., Koch, S., Jordan, W., & Pendavis, J. (1987). Twenty by twenty: A two-decade history of 20 members of the 1965 Georgia governor's honors program. *Gifted Child Today, 10*(5), 2–16.

Goldsmith, L. T. (1987). Girl prodigies: Some evidence and some speculations. *Roeper Review, 10*(2), 74–82.

Gowan, J. C., Khatena, J., & Torrance, E. P. (1979). *Educating the ablest.* Itasca, Ill.: F. E. Peacock Publishers.

Gross, M., & Kirsten, S. (1987). Linking education and community: Marvern, Australia. *Gifted Child Today, 10*(4), 44–45.

Guilford, J. P. (1950). Creativity. *American Psychologist, 5,* 444–54.

Guilford, J. P. (1956). Structure of intellect. *Psychological Bulletin, 53,* 267–93.

Guilford, J. P. (1959). Three faces of intellect. *American Psychologist, 14,* 469–79.

Haeger, W., & Feldhusen, J. (1987). *Developing a mentor program.* East Aurora, N.Y.: DOK.

Hendricks, J., & Scott, M. (1987). Mentor companions in curiosity: A program for accepting and encouraging curiosity in young gifted children. *Creative Child and Adult Quarterly, 12*(2), 119–23.

Hollinger, C. L., & Fleming, E. S. (1988). Gifted and talented women: Antecedents and correlates of life satisfaction. *Gifted Child Quarterly, 32*(2), 254–59.

Hollingsworth, P. L. (1987). *The University of Tulsa School for Gifted Children.* Tulsa, Okla.: The School.

Irvine, D. J. (1987). A three-dimensional model for individualizing instruction for gifted students. Paper presented at the Seventh World Conference on Gifted and Talented Children, Salt Lake City, Utah.

Karnes, M. B. (1978). Identifying and programming for young gifted/talented handicapped children. In A. Fink (Ed.), *International perspectives on future special education.* Reston, Va.: Council for Exceptional Children.

Karnes, M. B. (1979). Young handicapped children can be gifted and talented. *Journal for the Education of the Gifted, 2*(3), 157–72.

Karnes, M. B., & Bertschi, J. D. (1978). Identifying and educating gifted/talented nonhandicapped and handicapped preschoolers. *Teaching Exceptional Children, 10,* 114–19.

Kaufman, A., & Kaufman, N. (1983). *Kaufman assessment battery for children: Sampler manual.* Circle Pines, Minn.: American Guidance Service.

Kerr, B. A. (1985). Smart girls, gifted women. Columbus: Ohio Psychology Publishing Co.

Khatena, J. (1982). Myth: Creativity is too difficult to measure. *Gifted Child Quarterly, 26*(1), 21–23.

Klausmeier, K. (1986). Enrichment: An educational imperative for meeting the needs of gifted students. In C. J. Maker (Ed.), *Critical issues in gifted education: Defensible programs for the gifted.* Rockville, Md.: Aspen Publishers, Inc.

Kitano, M. K., & Kirby, D. F. (1986). *Gifted education: A comprehensive view.* Boston: Little, Brown and Company.

Klausmeier, K., Mishra, S. P., & Maker, C. J. (1987). Identification of gifted learners: A national survey of assessment practices and training needs of school psychologists. *Gifted Child Quarterly, 31*(3), 135–37.

Koopmans-Dayton, J. D., & Feldhusen, J. F. (1987). A resource guide for parents of gifted preschoolers. *The Gifted Child Today, 10*(6), 2–7.

Kramer, L. R. (1987a). *Differences in learning and achieving in self-contained and resource-room programs for the gifted.* Paper presented at the annual conference of the American Education Research Association, Washington, D.C.

Kramer, L. R. (1987b). *Self-contained and resource-room programs for the gifted: Factors influencing effectiveness.* Paper presented at the annual meeting of the American Education Research Association, Washington, D.C.

Landers, S. (1986, April 10). Atypical gifted students often excluded from programs researchers say. *Education Daily,* 6.

Laycock, F. (1979). *Gifted children.* Glenview, Ill.: Scott, Foresman & Co.

Leroux, J. A., & DeFazio, P. (1987). University programs for high-ability adolescents. Paper presented at the annual meeting of the American Education Research Association, Washington, D. C.

MacKinnon, D. W. (1962). The nature and nurture of creative talent. *American Psychologist, 17*(7), 484–95.

McAuliff, J. H., & Stoskin, L. (1987). Synectic: The creative connection; Maryland, United States. *Gifted Child Today, 10*(4), 18–20.

Meeker, M. N. (1978). Nondiscriminatory testing procedures to assess giftedness in Black, Chicano, Navajo, and Anglo children. In A. Y. Baldwin, G. H. Gear, & L. J. Lucito (Eds.), *Educational planning for the gifted.* Reston, Va.: Council for Exceptional Children.

Mercer, J. R., & Lewis, J. F. (1978). Using the system of multicultural pluralistic assessment (SOMPA) to identify the gifted minority child. In A. Y. Baldwin, G. H. Gear, & L. J. Lucito (Eds.), *Educational planning for the gifted.* Reston, Va.: Council for Exceptional Children.

Olszewski-Kubilius, P. (1989). Development of academic talent: The role of summer programs. In J. L. VanTassel-Baska & P. Olszewski-Kubilius (Eds.), *Patterns of influence on gifted learners.* New York: Teachers College Press.

Olszewski-Kubilius, P. M., Kulieke, M. J., & Krasney, N. (1988). Personality dimensions of gifted adolescents: A review of the empirical literature. *Gifted Child Quarterly, 32*(4), 347–52.

Parke, B. N. (1989). *Gifted students in the regular classroom.* Boston: Allyn and Bacon.

Purcell, C. (1978). *Gifted and talented children's education act of 1978.* Washington, D. C.: U.S. Government Printing Office.

Renzulli, J. S. (1978). What makes giftedness? Reexamining a definition. *Phi Delta Kappan, 60*(3), 180–84, 261.

Renzulli, J. S., Reis, S. M., & Smith, L. M. (1981). *The revolving door identification model.* Wethersfield, Conn.: Creative Learning Press.

Renzulli, J. S., Smith, L. H., White, A. J., Callahan, C. M., & Hartman, R. K. (1976). *Scales for rating the behavioral characteristics of superior students.* Wethersfield, Conn.: Creative Learning Press.

Renzulli, J. S., & VanTassel-Baska, J. (1987). Point–counterpoint: The positive side of pull-out programs and the ineffectiveness of the pull-out program model in gifted education: A minority perspective. *Journal for the Education of the Gifted, 10*(4), 245–69.

Sanborn, M. P. (1979). Career development: Problems of gifted and talented students. In N. Colangelo & R. T. Zaffrann (Eds.), *New voices in counseling the gifted.* Dubuque, Iowa: Kendall Hunt Publishing Co.

Seeley, K. (1985). Facilitators for gifted learners. In J. Feldhusen (Ed.), *Toward excellence in gifted education.* Denver: Love Publishing Company.

Silverman, L. K. (1986). What happens to the gifted girls? In C. J. Maker (Ed.), *Critical issues in gifted education: Defensible programs for the gifted.* Rockville, Md.: Aspen Publishers, Inc.

Silverman, L. K. (1989). Career counseling for the gifted. In J. L. VanTassel-Baska & P. M. Olszewski-Kubilius (Eds.), *Patterns of influence on gifted learners.* New York: Teachers College Press.

Shaughnessy, M., & Neely, R. (1987). Parenting the prodigies: What if your child is highly verbal or mathematically precocious? *Creative Child and Adult Quarterly, 12*(1), 7–20.

Solano, D. H., & George, W. L. (1976). College courses for the gifted. *Gifted Child Quarterly, 20*(3), 274–85.

Stanley, J. C. (1977). Rationale of the study of mathematically precocious youth (SMPY) during its first years of promoting educational acceleration. In J. C. Stanley, W. C. George, & C. H. Solano (Eds.), *The gifted and the creative: A fifty-year perspective.* Baltimore: John Hopkins University Press.

Sternberg, R. J. (1981). A componential theory of intellectual giftedness. *Gifted Child Quarterly, 25*, 86–93.

Sternberg, R. J. (1987). *Beyond I Q.* New York: Cambridge University Press.

Taffel, A. (1987). Fifty years of developing the gifted in science and mathematics. *Roeper Review, 10*(1), 21–24.

Taylor, C. W., & Ellison, R. L. (1966). *Manual for alphabiographical inventory.* Salt Lake City, Utah: Institute for Behavioral Research in Creativity.

Taylor, C. W., & Ellison, R. L. (1983). Searching for talent resources. *Gifted Child Quarterly, 27*(3), 99–106.

Terman, L. M. (1925). *Genetic studies of genius, vol. 1: Mental and physical traits of a thousand gifted children.* Stanford, Cal.: Stanford University Press.

Thomas, T. A. (1987). *CSUS academic talent search follow-up report: After the first four years.* Paper presented at the annual meeting of the American Education Research Association, Washington, D.C.

Torrance, E. P. (1961). Problems of highly creative children. *Gifted Child Quarterly, 5*, 31–34.

Torrance, E. P. (1965). *Gifted children in the classroom.* New York: Macmillan Co.

Torrance, E. P. (1966). *Torrance tests of creative thinking.* Bensenville, Ill.: Scholastic Testing Service.

Torrance, E. P. (1968). Finding hidden talent among disadvantaged children. *Gifted and Talented Quarterly, 12*, 131–37.

Torrance, E. P. (1971). Are the Torrance tests of creative thinking biased against or in favor of disadvantaged groups? *Gifted Child Quarterly, 15*(2), 75–80.

Torrance, E. P. (1977). Creativity gifted and disadvantaged gifted. In J. C. Stanley, W. C. George, & C. H. Solano (Eds.), *The gifted and the creative: A fifty-year perspective.* Baltimore: Johns Hopkins University Press.

VanTassel-Baska, J. (1988). *Comprehensive curriculum for gifted learners.* Boston: Allyn and Bacon.

VanTassel-Baska, J. (1989a). Acceleration. In C. J. Maker (Ed.), *Critical issues in gifted education: Defensible programs for the gifted.* Rockville, Md.: Aspen Publishers, Inc.

VanTassel-Baska, J. (1989b). Counseling the gifted. In J. Feldhusen, J. VanTassel-Baska, & K. Seeley (Eds.), *Excellence in educating the gifted.* Denver: Love Publishing Company.

VanTassel-Baska, J. (1989c). The disadvantaged gifted. In J. Feldhusen, J. VanTassel-Baska, & K. Seeley (Eds.), *Excellence in educating the gifted.* Denver: Love Publishing Company.

VanTassel-Baska, J., & Chepko-Sade, D. (1986). *An incidence study of disadvantaged gifted students in the Midwest.* Evanston, Ill.: Northwestern University Center for Talent Development.

Wallach, M. A. (1976). Tests tell us little about talent. *American Scientist, 64*, 57.

Whitmore, J. R., & Maker, C. J. (1985). *Intellectual giftedness in disabled persons.* Rockville, Md.: Aspen Systems Corporation.

Williams, F. E. (1988). A magic circle. *Gifted Child Today, 11*(1), 2–5.

Chapter 14

Abrams, J. C., & Kaslow, F. (1977). Family systems and the learning-disabled child: Intervention and treatment. *Journal of Learning Disabilities, 10*, 86–90.

Adler, J. (1987, March 17). Cause for concern—And optimism. *Newsweek,* 63–66.

Atkins, D. V. (1987). Siblings of the hearing-impaired: Perspectives for parents. *Volta Review, 89*(5), 32–45.

Baker, B. E. (1970). The effectiveness of parent modalities in the treatment of children with learning disabilities. *Dissertation Abstracts International, 31* (1929A–2541A), 2166A.

Barsh, R. H. (1968). *The parent of the handicapped child: The study of child-rearing practices.* Springfield, Ill.: Charles C. Thomas.

Beckman-Bell, P. (1981). Child-related stress in families of handicapped children. *Topics in Early Childhood Special Education, 1*(3), 45–54.

Berns, J. H. (1980). Grandparents of handicapped children. *Social Work, 15*(3), 238–9.

Blacher, J. (1984). Sequential stages of parental adjustment to the birth of a child with handicaps: Fact or artifact? *Mental Retardation, 22*(2), 55–68.

Blackard, M. K., & Barsh, E. T. (1982). Parents' and professionals' perceptions of the handicapped child's impact on the family. *Journal of the Association for the Severely Handicapped, 7*, 62–70.

Blatt, B. (1988). *Conquest of mental retardation.* Austin, Tex.: Pro-Ed.

Bristol, M. M., & Gallagher, J. J. (1982). A family focus for intervention. In E. T. Ramey & P. L. Trohanis (Eds.), *Finding and educating high-risk and handicapped infants.* Baltimore: University Park Press.

Bristor, M. W. (1984). The birth of a handicapped child—A wholistic model for grieving. *Family Relations, 33*, 25–32.

Buscaglia, L. (1975). *The disabled and their parents: A counseling challenge.* Thorofare, N.J.: Charles B. Slack.

Busk, H. H. (1985). Setting the platitudes straight. *Exceptional Parents, 15*(7), 23–8.

Cartwright, C. A. (1981). Effective programs for parents of young handicapped children. *Topics in Early Childhood Special Education, 3*, 1–9.

Chandler, L. K., Fowler, S. A., & Lubeck, R. C. (1985). Assessing family needs: The first step in providing family-focused intervention. Washington, D.C.: Special Education Programs (ED/OSERS).

Chinn, P. C., Winn, J., & Walter, R. H. *Two-way talking with parents of special children: A process of positive communication.* St. Louis, Mo.: C. V. Mosby.

Cleveland, M. (1980). Family adaptation to traumatic spinal-cord injury: Response to crisis. *Family Therapy, 29*(4), 558–65.

Cobb, P. S. (1987). Creating respite-care programs. *Exceptional Parent, 15*(5), 31–3.

Crnic, K., Greenberg, M., Ragozin, A., Robinson, N., & Basham, R. (1983). Effects of stress and social support on mothers of premature and full-term infants. *Child Development, 54*, 209–17.

D'Arcy, E. (1968). Congenital defects: Mothers' reactions to first information. *British Medical Journal, 3*, 796–98.

Davis, R. D. (1967). Family processes in mental retardation. *American Journal of Psychiatry, 124*(3), 340–50.

Dougan, T., Isbell, L., & Vyas, P. (1979). *We have been there: A guide book for parents of people with mental retardation.* Nashville, Tenn.: Abingdon Press.

Farber, B. (1962). Effects of a severely retarded child on the family. In E. P. Trapp & P. Himelskin (Eds.), *Readings on the exceptional child.* New York: Appleton-Century-Crofts.

Featherstone, H. (1980). *A difference in the family: Living with a disabled child.* New York: Penguin Books.

Forbes, E. (1987). My brother, Warren. *Exceptional Parent, 17*(5), 50–52.

Fotheringham, J. B., Skelton, M., & Hoddinott, B. A. (1971). *The retarded child and his family: The effects of home and institution* (Monograph Series No. 11). Toronto: Ontario Institute for Studies in Education.

Fowle, C. M. (1968). The effect of the severely mentally retarded child on his family. *American Journal of Mental Deficiency, 73*, 468–73.

Fox, M. A. (1975). The handicapped family. *Lancet, 2*, 400–401.

Fredericks, B. (1985). Parents/families of persons with severe mental retardation. In D. Bricker & J. Filler (Eds.), *Severe mental retardation: From theory to practice.* Reston, Va.: Council for Exceptional Children.

Freudenberger, J. J. (1977). Burn-out: Occupational hazard of the child-care worker. *Child Care Quarterly, 6*, 90–98.

Friedman, R. (1978). Using the family and school in the treatment of learning disabilities. *Journal of Learning Disabilities, 11*, 378–82.

Gallagher, J. R., Beckman-Bell, P., & Cross, A. H. (1983). Families of handicapped children: Sources of stress and its amelioration. *Exceptional Children, 50*, 10–19.

Gardner, J. F., & Markowitz, R. K. (1986). *Maryland family support services consortium, final report.* Baltimore: Maryland State Planning Council on Developmental Disabilities.

Gorham, K. A. (1975). A lost generation of parents. *Exceptional Children, 41,* 521–25.

Gorham, K. A., DesJardins, C., Page, R., Pettis, E., & Scheiber, B. (1975). Effect on parents. In N. Hobbs (Ed.), *Issues in the classification of children.* San Francisco: Jossey-Bass.

Grossman, F. K. (1972a). *Brothers and sisters of retarded children.* Syracuse, N.Y.: Syracuse University Press.

Grossman, F. K. (1972b). Brothers and sisters of retarded children. *Psychology Today, 5,* 102–4.

Hackney, H. (1981). The child, the family, and the school. *Gifted Child Quarterly, 25,* 51–54.

Haynes, U. (1977). *A developmental approach to case finding.* Rockville, Md.: U.S. Department of Health, Education, and Welfare.

Hetrick, E. W. (1979). Training of parents of learning-disabled children in facilitative communication skills. *Journal of Learning Disabilities, 12,* 275–77.

Heward, W. L., Dardig, J. C., and Rossett, A. (1979). *Working with parents of handicapped children.* Columbus, Ohio: Charles E. Merrill Publishing.

Howard, J. (1978). The influence of children's developmental dysfunctions on marital quality and family interaction. In R. M. Lerner & G. B. Spanier (Eds.), *Child influences on marital and family interaction: A life-span perspective.* New York: Academic Press.

Hutchinson, E. F. (1982). Wheelchairs. *The Exceptional Parent, 12*(1), 7, 60.

I'm not going to be John's baby sitter forever: Sibling, planning, and the disabled (1987, November). *Exceptional Parent,* 60–64.

Jogis, J. L. (1975). To be spoken sadly. In L. Buscaglia (Ed.), *The disabled and their parents: A counseling challenge.* Thorofare, N.J.: Charles B. Slack.

Klein, S. D. (1972). Brother to sister, sister to brother. *Exceptional Parent, 2,* 10–15, 26–27.

Koch, R. C., & Dobson, J. C. (1971). *The mentally retarded child and his family.* New York: Brunner/Mazel.

Kotze, J. M. A. (1986). Educational aid to parents of young handicapped children. Paper presented at the World Conference of O.M.E.P. World Organization for Preschool Education, Jerusalem, Israel.

Kraft, S. P., & Snell, M. A. (1980). Parent-teacher conflict: Coping with parental stress. *The Pointer, 24*(2), 29–37.

Kroth, R. L. (1987). Mixed or missed messages between parents and professionals. *Volta Review, 89*(1), 1–10.

Lamb, M. E. (1983). Fathers of exceptional children. In M. Seligman (Ed.), *The family with a handicapped child: Understanding and treatment.* New York: Grune & Stratton.

Lamb, C. B. (1980). Fostering acceptance of a disabled sibling through books. *The Exceptional Parent, 10*(1), 12–13.

Lavelle, N., & Keogh, B. K. (1980). Expectations and attributions of parents of handicapped children. In J. J. Gallagher (Ed.), *New directions for exceptional children, parents, and families of handicapped children.* San Francisco: Jossey-Bass.

Leigh, I. W. (1987). Parenting and the hearing-impaired. *Volta Review, 89*(5), 11–21.

Leigh, J. (1975). What we know about counseling the disabled and their parents: A review of the literature. In L. Buscaglia (Ed.), *The disabled and their parents: A counseling challenge.* Thorofare, N.J.: Charles B. Slack.

Lettick, S. (1979). Ben. In R. Sullivan (Ed.), Siblings of autistic children. *Journal of Autism and Developmental Disorders, 9*(3), 287–98.

Lipsky, D. K. (1987). *Family support for families with a disabled member* (Monograph No. 39). New York: World Rehabilitation Fund, Inc.

Love, H. (1973). *The mentally retarded child and his family.* Springfield, Ill.: Charles C. Thomas.

Luterman, D. (1987). *Deafness in the family.* Boston: Little, Brown & Co.

Maslach, C. (1978). Job Burn-out: How people cope. *Public Welfare, 36,* 56–8.

McAndrew, I. (1976). Children with a handicap and their families. *Child: Care, Health, and Development, 2*(4), 213–38.

McKinney, J. D., & Hocutt, A. M. (1982). Public school involvement of parents and learning-disabled children and average learners. *Exceptional Education Quarterly, 3*(2), 64–73.

McPhee, N. (1982). A very special magic: A grandparent's delight. *Exceptional Parent, 12*(3), 13–16.

Muir-Hutchinson, L. (1987). Working with professionals. *Exceptional Parent, 17*(5), 8–10.

Murphy, A. T. (1979). The families of handicapped children: Context for disability. *Volta Review, 81,* 265–79.

Pagel, S., & Price, J. (1980). Strategies to alleviate teacher stress. *Pointer, 24*(2), 45–53.

Peterson, N. L. (1987). *Early intervention for handicapped and at-risk children: An introduction to early-childhood special education.* Denver: Love Publishing Company.

Pieper, E. (1976). Grandparents can help. *The Exceptional Parent, 6*(2), 7–10.

Pueschel, S. M. The impact on the family: Living with the handicapped child. *Issues in Law and Medicine, 2*(3), 171–87.

Rich, A. (1984). My family and I. *Exceptional Parent, 14*(5), C2.

Rose, H. W. (1987). *Something's wrong with my child.* Springfield, Ill.: Charles C. Thomas.

Ross, A. O. (1964). *The exceptional child in the family.* New York: Grune & Stratton.

Salkever, M. (1981). Tammy: A part of our family. *Exceptional Parent, 11*(5), 11–16.

Scagliotta, E. G. (1974). Contributions of the learning-disabled child to family life. In D. Kronick (Ed.), *Learning disabilities: Its implications to a responsible society.* San Rafael, Cal.: Academy Therapy Publications.

Schell, G. C. (1981). The young handicapped child: A family perspective. *Topics in Early Childhood Special Education, 1*(3), 21–28.

Seligman, M. (1979). *Strategies for helping parents of handicapped children.* New York: The Free Press.

Seligman, M., & Seligman, D. A. (1980). The professional's dilemma: Learning to work with parents. *The Exceptional Parent, 10*(5), 511–3.

Shelton, M. (1972). Areas of parental concern about retarded children. *Mental Retardation, 2,* 38–41.

Shelton, T. L., Jeppson, E. S., & Johnson, B. H. (1987). *Family-centered care for children with special health-care needs.* Washington, D.C.: Association for the Care of Children's Health.

Sherman, B. R. (1988). Predictors of the decision to place developmentally disabled family members in residential care. *American Journal of Mental Retardation, 92*(4), 344–51.

Shontz, F. (1965). Reactions to crisis. *Volta Review, 67,* 364–70.

Smith, J., & Cline, D. (1980). Quality Programs. *The Pointer, 24*(2), 80–87.

Somers, M. N. (1987). Parenting in the 1980s: Programming perspectives and issues. *Volta Review, 89*(5), 68–77.

Sullivan, R. (1979). Siblings of autistic children. *Journal of Autism and Developmental Disorders, 9*(3), 287–98.

Tew, B. F., Lawrence, M., Payne, H., & Townsley, K. (1977). Marital stability following the birth of a child with spina bifida. *British Journal of Psychiatry, 131,* 77–82.

Tjossem, T. D. (1976). *Intervention strategies for high-risk infants and young children.* Baltimore: University Park Press.

Turnbull, A. P., & Turnbull, H. R., III. (1978). *Parents Speak Out.* Columbus, Ohio: Charles E. Merrill Publishing.

Turnbull, A. P., & Turnbull, H. R., III. (1986). *Families and professionals: Creating an exceptional partnership.* Columbus, Ohio: Charles E. Merrill Publishing.

Turnbull, A. P., Strickland, B., & Goldstein, S. (1978). Parental involvement in developing and implementing the IEP: Training professionals and parents. *Education and Training of the Mentally Retarded, 13,* 414–23.

Tynan, D. D., & Fritsch, R. E. (1987). *Stress associated with handicapped children: Guidelines for family management.* (ERIC Document Reproduction Service, No. ED–285–314).

Volpe, J. J., & Koenigsberger, R. (1981). Neurologic disorders. In G. B. Avery (Ed.), *Neonatology, pathophysiology, and management of the newborn* (2nd ed.). Philadelphia: J. B. Lippincott Co.

Webster, E. J. (1977). *Counseling with parents of handicapped children:*

Guidelines for improving communications. New York: Grune & Stratton.

Welsh, M. M., & Odum, C. S. H. (1981). Parent involvement in the education of the handicapped child: A review of the literature. *Journal of the Division for Early Childhood, 3,* 15–23.

West, E. (1981). My child is blind—Thoughts on family life. *Exceptional Parent, 11*(1), S9–S12.

When I grow up, I'm never coming back! The adolescent and the family (1988, March). *Exceptional Parent* 62–67.

Wunderlich, C. (1977). *The mongoloid child: Recognition and care.* Tucson: University of Arizona Press.

Chapter 15

Baca, L. M., & Cervantes, H. T. (1984). *The bilingual special education interface.* St. Louis, Mo.: C. V. Mosby.

Barresi, J. G. (1982). Educating handicapped migrants: Issues and options. *Exceptional Children, 48,* 473–88.

Bedell, F. D. (1989). Testimony delivered at hearings conducted by the National Council on the Handicapped. June 7 and 8, Washington, D.C.

Brooks-Gunn, J., & Furstenberg, F. F. (1986). The children of adolescent mothers: Physical, academic, and psychological outcomes. *Developmental Review, 6,* 224–51.

Bryen, D. N. (1974). Special education and the linguistically different child. *Exceptional Children, 40,* 593.

Burt, C. (1921). *Mental and scholastic tests.* London: King.

Cattell, R. B. (1940). A culture-free intelligence test, I. *Journal of Educational Psychology, 31,* 161–80.

Cattell, R. B., Feingold, S. N., & Sarason, S. B. (1941). A culture-free intelligence test, II. Evaluation of cultural influences on test performance. *Journal of Educational Psychology, 32,* 81–100.

Chinn, P. C. (1979). The exceptional minority child: Issues and some answers. *Exceptional Children, 45,* 532–36.

Chinn, P. C., & Hughes, S. (1987). Representation of minority students in special education classes. *Remedial and Special Education, 8*(4), 41–46.

Chinn, P. C., & McCormick, L. (1986). Cultural diversity and exceptionality. In N. G. Haring and L. McCormick (Eds.), *Exceptional children and youth* (4th ed.) (pp. 95–117). Columbus, Ohio: Charles E. Merrill Publishing Co.

Collier, C., & Hoover, J. J. (1987). Sociocultural considerations when referring minority children for learning disabilities. *Learning Disabilities Focus, 3,* 39–45.

Correa, V. I. (1987). Working with Hispanic parents of visually impaired children: Cultural implications. *Journal of Visual Impairment and Blindness, 81,* 260–64.

Diana v. State Board of Education (1970, 1973). C–70, 37 RFP. (N.D. Cal., 1970, 1973).

Drew, C. J. (1973). Criterion-referenced and norm-referenced assessment of minority group children. *Journal of School Psychology, 11,* 323–29.

Drew, C. J., Logan, D. R., & Hardman, M. L. (1988). *Mental retardation: A life-cycle approach* (4th ed.). Columbus, Ohio: Charles E. Merrill Publishing Co.

Elbert, J. C. (1984). Training in child diagnostic assessment: A survey of clinical psychology graduate programs. *Journal of Clinical Child Psychology, 13,* 122–33.

Erickson, J. G., & Walker, C. L. (1983). Bilingual exceptional children: What are the issues? In D. R. Omark & J. G. Erickson (Eds.), *The bilingual exceptional child* (pp. 4–22). San Diego: College-Hill Press, Inc.

Field, T. (1980). Interactions of preterm and term infants with their lower and middle class teenage and adult mothers. In T. Field, S. Goldberg, D. Stern, & A. Sostek (Eds.), *High-risk infants and children: Adult and peer interactions.* New York: Academic Press.

Fishgrund, J. E., Cohen, O. P., & Clarkson, R. L. (1987). Hearing-impaired children in Black and Hispanic families. *Volta Review, 89*(5), 59–67.

Folb, E. A. (1980). *Runnin' down some lines: The language and culture of black teenagers.* Cambridge, Mass.: Harvard University Press.

Frith, G. H. (1982). Educating migrant students: The paraprofessional component. *Exceptional Children, 48,* 506–7.

Garcia, R. L. (1978). *Fostering a pluralistic society through multiethnic education.* Bloomington, Ind.: Phi Delta Kappa Educational Foundation.

Gelfand, D. M., Jenson, W. R., & Drew, C. J. (1988). *Understanding child behavior disorders* (2nd ed.). New York: Holt, Rinehart, & Winston.

Gollnick, D. M., & Chinn, P. C. (1986). *Multicultural education in a pluralistic society* (2nd ed.). Columbus, Ohio: Charles E. Merrill Publishing Co.

Heath, F., & Heath, B., *Language in the U.S.A.* Cited by Ovando, C. J. (1989). Language diversity and education. In J. A. Banks and C. A. Banks (Eds.), *Multicultural education: Issues and perspectives.* Boston: Allyn and Bacon.

Heward, W. L., & Orlansky, M. D. (1988). *Exceptional children* (3rd ed.). Columbus, Ohio: Charles E. Merrill Publishing Co.

Hilliard, A. (1980). Cultural diversity and special education. *Exceptional Children, 46,* 584–88.

Hunter, B. (1982). Policy issues in special education for migrant students. *Exceptional Children, 48,* 469–72.

Kaufman, A. S. (1979). *Intelligence testing with the WISC-R.* New York: Wiley/Interscience.

Larry P. v. Riles (1972). C–71–2270 US.C, 343 F. Supp. 1306 (N.D. Cal. 1972).

Larry P. v. Riles (1979). 343 F. Supp. 1306, 502 F. 2d 963 (N.D. Cal. 1979).

Leung, B. (1987). Cultural considerations in working with Asian parents. Paper presented at the conference of the National Center for Clinical Infant Programs, Los Angeles.

Lopez, S. (1988). The empirical basis of ethnocultural and linguistic bias in mental health evaluations of Hispanics. *American Psychologist, 43,* 1095–96.

Luftig, R. L. (1989). *Assessment of learners with special needs.* Boston: Allyn and Bacon.

Magrab, P. R., Sostek, A. M., & Powell, B. A. (1984). Prevention in the prenatal period. In M. C. Roberts & L. Peterson (Eds.), *Prevention of problems in childhood: Psychological research and applications.* New York: Wiley-Interscience.

Maheady, L., Towne, R., Algozzine, B., Mercer, J., & Ysseldyke, J. (1983). Minority overrepresentation: A case for alternative practices prior to referral. *Learning Disability Quarterly, 6,* 448–56.

Malgady, R. G., Rogler, L. H., & Constantino, G. (1987). Ethnocultural and linguistic bias in mental health evaluation of Hispanics. *American Psychologist, 42,* 228–34.

Manion, M. L., & Bersani, H. A. (1987). Mental retardation as a Western sociological construct: A crosscultural analysis. *Disability, Handicap, and Society, 2,* 231–45.

Mattes, L. J., & Omark, D. R. (1984). *Speech and language assessment for the bilingual handicapped.* San Diego: College-Hill Press, Inc.

McDavis, R. J. (1980). The black client. In N. A. Vacc & J. P. Wittmer (Eds.), *Let me be me: Special populations and the helping profession* (pp. 151–74). Muncie, Ind.: Accelerated Development.

Merton, R. K. (1948). The self-fulfilling prophecy. *Antioch Review, 8,* 193–210.

Merton, R. K. (1987). Three fragments from a sociologist's notebooks: Establishing the phenomenon, specified ignorance, and strategic research materials. *Annual Review of Sociology, 13,* 1–28.

Miller-Jones, D. (1989). Culture and testing. *American Psychologist, 44,* 360–66.

Morrow, R. D. (1987). Cultural differences—Be aware! *Academic Therapy, 23,* 143–49.

National Center for Health Statistics (1982, May 12). *Vital and health statistics* (Advance Data No. 79, Supplemental Exhibit 4). Washington, D.C.: U.S. Government Printing Office.

Office of Civil Rights (1986). *The 1984 elementary and secondary school civil rights survey.* Washington, D. C.: U.S. Department of Education.

Patton, J. R., Payne, J. S., Kauffman, J. M., Brown, G. B., & Payne, R. A. (1987). *Exceptional children in focus.* Columbus, Ohio: Charles E. Merrill Publishing Co.

Pepper, F. C. (1976). Teaching the American Indian child in mainstream settings. In R. L. Jones (Ed.), *Mainstreaming and the minority child* (pp. 133–58). Reston, Va.: Council for Exceptional Children.

Prasse, D. P., & Reschly, D. J. (1986). Larry P.: A case of segregation, testing, or program efficacy? *Exceptional Children, 52,* 333–46.

Pyecha, J. N., & Ward, L. A. (1982). A study of the implementation of Public Law 94–142 for handicapped migrant children. *Exceptional Children, 48,* 490–500.

Raven, J. C. (1938). *Guide to using the progressive matrices.* London: H. H. Lewis and Co.

Reynolds, C. R. (1987). Race bias in testing. In R. J. Corsini (Ed.), *Concise encyclopedia of psychology* (pp. 953–54). New York: John Wiley & Sons.

Reynolds, C. R., & Brown, R. T. (1984). *Perspectives on bias in mental testing.* New York: Plenum.

Roberts, E., & DeBlassie, R. R. (1983). Test bias and the culturally different early adolescent. *Adolescence, 18,* 837–43.

Rodriguez, F. (1982). Mainstreaming a multicultural concept into special education: Guidelines for teacher trainers. *Exceptional Children, 49,* 220–27.

Rosenthal, R. (1987). Pygmalion effects: Existence, magnitude, and social importance. *Educational Researcher, 16*(9), 37–41.

Rosenthal, R., & Jacobson, L. (1968a). *Pygmalion in the classroom: Teacher expectation and pupils' intellectual development.* New York: Holt, Rinehart, & Winston.

Rosenthal, R., & Jacobson, L. (1968b). Self-fulfilling prophecies in the classroom: Teachers' expectations as unintended determinants of pupils' intellectual competence. In M. Deutsch, I. Katz, & A. R. Jensen (Eds.), *Social class, race, and psychological development* (pp. 219–53). New York: Holt, Rinehart, & Winston.

Rosenthal, R., & Jacobson, L. (1968c). Teacher expectations for the disadvantaged. *Scientific American, 218,* 19–23.

Salend, S. J., Michael, R. J., & Taylor, M. (1984). Competencies necessary for instructing migrant handicapped students. *Exceptional Children, 51,* 50–55.

Schildroth, A. N. (1986). Residential schools for deaf students: A decade in review. In A. N. Schildroth & M. A. Karchmer (Eds.), *Deaf children in America* (pp. 83–104). San Diego: College-Hill Press, Inc.

Skowronski, J. J., & Carlston, D. E. (1989). Negativity and extremity biases in impression formation: A review of explanations. *Psychological Bulletin, 105,* 131–42.

Slate, N. M. (1983). Nonbiased assessment of adaptive behavior: Comparison of three instruments. *Exceptional Children, 50,* 67–70.

Smith, R. D. (1987). Multicultural considerations: Working with families of developmentally disabled and high-risk children; The Hispanic perspective. Paper presented at the conference of the National Center for Clinical Infant Programs, Los Angeles.

Tucker, J. A. (1980). Ethnic proportions in classes for the learning disabled: Issues in nonbiased assessment. *Journal of Special Education, 14,* 93–105.

Turner, A. (1987). Multicultural considerations: Working with families of developmentally disabled and high-risk children; The Black perspective. Paper presented at the conference of the National Center for Clinical Infant Programs, Los Angeles.

U.S. Bureau of the Census (1985). *Current population reports* (Series P-60, No. 149). Washington, D.C.: U.S. Government Printing Office.

U.S. Department of Education (1989). *To assure the free appropriate public education of all handicapped children.* Eleventh Annual Report to Congress on the implementation of Education of the Handicapped Act. Washington, D.C.: The Department.

White, J. (1984). *The psychology of Blacks: An Afro-American perspective.* Englewood Cliffs, N.J.: Prentice-Hall.

Willig, A. C., & Greenberg, H. F. (1986). *Bilingualism and learning disabilities: Policy and practice for teachers and administrators.* New York: American Library.

Wineburg, S. S. (1987). The self-fulfillment of the self-fulfilling prophecy. *Educational Researcher, 16*(9), 28–37.

Wood, F. H., Johnson, J. L., & Jenkins, J. R. (1986). The *Lora* case: Nonbiased referral, assessment, and placement procedures. *Exceptional Children, 52,* 323–31.

Wright, P., & Santa Cruz, R. (1983). Ethnic composition of special education programs in California. *Learning Disability Quarterly, 6,* 387–94.

Yacobacci-Tam, P. (1987). Interacting with the culturally different family. *Volta Review, 89*(5), 46–58.

Author Index

Subject Index